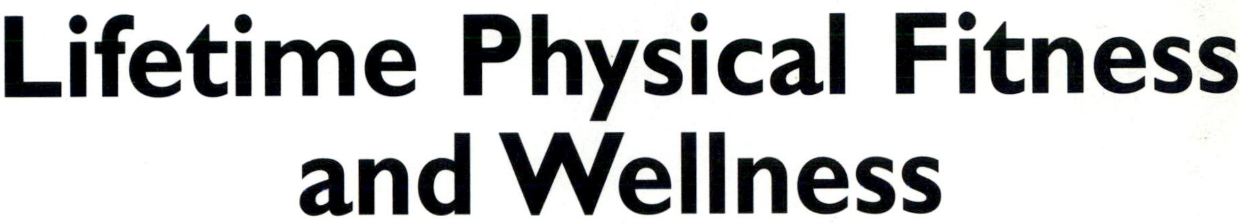

# Lifetime Physical Fitness and Wellness

## A Personalized Program

**FOURTH EDITION**

Werner W. K. Hoeger
Boise State University

Sharon A. Hoeger

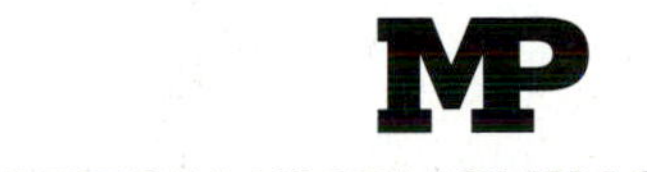

**MORTON PUBLISHING COMPANY**
925 W. Kenyon, Unit 12
Englewood, Colorado 80110

Interior Design: Joanne R. Saliger
Cover Design: Bob Schram, Bookends.
Illustrator: Jennifer Johnson
Copy Editor: Carolyn Acheson
Typography: Ash Street Typecrafters, Inc.



Printed in the United States of America

10 9 8 7 6 5 4 3

ISBN: 0-89582-291-1

# Preface

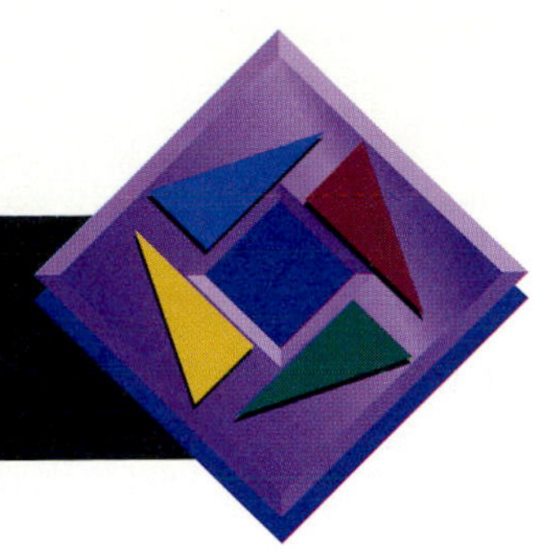

The current American way of life does not provide the human body with sufficient physical exercise to maintain adequate health. Further, many present lifestyle patterns are such a serious threat to our health that they actually increase the deterioration rate of the human body and often lead to premature illness and mortality.

Although people in the United States are firm believers in the benefits of physical activity and positive lifestyle habits as a means to promote better health, most do not reap these benefits because they simply do not know how to implement a sound physical fitness and wellness program that will indeed yield the desired results.

Scientific evidence has clearly shown that improving the quality and most likely the longevity of our lives is a matter of personal choice. The biggest challenge that we are faced with at the end of this century is to teach individuals how to take control of their personal health habits to insure a better, healthier, happier, and more productive life. The information presented in this book has been written with this objective in mind, providing you with the opportunity to initiate your own healthy lifestyle program.

As you work through the different chapters in this book, you will be able to develop and regularly update your own lifetime program to improve the various components of physical fitness and wellness. The emphasis is on teaching you how to take control of your personal health and lifestyle habits, so that you can make a constant and deliberate effort to stay healthy and realize your highest potential for well-being.

## New and Enhanced Features of the Fourth Edition

The chapters in this edition of Lifetime Physical Fitness & Wellness have been revised and updated to conform with advances and recommendations made since the publication of the third edition. The most significant changes in this new edition are:

- The cardiovascular endurance chapter has been divided into two chapters, one for assessment and one for prescription. A Twelve-Minute Swim Test and an Exercise Readiness Questionnaire have been added to the assessment chapter. The questionnaire helps evaluate students' readiness for exercise based on four categories of evaluation: mastery (self-control), attitude, health, and commitment.

  An entire section on aerobic activity choices has been included in the cardiovascular endurance prescription chapter. This introduction to the most popular forms of aerobic activities will enhance the development and implementation of cardiovascular fitness programs. A Fitness Ratings of Aerobic Activities chart has also been incorporated to this chapter.
- The U.S. Health Objectives for the Year 2000 are included in Chapter 1. These health objectives clearly emphasize the need for health promotion and disease prevention, personal responsibility, and health benefits for all people in the United States.
- Grip and Abdominal Crunch Strength Tests and information on anabolic steroids and plyometrics were added to the muscular strength chapter.

- The Body Mass Index (BMI) has been added to the body composition chapter. Along with the Waist-to-Hip Ratio, these tests are used to screen individuals who might be at higher risk for disease due to high fat content.
- The nutrition chapter has been completely revised and now contains information on the Food Guide Pyramid, new food labels, the effect of phytochemicals in the prevention of disease, energy (ATP) production, the role of glycogen in the body, carbohydrate loading, and amino acid supplements.
- A broader discussion of the terms obesity, overweight, recommended weight, and "tolerable" weight is included in the weight loss chapter. Such information helps students make an informed decision as to what constitutes a realistic target weight.
- Revisions were made to the Cardiovascular Disease Prevention chapter to incorporate recent advances in this area.
- An enhanced discussion on the development of cancer, the role of the enzyme telomerase in cancer cell division, and the action of phytochemicals in fighting this disease are included in the Cancer Prevention chapter.
- Enhancements to the stress management chapter include concepts on stress vulnerability and time management.
- Information on HIV and AIDS has been greatly enhanced in Chapter 13.
- New color photography and many outstanding new graphs have been added throughout the book.

## SUPPLEMENTS

The following ancillaries are provided free of charge to all qualified **Lifetime Physical Fitness & Wellness** adopters:

- One of the most **comprehensive computer software packages** available with any fitness/ wellness textbook. The software includes a *Fitness and Wellness Profile, a Personalized Cardiovascular Exercise Prescription*, a *Nutrient Analysis*, and a weekly and monthly *Exercise Log*. This software package helps provide a more meaningful experience to all participants and greatly decreases the workload of course instructors.

  A new feature of the fourth edition is the *Nutrient Analysis Data Base Enhancer* software. This software allows instructors to add food items to the already existing data base available with the book.
- A **video** containing a detailed explanation of many of the fitness assessment test items used in the book. Instructors can use this video to help familiarize themselves with the proper test protocols for each fitness test. This audio-visual aid contains the following test items: 1.5-Mile Run Test, Step Test, Astrand-Ryhming Test, Muscular Strength and Endurance Test, Muscular Endurance Test, Strength-to-Body Weight Ratio Test, Modified Sit-and-Reach Test, Body Rotation Test, Shoulder Rotation Test, Skinfold Thickness Test, and Girth Measurements Test.
- The Physical Fitness and Wellness Computerized Testbank with the following options: (a) over 800 multiple choice questions, (b) capability to add/or edit test questions, (c) previously generated tests can be recalled — creating new exam versions because multiple choice answers can be rotated with each new test generated, and (d) capability to generate tests using a LaserJet printer.
- Sixty-four color **overhead transparency acetates** of the book's most important illustrations and figures to facilitate class instruction and help explain key fitness and wellness concepts.
- An **instructor's manual** to aid with the implementation of your physical fitness and wellness course.

# Acknowledgments

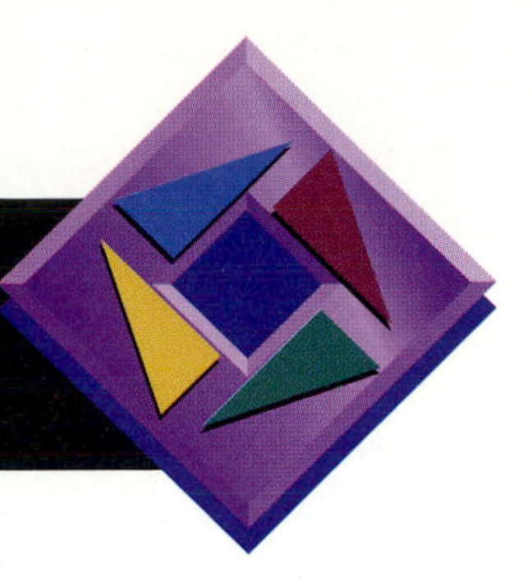

We wish to express our gratitude to colleagues throughout the country who evaluated the third edition of *Lifetime Physical Fitness and Wellness.* The feedback received greatly enhanced the preparation of this edition.

Special thanks to all of the following individuals who helped with the photography in this new edition: Jason Brooks Aberg, Heather Lloyd, Julie Wagner, Jennifer Blackman, Dr. Sherman Button, Nancy Button, Bernhard Hoeger, Michelle Puetz, Amy Gibson, Phyllis Sawyer, Leland and Norma Hansen, Jim Moore, Brad Page, Scott Whiles, Jamie Korte, Neil Edwards, Julie Hammons, Brad Thompson, Monika Gangwer, Dan Barber, Cherianne Caulkins, Debra Cunningham, Michelle Chupurdia, and Sally O'Donnell.

# Contents

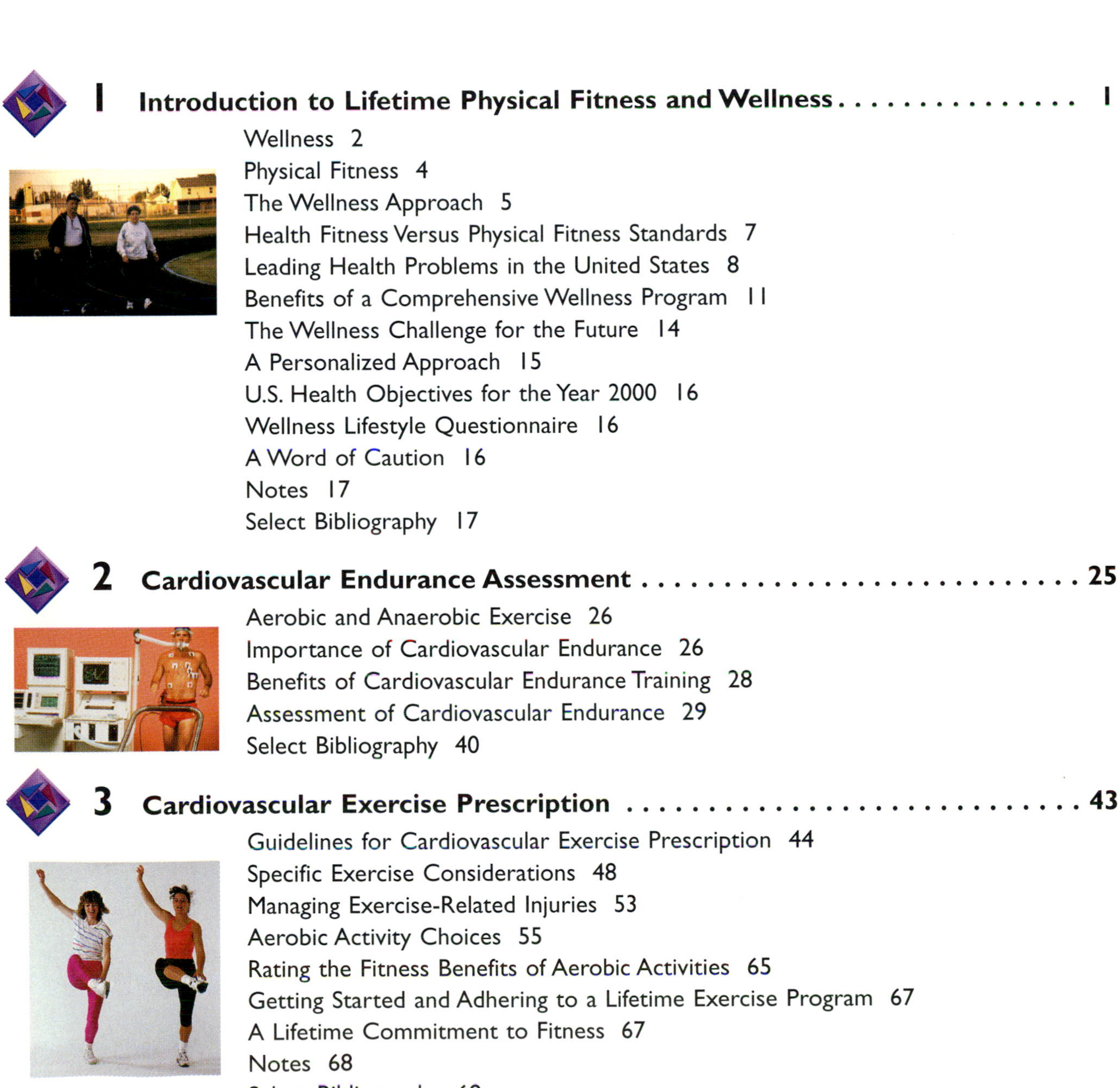

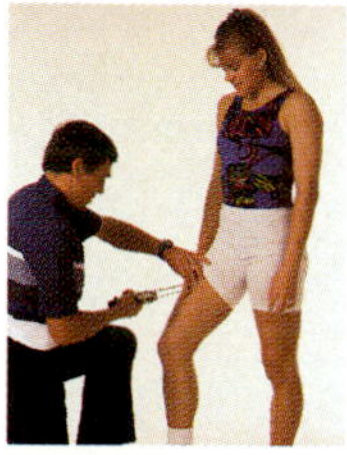

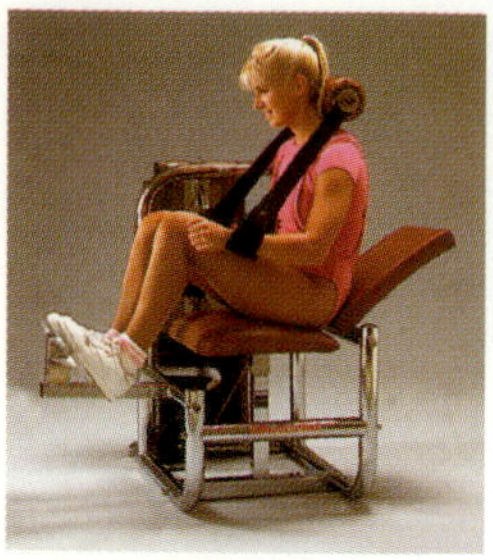

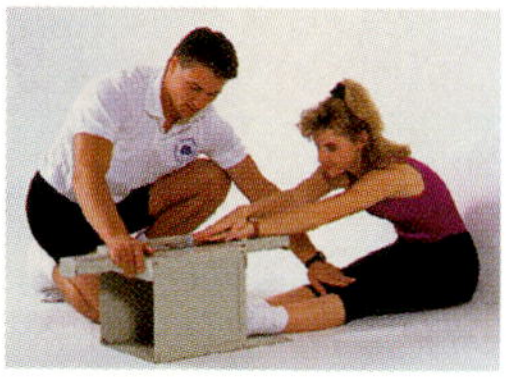

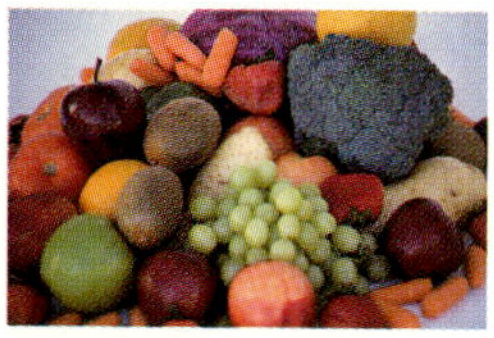

# Introduction to Lifetime Physical Fitness and Wellness

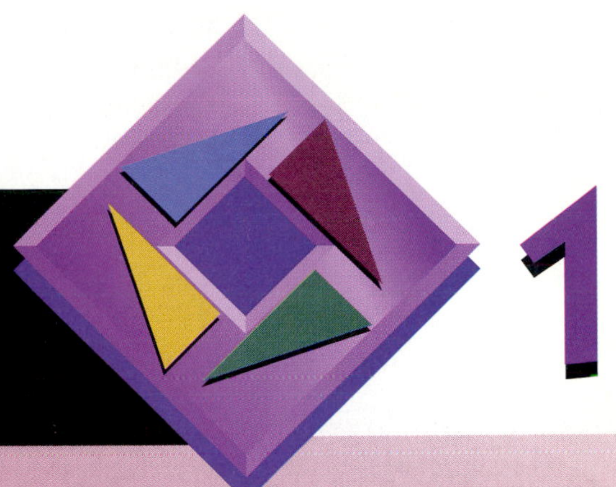


## Key Concepts

Wellness
Physical fitness
Health-related fitness
Skill-related fitness
Chronic diseases
Epidemiology
Health care costs
Personalized approach
Year 2000 Health Objectives

## Objectives

- Define wellness, list its dimensions, and identify components of wellness.
- Define physical fitness and list health-related and skill-related fitness components.
- Learn the differences between physical fitness and wellness.
- Differentiate health standards and physical fitness standards.
- Identify the major health problems in the United States.
- Understand the benefits and the significance of participating in a lifetime fitness and wellness program.
- Identify lifestyle factors that enhance health and longevity.
- Recognize risk factors that may interfere with safe exercise participation.

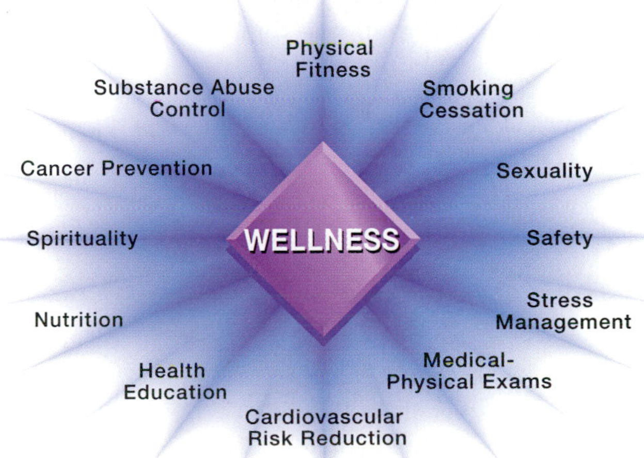

Movement and physical activity are basic functions for which the human organism was created. Advances in modern technology, however, have nearly eliminated the need for physical activity in almost everyone's daily life. Physical activity is no longer a natural part of our existence. We now live in an automated society, one in which most of the activities that used to require strenuous physical exertion can be accomplished by machines with the simple pull of a handle or push of a button.

The available scientific evidence shows that physical inactivity and a sedentary lifestyle seriously threaten our health and hasten the deterioration rate of the human body. Physically active people live longer than their inactive counterparts, even if they start to become active later in life. Current estimates for the United States indicate that more than 250,000 deaths yearly are the result of lack of regular physical activity.[1]

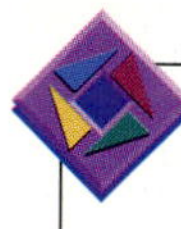

*Physical inactivity and a sedentary lifestyle seriously threaten our health and hasten the deterioration rate of the human body.*

With the advances in technology, three additional factors have changed our lives significantly and have negatively affected human health: nutrition, stress, and environment. Fatty foods, sweets, alcohol, tobacco, excessive stress, and environmental hazards (wastes, noise, air pollution, and the like) have detrimental effects on people.

At the beginning of the 20th century, the most common health problems in the United States were infectious diseases including tuberculosis, diphtheria, influenza, kidney disease, polio, and other diseases of infancy. Progress in the field of medicine largely eliminated these diseases. As the American people started to enjoy the "good life" (sedentary living, alcohol, fatty foods, excessive sweets, tobacco, drugs), however, a parallel increase was seen in chronic diseases such as hypertension, atherosclerosis, coronary disease, strokes, diabetes, cancer, emphysema, and cirrhosis of the liver. (Figure 1.1 illustrates the changing profile over time).

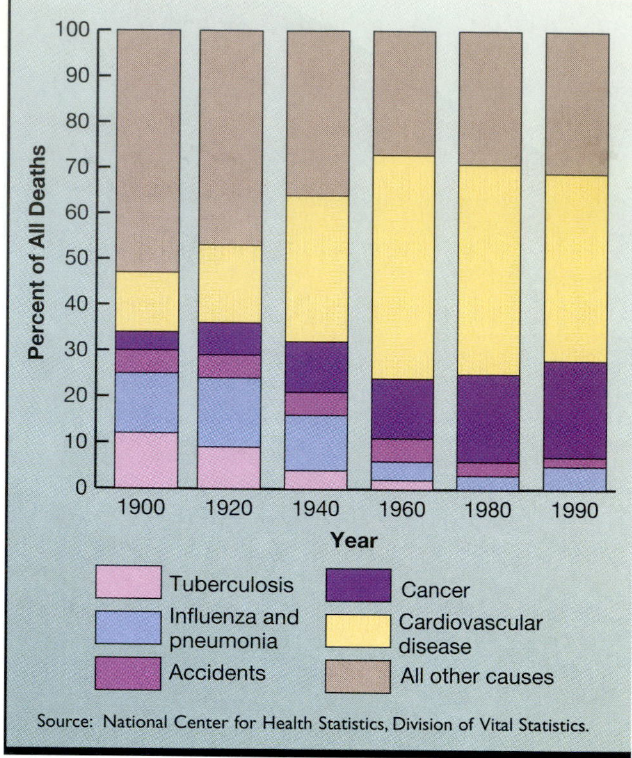


**FIGURE 1.1** ◆ Leading causes of death in the United States.

As the incidence of chronic diseases increased, prevention emerged as the best medicine. Consequently, a new fitness and wellness trend gradually took root and grew over the last two and a half decades. People began to realize that good health is largely self-controlled and that the leading causes of premature death and illness in the United States could be prevented by adhering to positive lifestyle habits.

## WELLNESS

Most people recognize that participating in a fitness program improves quality of life. In recent years, however, we came to realize that improving physical fitness alone was not always enough to lower the risk for disease and ensure better health.

For example, individuals who run 3 miles a day, lift weights regularly, participate in stretching exercises, and watch their body weight can be classified readily as having good or excellent fitness. If these same people, however, have high blood pressure, smoke, are under constant stress, consume too much alcohol, and eat too many fatty foods, they are at risk for cardiovascular disease and may not be aware of it. The characteristics that predict which people may develop a certain disease are called *risk factors*.

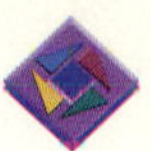

One of the best examples that good fitness does not always provide a risk-free guarantee of a healthy and productive life was the tragic death in 1984 of Jim Fixx, author of *The Complete Book of Running*. At the time of his death by heart attack, Fixx was 52 years old. He had been running between 60 and 80 miles a week and had believed that people at his high fitness level could not die from heart disease.

At age 36 Jim Fixx smoked two packs of cigarettes per day, weighed about 215 pounds, did not participate in regular cardiovascular exercise, and had a family history of heart disease. His father, having had a first heart attack at age 35, later died at age 43.

Perhaps in an effort to lessen his risk for heart disease, Fixx began to raise his level of fitness. He started to jog, lost 50 pounds, and quit smoking cigarettes.[2] On several occasions, though, Fixx declined to have an exercise electrocardiogram (ECG) (see Chapter 9), which most likely would have revealed his cardiovascular problem. His unfortunate death is a tragic example that exercise programs by themselves will not make high-risk people immune to heart disease, though they may delay the onset of a serious or fatal problem.

Good health, therefore, no longer is viewed as simply the absence of illness. The notion of good health has evolved notably in the last few years and continues to change as scientists learn more about lifestyle factors that bring on illness and affect wellness. Once the idea took hold that fitness by itself would not always decrease the risk for disease and ensure better health, the wellness concept developed in the 1980s.

*Wellness* is defined as *the constant and deliberate effort to stay healthy and achieve the highest potential for well-being*. Wellness is an all-inclusive umbrella covering a variety of health related factors. Wellness living requires the implementation of positive programs to change behavior and thereby improve health and quality of life, prolong life, and achieve total well-being.

To enjoy a wellness lifestyle, a person needs to practice behaviors that will lead to positive outcomes in five dimensions of wellness: physical, emotional, intellectual, social, and spiritual. These dimensions are interrelated; one frequently affects the others. For example, a person who is 'emotionally down' often has no desire to exercise, study, socialize with friends, or attend church.

In looking at the five dimensions of wellness (Figure 1.2), high-level wellness clearly goes beyond the absence of disease and optimal fitness. Wellness incorporates components such as fitness, proper nutrition, stress management, disease prevention, social support, self-worth, nurturance (sense of being needed), spirituality, smoking cessation, personal safety, substance control, regular physical examinations, health education, and environmental support (see Figure 1.3).

For a wellness way of life, individuals not only must be physically fit and manifest no signs of disease, but they also must have no risk factors for disease (such as hypertension, abnormal cholesterol levels, cigarette smoking, negative stress, faulty nutrition, careless sex). The relationship between adequate fitness and wellness is illustrated in the wellness continuum in Figure 1.4 Even though an individual tested in a fitness center may demonstrate adequate or even excellent fitness, indulgence in unhealthy lifestyle behaviors still will increase the risk for chronic diseases and decrease the person's well-being.

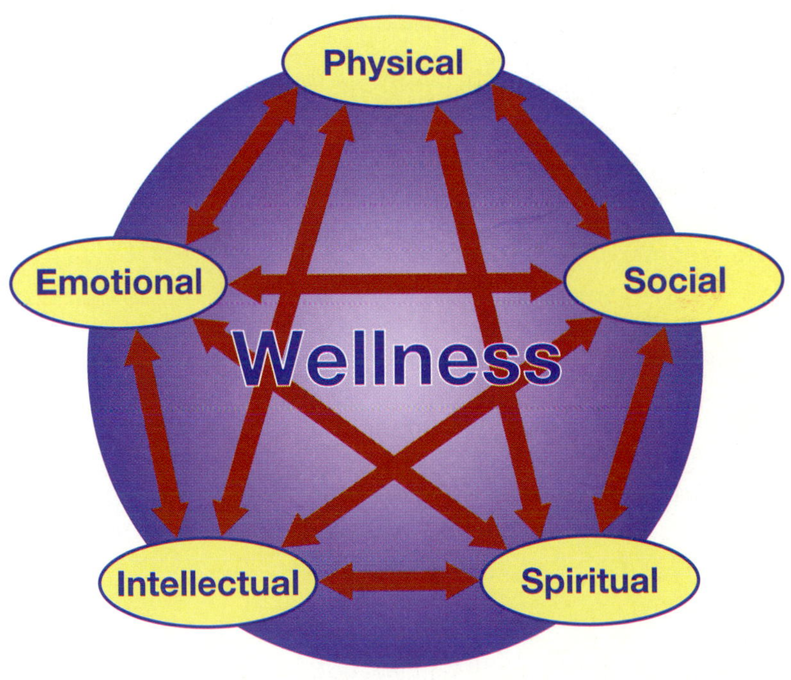


**FIGURE 1.2** ◆ Dimensions of wellness.

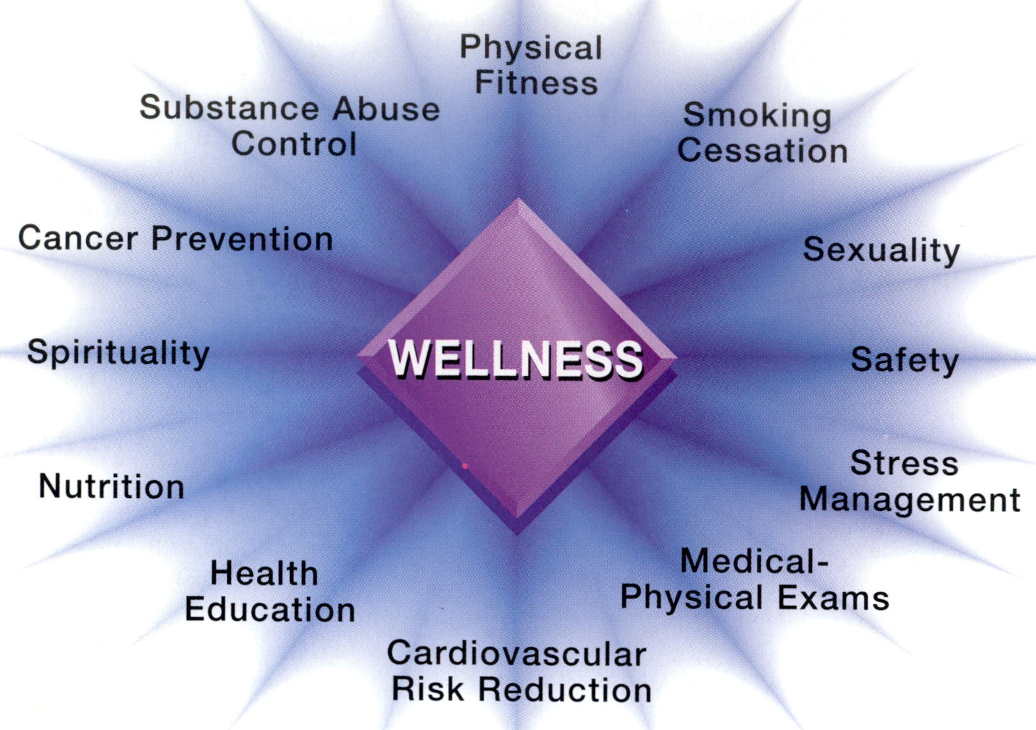
Physical Fitness
Substance Abuse Control
Smoking Cessation
Cancer Prevention
Sexuality
WELLNESS
Spirituality
Safety
Nutrition
Stress Management
Health Education
Medical-Physical Exams
Cardiovascular Risk Reduction

**FIGURE 1.3** ◆ Wellness components.

## PHYSICAL FITNESS

Physical fitness has been defined in several ways and has meant different things to different people. Initially, health care practitioners defined fitness simply as the absence of disease. Many athletic coaches perceived fitness as the ability to perform certain sports skills. Perhaps the most comprehensive definition of physical fitness is that of the American Medical Association, which has defined physical fitness as *the general capacity to adapt and respond favorably to physical effort*. Individuals are physically fit when they can meet the ordinary as well as the unusual demands of daily life safely and effectively without being overly fatigued, and still have energy left for leisure and recreational activities.

As the fitness concept grew during the 1970s, it became clear that no single test was sufficient to assess overall fitness. A battery of tests was necessary because several specific components have to be established to determine an individual's overall level of fitness.

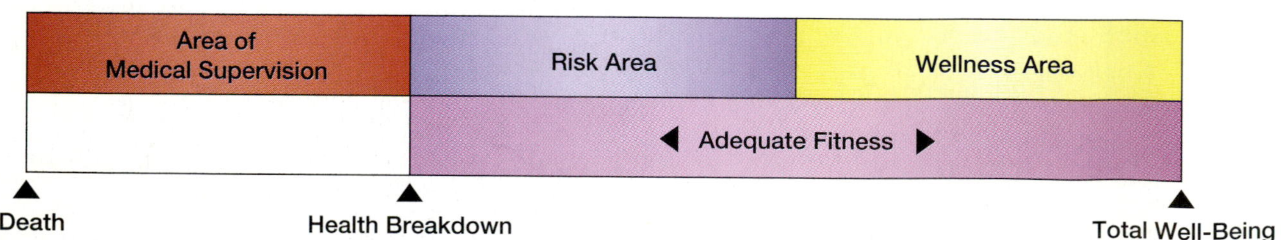


**FIGURE 1.4** ◆ Wellness continuum.

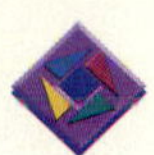

Physical fitness can be classified into health-related and motor skill-related fitness. The four *health-related fitness components* are: cardiovascular (aerobic) endurance, muscular strength and endurance, muscular flexibility, and body composition, as depicted in Figure 1.5. The motor skill-related components of fitness are more important in athletics. In addition to the four components just mentioned, motor skill-related fitness includes agility, balance, coordination, power, reaction time, and speed. Although these components are important in achieving success in athletics, they are not crucial for developing better health. In terms of preventive medicine, the main emphasis of fitness programs should be placed on the health-related components. That is the focus of this book.

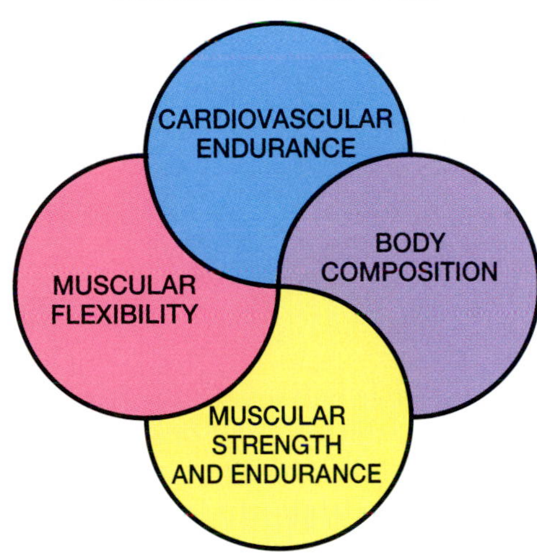


**FIGURE 1.5** ◆

## THE WELLNESS APPROACH

During the late 1960s and in the 1970s, we began to realize that good fitness is important in the fight against chronic diseases, particularly those of the cardiovascular system. Because of more participation in fitness programs in the last few years, cardiovascular mortality rates have dropped. The rate started to decline in about 1963, and between 1970 and 1988 heart disease had dropped by 34%. This decrease is credited to higher levels of wellness and better health care in the country. More than half of the decline is attributed to better diet and fewer people smoking.

Furthermore, several studies have shown an inverse relationship between exercise and premature cardiovascular mortality rates. In a study conducted among 16,936 Harvard alumni linking physical activity habits and mortality rates,[3] as the amount of weekly physical activity increased, the risk of cardiovascular deaths decreased. The largest drop in cardiovascular deaths was observed among alumni who used up more than 2,000 calories per week through physical activity. Figure 1.6 graphically illustrates the study results.

A major study published in the *Journal of the American Medical Association*, based on data from 13,344 people followed over an average of 8 years, substantiated the findings of the Harvard alumni study.[4] Conducted by Dr. Steven N. Blair and co-researchers at the Institute of Aerobics Research in Dallas, Texas, study results confirm that the level of cardiovascular fitness is related to mortality from all causes. As shown in Figure 1.7, the higher the level of cardiovascular fitness, the longer the lifespan. Death rate from all causes for the least fit (group 1) men was 3.4 times higher than for the most fit men. For the least fit women, the death

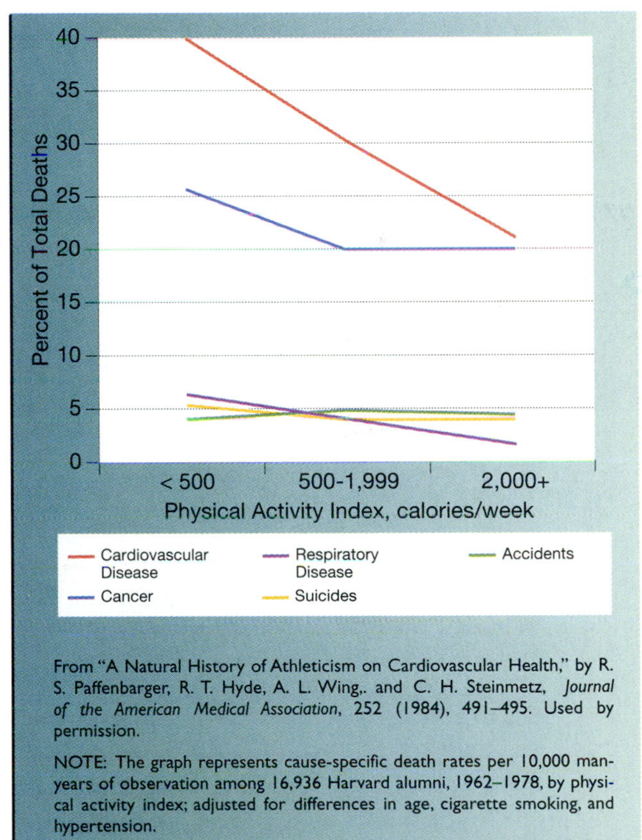


From "A Natural History of Athleticism on Cardiovascular Health," by R. S. Paffenbarger, R. T. Hyde, A. L. Wing,. and C. H. Steinmetz, *Journal of the American Medical Association*, 252 (1984), 491–495. Used by permission.

NOTE: The graph represents cause-specific death rates per 10,000 man-years of observation among 16,936 Harvard alumni, 1962–1978, by physical activity index; adjusted for differences in age, cigarette smoking, and hypertension.

**FIGURE 1.6** ◆ Death rates among Harvard alumni by physical activity index.

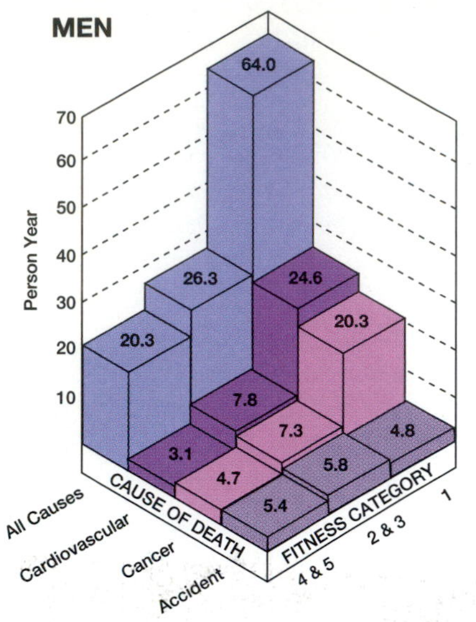


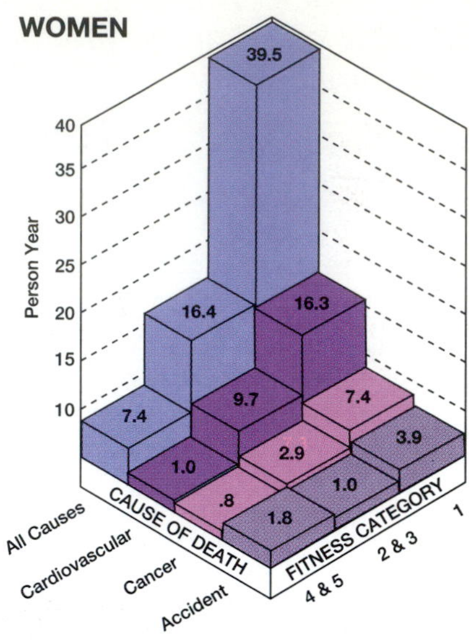


Least fit group = 1 Most fit group = 5

Based on data from "Physical Fitness and All-Cause Mortality: A Prospective Study of Healthy Men and Women, by S. N. Blair, H. W. Kohl III, R. S. Paffenbarger, Jr., D. G. Clark, K. H. Cooper, and L. W. Gibbons. *Journal of the American Medical Association,* 262 (1989), 2395–2401.

NOTE: Age-adjusted cause-specific death rates per 10,000 person-years of follow-up (1970–1985) by physical fitness groups in men and women in the Aerobics Center longitudinal study in Dallas, Texas. Fitness group 1 is the least fit group, fitness group 5 is the most fit group (one person-year indicates one person followed up 1 year later.

**FIGURE 1.7** ◆ Death rates by physical fitness groups.

rate was 4.6 times higher than for the most fit women.

This study also reported a much lower rate of premature death, even at moderate fitness levels that most adults can achieve easily. People are protected even more when they combine higher fitness levels with reduction in other risk factors such as hypertension, serum cholesterol, cigarette smoking, and excessive body fat.

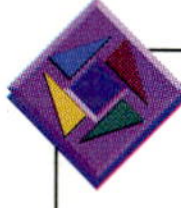

*Several major research studies have established a clear inverse relationship between exercise and premature cardiovascular mortality.*

In another major research study conducted in the 1980s, a healthy lifestyle was shown to contribute to some of the lowest mortality rates ever reported in the literature.[5] As illustrated in Figure 1.8, compared with the general White population, this group of 5,231 men and 4,631 women (wives) had much lower cancer, cardiovascular, and overall death rates.

Healthy lifestyle habits include abstaining from tobacco, alcohol, caffeine, and drugs, and adhering to a well-balanced diet, based on grains, fruits, and vegetables, and moderate consumption of poultry and red meat. The investigators in this study looked at three general health habits among the participants: lifetime abstinence from smoking, regular physical activity, and sleep.

Men in this study had one-third the death rate from cancer, one-seventh the death rate from cardiovascular disease, and one-fifth the rate of overall mortality. The wives had about half the rate of cancer and overall mortality and a third the death rate from cardiovascular disease, as shown in Figure 1.7. With reference to Figure 1.9, life expectancy for 25-year-olds who adhered to the three health habits were 85 and 86 years, respectively, as compared to 74 and 80 for the average U.S. White man and woman.

From this study we can conclude that people who adhere to a lifetime healthy lifestyle indeed will reap healthy rewards. Better health leads to improvement in quality of life. The additional 6 to 11 years of "golden" life are precious to those who maintain a lifetime wellness program.

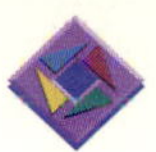

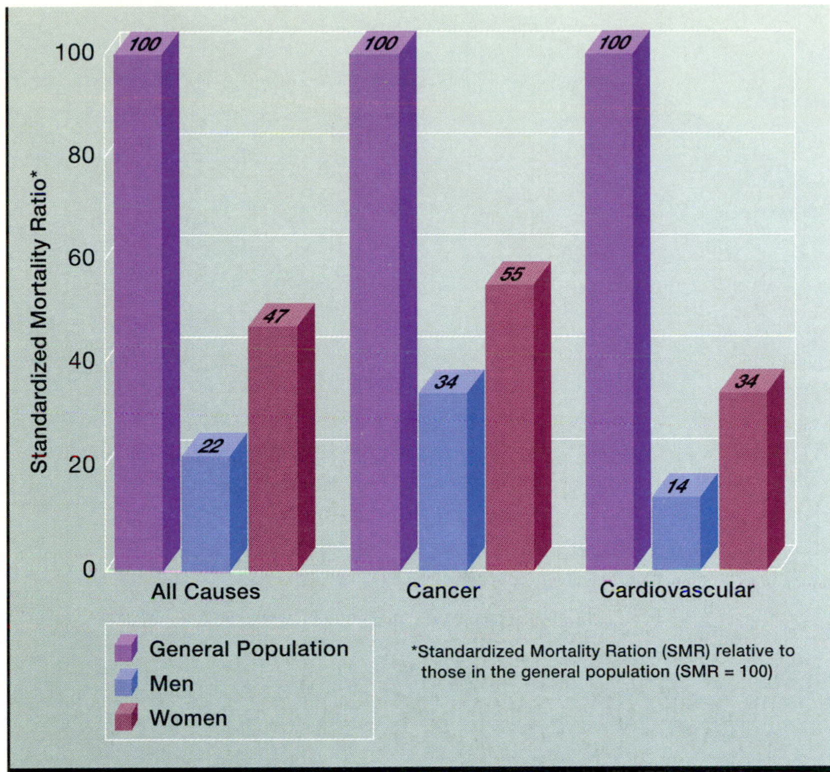


**FIGURE 1.8** ◆ Effects of a healthy lifestyle on all causes, cancer, and cardiovascular death rates in White men and women.

## HEALTH FITNESS VERSUS PHYSICAL FITNESS STANDARDS

Throughout the discussion of health-related fitness assessment in Chapters 2, 4, 5, and 6, several tests are identified to assess fitness. A meaningful debate regarding age- and gender-related fitness standards for the general population has resulted in two standards: a health fitness standard and a physical fitness standard.

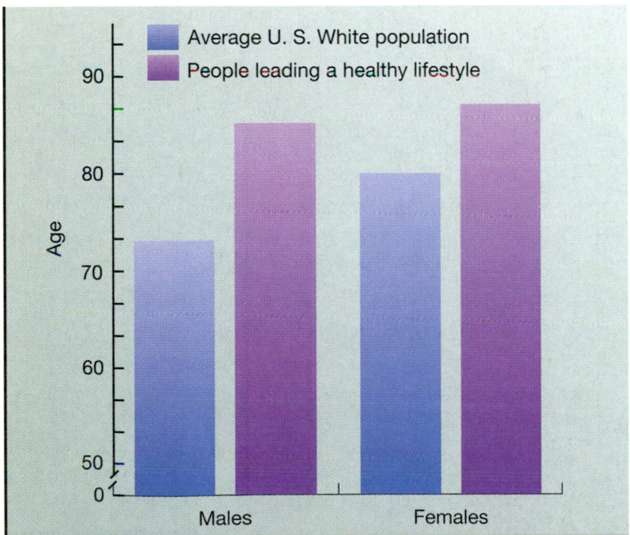


**FIGURE 1.9** ◆ Life expectancy for 25-year-olds adhering to a lifetime healthy lifestyle program versus average U.S. White population.

### Health Fitness Standards

As illustrated in Figure 1.10, although *fitness* improvements (Max $VO_2$ — see next page) with a moderate aerobic exercise program are not as notable, significant *health* benefits are reaped with such a program. These benefits are quite striking and only slightly greater health benefits are obtained with a more intense exercise program. Benefits include a reduction in blood lipids, lower blood pressure, lower risk for diabetes, weight loss, stress release, and lower risk for disease and premature mortality.

The health fitness standards proposed here are based on epidemiological* data linking minimum fitness values to disease prevention and health. These standards seem to be the lowest fitness requirements for maintaining good health, decreasing the risk for chronic diseases, and lowering the incidence of muscular-skeletal injuries.

* Epidemiology is the study of diseases that affect many individuals within a population.

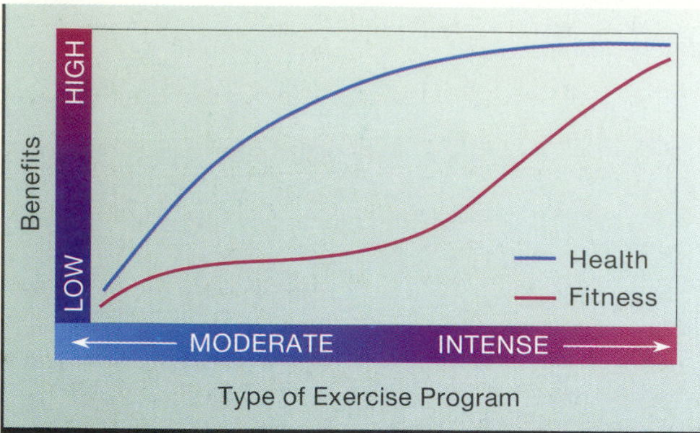


**FIGURE 1.10** ◆ Health and fitness benefits based on the type of aerobic fitness program.

Attaining the health fitness standards requires only moderate amounts of physical activity. For example, a 2-mile walk in less than 30 minutes, five to six times per week, seems to be sufficient to achieve the health-fitness standard for cardiovascular endurance.

Cardiovascular endurance is measured in terms of the maximal amount of oxygen the body is able to utilize per minute of physical activity (see Chapter 2). Maximal oxygen uptake commonly is expressed in milliliters of oxygen per kilogram of body weight per minute (ml/kg/min). Individual values can range from about 10 ml/kg/min in cardiac patients to approximately 80 to 90 ml/kg/min in world-class runners and cross-country skiers.

Data from the research study presented in Figure 1.7 indicate that maximal oxygen uptake values of 35 and 32.5 ml/kg/min for men and women, respectively, may be sufficient to lower the risk for all-cause mortality significantly. Although greater improvements in fitness yield a slightly lower risk for premature death, the largest drop is seen between the least fit (group 1) and the moderately fit (groups 2 and 3). Therefore, the 35 and 32.5 ml/kg/min values could be selected as the health fitness standards.

### Physical Fitness Standards

Physical fitness standards are set higher than the health fitness norms and require a more vigorous exercise program. Many experts believe that people who meet the criteria of "good" physical fitness should be able to do moderate to vigorous physical activity without undue fatigue and to maintain this capability throughout life. In this context, physically fit people of all ages will have the freedom to enjoy most of life's daily and recreational activities to their fullest potential. Current health fitness standards may not be enough to achieve these objectives.

Sound physical fitness gives the individual a degree of independence throughout life that many people in the United States no longer enjoy. Most older people should be able to carry out activities similar to those they conducted in their youth, though not with the same intensity. Although a person does not have to be an elite athlete, activities such as changing a tire, chopping wood, climbing several flights of stairs, playing a vigorous game of basketball, mountain biking, playing soccer with grandchildren, walking several miles around a lake, and hiking through a national park require more than the current "average fitness" level of the American people.

If the main objective of the fitness program is to lower the risk for disease, attaining the health fitness standards may be enough to ensure better health. On the other hand, if the individual wants to participate in moderate to vigorous fitness activities, achieving a high physical fitness standard is recommended. For the purposes of this book, both health fitness and physical fitness standards are given for each fitness test. The individual then has to decide the personal objectives for the fitness program.

## LEADING HEALTH PROBLEMS IN THE UNITED STATES

The most prominent causes of death in the United States today are basically lifestyle-related (see Figure 1.11). Current statistics indicate that approximately 70% of all deaths in the United States are caused by cardiovascular disease and cancer. Nearly 80% of these deaths could be prevented through a healthy lifestyle. The third cause of death, chronic and obstructive pulmonary disease, is related largely to tobacco use. Accidents are the fourth leading cause of death. Even though not all accidents are preventable, many are. Fatal accidents often are related to abusing drugs and not wearing seat belts.

Based on current figures, more than half of disease is lifestyle-related, a fifth is attributed to the environment, and a tenth is influenced by the

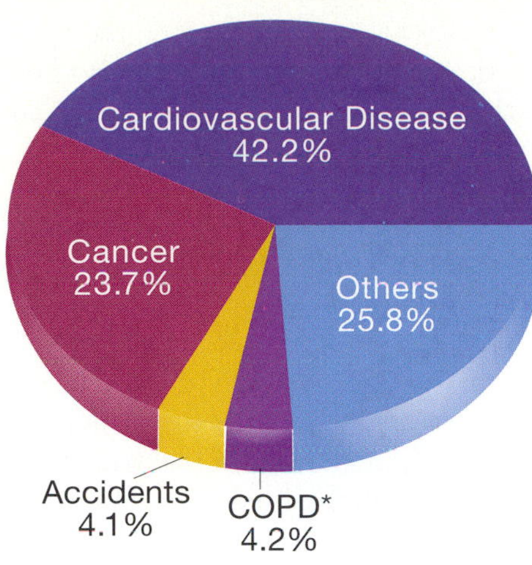


*Source:* Advance Report of Final Mortality Statistics, 1991. *Monthly Vital Statistics Report, National Center for Health Statistics.* U.S. Department of Health and Human Services, 1993.

**FIGURE 1.11** ◆ Leading causes of death in the United States: 1991.

health care the individual receives. Only 16% is related to genetic factors. Thus, the individual controls 84% of disease and quality of life (see Figure 1.12). Further, according to estimates, 83% of deaths before age 65 are preventable. In essence, most Americans are threatened by the very lives they lead today.

## Cardiovascular Disease

The most prevalent degenerative diseases in the United States are those of the cardiovascular system (see Figure 1.1). Almost half of all deaths in this country are attributed to heart and blood vessel disease.

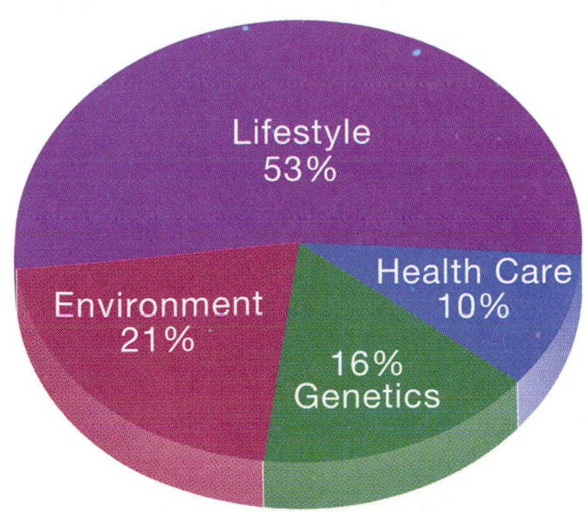


**FIGURE 1.12** ◆ Factors that affect health and well-being.

In 1994, according to estimates by the American Heart Association,[6] more than 54 million Americans were afflicted with diseases of the cardiovascular system, including 50 million with hypertension and 6.3 million with coronary heart disease. Many of these people have more than one type of cardiovascular disease.

In addition, the 1994 estimated cost of heart and blood vessel disease exceeded $128 billion. Heart attacks alone cost American industry approximately 132 million workdays annually, including $15 billion in lost productivity because of physical and emotional disability. About half of the people who die are men in their most productive years, between ages 40 and 65. The American Heart Association estimates that more than $700 million a year is spent in replacing employees who have had heart attacks.

About a million and a half people have heart attacks each year. Half a million of those people die as a consequence. About half the time the first symptom of coronary heart disease is the heart attack itself, and 40% of those who have a first heart attack die within the first 24 hours. In one of every five cardiovascular deaths, sudden death is the initial symptom.

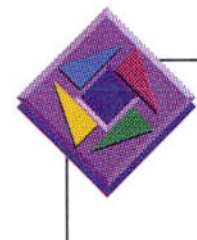

*The most prominent causes of death in the United States today are lifestyle-related.*

Most coronary heart disease risk factors are reversible and preventable. They can be controlled by modifying the lifestyle (see Chapter 9).

## Cancer

The second leading cause of death in the United States is cancer. Unlike cardiovascular disease, the mortality rate for cancer has increased steadily over the last few decades (see Figure 1.1). Even though cancer is not the number-one killer, it certainly is the number-one health fear of the American people.

Cancer is defined as *an uncontrolled growth and spread of abnormal cells in the body.* Some cells grow into a mass of tissue called a tumor, which can be either benign or malignant. A malignant tumor is considered a cancer. If the spread of cells is not controlled or checked, death is the inevitable result.

Approximately 23% of all deaths in the United States were from cancer. About 538,000 people died from this disease in 1994, and an estimated 1,208,000 new cases were reported the same year.[7] The overall medical costs for cancer were estimated to be in excess of $104 billion for 1990. Table 1.1 shows the 1994 estimated new cases and deaths for major sites of cancer, excluding nonmelanoma skin cancer (cancer that does not spread to other regions of the body) and carcinoma in situ (encapsulated tumor that is found at an early stage and has not spread).

Testing procedures for early detection of cancer, as well as treatment modalities, are changing and improving continuously. More than 8 million Americans with a history of cancer now are alive, and close to 5 million of them can be considered cured. The American Cancer Society maintains that the most influential factor in fighting cancer today is prevention through health education programs. Evidence indicates that as much as 80% of all human cancer can be prevented through positive lifestyle behaviors.

The basic recommendations for preventing cancer include a diet high in fruits and vegetables, high in fiber, high in vitamins A and C, and low in fat. Alcohol and salt-cured, smoked, and nitrite-cured foods should be consumed in moderation. Cigarette smoking and tobacco use in general should be eliminated, and obesity should be avoided. A comprehensive cancer prevention program is presented in Chapter 10.

## Chronic Obstructive Pulmonary Disease

Chronic obstructive pulmonary disease (COPD) refers to diseases that limit air flow, such as chronic bronchitis, emphysema, and a reactive airway component similar to that of asthma. The incidence of COPD increases proportionately with cigarette smoking (or other forms of tobacco use) and exposure to certain types of industrial pollution. In the case of emphysema, genetic factors also may play a role.

## Accidents

Most people do not consider accidents a health problem, but accidents are the fourth leading cause of death in the United States, affecting the total well-being of millions of Americans each year. Accident prevention and personal safety also are part of a health enhancement program aimed at achieving a higher quality of life. Proper nutrition,

**TABLE 1.1**
**Estimated Deaths and New Cases for Major Sites of Cancer: 1994**

| | Estimated New Cases | | | Estimated Deaths | | |
|---|---|---|---|---|---|---|
| | Total | Male | Female | Total | Male | Female |
| Lung | 161,000 | 101,000 | 60,000 | 143,000 | 92,000 | 51,000 |
| Colon-Rectum | 157,500 | 79,000 | 78,500 | 60,500 | 30,000 | 30,500 |
| Breast* | 175,900 | 900 | 175,000 | 44,800 | 300 | 44,500 |
| Prostate | 122,000 | 122,000 | — | 32,000 | 32,000 | — |
| Pancreas | 28,200 | 13,700 | 14,500 | 25,200 | 12,100 | 13,200 |
| Urinary | 75,500 | 52,800 | 22,700 | 20,100 | 12,700 | 7,400 |
| Leukemia | 28,000 | 15,800 | 12,200 | 18,100 | 9,800 | 8,300 |
| Ovary | 20,700 | — | 20,700 | 12,500 | — | 12,500 |
| Uterus** | 46,000 | — | 46,000 | 10,000 | — | 10,000 |
| Oral | 30,800 | 20,600 | 10,200 | 8,150 | 5,275 | 2,875 |
| Skin*** | 32,000 | 17,000 | 15,000 | 8,500 | 5,400 | 3,100 |

* Invasive cancer only
** New cases total over 50,000 if carcinoma in situ is included
*** Estimates are over 600,000 if new cases of nonmelanoma are included.

Source: *1994 Cancer Facts and Figures*. American Cancer Society.

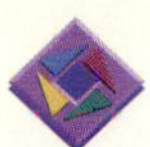

exercise, abstinence from cigarette smoking, and stress management are of little help if the person is involved in a disabling or fatal accident caused by distraction, a single reckless decision, or not wearing safety seat belts properly.

Accidents do not just happen. We cause accidents, and we are victims of accidents. Although some factors in life — earthquakes, tornadoes, and airplane crashes — are completely beyond our control, more often than not personal safety and accident prevention are a matter of common sense. Most accidents are the result of poor judgment and confused mental states. Frequently accidents happen when we are upset, not paying attention to the task with which we are involved, or abusing alcohol and other drugs.

Alcohol abuse is the number-one cause of all accidents. Alcohol intoxication is the leading cause of fatal automobile accidents. Other drugs commonly abused in society alter feelings and perceptions, cause mental confusion, and impair judgment and coordination, greatly increasing the risk for accidental morbidity and mortality (see Chapter 13).

As an aid, a "Health Protection Plan for Environmental Hazards, Crime Prevention, and Personal Safety" is given in Appendix C. By following the recommendations in this questionnaire, you can further enhance your personal safety and well-being.

## BENEFITS OF A COMPREHENSIVE WELLNESS PROGRAM

A most inspiring story illustrating what fitness can do for a person's health and well-being is that of George Snell from Sandy, Utah. At age 45, Snell weighed approximately 400 pounds, his blood pressure was 220/180, he was blind because of diabetes he did not know he had, and his blood glucose level was 487.

Snell had determined to do something about his physical and medical condition, so he started a walking/jogging program. After about 8 months of conditioning, Snell had lost almost 200 pounds, his eyesight had returned, his glucose level was down to 67, and he was taken off medication. Two months later, less than 10 months after beginning his personal exercise program, he completed his first marathon, a running course of 26.2 miles.

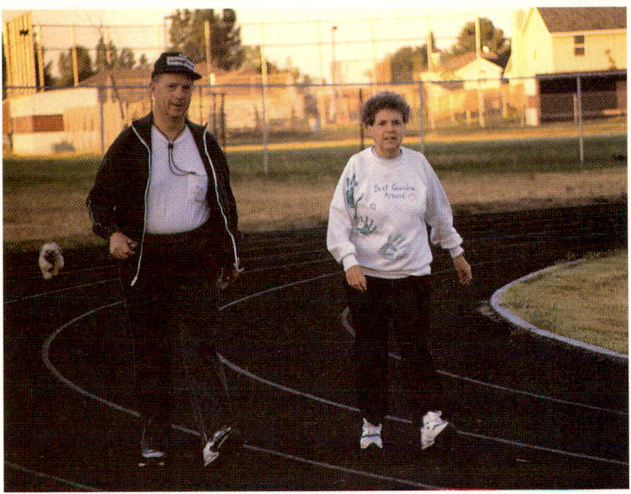

*Regular participation in a lifetime exercise program increases quality of life and longevity.*

### Health Benefits

Most people exercise because it improves their personal appearance and makes them feel good about themselves. Although many benefits accrue from participating in a regular fitness and wellness program and active people generally live longer, the greatest benefit of all is that physically fit individuals enjoy a better quality of life. These people live life to its fullest, with fewer health problems than inactive individuals who also may indulge in negative lifestyle patterns. Although compiling an all-inclusive list of the benefits reaped through fitness and wellness program participation is difficult, the following list provides a summary of many of these benefits.

1. Improves and strengthens the cardiovascular system (by facilitating oxygen supply to all parts of the body, including the heart, muscles, and brain).
2. Maintains better muscle tone, muscular strength and endurance.
3. Improves muscular flexibility.
4. Helps maintain recommended body weight.
5. Improves posture and physical appearance.
6. Lowers the risk for chronic diseases and illness (such as coronary heart disease, cancer, and strokes).
7. Decreases the mortality rate from chronic diseases.
8. Thins the blood so it is less likely to clot (decreasing the risk for coronary heart disease and strokes).

9. Lowers blood pressure.
10. Helps prevent diabetes.
11. Helps people sleep better.
12. Helps prevent chronic back pain.
13. Relieves tension and helps in coping with life stresses.
14. Raises levels of energy and job productivity.
15. Extends longevity and slows down the aging process.
16. Improves self-image and morale and helps fight depression.
17. Motivates toward positive changes in lifestyle (better nutrition, stopping smoking, alcohol and drug abuse control).
18. Speeds recovery time following physical exertion.
19. Speeds recovery following injury and disease.
20. Regulates and improves overall body functions.
21. Improves physical stamina and counteracts chronic fatigue.
22. Improves quality of life; makes people feel better and live a healthier and happier life.

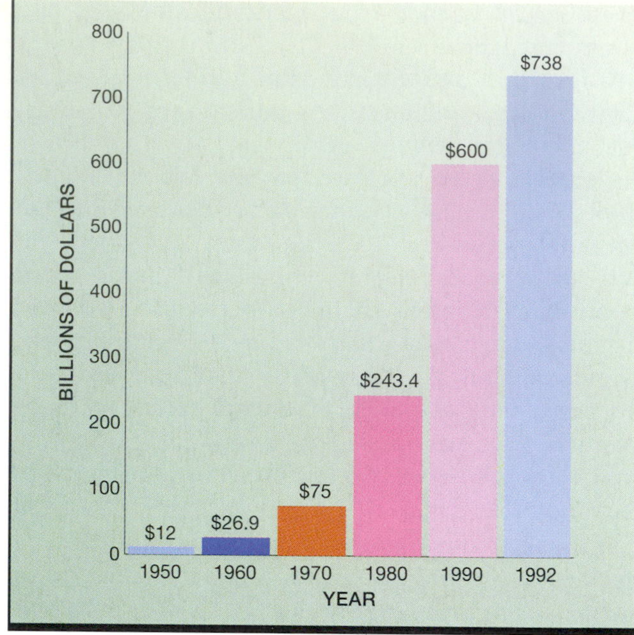


**FIGURE 1.13** ◆ U.S. health care cost increments since 1950.

## Economic Benefits

The economic impact of sedentary living has left a strong impression on the nation's economy. As the need for physical exertion steadily decreased during the last century, the nation's health-care expenditures increased dramatically. Health-care costs in the United States rose from $12 billion in 1950 to approximately $738 billion in 1992 (Figure 1.13). If the rate of escalation continues, health-care expenditures will reach $1.6 trillion by the year 2002. The 1992 figure represents more than 12% of the gross national product (GNP). It is projected to reach about 18% by the year 2002 and 37% by 2030. Furthermore, and as illustrated in Figure 1.14, the 1989 average health-care cost per person in the United States ($2,354) was almost twice as high as for most other industrialized nations.

Strong scientific evidence now links participation in fitness and wellness programs not only to better health but also to lower medical costs and higher job productivity. Most of this research is being conducted and reported by organizations that already have implemented fitness or wellness programs. Approximately half of the health-care expenditures in the United States are being absorbed by American business and industry. In 1989 business spending on health insurance premiums and health care for employees and former employees was more than 100% of after-tax profits by all U.S. companies combined.

As a result of the recent staggering rise in medical costs, many organizations are beginning to realize that keeping employees healthy costs less than treating them once they are sick. Containing the costs of health care through fitness and wellness programs has become a major issue for many organizations around the country. Let's examine the evidence.

The backache syndrome, usually the result of physical degeneration (inelastic and weak muscles), costs American industry more than $1 billion a year in lost productivity and services. An additional $250 million is spent in workers compensation. The Adolph Coors Company in Golden, Colorado, which offers a wellness program for employees and their families, reported savings of more than $319,000 in 1983 alone through a preventive and rehabilitative back injury program.

The Prudential Insurance Company of Houston, Texas, released the findings of a study conducted on its 1,386 employees. Those who participated for at least one year in the company's fitness program averaged 3.5 days of disability, compared to 8.6 days for nonparticipants. A further breakdown by level of fitness showed no disability days for those in the high-fitness group,

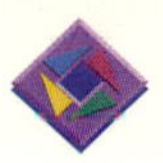

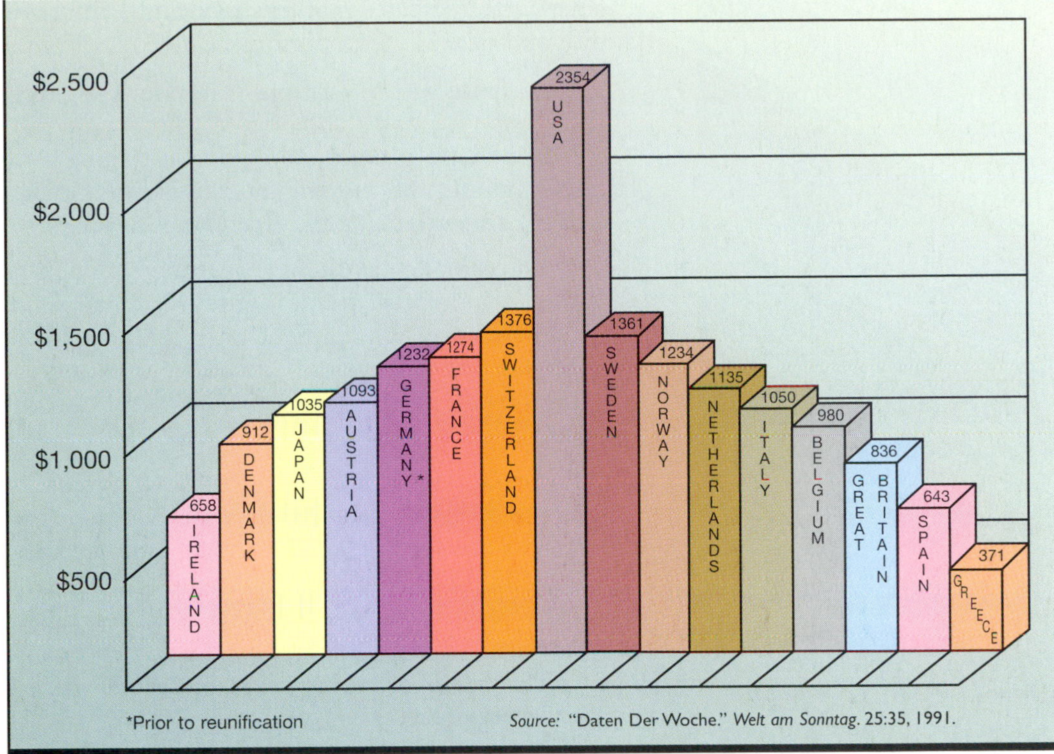


**FIGURE 1.14** ◆ 1989 Average health care costs per person for selected countries.

1.6 days for the good-fitness group, and 4.1 days for the fair-fitness group.

Since 1979 the Mesa Petroleum Company in Amarillo, Texas, has offered an on-site fitness program to its employees and their family members. A company health care analysis showed the average medical costs per person to be 150% higher for the nonparticipating than for the fitness-participating group. This represented a yearly reduction of $200,000 in medical expenses. Sick leave time also was significantly less for the physically active group — 27 hours per year, compared to 44 for the inactive group.

A similar study, conducted by Tenneco Incorporated in Houston, also showed a significant reduction in medical-care costs for men and women who participated in an exercise program. Annual medical care costs for male and female nonexercisers were 79% and 140% higher than the exercisers'. Sick leave was reduced in the men and women participants.

Furthermore, a survey of the more than 3,000 employees at Tenneco found that job productivity is related to fitness. The company reported that individuals with high job performance ratings also rated high in exercise participation.

Strong data also are coming in from Europe. Research in Germany reported 68.6% less absenteeism among workers with cardiovascular symptoms who participated in a fitness program. The law also mandates that corporations employing workers for sedentary jobs must provide an in-house facility for physical exercise.

The Goodyear Company in Norrkoping, Sweden, indicated a 50% reduction in absenteeism following implementation of a fitness program. Studies in the former Soviet Union report expanded physical work capacity and motor coordination, lower incidence of disease, shorter duration of illness, and fewer relapses among individuals participating in industrial fitness programs.

Another reason some organizations are offering wellness programs to their employees — overlooked by many because it does not seem to affect the bottom line directly — is simply concern by top management for the physical well-being of employees. Whether the program lowers medical costs is not the main issue. The only reason that really matters to top management is that wellness programs help individuals feel better about themselves and improve their quality of life.

Such is the case of Mannington Mills Corporation, which invested $1.8 million in an on-site fitness center. The return on investment is secondary to the company's interest in happier and healthier employees. The center also is open to dependents and retirees. As a result of this program, Mannington Mills believes the participants — about half of

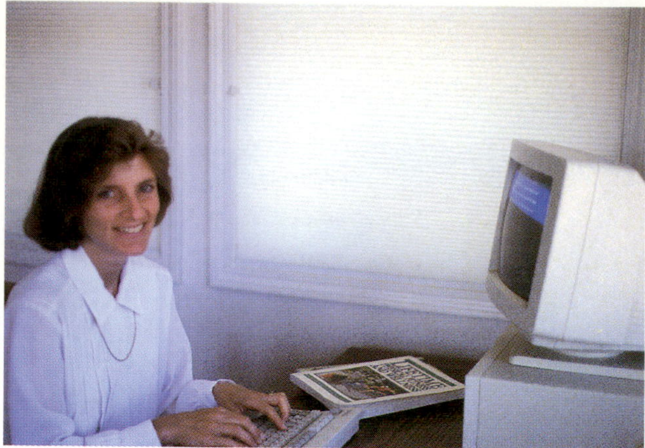

*Higher fitness leads to greater job productivity.*

the 1,600 people who are eligible — can enjoy life to its fullest potential, and the employees most likely will be more productive simply because of the company's caring attitude.

In addition to the financial and physical benefits, some corporations are offering wellness programs as an incentive to attract, hire, and retain employees. Many companies are taking a hard look at the fitness and health level of potential employees and are using this information in their screening process. Some organizations refuse to hire smokers or overweight individuals.

Other executives believe that an on-site health promotion program is the best fringe benefit they can offer at their corporation. Young executives are looking for organizations such as these, not only for the added health benefits but also because the head corporate officers are showing an attitude of concern and care.

## THE WELLNESS CHALLENGE FOR THE FUTURE

Because a better and healthier life is something every person should strive for, our biggest challenge as we look to the turn of the century is to teach people how to take control of their personal health habits and adhere to a positive lifestyle. Considering the wealth of information available on the benefits of fitness and wellness programs, improving the quality and possible length of our lives is a matter of personal choice.

Research indicates that to significantly improve health and extend life, a person should:

1. **Participate in a lifetime exercise program.** Exercise regularly three to six times a week. The exercise program should consist of 20 to 30 minutes of aerobic exercise, along with some strengthening and stretching exercises.
2. **Do not smoke cigarettes.** Cigarette smoking is the largest preventable cause of illness and premature death in the United States. When considering all related deaths, smoking is responsible for about 450,000 unnecessary deaths each year.
3. **Eat right.** Eat a good breakfast and two additional well-balanced meals every day. Unless snacks consist of healthy foods, refrain from snacking between meals. Avoid eating too many calories and foods with a lot of sugar, fat, and sodium (salt). Increase your daily consumption of fruits, vegetables, and whole-grain products.
4. **Maintain recommended body weight.** Maintain proper body weight through adequate nutrition and exercise. This is important in preventing chronic diseases and in developing a higher level of fitness.
5. **Get enough rest.** Sleep 7 to 8 hours each night.
6. **Lower stress levels.** Reduce your vulnerability to stress and practice stress management techniques as needed.
7. **Be wary of alcohol.** Drink alcohol moderately or not at all. Alcohol abuse leads to mental, emotional, physical, and social problems.
8. **Surround yourself with healthy friendships.** Unhealthy friendships contribute to destructive behaviors and low self-esteem. Associating with people who strive to maintain good fitness and health reinforces a positive outlook in life and encourages positive behaviors. Constructive social interactions enhance well-being.
9. **Be informed about the environment.** Seek clean air, clean water, and a clean environment. Be aware of pollutants and occupational hazards: asbestos fibers, nickel dust, chromate, uranium dust, and so on. Take precautions when using pesticides and insecticides.
10. **Take personal safety measures.** Although not all accidents are preventable, many are. Taking

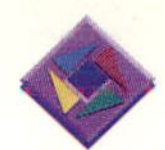

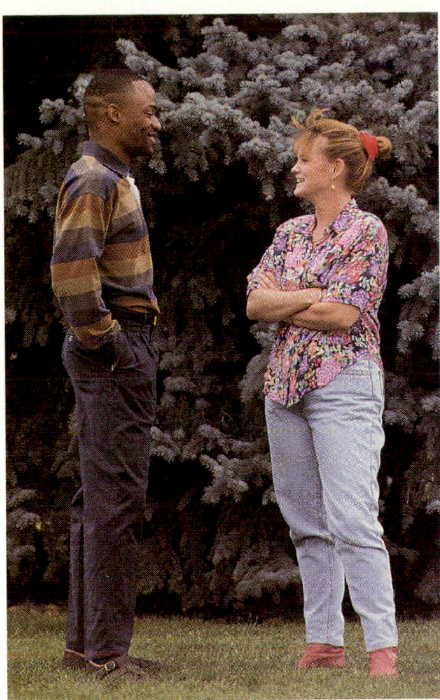

*Positive social interactions enhance wellness.*

simple precautionary measures, such as using seat belts and keeping electrical appliances away from water (see Appendix C), lessens the risk for avoidable accidents.

Thanks to current scientific data and the fitness and wellness movement of the past two decades, most Americans now see a need to participate in programs that improve and maintain health. Many people still are not taking part, though, because they are unaware of the basic principles for safe and effective participation in exercise. Others are exercising incorrectly and therefore are not reaping the full benefits of their program.

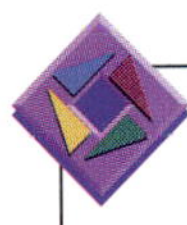

*Lifestyle choices that you make now will have an impact on how well you live the rest of your life.*

Almost half the adult population in the United States claims to participate in some sort of physical activity. Slightly more than 10% reports daily aerobic activity lasting more than 30 minutes. Aerobic activities are the most popular form of exercise, so even a lower percentage of the population probably engages in and derives benefits from strength and flexibility programs. In addition, an estimated half or more of the adult population in the United States has a weight problem and a third of all adults are considered obese (20% or more above recommended weight).

## A PERSONALIZED APPROACH

Because fitness and wellness needs vary significantly from one person to the other, all exercise and wellness prescriptions must be personalized to obtain best results. This book provides the necessary guidelines to develop a personal lifetime program to improve fitness and promote preventive health care and personal wellness. As you study this book and complete the respective fitness/wellness assignments, you will learn to:

- Determine whether medical clearance is needed for safe exercise participation.
- Assess the health-related components of fitness (cardiovascular endurance, muscular strength and endurance, muscular flexibility, and body composition).
- Write exercise prescriptions for cardiovascular endurance, muscular strength and endurance, and muscular flexibility.
- Conduct nutritional analyses and follow the recommendations for adequate nutrition.
- Write sound diet and weight-control programs.
- Determine the potential risk for cardiovascular disease, and implement a risk-reduction program.
- Follow a cancer risk-reduction program.
- Determine your levels of tension and stress, lessen your vulnerability to stress, and implement stress management programs.
- Implement a smoking cessation program, if applicable.
- Avoid chemical dependency, and know where to find assistance if needed.
- Learn the health consequences of sexually transmitted diseases, including AIDS, and guidelines for preventing STDs.
- Discover the relationship between fitness and aging.
- Write objectives to improve your fitness and wellness, and learn how to chart a wellness program for the future.
- Discern between myths and facts of exercise and health-related concepts.

## U.S. HEALTH OBJECTIVES FOR THE YEAR 2000

Every 10 years the U.S. Department of Health and Human Services releases a list of objectives for disease prevention and health promotion. From its onset in 1980, this 10-year plan has helped instill a new sense of purpose and focus for public health and preventive medicine.

The Year 2000 objectives, published in the document *Healthy People 2000: National Health Promotion and Disease Prevention Objectives* address three important points:

1. **Personal responsibility.** The need for individuals to become ever more health-conscious. Responsible and informed behaviors are the key to good health.
2. **Health benefits for all people.** Lower socioeconomic conditions and poor health often are interrelated. Extending the benefits of good health to all people is crucial to the health of the nation.
3. **Health promotion and disease prevention.** A shift from treatment to preventive techniques will drastically cut health care costs and help all Americans achieve a higher quality of life.

Development of the Year 2000 Health Objectives involved more than 10,000 people representing 300 national organizations, including the Institute of Medicine of the National Academy of Sciences, all state health departments, and the federal Office of Disease Prevention and Health Promotion. A summary of key objectives is provided in Figure 1.15 at the end of this chapter. Living the fitness and wellness principles provided in this book not only will enhance the quality of your life but also will allow you to be an active participant in achieving the Healthy People 2000 Objectives.

## WELLNESS LIFESTYLE QUESTIONNAIRE

Most people go to college to learn how to make a living, *but a fitness and wellness course will teach you how to live* — that is, how to truly live life to its fullest potential. Don't even think for a moment that success in life is measured by how much money you make. Making a good living will not help you unless you live a wellness lifestyle that will allow you to enjoy what you have.

Everyone would like to enjoy good health and wellness, but most people don't know how to reach this objective. Lifestyle is the most important factor affecting our personal well-being. While some people live long because of genetic factors, the quality of life during middle age and the "golden" years is basically related to wise choices initiated during youth and continued throughout life.

In a few short years, lack of wellness leads to a loss of vitality and gusto for life, as well as premature morbidity and mortality. The Wellness Lifestyle Questionnaire, given in Figure 1.17 at the end of this chapter, will provide an initial rating of your current efforts to stay healthy and well, and the components of a wellness lifestyle are discussed in subsequent chapters of this book.

Upon completing the questionnaire, select the areas where you think you will need the most improvement. Although you need to pay attention to all aspects of wellness, initially work on those lifestyle factors in which definite improvements are required. Lifestyle choices that you make now will have an impact on how well you live the rest of your life.

## A WORD OF CAUTION

Even though exercise testing and participation is relatively safe for most apparently healthy individuals under age 45, how the cardiovascular system

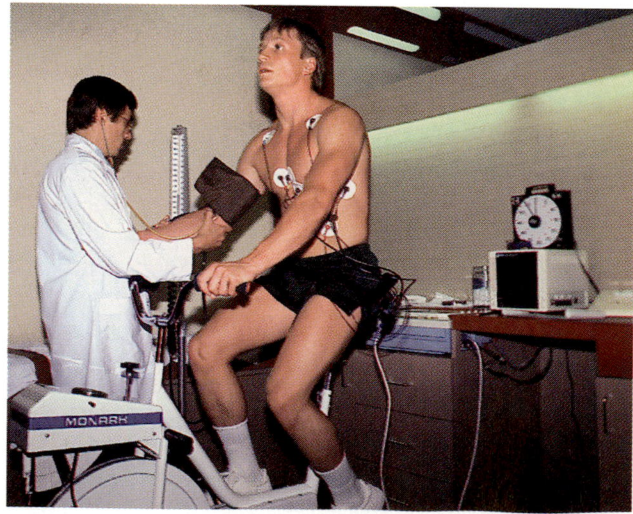


*Exercise electrocardiogram. An exercise tolerance test with twelve-lead electrocardiographic monitoring may be required of some individuals prior to initiating an exercise program.*

will react to higher levels of physical activity cannot be totally predicted. Consequently, a person takes a small but real risk of certain bodily changes occurring during exercise testing or participation. These include abnormal blood pressure, irregular heart rhythm, fainting, and, in rare instances, a heart attack or cardiac arrest.

Before you begin an exercise program or participate in any exercise testing, you should fill out the questionnaire in Figure 1.16. If your answer to any of the questions is *yes*, you should see a physician before participating in a fitness program. Exercise testing and participation is not wise under some of the conditions listed in this questionnaire and may require a stress electrocardiogram (ECG) test. If you have any questions regarding your current health status, consult your doctor before initiating, continuing, or increasing your level of physical activity.

## NOTES


1. U.S. Centers for Disease Control and Prevention and American College of Sports Medicine, "Summary Statement: Workshop on Physical Activity and Public Health," *Sports Medicine Bulletin*, 28(4), 7.
2. S. P. Van Camp, "The Fixx Tragedy: A Cardiologist's Perspective," *Physician and Sports Medicine* 12:9 (1984), 153-155.
3. R. S. Paffenbarger, Jr., R. T. Hyde, A. L. Wing, and C. H. Steinmetz, "A Natural History of Athleticism and Cardiovascular Health," *Journal of the American Medical Association,* 252 (1984), 491-495.
4. S. N. Blair, H. W. Kohl III, R. S. Paffenbarger, Jr., D. G. Clark, K. H. Cooper, and L. W. Gibbons, "Physical Fitness and All-Cause Mortality: A Prospective Study of Healthy Men and Women," *Journal of the American Medical Association,* 262 (1989), 2395-2401.
5. J. E. Enstrom, "Health Practices and Cancer Mortality Among Active California Mormons," *Journal of the National Cancer Institute,* 81 (1989), 1807-1814.
6. American Heart Association, *Heart and Stroke Facts*: 1994 (Dallas: AHA, 1993).
7. American Cancer Society, *1994 Cancer Facts and Figures* (New York: ACS, 1994).


## SELECT BIBLIOGRAPHY


Allsen, P. E., J. M. Harrison, and B. Vance. *Fitness for Life: An Individualized Approach*. Dubuque, IA: Wm C. Brown, 1993.

American College of Sports Medicine. "The Recommended Quantity and Quality of Exercise for Developing and Maintaining Cardiorespiratory and Muscular Fitness in Healthy Adults." *Medicine and Science in Sports and Exercise,* 22 (1990), 265-274.

Blair, S., D. Jacobs, and K. Powell. "Relationships Between Exercise or Physical Activity and Other Health Behaviors." *Public Health Reports,* 100 (1985), 172-180.

Davies, N. E., and L. H. Felder. "Applying Brakes to the Runaway American Health Care System." *Journal of the American Medical Association,* 263 (1990), 73-76.

Duncan, D. F., and R. S. Gold. "Reflections: Health Promotion — What Is It?" *Health Values,* 10:3 (1986), 47-48.

Gettman, L. R. "Cost/Benefit Analysis of a Corporate Fitness Program." *Fitness in Business,* 1:1 (1986), 11-17.

Hatziandreu, E. L., J. P. Koplan, M. C. Weinstein, C. J. Caspersen, and K. E. Warner. "A Cost-Effectiveness Analysis of Exercise as a Health Promotion Activity." *American Journal of Public Health,* 78 (1988), 1417-1421.

Hoeger, W. W. K. *Principles and Labs for Physical Fitness and Wellness* Englewood, CO: Morton Publishing, 1994.

Koplan, J. P., C. J. Caspersen, and K. E. Powell." Physical Activity, Physical Fitness, and Health: Time to Act." *Journal of the American Medical Association,* 262 (1989), 24-37.

Smith, L. K. "Cost-Effectiveness of Health Promotion Programs." *Fitness Management,* 2 (1986), 12-15.

"New Fitness Data Verifies: Employees Who Exercise Are Also More Productive." *Athletic Business,* 8:12 (1984), 24-30.

Wilmore, J. H. "Design Issues and Alternatives in Assessing Physical Fitness Among Apparently Healthy Adults in a Health Examination Survey of the General Population." In F. Drury (Editor), *Assessing Physical Fitness and Activity in General Population Studies.* Washington, DC: U.S. Public Health Service, National Center for Health Statistics, 1988.

Wright, C. C. "Cost Containment Through Health Promotion Programs." *Journal of Occupational Medicine,* 22 (1980), 36-39.

## HEALTHY PEOPLE 2000: SELECTED HEALTH OBJECTIVES FOR THE YEAR 2000

I. Physical Activity and Fitness

1. Increase the proportion of people who engage regularly, preferably daily, in *light* to *moderate* physical activity for at least 30 minutes per day.
2. Increase the proportion of people who engage in *vigorous* physical activity that promotes the development and maintenance of cardiorespiratory fitness 3 or more days per week for 20 or more minutes per occasion.
3. Increase the proportion of people who regularly perform physical activities that enhance and maintain muscular strength, muscular endurance, and flexibility.
4. Reduce the proportion of people who engage in no leisure-time physical activity.
5. Reduce overweight to a prevalence of no more than 20% among people aged 20 and older and no more than 15% among adolescents aged 12 through 19.
6. Increase to at least 50% the proportion of overweight people aged 12 and older who have adopted sound dietary practices combined with regular physical activity to attain an appropriate body weight.

II. Nutrition

1. Reduce dietary fat intake to an average of 30% of calories or less and average saturated fat intake to less than 10% of calories among people aged 2 and older.
2. Increase complex carbohydrate and fiber-containing foods in the diets of adults to 5 or more daily servings for vegetables and fruits, and to 6 or more daily servings for grain products.
3. Increase calcium consumption in the diet.
4. Reduce iron deficiency among children ages 1 through 4 and women of childbearing age.
5. Decrease salt and sodium intake in the diet.
6. Increase to at least 85% the proportion of people aged 18 and older who use food labels to make nutritious selections.

III. Chronic Diseases

1. Increase years of healthy life to at least 65 years.
2. Reduce coronary heart disease deaths.
3. Reduce the mean serum cholesterol level among adults to no more than 200 mg/dL.
4. Increase the proportion of adults with high blood cholesterol who are aware of their condition and are taking action to reduce their blood cholesterol to recommended levels.
5. Increase the proportion of people with high blood pressure whose blood pressure is under control.
6. Increase the proportion of people with high blood pressure who are taking action to help control their blood pressure.
7. Reverse the rise in cancer deaths.
8. Slow the rise in lung cancer deaths.
9. Reduce the rate of breast cancer deaths.
10. Reduce colorectal cancer deaths.
11. Reduce diabetes-related deaths.
12. Reduce the proportion of people with asthma who experience limitation in activity.
13. Reduce deaths from cirrhosis of the liver.
14. Reduce hip fractures among older adults.
15. Reduce limitation in activity because of chronic back conditions.
16. Reduce the proportion of people who experience a limitation in major activity because of chronic conditions.

IV. Mental Health and Disorders

1. Reduce the prevalence of mental disorders.
2. Reduce the suicide rate.
3. Reduce the proportion of people who experience adverse health effects from stress.
4. Decrease the proportion of people who experience stress who do not take steps to reduce or control their stress.

V. Tobacco

1. Reduce the incidence of cigarette smoking.
2. Reduce the initiation of cigarette smoking by children and youth.
3. Reduce the proportion of children who are exposed regularly to tobacco smoke at home.
4. Reduce use of smokeless tobacco.
5. Increase the proportion of worksites with a formal smoking policy that prohibits or severely restricts smoking at the workplace.

VI. Alcohol and Other Drugs

1. Reduce the proportion of young people who have used alcohol, marijuana, and cocaine.
2. Reduce the proportion of high school seniors and college students engaging in recent occasions of heavy drinking of alcoholic beverages.
3. Reduce alcohol consumption by people aged 14 and older to an annual average of no more than 2 gallons of ethanol per person.
4. Increase the proportion of high school seniors who associate risk of physical or psychological harm with the heavy use of alcohol, occasional use of marijuana, and experimentation with cocaine.
5. Reduce the proportion of male high school seniors who use anabolic steroids.
6. Reduce deaths caused by alcohol-related motor vehicle crashes.
7. Reduce drug-related deaths.
8. Increase the proportion of all intravenous drug abusers who are in drug abuse treatment programs.
9. Increase the proportion of intravenous drug abusers not in treatment who use only uncontaminated drug paraphernalia ("works").

VII. AIDS, HIV Infection, and Sexually Transmitted Diseases

1. Confine annual incidence of diagnosed AIDS cases to no more than 98,000 cases.
2. Confine the prevalence of HIV infection to no more than 800 per 100,000 people.
3. Increase the proportion of sexually active, unmarried people who used a condom at last sexual intercourse.
4. Reduce the incidence of gonorrhea.
5. Reduce the incidence of chlamydia.
6. Reduce the incidence of primary and secondary syphilis.
7. Reduce the incidence of genital herpes and genital warts.
8. Reduce the incidence of pelvic inflammatory disease.
9. Reduce the incidence of sexually transmitted hepatitis B infection.

VIII. Family Planning

1. Reduce the number of pregnancies that are unintended.
2. Reduce the proportion of adolescents who have engaged in sexual intercourse.
3. Increase the proportion of sexually active, unmarried people aged 19 and younger who use contraception, especially combined-method contraception that both effectively prevents pregnancy and provides barrier protection against disease.

IX. Unintentional Injuries

1. Reduce deaths caused by unintentional injuries.
2. Increase use of occupant protection systems, such as safety belts, inflatable safety restraints, and child safety seats among motor vehicle occupants.
3. Increase use of helmets among motorcyclists and bicyclists.

* Adapted from U.S. Department of Health and Human Services, Public Health Service. *Healthy People 2000: National Health Promotion and Disease Prevention Objectives.* (Boston: Jones and Bartlett Publishers, 1992). Refer to this publication for further information on these objectives.

**FIGURE 1.15** ◆

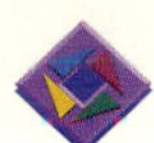

# HEALTH HISTORY QUESTIONNAIRE

Although exercise testing and exercise participation are relatively safe for most apparently healthy individuals under, the reaction of the cardiovascular system to increased physical activity cannot always be totally predicted. Consequently, a person takes a small but real risk of certain changes occurring during exercise testing or participation. These changes may include abnormal blood pressure, irregular heart rhythm, fainting, and, in rare instances, a heart attack or cardiac arrest.

Therefore, it is imperative that you provide honest answers to this questionnaire. Exercise may be ill-advised under some of the conditions listed below; others simply may require special consideration. **If any of the conditions apply, consult your physician before you participate in an exercise program.** Also, promptly report to your instructor any exercise-related abnormalities that you may experience during exercise participation.

A. Have you ever had or do you now have any of the following conditions:

☐ 1. Myocardial infarction
☐ 2. Coronary artery disease
☐ 3. Congestive heart failure
☐ 4. Elevated blood lipids (cholesterol and triglycerides)
☐ 5. Chest pain at rest or during exertion
☐ 6. Shortness of breath
☐ 7. Abnormal resting or stress electrocardiogram
☐ 8. Uneven, irregular, or skipped heartbeats (including racing or fluttering heart)
☐ 9. Blood embolism
☐ 10. Thrombophlebitis
☐ 11. Rheumatic heart fever
☐ 12. Elevated blood pressure
☐ 13. Stroke
☐ 14. Diabetes
☐ 15. Family history of coronary heart disease, syncope, or sudden death before age 60
☐ 16. Any other heart problem that makes exercise unsafe

B. Do you have any of the following conditions:

☐ 1. Arthritis, rheumatism, or gout
☐ 2. Chronic low back pain
☐ 3. Any other joint, bone, or muscle problems
☐ 4. Any respiratory problems
☐ 5. Obesity (more than 30% overweight)
☐ 6. Anorexia
☐ 7. Bulimia
☐ 8. Mononucleosis
☐ 9. Any physical disability that could interfere with safe participation in exercise

C. Do any of the following conditions apply:

☐ 1. Do you smoke cigarettes?
☐ 2. Are you taking any prescription drug?
☐ 3. Men: Are you 40 or older?
☐ 3. Women: Are you 50 or older?

D Do you have any other concern regarding your ability to safely participate in an exercise program? If so, explain:

________________________________________

________________________________________

Student's Signature: ____________________ Date: ____________

**FIGURE 1.16** ◆

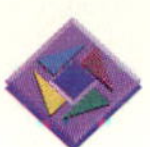

## WELLNESS LIFESTYLE QUESTIONNAIRE

Please circle the appropriate answer to each question and total your points as indicated at the end of the questionnaire. Circle 5 if the statement is ALWAYS true, 4 if the statement is FREQUENTLY true, 3 if the statement is OCCASIONALLY true, 2 if the statement is SELDOM true, 1 if the statement is NEVER true.

1. I am able to identify the situations and factors that overstress me. 5 4 3 2 1
2. I eat only when I am hungry. 5 4 3 2 1
3. I don't take tranquilizers or other drugs to relax. 5 4 3 2 1
4. I support efforts in my community to reduce environmental pollution. 5 4 3 2 1
5. I avoid buying foods with artificial colorings. 5 4 3 2 1
6. I rarely have problems concentrating on what I'm doing because of worrying about other things. 5 4 3 2 1
7. My employer (school) takes measures to ensure that my work (study) place is safe. 5 4 3 2 1
8. I try not to use medications when I feel unwell. 5 4 3 2 1
9. I am able to identify certain bodily responses and illnesses as my reactions to stress. 5 4 3 2 1
10. I question the use of diagnostic x-rays. 5 4 3 2 1
11. I try to alter personal living habits that are risk factors for heart disease, cancer, and other lifestyle diseases. 5 4 3 2 1
12. I avoid taking sleeping pills to help me sleep. 5 4 3 2 1
13. I try not to eat foods with refined sugar or corn sugar ingredients. 5 4 3 2 1
14. I accomplish goals I set for myself. 5 4 3 2 1
15. I stretch or bend for several minutes each day to keep my body flexible. 5 4 3 2 1
16. I support immunization of all children for common childhood diseases. 5 4 3 2 1
17. I try to prevent friends from driving after they drink alcohol. 5 4 3 2 1
18. I minimize extra salt intake. 5 4 3 2 1
19. I don't mind when other people and situations make me wait or lose time. 5 4 3 2 1
20. I walk four or fewer flights of stairs rather than take the elevator. 5 4 3 2 1
21. I eat fresh fruits and vegetables. 5 4 3 2 1
22. I use dental floss at least once a day. 5 4 3 2 1
23. I read product labels on foods to determine their ingredients. 5 4 3 2 1
24. I try to maintain a normal body weight. 5 4 3 2 1
25. I record my feelings and thoughts in a journal or diary. 5 4 3 2 1
26. I have no difficulty falling asleep. 5 4 3 2 1
27. I engage in some form of vigorous physical activity at least three times a week. 5 4 3 2 1

*(Continued)*

* *Health & Wellness*, fourth edition, by Edlin and Golanty © 1992, Boston: Jones and Bartlett Publishers. Reprinted by permission.

**FIGURE 1.17** ◆

28. I take time each day to quiet my mind and relax. 5 4 3 2 1
29. I am willing to make and sustain close friendships and intimate relationships. 5 4 3 2 1
30. I obtain an adequate daily supply of vitamins from my food or vitamin supplements. 5 4 3 2 1
31. I rarely have tension or migraine headaches, or pain in the neck or shoulders. 5 4 3 2 1
32. I wear a safety belt when driving. 5 4 3 2 1
33. I am aware of the emotional and situational factors that lead me to overeat. 5 4 3 2 1
34. I avoid driving my car after drinking any alcohol. 5 4 3 2 1
35. I am aware of the side effects of the medicines I take. 5 4 3 2 1
36. I am able to accept feelings of sadness, depression, and anxiety, knowing that they are almost always transient. 5 4 3 2 1
37. I would seek several additional professional opinions if my doctor were to recommend surgery for me. 5 4 3 2 1
38. I agree that nonsmokers should not have to breathe the smoke from cigarettes in public places. 5 4 3 2 1
39. I agree that pregnant women who smoke harm their babies. 5 4 3 2 1
40. I think I get enough sleep. 5 4 3 2 1
41. I ask my doctor why a certain medication is being prescribed and inquire about alternatives. 5 4 3 2 1
42. I am aware of the calories expended in my activities. 5 4 3 2 1
43. I am willing to give priority to my own needs for time and psychological space by saying "no" to others' requests of me. 5 4 3 2 1
44. I walk instead of drive whenever feasible. 5 4 3 2 1
45. I eat a breakfast that contains about one-third of my daily need for calories, proteins, and vitamins. 5 4 3 2 1
46. I prohibit smoking in my home. 5 4 3 2 1
47. I remember and think about my dreams. 5 4 3 2 1
48. I seek medical attention only when I have symptoms or believe that some (potential) condition needs checking, rather than have routine yearly checkups. 5 4 3 2 1
49. I endeavor to make my home accident-free. 5 4 3 2 1
50. I ask my doctor to explain the diagnosis of my problem until I understand all that I care to. 5 4 3 2 1
51. I try to include fiber or roughage (whole grains, fresh fruits and vegetables, or bran) in my daily diet. 5 4 3 2 1
52. I can deal with my emotional problems without alcohol or other mood-altering drugs. 5 4 3 2 1
53. I am satisfied with my school/work. 5 4 3 2 1
54. I require children riding in my car to be in infant seats or in shoulder harnesses. 5 4 3 2 1
55. I try to associate with people who have a positive attitude about life. 5 4 3 2 1

**FIGURE 1.17** ◆ *(Continued)*

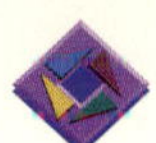

56. I try not to eat snacks of candy, pastries, and other "junk" foods. 5 4 3 2 1

57. I avoid people who are "down" all the time and bring down those around them. 5 4 3 2 1

58. I am aware of the calorie content of the foods I eat. 5 4 3 2 1

59. I brush my teeth after meals. 5 4 3 2 1

60. (for women only) I routinely examine my breasts. 5 4 3 2 1

(for men only) I am aware of the signs of testicular cancer. 5 4 3 2 1

**How to Score**

Enter the numbers you've circled next to the question number and total your score for each category. Then determine your degree of wellness for each category using the wellness status key.

| Emotional health | Fitness and body care | Environmental health | Stress | Nutrition | Medical self-responsibility |
|---|---|---|---|---|---|
| 6____ | 15____ | 4____ | 1____ | 2____ | 8____ |
| 12____ | 20____ | 7____ | 3____ | 5____ | 10____ |
| 25____ | 22____ | 17____ | 9____ | 13____ | 11____ |
| 26____ | 24____ | 32____ | 14____ | 18____ | 16____ |
| 36____ | 27____ | 34____ | 19____ | 21____ | 35____ |
| 40____ | 33____ | 38____ | 28____ | 23____ | 37____ |
| 47____ | 42____ | 39____ | 29____ | 30____ | 41____ |
| 52____ | 44____ | 46____ | 31____ | 45____ | 48____ |
| 55____ | 58____ | 49____ | 43____ | 51____ | 59____ |
| 57____ | 59____ | 54____ | 53____ | 56____ | 60____ |
| Total____ | Total____ | Total____ | Total____ | Total____ | Total____ |

**Wellness Status**

To assess your status in each of the six categories, compare your total score in each to the following key: 0-34 Need improvement; 35-44 Good; 45-50 Excellent.

**FIGURE 1.17** ◆ *(Continued)*

# Cardiovascular Endurance Assessment

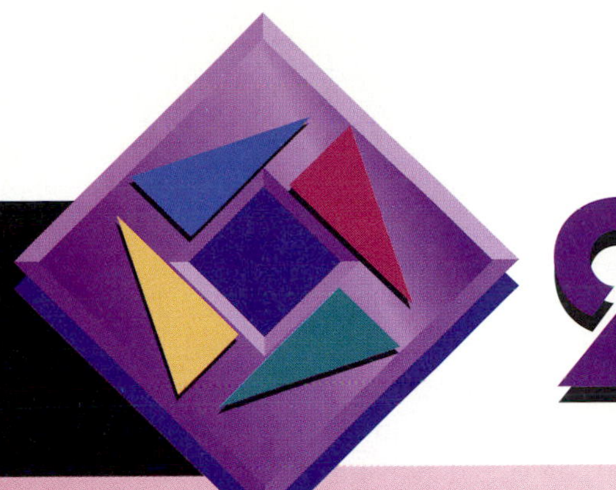


## Key Concepts

Cardiovascular endurance
Aerobic exercise
Anaerobic exercise
Maximal oxygen uptake (Max $VO_2$)
Maximal exercise
Submaximal exercise
Exercise readiness

## Objectives

- Understand the importance of adequate cardiovascular endurance in maintaining good health and well-being.
- Define cardiovascular endurance and the benefits of cardiovascular endurance training.
- Define aerobic and anaerobic exercise.
- Be able to assess cardiovascular endurance using five different maximal oxygen uptake estimation protocols (1.5-Mile Run Test, 1.0-Mile Walk Test, Step Test, Astrand-Ryhming Test, and 12-Minute Swim Test).
- Learn to interpret cardiovascular endurance assessment test results according to health fitness and physical fitness standards.
- Determine readiness to start an exercise program.

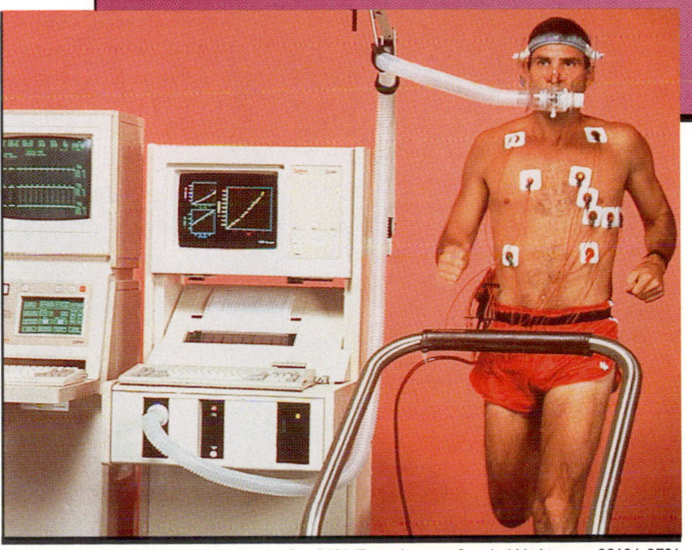

Photo Courtesy of Quinton Instrument Co., 2121 Terry Avenue, Seattle, Washington 98121-2791

Cardiovascular endurance has been defined as *the ability of the lungs, heart, and blood vessels to deliver adequate amounts of oxygen to the cells to meet the demands of prolonged physical activity*. As a person breathes, part of the oxygen in the air is taken up in the lungs and transported in the blood to the heart. The heart then is responsible for pumping the oxygenated blood through the circulatory system to all organs and tissues of the body. At the cellular level, oxygen is used to convert food substrates*, primarily carbohydrates and fats, into energy necessary to conduct body functions and maintain constant internal equilibrium. During physical exertion more energy is needed to perform the activity. As a result, the heart, lungs, and blood vessels have to deliver more oxygen to the cells to supply the required energy.

* Substrates are the bases on which an organism lives, or substances that are acted upon in the body.

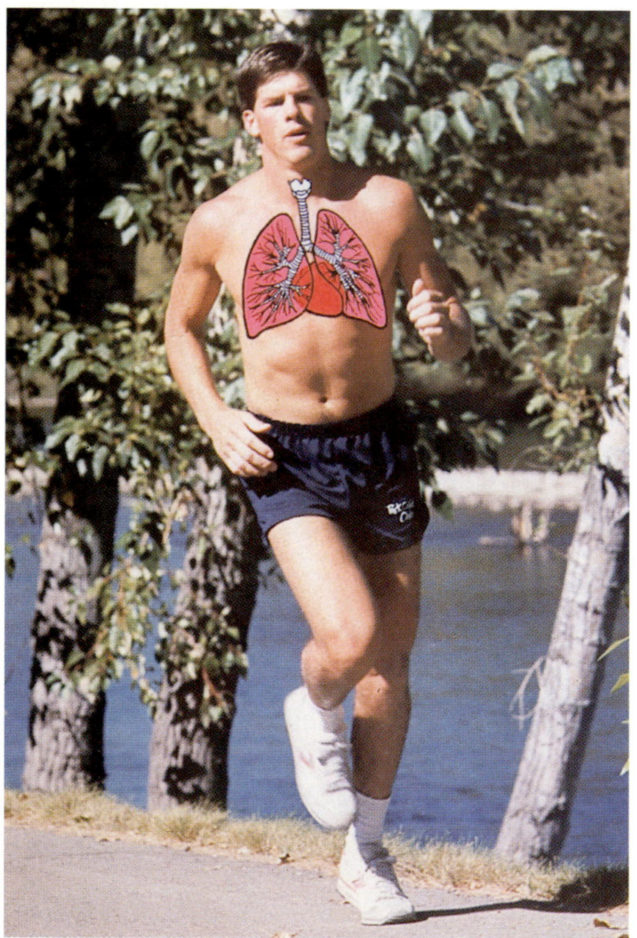

*Cardiovascular endurance is the ability of the lungs, heart, and blood vessels to deliver adequate amounts of oxygen to the cells to meet the demands of prolonged physical activity.*

During prolonged exercise an individual with a high level of cardiovascular endurance is able to deliver the required amount of oxygen to the tissues with relative ease. The cardiovascular system of a person with a low level of endurance has to work much harder, as the heart has to pump more often to supply the same amount of oxygen to the tissues and, consequently, fatigues faster. Hence, a higher capacity to deliver and utilize oxygen (oxygen uptake) indicates a more efficient cardiovascular system.

## AEROBIC AND ANAEROBIC EXERCISE

Cardiovascular endurance activities often are called aerobic exercises. The word *aerobic* means "with oxygen." Whenever an activity requires oxygen to produce energy, it is considered an aerobic exercise. Examples of cardiovascular or aerobic exercises are walking, jogging, swimming, cycling, cross-country skiing, water aerobics, rope skipping, and aerobics.

*Anaerobic* activities, on the other hand, are carried out "without oxygen." The intensity of anaerobic exercise is so high that oxygen is not utilized to produce energy. Because energy production is limited in the absence of oxygen, these activities can be carried out for only short periods (2 to 3 minutes). The higher the intensity of the activity, the shorter the duration.

Activities such as the 100, 200, and 400 meters in track and field, the 100 meters in swimming, gymnastics routines, and strength training are good examples of anaerobic activities. Anaerobic activities do not contribute much to development of the cardiovascular system. Only aerobic activities will help increase cardiovascular endurance.

## IMPORTANCE OF CARDIOVASCULAR ENDURANCE

Physical activity is no longer a natural part of our existence. We live in an automated world, one in which most of the activities that used to require strenuous physical exertion can be done by machines. For instance, most people drive their automobiles to a store only a few blocks away and then spend a couple of minutes driving around the

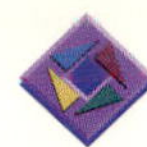

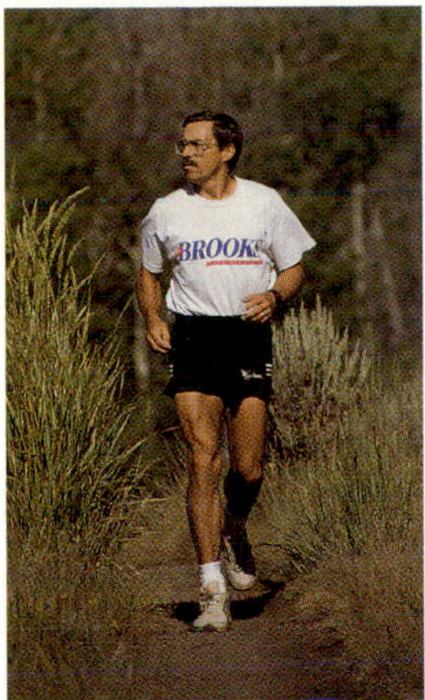

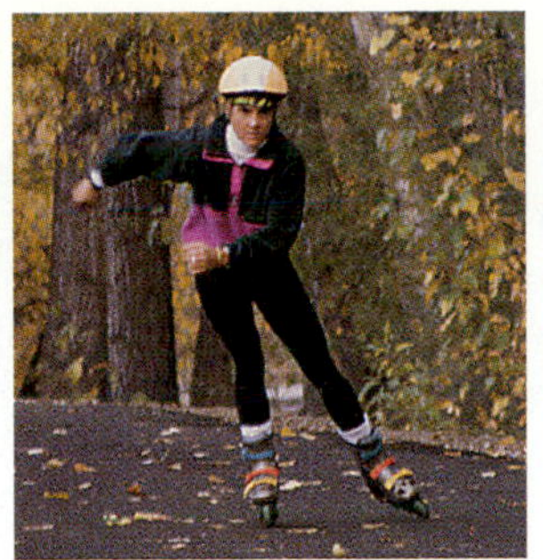

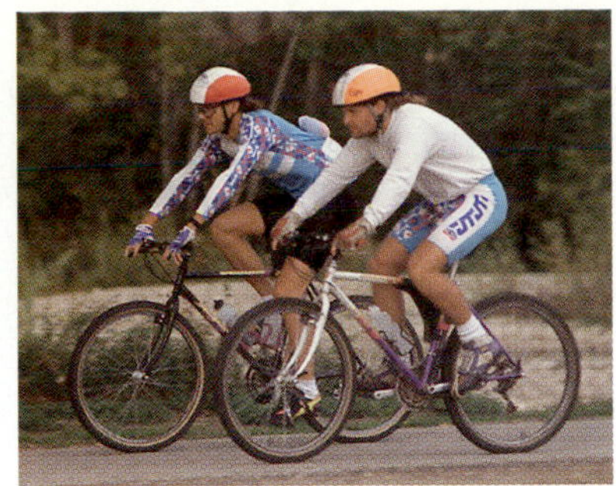

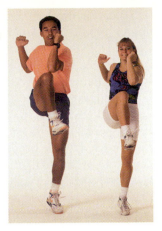

**SAMPLE AEROBIC ACTIVITIES**

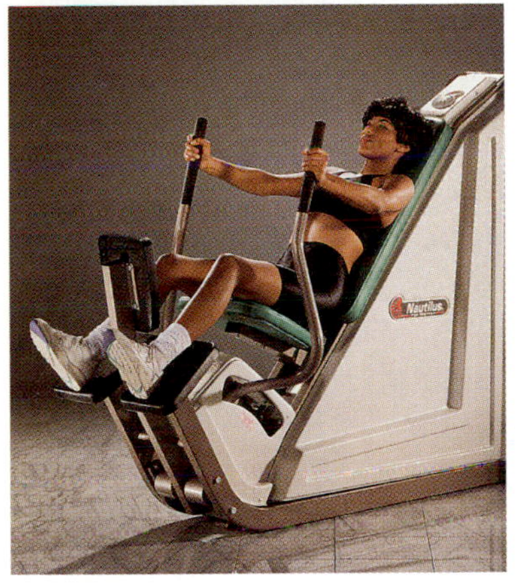

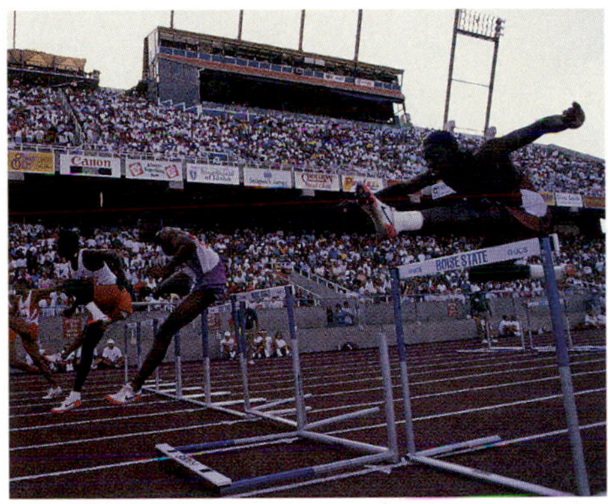

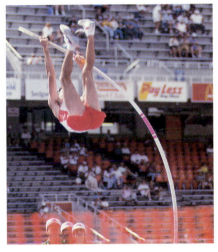

**SAMPLE ANAEROBIC ACTIVITIES**

parking lot to find a spot 10 yards closer to the store's entrance. They do not even have to carry out the groceries. A youngster working at the store usually takes them out in a cart and places them in the vehicle.

Similarly, during a visit to a multilevel shopping mall, almost everyone chooses to ride the escalators instead of taking the stairs. Automobiles, elevators, escalators, telephones, intercoms, remote controls, electric garage door openers — all are modern-day amenities that minimize the amount of movement and effort required of the human body.

Among the most harmful effects of modern-day technology is an increase in chronic conditions related to a lack of physical activity. These include hypertension, heart disease, chronic low back pain, and obesity. They are referred to as *hypokinetic diseases*. "Hypo" means low or little, and "kinetic" implies motion. Lack of adequate physical activity

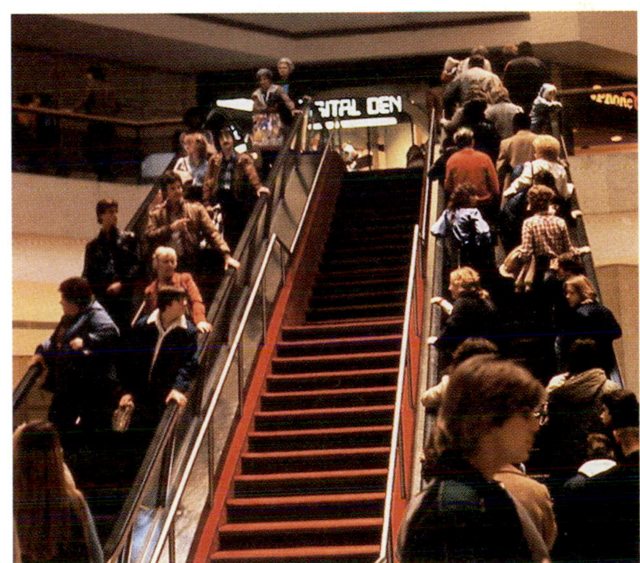

*Advances in modern technology have almost completely eliminated the need for physical activity, significantly enhancing the deterioration rate of the human body.*

is a fact of modern life that most people can no longer avoid. To enjoy modern technology and still expect to live life to its fullest, however, a personalized lifetime exercise program must become a part of daily living.

A sound cardiovascular endurance program greatly contributes to good health. Of the four components of physical fitness, cardiovascular endurance is the single most important. Certain amounts of muscular strength and flexibility are necessary in daily activities to lead a normal life. Even so, a person can get away without having large amounts of strength and flexibility but cannot do without a good cardiovascular system.

The "typical" American is not a good role model when cardiovascular endurance is concerned. Only about a tenth of the adult population exercises vigorously enough to meet the physical fitness standard for cardiovascular fitness. About 40% is able to meet the health-fitness standard.

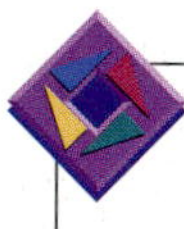

*Cardiovascular endurance is the most important component of health-related fitness.*

Aerobic exercise is especially important in preventing coronary heart disease. A poorly conditioned heart that has to pump more often just to keep a person alive is subject to more wear-and-tear than a well-conditioned heart. In situations where strenuous demands are placed on the heart, such as doing yard work, lifting heavy objects or weights, or running to catch a train, the unconditioned heart may not be able to sustain the strain. In addition, regular participation in cardiovascular endurance activities helps achieve and maintain recommended body weight, the fourth component of health-related physical fitness.

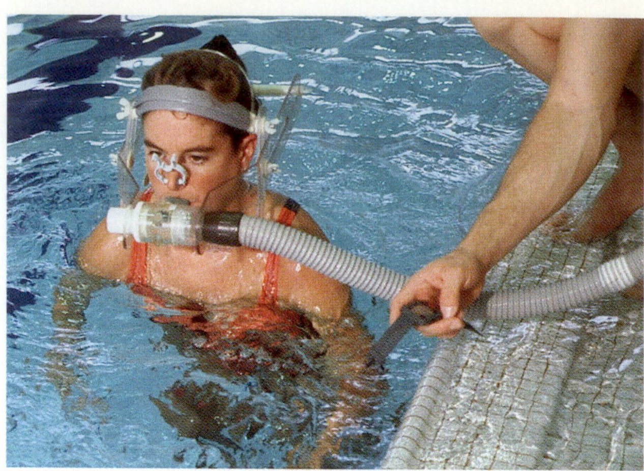

*Oxygen uptake assessment during a water aerobics exercise test.*

## BENEFITS OF CARDIOVASCULAR ENDURANCE TRAINING

Everyone who participates in a cardiovascular or aerobic exercise program can expect a number of physiological adaptations from training. Among these benefits are:

1. *A higher maximal oxygen uptake (Max $VO_2$).* The amount of oxygen the body is able to use during physical activity increases significantly. This allows the individual to exercise longer and at a higher rate before becoming fatigued.

   Small increases in Max $VO_2$ can be observed in as few as 2 to 3 weeks of aerobic training. Depending on the initial fitness level, Max $VO_2$ may increase as much as 30%, although higher increases have been reported in people with very low initial levels of fitness.

2. *An increase in the oxygen-carrying capacity of the blood.* As a result of training, the red blood cell count goes up. Red blood cells contain hemoglobin, which transports oxygen in the blood.

3. *A decrease in resting heart rate and an increase in cardiac muscle strength.* During resting conditions, the heart ejects between 5 and 6 liters of blood per minute (a liter is slightly larger than a quart). This amount of blood, also referred to as *cardiac output*, meets the energy demands in the resting state.

   Like any other muscle, the heart responds to training by increasing in strength and size. As the heart gets stronger, the muscle can produce a more forceful contraction, which causes more blood to be ejected with each beat (stroke volume), yielding a lower heart rate. This lower heart rate also allows the heart to rest longer between beats. Average resting and maximal cardiac outputs, stroke volumes, and heart rates for sedentary, trained, and highly trained (elite) males are shown in Table 2.1.

   Resting heart rates frequently are lowered by 10 to 20 beats per minute (bpm) after only 6 to

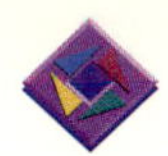

**TABLE 2.1**
**Average Cardiovascular Differences Between Sedentary, Trained, and Highly Trained Males**

| | RESTING | | | MAXIMAL | | |
|---|---|---|---|---|---|---|
| | $\dot{Q}$ (L/min) | SV (ml) | HR (bpm) | $\dot{Q}$ (L/min) | SV (ml) | HR (bpm) |
| Sedentary | 5 | 68 | 74 | 20 | 100 | 200 |
| Trained | 5 | 90 | 56 | 30 | 150 | 200 |
| Highly Trained | 5 | 110 | 45 | 35 | 175 | 200 |

$\dot{Q}$ = cardiac output
SV = stroke volume
HR = heart rate
L/min = liters per minute
ml = milliliters
bpm = beats per minute

8 weeks of training. A reduction of 20 bpm saves the heart about 10,483,200 beats per year. The average heart beats between 70 and 80 bpm. As seen in Table 2.1, resting heart rates in highly trained athletes are often around 45 bpm.

4. *A lower heart rate at given workloads.* When compared with untrained individuals, a trained person has a lower heart rate response to a given task. This is because of the greater efficiency of the cardiovascular system. Individuals also are surprised to find that, following several weeks of training, a given workload (let's say a 10-minute mile) elicits a much lower heart rate response as compared to the response when training first started.

5. *An increase in the number and size of the mitochondria.* All energy necessary for cell function is produced in the mitochondria. As the size and number increase, so does the potential to produce energy for muscular work.

6. *An increase in the number of functional capillaries.* These smaller blood vessels allow for the exchange of oxygen and carbon dioxide between the blood and the cells. As more vessels open up, more gas exchange can take place, delaying the onset of fatigue during prolonged exercise. This increase in capillaries also speeds up the rate at which waste products of cell metabolism can be removed. Increased capillarization also is seen in the heart, which enhances oxygen delivery capacity to the heart muscle itself.

7. *Faster recovery time.* Trained individuals recover more rapidly after exercising. A fit system is able to restore more quickly any internal equilibrium disrupted during exercise.

8. *Lower blood pressure and blood lipids.* A regular aerobic exercise program leads to lower blood pressure and fats such as cholesterol and triglycerides, all of which have been linked to the formation of atherosclerotic plaque, which obstructs the arteries. This decreases the risk of coronary heart disease (see Chapter 9). High blood pressure also is a leading risk factor for strokes.

9. More fat-burning enzymes. The role of fat-burning enzymes is significant because fat is lost primarily by burning it in muscle. As the concentration of the enzymes increases, so does the ability to burn fat.

## ASSESSMENT OF CARDIOVASCULAR ENDURANCE

The level of cardiovascular endurance, cardiovascular fitness, or aerobic capacity is determined by the maximal amount of oxygen (Max $VO_2$) the human body is able to utilize per minute of physical activity. This value can be expressed in liters per minute (L/min) or milliliters per kilogram per minute (ml/kg/min). The relative value in ml/kg/min is used most often because it considers total body mass (weight). When comparing two individuals with the same absolute value, the one with the lesser body mass will have a higher relative value, indicating that more oxygen is available to each kilogram (2.2 pounds) of body weight. Because all tissues and organs of the body need oxygen to function, a higher oxygen consumption indicates a more efficient cardiovascular system.

The most precise way to determine maximal oxygen uptake is through *direct gas analysis.* This is done by using a metabolic cart through which the amount of oxygen consumption can be measured directly. This type of equipment is not available in most health/fitness centers. Therefore, several alternative methods of estimating maximal oxygen uptake have been developed using limited equipment.

Even though most cardiovascular endurance tests probably are safe to administer to apparently healthy individuals (those with no major coronary risk factors or symptoms), the American College of Sports Medicine recommends that a physician be present for all maximal exercise tests on apparently healthy men over age 40 and women over age 50. *A maximal test is any test that requires the participant's all-out or nearly all-out effort.* For submaximal exercise tests a physician should be present when testing higher risk/symptomatic individuals or diseased people, regardless of the participant's current age.

Five exercise tests used to assess cardiovascular fitness are introduced in this chapter: 1.5-Mile Run Test, 1.0-Mile Walk Test, Step Test, Astrand-Ryhming Test, and 12-Minute Swim Test. The test procedures are explained in detail in Figures 2.1, 2.2, 2.3, 2.4, and 2.5, respectively. Depending on time, facilities, and individual physical limitations, you may do one or more of these tests. For example, people who can't jog or walk could take the bike test or the swim test. Because these are different tests, they will not necessarily yield the exact same results. Therefore, to make valid comparisons, you should take the same test when doing pre- and post-assessments.

## 1.5-Mile Run Test

This test is used most often to predict cardiovascular fitness according to the time the person takes to run or walk a 1.5-mile course (see Figure 2.1). Max $VO_2$ is estimated based on the time the person takes to cover the distance (see Table 2.2).

The only equipment necessary to conduct this test is a stopwatch and a track or premeasured 1.5-mile course. This perhaps is the easiest test to do, but a note of caution is in order: As the objective is to cover the distance in the shortest time, it is considered a maximal exercise test. The 1.5-Mile Run Test should be limited to conditioned individuals who have been cleared for exercise. The test is not recommended for unconditioned beginners or for men over age 40 and women over age 50 without proper medical clearance, symptomatic individuals, and those with known disease or coronary heart disease risk factors. A program of at least 6 weeks of aerobic training is recommended before unconditioned individuals take this test.

### 1.5 MILE RUN TEST

1. Make sure that you qualify for this test. This test is not advised for unconditioned beginners, individuals with symptoms of heart disease, and those with known heart disease or risk factors.
2. Select the testing site. Find a school track (each lap is one-fourth of a mile) or a premeasured 1.5-mile course.
3. Have a stopwatch available to determine your time.
4. Conduct a few warm-up exercises before the test. Do some stretching exercises, some walking, and slow jogging.
5. Start the test and try to cover the distance in the fastest time possible (walking or jogging). Time yourself during the run to see how fast you have covered the distance. If any unusual symptoms arise during the test, do not continue. Stop immediately and retake the test after another 6 weeks of aerobic training.
6. At the end of the test, cool down by walking or jogging slowly for another 3 to 5 minutes. Do not sit or lie down after the test.
7. According to your performance time, look up your estimated maximal oxygen uptake Max $VO_2$ in Table 2.2.
8. Example: A 20-year-old female runs the 1.5-mile course in 12 minutes and 40 seconds. Table 2.2 shows a Max $VO_2$ of 39.8 ml/kg/min for a time of 12:40. According to Table 2.8, this maximal oxygen uptake would place her in the good cardiovascular fitness category.

**FIGURE 2.1** ◆ Procedure for the 1.5-Mile Run Test.

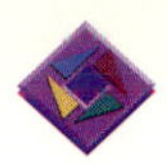

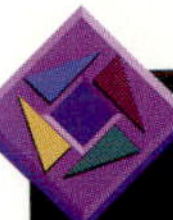

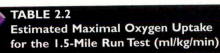

**TABLE 2.2**
**Estimated Maximal Oxygen Uptake for the 1.5-Mile Run Test (ml/kg/min)**

| Time | Max $VO_2$ | Time | Max $VO_2$ |
|---|---|---|---|
| 6:10 | 80.0 | 12:40 | 39.8 |
| 6:20 | 79.0 | 12:50 | 39.2 |
| 6:30 | 77.9 | 13:00 | 38.6 |
| 6:40 | 76.7 | 13:10 | 38.1 |
| 6:50 | 75.5 | 13:20 | 37.8 |
| 7:00 | 74.0 | 13:30 | 37.2 |
| 7:10 | 72.6 | 13:40 | 36.8 |
| 7:20 | 71.3 | 13:50 | 36.3 |
| 7:30 | 69.9 | 14:00 | 35.9 |
| 7:40 | 68.3 | 14:10 | 35.5 |
| 7:50 | 66.8 | 14:20 | 35.1 |
| 8:00 | 65.2 | 14:30 | 34.7 |
| 8:10 | 63.9 | 14:40 | 34.3 |
| 8:20 | 62.5 | 14:50 | 34.0 |
| 8:30 | 61.2 | 15:00 | 33.6 |
| 8:40 | 60.2 | 15:10 | 33.1 |
| 8:50 | 59.1 | 15:20 | 32.7 |
| 9:00 | 58.1 | 15:30 | 32.2 |
| 9:10 | 56.9 | 15:40 | 31.8 |
| 9:20 | 55.9 | 15:50 | 31.4 |
| 9:30 | 54.7 | 16:00 | 30.9 |
| 9:40 | 53.5 | 16:10 | 30.5 |
| 9:50 | 52.3 | 16:20 | 30.2 |
| 10:00 | 51.1 | 16:30 | 29.8 |
| 10:10 | 50.4 | 16:40 | 29.5 |
| 10:20 | 49.5 | 16:50 | 29.1 |
| 10:30 | 48.6 | 17:00 | 28.9 |
| 10:40 | 48.0 | 17:10 | 28.5 |
| 10:50 | 47.4 | 17:20 | 28.3 |
| 11:00 | 46.6 | 17:30 | 28.0 |
| 11:10 | 45.8 | 17:40 | 27.7 |
| 11:20 | 45.1 | 17:50 | 27.4 |
| 11:30 | 44.4 | 18:00 | 27.1 |
| 11:40 | 43.7 | 18:10 | 26.8 |
| 11:50 | 43.2 | 18:20 | 26.6 |
| 12:00 | 42.3 | 18:30 | 26.3 |
| 12:10 | 41.7 | 18:40 | 26.0 |
| 12:20 | 41.0 | 18:50 | 25.7 |
| 12:30 | 40.4 | 19:00 | 25.4 |

Source: Adapted from "A Means of Assessing Maximal Oxygen Intake," by K. H. Cooper, *Journal of the American Medical Association* 203 (1968), 201–204; *Health and Fitness Through Physical Activity*, by M. L. Pollock et al. (New York: John Wiley & Sons, 1978); and *Training for Sport and Activity*, by J. H. Wilmore (Boston: Allyn and Bacon, 1982).

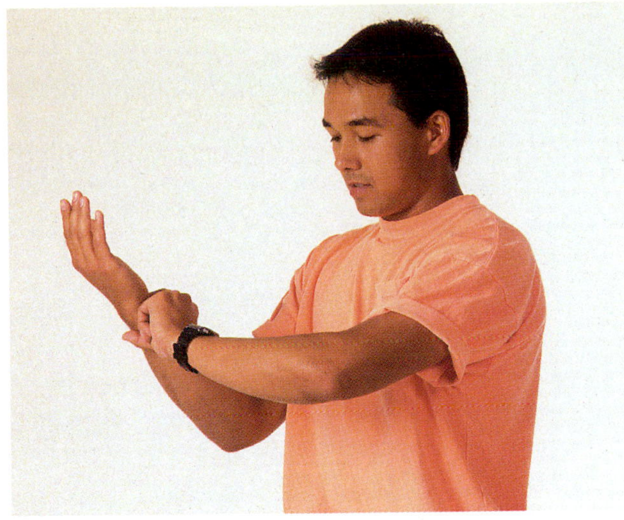

*Pulse taken at the radial artery.*

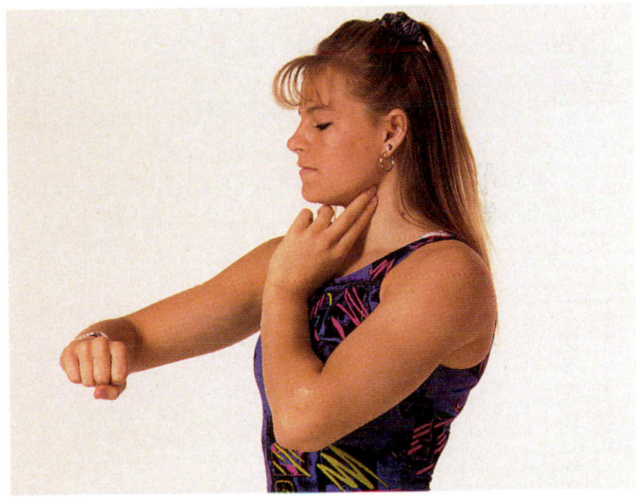

*Pulse taken at the carotid artery.*

## 1.0-Mile Walk Test

This test can be used by individuals who are unable to run because of low fitness levels or injuries. All that is required is a brisk 1.0-mile walk that will elicit an exercise heart rate of at least 120 beats per minute at the end of the test.

You will need to know how to take your heart rate by counting your pulse. This can be done on the wrist by placing two fingers over the radial artery (inside the wrist on the side of the thumb) or over the carotid artery in the neck just below the jaw, next to the voice box.

Max $VO_2$ is estimated according to a prediction equation that requires the following data: 1.0-mile walk time, exercise heart rate at the end of the walk, age, sex, and body weight in pounds. The procedure for this test and the equation are given in Figure 2.2.

## 1.0 MILE WALK TEST

1. Select the testing site. Use a 440-yard track (4 laps to a mile) or a premeasured 1.0-mile course.
2. Prior to the test, determine your body weight in pounds.
3. Have a stopwatch available to determine total walking time and exercise heart rate.
4. Walk the 1.0-mile course at a brisk pace (the exercise heart rate at the end of the test should be above 120 beats per minute).
5. At the end of the 1.0-mile walk, check your walking time and immediately count your pulse for 10 seconds. Multiply the 10-second pulse count by 6 to obtain the exercise heart rate in beats per minute.
6. Convert the walking time from minutes and seconds to minute units. Because there are 60 seconds in 1 minute, divide the seconds by 60 to obtain the fraction of a minute. For instance, a walking time of 12 minutes and 15 seconds would equal $12 + (15 \div 60)$, or 12.25 minutes.
7. To obtain the estimated maximal oxygen uptake (Max $VO_2$) in ml/kg/min, plug your values in the following equation:

   $$\text{Max } VO_2 = 132.853 - (.0769 \times W) - (.3877 \times A) + (6.315 \times G) - (3.2649 \times T) \times (.1565 \times HR)$$

   Where:

   W = Weight in pounds
   A = Age in years
   G = Gender (use 0 for women and 1 for men)
   T = Total time for the 1-mile walk in minutes (see item 6 above)
   HR = Exercise heart rate in beats per minute at the end of the one-mile walk

   *Example:* A 19-year-old female who weighs 140 pounds completed the 1-mile walk in 14 minutes 39 seconds and with an exercise heart rate of 148 beats per minute. The estimated Max $VO_2$ would be:

   W = 140 lbs
   A = 19
   G = 0 (female gender = 0)
   T = $14{:}39 = 14 + (39 \div 60) = 14.65$ min
   HR = 148 bpm

   $$\text{Max } VO_2 = 132.853 - (.0769 \times 140) - (.3877 \times 19) + (6.315 \times 0) - (3.2649 \times 14.65) - (.1565 \times 148)$$

   $$\text{Max } VO_2 = 43.7 \text{ ml/kg/min}$$

8. If you take the 1.0-Mile Walk Test, you may use the spaces below to record your data and solve the equation for your own Max $VO_2$.

   W = ____________ lbs

   A = ____________

   G = ____________ (female gender = 0)

   T = ______:______ = (min) + ( (sec) ÷ 60) = min

   HR = ____________ bpm

   Max $VO_2$ = 132.853 – (.0769 × ) – (.3877 × ) + (6.315 × ) – (3.2649 × ) – (.1565 × )

   Max $VO_2$ = 132.853 – ( ) – ( ) + ( ) – ( ) – ( )

   Max $VO_2$ = ml/kg/min

Source: "Estimation of $VO_{2max}$ from a One-Mile Track Walk, Gender, Age, and Body Weight," by G. Kline et al., *Medicine and Science in Sports and Exercise* 19:3 (1987), 253–259. 

**FIGURE 2.2** ◆ Procedure for the 1.0-Mile Walk Test.

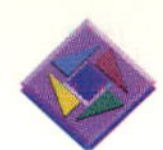

## Step Test

The Step Test requires little time and equipment and most people can take it, as a submaximal workload is used to estimate Max $VO_2$. Symptomatic and diseased individuals should not take this test. Significantly overweight individuals and those with joint problems in the lower extremities may have difficulty performing the test.

The actual test takes only 3 minutes. A 15-second recovery heart rate is taken between 5 and 20 seconds following the test (see Figure 2.3 and Table 2.3). The equipment required is a bench or gymnasium bleacher 16¼ inches high, a stopwatch, and a metronome.

You will also need to know how to take your heart rate by counting your pulse (explained under the 1.0-Mile Walk Test). By teaching people to take their own heart rate, a large group of people can be tested at once, using gymnasium bleachers.

### STEP TEST

Conduct the test with a bench or gymnasium bleacher 16¼ inches high.

Perform the stepping cycle to a four-step cadence (up-up-down-down). Men: Perform 24 complete step-ups per minute, regulated with a metronome set at 96 beats per minute. Women: Perform 22 step-ups per minute, or 88 beats per minute on the metronome.

1. Allow a brief practice period of 5 to 10 seconds to familiarize yourself with the stepping cadence.
2. Begin the test and perform the step-ups for exactly 3 minutes.
3. After 3 minutes, remain standing and take your heart rate (HR) for a 15-second interval from 5 to 20 seconds into recovery. Convert recovery HR to beats per minute (multiply 15-second HR by 4).
4. Estimate maximal oxygen uptake Max $VO_2$ in ml/kg/min according to the following equations:

   Men:

   $\text{Max VO}_2 = 111.33 - (0.42 \times \text{recovery HR in bpm})$

   Women:

   $\text{Max VO}_2 = 65.81 - (0.1847 \times \text{recovery HR in bpm})$

   *Example:* Recovery 15-second HR for a male following the 3-minute step test is found to be 39 beats. Max $VO_2$ is estimated as follows:

   15-second HR = 39 beats

   Minute HR = $39 \times 4 = 156$ bpm

   $\text{Max VO}_2 = 111.33 - (0.42 \times 156)$

   $\text{Max VO}_2 = 45.81$ ml/kg/min
5. Max $VO_2$ also can be obtained according to recovery heart rates in Table 2.3.

Source: *Exercise Physiology: Energy, Nutrition, and Human Performance*, by W. D. McArdle et al. (Philadelphia: Lea & Febiger, 1991).

**FIGURE 2.3** ◆ Procedure for the Step Test.

**TABLE 2.3**
**Predicted Maximal Oxygen Uptake for Step Test (ml/kg/min)**

| 15-Sec HR[a] | HR-bpm[b] | Max $VO_2$ Men | Max $VO_2$ Women |
|---|---|---|---|
| 30 | 120 | 60.9 | 43.6 |
| 31 | 124 | 59.3 | 42.9 |
| 32 | 128 | 57.6 | 42.2 |
| 33 | 132 | 55.9 | 41.4 |
| 34 | 136 | 54.2 | 40.7 |
| 35 | 140 | 52.5 | 40.0 |
| 36 | 144 | 50.9 | 39.2 |
| 37 | 148 | 49.2 | 38.5 |
| 38 | 152 | 47.5 | 37.7 |
| 39 | 156 | 45.8 | 37.0 |
| 40 | 160 | 44.1 | 36.3 |
| 41 | 164 | 42.5 | 35.5 |
| 42 | 168 | 40.8 | 34.8 |
| 43 | 172 | 39.1 | 34.0 |
| 44 | 176 | 37.4 | 33.3 |
| 45 | 180 | 35.7 | 32.6 |
| 46 | 184 | 34.1 | 31.8 |
| 47 | 188 | 32.4 | 31.1 |
| 48 | 192 | 30.7 | 30.3 |
| 49 | 196 | 29.0 | 29.6 |
| 50 | 200 | 27.3 | 28.9 |

[a] HR = heart rate
[b] bpm = beats per minute

## Astrand-Ryhming Test

Because of its simplicity and practicality, the Astrand-Ryhming Test has become one of the most popular tests used to estimate Max $VO_2$ in the laboratory setting. The test is conducted on a bicycle ergometer, and, similar to the Step Test, it requires only submaximal workloads and little time to administer.

The cautions for the Step Test also apply to the Astrand-Ryhming Test. Nevertheless, because participants do not have to support their own body weight while riding the bicycle, overweight individuals and those with limited joint problems in the lower extremities can take this test.

The bicycle ergometer to be used for this test should allow for the regulation of workloads (see the test procedure in Figure 2.4 and Tables 2.4, 2.5, and 2.6). Besides the bicycle ergometer, a stopwatch and an additional technician to monitor the heart rate are needed to conduct the test.

The heart rate is taken every minute for 6 minutes. At the end of the test, the heart rate should be in the range given for each workload in Table 2.5 (generally between 120 and 170 beats per minute).

When administering the test to older people, good judgment is essential. Low workloads should be used, because if the higher heart rates are reached (around 150 to 170 bpm), these individuals could be working near or at their maximal capacity, making the test unsafe without adequate medical supervision. When choosing workloads for older people, final exercise heart rates should not exceed 130 to 140 bpm.

### ASTRAND-RYHMING TEST

1. Adjust the bike seat so the knees are almost completely extended as the foot goes through the bottom of the pedaling cycle.
2. During the test, keep the speed constant at 50 revolutions per minute for the test duration of 6 minutes.
3. Select the appropriate workload for the bike based on age, weight, health, and estimated fitness level. For unconditioned individuals: women, use 300 kpm (kilopounds per meter) or 450 kpm; men, 300 kpm or 600 kpm. Conditioned adults: women, 450 kpm or 600 kpm; men, 600 kpm or 900 kpm.*
4. Ride the bike for 6 minutes and check the heart rate every minute, during the last 10 seconds of each minute. Determine heart rate by recording the time it takes to count 30 pulse beats, and then converting to beats per minute using Table 2.4.
5. Average the final two heart rates (fifth and sixth minutes). If these two heart rates are not within five beats per minute of each other, continue the test for another few minutes until this is accomplished. If the heart rate continues to climb significantly after the sixth minute, stop the test and rest for 15 to 20 minutes. You then may retest, preferably at a lower workload. The final average heart rate should also fall between the ranges given for each workload in Table 2.5 (e.g., men: 300 kpm = 120 to 140 beats per minute; 600 kpm = 120 to 170 beats per minute).
6. Based on the average heart rate of the final 2 minutes and your workload, look up the maximal oxygen uptake (Max $VO_2$) in Table 2.5 (e.g., men: 600 kpm and average heart rate = 145, Max $VO_2$ = 2.4 liters/minute).
7. Correct Max $VO_2$ using the correction factors found in Table 2.6 (e.g., Max $VO_2$ = 2.4 and age 35, correction factor = .870. Multiply 2.4 × .870 and final corrected Max $VO_2$ = 2.09 liters/minute).
8. To obtain Max $VO_2$ in ml/kg/min, multiply the Max $VO_2$ by 1,000 (to convert liters to milliliters) and divide by body weight in kilograms (to obtain kilograms, divide your body weight in pounds by 2.2046).
9. Example: Corrected Max $VO_2$ = 2.09 liters/minute

   Body weight = 132 pounds or 60 kilograms (132 ÷ 2.2046 = 60)

   $$\text{Max } VO_2 = \frac{2.09 \times 1{,}000}{60} = 34.8 \text{ ml/kg/min}$$

* On the Monarch bicycle ergometer when riding at a speed of fifty revolutions per minute, a load of 1 kp = 300 kpm, 1.5 kp = 450 kpm, 2 kp = 600 kpm, and so forth, with increases of 150 kpm to each half kp.

**FIGURE 2.4** ◆ Procedure for the Astrand-Ryhming test.

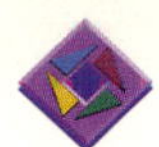

**TABLE 2.4**
**Conversion of Time for 30 Pulse Beats to Pulse Rate Per Minute**

| sec. | bpm | sec. | bpm | sec. | bpm | sec. | bpm | sec. | bpm | sec. | bpm |
|---|---|---|---|---|---|---|---|---|---|---|---|
| 22.0 | 82 | 19.6 | 92 | 17.2 | 105 | 14.8 | 122 | 12.4 | 145 | 10.0 | 180 |
| 21.9 | 82 | 19.5 | 92 | 17.1 | 105 | 14.7 | 122 | 12.3 | 146 | 9.9 | 182 |
| 21.8 | 83 | 19.4 | 93 | 17.0 | 106 | 14.6 | 123 | 12.2 | 148 | 9.8 | 184 |
| 21.7 | 83 | 19.3 | 93 | 16.9 | 107 | 14.5 | 124 | 12.1 | 149 | 9.7 | 186 |
| 21.6 | 83 | 19.2 | 94 | 16.8 | 107 | 14.4 | 125 | 12.0 | 150 | 9.6 | 188 |
| 21.5 | 84 | 19.1 | 94 | 16.7 | 108 | 14.3 | 126 | 11.9 | 151 | 9.5 | 189 |
| 21.4 | 84 | 19.0 | 95 | 16.6 | 108 | 14.2 | 127 | 11.8 | 153 | 9.4 | 191 |
| 21.3 | 85 | 18.9 | 95 | 16.5 | 109 | 14.1 | 128 | 11.7 | 154 | 9.3 | 194 |
| 21.2 | 85 | 18.8 | 96 | 16.4 | 110 | 14.0 | 129 | 11.6 | 155 | 9.2 | 196 |
| 21.1 | 85 | 18.7 | 96 | 16.3 | 110 | 13.9 | 129 | 11.5 | 157 | 9.1 | 198 |
| 21.0 | 86 | 18.6 | 97 | 16.2 | 111 | 13.8 | 130 | 11.4 | 158 | 9.0 | 200 |
| 20.9 | 86 | 18.5 | 97 | 16.1 | 112 | 13.7 | 131 | 11.3 | 159 | 8.9 | 202 |
| 20.8 | 87 | 18.4 | 98 | 16.0 | 113 | 13.6 | 132 | 11.2 | 161 | 8.8 | 205 |
| 20.7 | 87 | 18.3 | 98 | 15.9 | 113 | 13.5 | 133 | 11.1 | 162 | 8.7 | 207 |
| 20.6 | 87 | 18.2 | 99 | 15.8 | 114 | 13.4 | 134 | 11.0 | 164 | 8.6 | 209 |
| 20.5 | 88 | 18.1 | 99 | 15.7 | 115 | 13.3 | 135 | 10.9 | 165 | 8.5 | 212 |
| 20.4 | 88 | 18.0 | 100 | 15.6 | 115 | 13.2 | 136 | 10.8 | 167 | 8.4 | 214 |
| 20.3 | 89 | 17.9 | 101 | 15.5 | 116 | 13.1 | 137 | 10.7 | 168 | 8.3 | 217 |
| 20.2 | 89 | 17.8 | 101 | 15.4 | 117 | 13.0 | 138 | 10.6 | 170 | 8.2 | 220 |
| 20.1 | 90 | 17.7 | 102 | 15.3 | 118 | 12.9 | 140 | 10.5 | 171 | 8.1 | 222 |
| 20.0 | 90 | 17.6 | 102 | 15.2 | 118 | 12.8 | 141 | 10.4 | 173 | 8.0 | 225 |
| 19.9 | 90 | 17.5 | 103 | 15.1 | 119 | 12.7 | 142 | 10.3 | 175 | | |
| 19.8 | 91 | 17.4 | 103 | 15.0 | 120 | 12.6 | 143 | 10.2 | 176 | | |
| 19.7 | 91 | 17.3 | 104 | 14.9 | 121 | 12.5 | 144 | 10.1 | 178 | | |

sec. = seconds
bpm = beats per minute

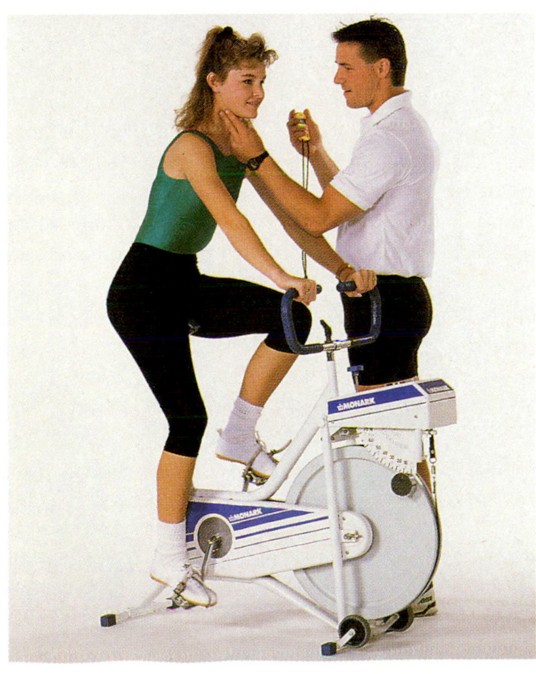

*Monitoring heart rate on carotid artery during the Astrand-Ryhming Test.*

**TABLE 2.5**
**Maximal Oxygen Uptake Estimates for the Astrand-Rhyming Test in L/min**

| Heart Rate | MEN | | | | | WOMEN | | | | |
|---|---|---|---|---|---|---|---|---|---|---|
| | 300 | 600 | 900 | 1200 | 1500 | 300 | 450 | 600 | 750 | 900 |
| 120 | 2.2 | 3.4 | 4.8 | | | 2.6 | 3.4 | 4.1 | 4.8 | |
| 121 | 2.2 | 3.4 | 4.7 | | | 2.5 | 3.3 | 4.0 | 4.8 | |
| 122 | 2.2 | 3.4 | 4.6 | | | 2.5 | 3.2 | 3.9 | 4.7 | |
| 123 | 2.1 | 3.4 | 4.6 | | | 2.4 | 3.1 | 3.9 | 4.6 | |
| 124 | 2.1 | 3.3 | 4.5 | 6.0 | | 2.4 | 3.1 | 3.8 | 4.5 | |
| 125 | 2.0 | 3.2 | 4.4 | 5.9 | | 2.3 | 3.0 | 3.7 | 4.4 | |
| 126 | 2.0 | 3.2 | 4.4 | 5.8 | | 2.3 | 3.0 | 3.6 | 4.3 | |
| 127 | 2.0 | 3.1 | 4.3 | 5.7 | | 2.2 | 2.9 | 3.5 | 4.2 | |
| 128 | 2.0 | 3.1 | 4.2 | 5.6 | | 2.2 | 2.8 | 3.5 | 4.2 | 4.8 |
| 129 | 1.9 | 3.0 | 4.2 | 5.6 | | 2.2 | 2.8 | 3.4 | 4.1 | 4.8 |
| 130 | 1.9 | 3.0 | 4.1 | 5.5 | | 2.1 | 2.7 | 3.4 | 4.0 | 4.7 |
| 131 | 1.9 | 2.9 | 4.0 | 5.4 | | 2.1 | 2.7 | 3.4 | 4.0 | 4.6 |
| 132 | 1.8 | 2.9 | 4.0 | 5.3 | | 2.0 | 2.7 | 3.3 | 3.9 | 4.5 |
| 133 | 1.8 | 2.8 | 3.9 | 5.3 | | 2.0 | 2.6 | 3.2 | 3.8 | 4.4 |
| 134 | 1.8 | 2.8 | 3.9 | 5.2 | | 2.0 | 2.6 | 3.2 | 3.8 | 4.4 |
| 135 | 1.7 | 2.8 | 3.8 | 5.1 | | 2.0 | 2.6 | 3.1 | 3.7 | 4.3 |
| 136 | 1.7 | 2.7 | 3.8 | 5.0 | | 1.9 | 2.5 | 3.1 | 3.6 | 4.2 |
| 137 | 1.7 | 2.7 | 3.7 | 5.0 | | 1.9 | 2.5 | 3.0 | 3.6 | 4.2 |
| 138 | 1.6 | 2.7 | 3.7 | 4.9 | | 1.8 | 2.4 | 3.0 | 3.5 | 4.1 |
| 139 | 1.6 | 2.6 | 3.6 | 4.8 | | 1.8 | 2.4 | 2.9 | 3.5 | 4.0 |
| 140 | 1.6 | 2.6 | 3.6 | 4.8 | 6.0 | 1.8 | 2.4 | 2.8 | 3.4 | 4.0 |
| 141 | | 2.6 | 3.5 | 4.7 | 5.9 | 1.8 | 2.3 | 2.8 | 3.4 | 3.9 |
| 142 | | 2.5 | 3.5 | 4.6 | 5.8 | 1.7 | 2.3 | 2.8 | 3.3 | 3.9 |
| 143 | | 2.5 | 3.4 | 4.6 | 5.7 | 1.7 | 2.2 | 2.7 | 3.3 | 3.8 |
| 144 | | 2.5 | 3.4 | 4.5 | 5.7 | 1.7 | 2.2 | 2.7 | 3.2 | 3.8 |
| 145 | | 2.4 | 3.4 | 4.5 | 5.6 | 1.6 | 2.2 | 2.7 | 3.2 | 3.7 |
| 146 | | 2.4 | 3.3 | 4.4 | 5.6 | 1.6 | 2.2 | 2.6 | 3.2 | 3.7 |
| 147 | | 2.4 | 3.3 | 4.4 | 5.5 | 1.6 | 2.1 | 2.6 | 3.1 | 3.6 |
| 148 | | 2.4 | 3.2 | 4.3 | 5.4 | 1.6 | 2.1 | 2.6 | 3.1 | 3.6 |
| 149 | | 2.3 | 3.2 | 4.3 | 5.4 | | 2.1 | 2.6 | 3.0 | 3.5 |
| 150 | | 2.3 | 3.2 | 4.2 | 5.3 | | 2.0 | 2.5 | 3.0 | 3.5 |
| 151 | | 2.3 | 3.1 | 4.2 | 5.2 | | 2.0 | 2.5 | 3.0 | 3.4 |
| 152 | | 2.3 | 3.1 | 4.1 | 5.2 | | 2.0 | 2.5 | 2.9 | 3.4 |
| 153 | | 2.2 | 3.0 | 4.1 | 5.1 | | 2.0 | 2.4 | 2.9 | 3.3 |
| 154 | | 2.2 | 3.0 | 4.0 | 5.1 | | 2.0 | 2.4 | 2.8 | 3.3 |
| 155 | | 2.2 | 3.0 | 4.0 | 5.0 | | 1.9 | 2.4 | 2.8 | 3.2 |
| 156 | | 2.2 | 2.9 | 4.0 | 5.0 | | 1.9 | 2.3 | 2.8 | 3.2 |
| 157 | | 2.1 | 2.9 | 3.9 | 4.9 | | 1.9 | 2.3 | 2.7 | 3.2 |
| 158 | | 2.1 | 2.9 | 3.9 | 4.9 | | 1.8 | 2.3 | 2.7 | 3.1 |
| 159 | | 2.1 | 2.8 | 3.8 | 4.8 | | 1.8 | 2.2 | 2.7 | 3.1 |
| 160 | | 2.1 | 2.8 | 3.8 | 4.8 | | 1.8 | 2.2 | 2.6 | 3.0 |
| 161 | | 2.0 | 2.8 | 3.7 | 4.7 | | 1.8 | 2.2 | 2.6 | 3.0 |
| 162 | | 2.0 | 2.8 | 3.7 | 4.6 | | 1.8 | 2.2 | 2.6 | 3.0 |
| 163 | | 2.0 | 2.8 | 3.7 | 4.6 | | 1.7 | 2.2 | 2.6 | 2.9 |
| 164 | | 2.0 | 2.7 | 3.6 | 4.5 | | 1.7 | 2.1 | 2.5 | 2.9 |
| 165 | | 2.0 | 2.7 | 3.6 | 4.5 | | 1.7 | 2.1 | 2.5 | 2.9 |
| 166 | | 1.9 | 2.7 | 3.6 | 4.5 | | 1.7 | 2.1 | 2.5 | 2.8 |
| 167 | | 1.9 | 2.6 | 3.5 | 4.4 | | 1.6 | 2.1 | 2.4 | 2.8 |
| 168 | | 1.9 | 2.6 | 3.5 | 4.4 | | 1.6 | 2.0 | 2.4 | 2.8 |
| 169 | | 1.9 | 2.6 | 3.5 | 4.3 | | 1.6 | 2.0 | 2.4 | 2.8 |
| 170 | | 1.8 | 2.6 | 3.4 | 4.3 | | 1.6 | 2.0 | 2.4 | 2.7 |

From *Acta Physiologica Scandinavica* by I. Astrand, 49 (1960) Supplementum 169, 45–60.

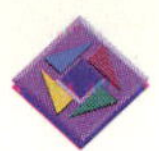

**TABLE 2.6**
**Age-Based Correction Factors for Maximal Oxygen Uptake**

| Age | Correction Factor | Age | Correction Factor | Age | Correction Factor | Age | Correction Factor |
|---|---|---|---|---|---|---|---|
| 14 | 1.11 | 25 | 1.00 | 39 | .838 | 53 | .726 |
| 15 | 1.10 | 26 | .987 | 40 | .830 | 54 | .718 |
| 16 | 1.09 | 27 | .974 | 41 | .820 | 55 | .710 |
| 17 | 1.08 | 28 | .961 | 42 | .810 | 56 | .704 |
| 18 | 1.07 | 29 | .948 | 43 | .800 | 57 | .698 |
| 19 | 1.06 | 30 | .935 | 44 | .790 | 58 | .692 |
| 20 | 1.05 | 31 | .922 | 45 | .780 | 59 | .686 |
| 21 | 1.04 | 32 | .909 | 46 | .774 | 60 | .680 |
| 22 | 1.03 | 33 | .896 | 47 | .768 | 61 | .674 |
| 23 | 1.02 | 34 | .883 | 48 | .762 | 62 | .668 |
| 24 | 1.01 | 35 | .870 | 49 | .756 | 63 | .662 |
| | | 36 | .862 | 50 | .750 | 64 | .656 |
| | | 37 | .854 | 51 | .742 | 65 | .650 |
| | | 38 | .846 | 52 | .734 | | |

Adapted from *Acta Physiologica Scandinavica* by I. Astrand, 49(1960), Supplementum 169, 45–60.

## 12-Minute Swim Test

Similar to the 1.5-Mile Run Test, the 12-Minute Swim Test is considered a maximal exercise test, and the same precautions apply. The objective is to swim as far as possible during the 12-minute test.

A swimming test (see Figure 2.5) is practical only for those who are planning to take part in a swimming program. Unlike land-based tests, predicting Max $VO_2$ through a swimming test is difficult. Differences in skill level, swimming conditioning, and body composition greatly affect the energy requirements (oxygen uptake) of swimming.

A skilled swimmer is able to swim more efficiently and expend much less energy than an unskilled swimmer. Improper breathing patterns cause premature fatigue. Overweight individuals are more buoyant in the water, and the larger surface area (body size) produces more friction against movement in the water.

Lack of conditioning affects swimming test results as well. An unconditioned skilled swimmer who is in good cardiovascular shape because of a

### 12-MINUTE SWIM TEST

1. Enlist a friend to time the test. The only other requisites are a stopwatch and a swimming pool. Do not attempt to do this test in an unsupervised pool.
2. Warm up by swimming slowly and doing a few stretching exercises before taking the test.
3. Start the test and swim as many laps as possible in 12 minutes. Pace yourself throughout the test, and do not swim to the point of complete exhaustion.
4. After completing the test, cool down by swimming another 2 or 3 minutes at a slower pace.
5. Determine the total distance you swam during the test, and look up your fitness category in Table 2.7.

**FIGURE 2.5** ◆ Procedure for the 12-Minute Swim Test.

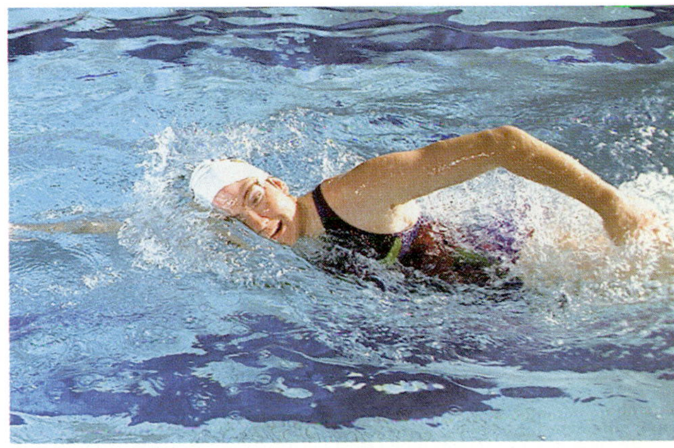

Swimming efficiency requires skill and proper conditioning.

regular jogging program will not perform as effectively in a swimming test. Swimming conditioning is important to perform adequately on this test.

Because of these limitations, Max $VO_2$ cannot be estimated for a swimming test and the fitness categories given in Table 2.7 are only estimated ratings. This test should be limited to people who cannot perform any of the other tests and whose primary aerobic exercise will be a swimming program. Unskilled and unconditioned swimmers can expect lower cardiovascular fitness ratings than those obtained with a land-based test.

**TABLE 2.7**
**Fitness Categories for the 12-Minute Swim Test**

| Distance (yards) | Fitness Categories |
|---|---|
| ≥700 | Excellent |
| 500–700 | Good |
| 400–500 | Average |
| 200–400 | Fair |
| ≤200 | Poor |

Adapted from *The Aerobics Program for Total Well-Being*, by K. H. Cooper (New York: Bantam Books, 1982).

## Interpreting Maximal Oxygen Uptake Results

After obtaining your Max $VO_2$, you can determine your current level of cardiovascular fitness by consulting Table 2.8. Locate the Max $VO_2$ in your age category, and on the top row you will find your present level of cardiovascular fitness.

For example, a 19-year-old male with a Max $VO_2$ of 35 ml/kg/min would be classified in the average cardiovascular fitness category. Once you have established your Max $VO_2$ and cardiovascular fitness category, record this information in Figure 2.6 in this chapter and in your Fitness and Wellness Profile in Appendix A. After you first undertake your personal cardiovascular exercise program, you may wish to retest yourself periodically to evaluate your progress.

## Exercise Readiness

Before proceeding to the next chapter on cardiovascular exercise prescription, and if you are not exercising now, you should ask yourself the following question: Are you willing to give exercise a try? A low percentage of the U. S. population is truly committed to exercise. Further, surveys indicate

**TABLE 2.8**
**Cardiovascular Fitness Classification According to Maximal Oxygen Uptake in ml/kg/min**

| | | FITNESS CLASSIFICATION | | | | |
|---|---|---|---|---|---|---|
| Gender | Age | Poor | Fair | Average | Good | Excellent |
| Men | ≤29 | ≤24.9 | 25–33.9 | 34–43.9 | 44–52.9 | ≥53 |
| | 30–39 | ≤22.9 | 23–30.9 | 31–41.9 | 42–49.9 | ≥50 |
| | 40–49 | ≤19.9 | 20–26.9 | 27–38.9 | 39–44.9 | ≥45 |
| | 50–59 | ≤17.9 | 18–24.9 | 25–37.9 | 38–42.9 | ≥43 |
| | 60–69 | ≤15.9 | 16–22.9 | 23–35.9 | 36–40.9 | ≥41 |
| Women | ≤29 | ≤23.9 | 24–30.9 | 31–38.9 | 39–48.9 | ≥49 |
| | 30–39 | ≤19.9 | 20–27.9 | 28–36.9 | 37–44.9 | ≥45 |
| | 40–49 | ≤16.9 | 17–24.9 | 25–34.9 | 35–41.9 | ≥42 |
| | 50–59 | ≤14.9 | 15–21.9 | 22–33.9 | 34–39.9 | ≥40 |
| | 60–69 | ≤12.9 | 13–20.9 | 21–32.9 | 33–36.9 | ≥37 |

High physical fitness standard

Health fitness standard

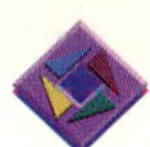

Name: ______________________________ Age: ____________

| Date | Test Used | Max $VO_2$ | Fitness Classification |
| --- | --- | --- | --- |
| | | | |
| | | | |
| | | | |
| | | | |
| | | | |
| | | | |

**FIGURE 2.6** ◆ Cardiovascular endurance report.

that more than half of the people who start exercising drop out during the first 6 months of the program. Sports psychologists are trying to find out why some people exercise habitually and many do not. All of the benefits of exercise cannot help unless people commit to a lifetime program of physical activity.

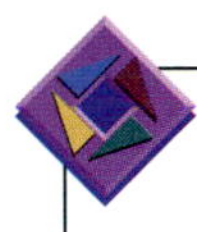

*If you are not exercising regularly, are you willing to stop contemplating and give exercise a try?*

The first step is to decide positively that you will try. Using Figure 2.7, you can list the advantages and disadvantages of incorporating exercise into your lifestyle. Your list may include things such as: It will make me feel better. I will lose weight. I will have more energy. It will lower risk for chronic diseases. Your list of disadvantages might include: I don't want to take the time. I'm too out of shape. There's no good place to exercise. I don't have the willpower to do it. When the reasons for exercise outweigh the reasons for not exercising, it will become easier to try.

The information provided in Figure 2.8 then can help you answer the question: Am I ready to start an exercise program? You are evaluated in four categories: mastery (self-control), attitude, health, and commitment. The higher you score in any category — mastery, for example — the more important that reason is for you to exercise.

Scores can vary from 4 to 16. A score of 12 and above is a strong indicator that that factor is important to you, whereas 8 and below is low. If you score 12 or more points in each category, your chances of initiating and sticking to an exercise program are good. If you do not score at least 12 points in three categories, your chances of succeeding at exercise may be slim. You need to be better informed about the benefits of exercise, and a retraining process may be helpful. More tips on how you can become committed to exercise are provided in the next chapter.

## SELECT BIBLIOGRAPHY

American College of Sports Medicine. *Guidelines for Exercise Testing and Prescription.* Philadelphia: Lea & Febiger, 1991.

American College of Sports Medicine. "The Recommended Quantity and Quality of Exercise for Developing and Maintaining Cardiorespiratory and Muscular Fitness in Healthy Adults." *Medicine and Science in Sports and Exercise,* 22 (1990), 265-274.

American Heart Association Committee on Exercise. *Exercise Testing and Training of Apparently Healthy Individuals: A Handbook for Physicians.* New York: AHA, 1972.

Astrand, I. *Acta Physiologica Scandinavica,* 49 (1960), Supplementum 169:45-60.

Astrand, P. O., and K. Rodahl. *Textbook of Work Physiology.* New York: McGraw-Hill, 1986.

Cooper, K. H. "A Means of Assessing Maximal Oxygen Intake." *Journal of the American Medical Association,* 203 (1968), 201-204.

Cooper, K. H. *The Aerobics Program for Total Well-Being.* New York: Mount Evans and Co., 1982.

Fox, E. L., R. W. Bowers, and H. L. Foss. *The Physiological Basis of Physical Education and Athletics.* Philadelphia: Saunders College Publishing, 1988.

Hoeger, W. W. K., and S. A. Hoeger. *Fitness & Wellness.* Englewood, CO: Morton Publishing, 1993.

Kline, G., et al. "Estimation of $VO_{2max}$ from a One-Mile Track Walk, Gender, Age, and Body Weight." *Medicine and Science in Sports and Exercise* 19:3 (1987), 253-259.

McArdle, W. D., F. I. Katch, and V. L. Katch. *Exercise Physiology: Energy, Nutrition and Human Performance.* Philadelphia: Lea & Febiger, 1991.

Wilmore, J. H., and D. L. Costill. *Training for Sport and Activity.* Dubuque, IA: Wm. C. Brown Publishers, 1988.

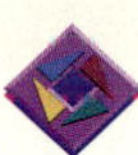

Name: ______________________ Date: ______________

Advantages of starting an exercise program

1. ______________________
2. ______________________
3. ______________________
4. ______________________
5. ______________________
6. ______________________
7. ______________________
8. ______________________

Disadvantages of starting an exercise program

1. ______________________
2. ______________________
3. ______________________
4. ______________________
5. ______________________
6. ______________________
7. ______________________
8. ______________________

**FIGURE 2.7** ◆ Advantages and disadvantages of adding exercise to your lifestyle.

## EXERCISE READINESS QUESTIONNAIRE

Name: ______________________________ Date: ______________

Carefully read each statement and circle the number that best describes your feelings in each statement. Please be completely honest with your answers.

| | Strongly Agree | Mildly Agree | Mildly Disagree | Strongly Disagree |
|---|---|---|---|---|
| 1. I can walk, ride a bike (or a wheelchair), swim, or walk in a shallow pool. | 4 | 3 | 2 | 1 |
| 2. I enjoy exercise. | 4 | 3 | 2 | 1 |
| 3. I believe exercise can lower the risk for disease and premature mortality. | 4 | 3 | 2 | 1 |
| 4. I believe exercise contributes to better health. | 4 | 3 | 2 | 1 |
| 5. I have participated previously in an exercise program. | 4 | 3 | 2 | 1 |
| 6. I have experienced the feeling of being physically fit. | 4 | 3 | 2 | 1 |
| 7. I can envision myself exercising. | 4 | 3 | 2 | 1 |
| 8. I am contemplating an exercise program. | 4 | 3 | 2 | 1 |
| 9. I am willing to stop contemplating and give exercise a try for a few weeks. | 4 | 3 | 2 | 1 |
| 10. I am willing to set aside time at least three times a week for exercise. | 4 | 3 | 2 | 1 |
| 11. I can find a place to exercise (the streets, a park, a YMCA, a health club). | 4 | 3 | 2 | 1 |
| 12. I can find other people who would like to exercise with me. | 4 | 3 | 2 | 1 |
| 13. I will exercise when I am moody, fatigued, and even when the weather is bad. | 4 | 3 | 2 | 1 |
| 14. I am willing to spend a small amount of money for adequate exercise clothing (shoes, shorts, leotards, or swimsuit). | 4 | 3 | 2 | 1 |
| 15. If I have any doubts about my present state of health, I will see a physician before beginning an exercise program. | 4 | 3 | 2 | 1 |
| 16. Exercise will make me feel better and improve my quality of life. | 4 | 3 | 2 | 1 |

**Scoring Your Test:**

This questionnaire allows you to examine your readiness for exercise. You have been evaluated in four categories: mastery (self-control), attitude, health, and commitment. Mastery indicates that you can be in control of your exercise program. Attitude examines your mental disposition toward exercise. Health provides evidence of the wellness benefits of exercise. Commitment shows dedication and resolution to carry out the exercise program. Write the number you circled after each statement in the corresponding spaces below. Add the scores on each line to get your totals. Scores can vary from 4 to 16. A score of 12 and above is a strong indicator that that factor is important to you, and 8 and below is low. If you score 12 or more points in each category, your chances of initiating and adhering to an exercise program are good. If you fail to score at least 12 points in three categories, your chances of succeeding at exercise may be slim. You need to be better informed about the benefits of exercise, and a retraining process may be required.

| | | | | | | | | | |
|---|---|---|---|---|---|---|---|---|---|
| Mastery: | 1. ______ | + | 5. ______ | + | 6. ______ | + | 9. ______ | = | ______ |
| Attitude: | 2. ______ | + | 7. ______ | + | 8. ______ | + | 13. ______ | = | ______ |
| Health: | 3. ______ | + | 4. ______ | + | 15. ______ | + | 16. ______ | = | ______ |
| Commitment: | 10. ______ | + | 11. ______ | + | 12. ______ | + | 14. ______ | = | ______ |

From *Fitness & Wellness*, by W. W. K. Hoeger and S. A. Hoeger (Englewood, CO: Morton Publishing, 1993).

**FIGURE 2.8** ◆

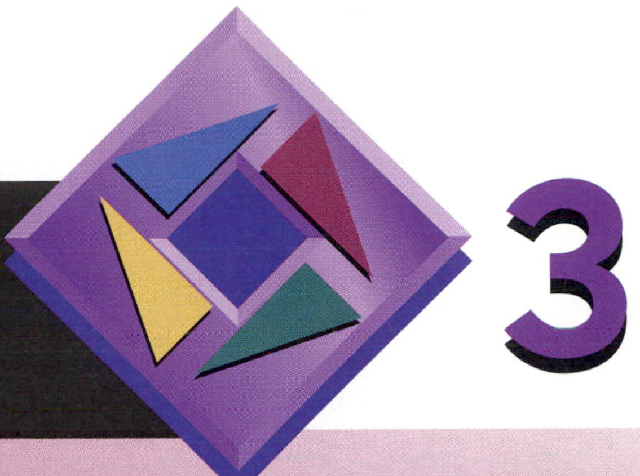

# 3 Cardiovascular Exercise Prescription

## Key Concepts

Cardiovascular endurance
Aerobic exercise
Exercise intensity
Cardiovascular training zone
Rate of perceived exertion (RPE)
MET
Heat stroke
ICE
Exercise intolerance
Exercise adherence

## Objectives

- Learn the principles that govern cardiovascular exercise: intensity, mode, duration, and frequency.
- Clarify misconceptions related to cardiovascular endurance training.
- Become familiar with concepts for preventing and treating injuries.
- Learn the benefits and advantages of selected aerobic activities.
- Learn basic skills to enhance adherence to exercise.

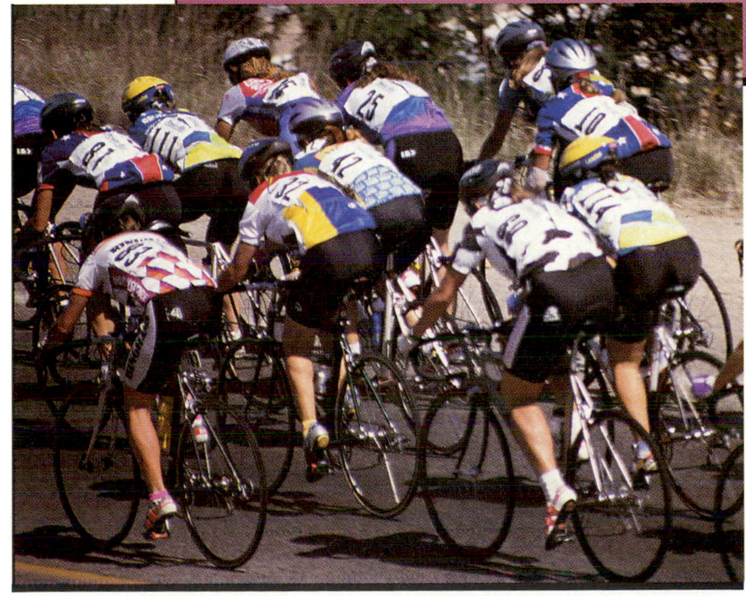

All too often individuals who exercise regularly and then take a cardiovascular endurance test are surprised to find that their maximal oxygen uptake is not as good as they think it is. Although these individuals may be exercising regularly, they most likely are not following the basic principles for cardiovascular exercise prescription. Therefore, they do not reap significant improvements in cardiovascular endurance.

## GUIDELINES FOR CARDIOVASCULAR EXERCISE PRESCRIPTION

To develop the cardiovascular system, the heart muscle has to be overloaded like any other muscle in the human body. Just as the biceps muscle in the upper arm is developed through strength-training exercises, the heart muscle has to be exercised to increase in size, strength, and efficiency. To better understand how the cardiovascular system can be developed, we have to be familiar with four basic principles: intensity, mode, duration, and frequency of exercise.

Before discussing the principles of cardiovascular prescription you should be aware that the American College of Sports Medicine recommends that apparently healthy men over age 40 and women over age 50 undergo a medical exam and a diagnostic exercise stress test prior to engaging in vigorous exercise.[1] The American College of Sports Medicine has defined vigorous exercise as an *exercise intensity above 60% of maximal oxygen uptake*. This intensity is the equivalent of exercise that provides a "substantial challenge" to the new participant or one that cannot be maintained for 20 continuous minutes.

### Intensity of Exercise

When trying to develop the cardiovascular system, intensity of exercise is the factor that perhaps is ignored most often. This principle refers to *how hard a person has to exercise to improve cardiovascular endurance*.

For muscles to develop, they have to be overloaded to a certain point. The training stimulus to develop the biceps muscle can be accomplished with curl-up exercises, but the stimulus for the cardiovascular system is provided by making the heart pump faster for a certain period of time. Cardiovascular development occurs when working between 50% and 85% of heart rate reserve.[2] Working closer to 85% of heart rate reserve yields quicker results. For this reason, many experts prescribe exercise between 70% and 85% for young people. The intensity of exercise can be calculated easily, and training can be monitored by checking your pulse.

#### Determining Training Intensity

To determine the intensity of exercise or cardiovascular training zone:

1. Estimate your maximal heart rate (MHR). The maximal heart rate depends on the person's age and can be estimated according to the formula: MHR = 220 minus age (220 – age)
2. Check your resting heart rate (RHR) sometime after you have been sitting quietly for 15 to 20 minutes. You may take your pulse for 30 seconds and multiply by 2, or take it for a full minute.
3. Determine the heart rate reserve (HRR). To do this, subtract the resting heart rate from the maximal heart rate (HRR = MHR – RHR). The heart rate reserve indicates the number of beats available to go from resting conditions to an all-out maximal effort.
4. Calculate the training intensities (TI) at 50%, 70%, and 85%. Multiply the heart rate reserve by the respective 50, 70, and 85 percentages, and then add the resting heart rate to these three figures (for example, 85% TI = HRR × .85 + RHR).

   *Example*: The 50%, 70%, and 85% training intensities for a 20-year-old person with a resting heart rate of 68 bpm is:

   MHR: 220 – 20 = 200 beats per minute (bpm)

   RHR = 68 bpm

   HRR: 200 – 68 = 132 beats

   50% TI = (132 × .50) + 68 = 134 bpm

   70% TI = (132 × .70) + 68 = 160 bpm

   85% TI = (132 × .85) + 68 = 180 bpm

   Cardiovascular training zone: 134 to 180 bpm

You can compute your own training intensity by using Figure 3.6 at the end of this chapter. The cardiovascular training zone indicates that whenever you exercise to improve the cardiovascular

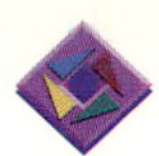

system, you should maintain your heart rate between the 50% and 85% training intensities to obtain adequate development. If you have been physically inactive, you should train around the 50% intensity during the first 4 to 6 weeks of the exercise program. After the first few weeks, you should exercise between 70% and 85% training intensity.

Following a few weeks of training, you may have a considerably lower resting heart rate (10 to 20 beats in 8 to 12 weeks). Therefore, you should recompute your target zone periodically. Once you have reached an ideal level of cardiovascular endurance, training in the 50% to 85% range will allow you to maintain your fitness level.

You should monitor your exercise heart rate regularly during the first few weeks of an exercise program to make sure you are training in the proper zone. Wait until you are about 5 minutes into your exercise session before taking your first rate. When you check your heart rate, count your pulse for 10 seconds and then multiply by 6 to get the per-minute pulse rate. Exercise heart rate will remain at the same level for about 15 seconds following exercise. After 15 seconds, your heart rate will drop rapidly. Do not hesitate to stop during your exercise bout to check your pulse. If the rate is too low, increase the intensity of exercise. If the rate is too high, slow down.

To develop the cardiovascular system, you do not have to exercise above the 85% rate. From a fitness standpoint, training above this percentage will not produce extra benefits and actually may be unsafe for some individuals. For unconditioned people and older adults, cardiovascular training should be around the 50% rate. This lower rate is recommended to avoid potential problems associated with high-intensity exercise.

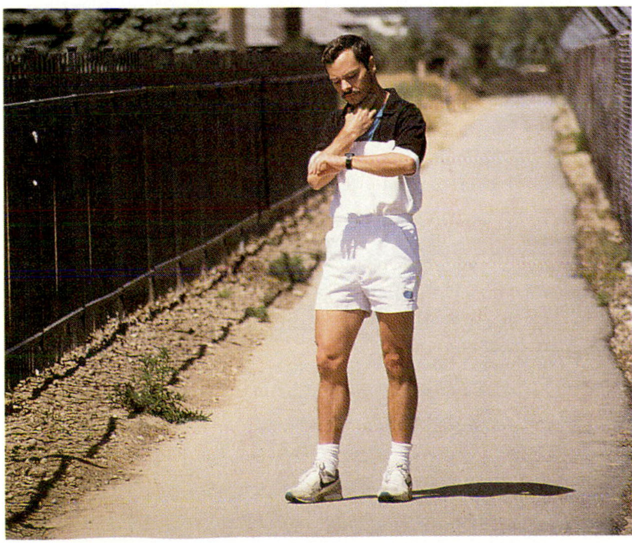

*Exercise heart rate should be checked regularly during the early stages of a new exercise program.*

### Health Fitness Versus Physical Fitness

Training benefits can be obtained by exercising at the 50% training intensity. Training at this lower percentage, however, may place a person in only an average or a "moderately fit" category (see Table 2.8, Chapter 2). As will be discussed under Specific Exercise Considerations, question 1, exercising at this lower intensity lowers the risk for cardiovascular mortality (health fitness) but does not allow the person to achieve a high cardiovascular fitness rating (physical fitness standard). The latter ratings are obtained by exercising closer to the 85% threshold.

### Rate of Perceived Exertion

Because many people do not check their heart rate during exercise, an alternative method of prescribing intensity of exercise has become more popular recently. This method uses a rate of perceived exertion (RPE) scale developed by Gunnar Borg. Using the scale in Figure 3.1, a person subjectively rates the perceived exertion or difficulty of exercise

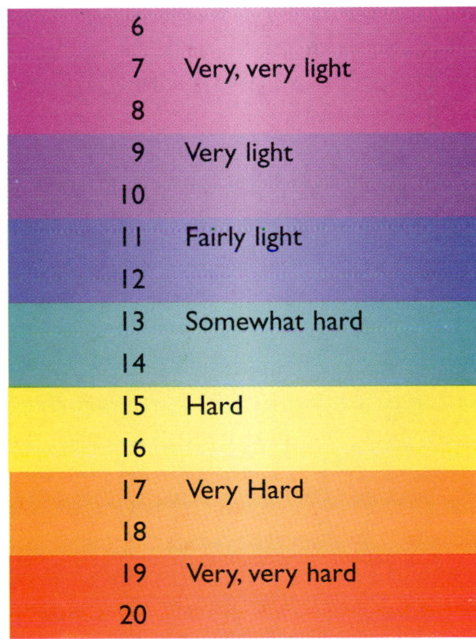

6
7 Very, very light
8
9 Very light
10
11 Fairly light
12
13 Somewhat hard
14
15 Hard
16
17 Very Hard
18
19 Very, very hard
20

From "Perceived Exertion: A Note on History and Methods," by Gunnar Borg, *Medicine and Science in Sports and Exercise*, 5 (1983), 90–93.

**FIGURE 3.1** ◆ Rate of Perceived Exertion Scale.

when training in the appropriate target zone. The exercise heart rate then is associated with the corresponding RPE value.

For example, if the training intensity requires a heart rate zone between 150 and 170 bpm, the person associates this with training between "hard" and "very hard." Some individuals, however, may perceive less exertion than others when training in the correct zone. Therefore, you have to associate your own inner perception of the task with the phrases on the scale. You then may proceed to exercise at that rate of perceived exertion.

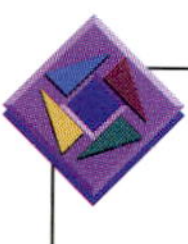

*Aerobic activities are rhythmic and continuous in nature and involve the major muscle groups of the body.*

You must be sure to cross-check your target zone with your perceived exertion in the first weeks of your exercise program. To help you develop this association, you should keep a regular record of your activities using the form provided in Figure 3.8 at the end of this chapter. After several weeks of training, you should be able to predict your exercise heart rate just by your own perceived exertion of the exercise session.

Whether you monitor the intensity of exercise by checking your pulse or through rate of perceived exertion, you should be aware that changes in normal exercise conditions will affect the training zone. For example, exercising on a hot/humid day or at high altitude increases the heart rate response to a given task, requiring adjustments in the intensity of your exercise.

## Mode of Exercise

The type of exercise that develops the cardiovascular system *has to be aerobic in nature*. Aerobic exercise involves the major muscle groups of the body, and it has to be rhythmic and continuous. As the amount of muscle mass involved during exercise increases, so does the effectiveness of the activity in providing cardiovascular development.

Once you have established your cardiovascular training zone, any activity or combination of activities that will get your heart rate up to that training zone and keep it there for as long as you exercise will give you adequate development. Examples of these activities are walking, jogging, aerobics, swimming, water aerobics, cross-country skiing, aero-belt exercise, rope skipping, cycling, racquetball, stair climbing, and stationary running or cycling.

The activity you choose should be based on your personal preferences, what you most enjoy doing, and your physical limitations. The amount of strength or flexibility you develop through various activities differs, but in terms of cardiovascular development, the heart doesn't know whether you are walking, swimming, or cycling. All the heart knows is that it has to pump at a certain rate, and as long as that rate is in the desired range, your cardiovascular fitness will improve.

From a health fitness point of view, training in the lower end of the cardiovascular zone will yield optimal health benefits. The closer the heart rate is to the higher end of the cardiovascular training zone, however, the greater will be the improvements in maximal oxygen uptake (high physical fitness).

## Duration of Exercise

The general recommendation is that a person *train between 20 and 60 minutes per session*. The duration is based on how intensely a person trains. If the training is done around 85%, 20 minutes are sufficient. At 50% intensity the person should train at least 30 minutes. As mentioned under Intensity of Exercise, unconditioned people and older adults should train at lower percentages; therefore, the activity should be carried out over a longer time.

Although most experts recommend 20 to 30 minutes of aerobic exercise per session, 1990 research published in the *American Journal of Cardiology* indicates that three 10-minute exercise sessions per day (separated by at least 4 hours), at approximately 70% of maximal heart rate, also produce training benefits.[3] Although the increases in maximal oxygen uptake with this program were not as large (57%) as those found in a group performing one continuous 30-minute bout of exercise per day, the researchers concluded that moderate-intensity exercise training, conducted for 10 minutes three times per day, benefits the cardiovascular system significantly.

Results of this study are meaningful because people often mention lack of time as the reason for not taking part in an exercise program. Many think they have to exercise at least 20 continuous minutes to get any benefits at all. Even though 20 to 30

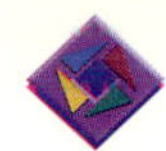

minutes are recommended, short, intermittent exercise bouts also are helpful to the cardiovascular system.

Exercise sessions always should be preceded by a 5-minute warm-up and followed by a 5-minute cool-down period (see Figure 3.2). The warm-up should consist of general calisthenics, stretching exercises, or exercising at a lower intensity level than the actual target zone. The cool-down entails gradually decreasing the intensity of exercise. Abruptly stopping causes blood to pool in the exercised body parts, diminishing the return of blood to the heart. Less blood return can cause dizziness and faintness or even bring on cardiac abnormalities.

## Frequency of Exercise

When starting an exercise program, three to five 20- to 30-minute training sessions per week are recommended to improve maximal oxygen uptake. When training is conducted more than 5 days a week, further improvements are minimal.

For individuals on a weight-loss program, 45- to 60-minute exercise sessions of low to moderate intensity, conducted 5 or 6 days per week, are recommended. Longer exercise sessions increase caloric expenditure for faster weight reduction (see Chapter 8).

Research also indicates that as few as three 20- to-30-minute training sessions per week, on nonconsecutive days, will maintain cardiovascular fitness (maximal oxygen uptake) as long as the heart rate is in the appropriate target zone. A summary of the cardiovascular exercise prescription guidelines according to the American College of Sports Medicine is provided in Figure 3.3.

| | |
|---|---|
| **Activity:** | Aerobic (examples: walking, jogging, cycling, swimming, aerobics, racquetball, soccer, stair climbing) |
| **Intensity:** | 50%–85% heart rate reserve |
| **Duration:** | 20–60 minutes of continuous aerobic activity |
| **Frequency:** | 3 to 5 days per week |

*Source:* The recommended quantity and quality of exercise for developing and maintaining cardiorespiratory and muscular fitness in healthy adults by the American College of Sports Medicine, *Medicine and Science in Sports and Exercise*, 22 (1990), 265–274.

**FIGURE 3.3** ◆ Cardiovascular exercise prescription guidelines.

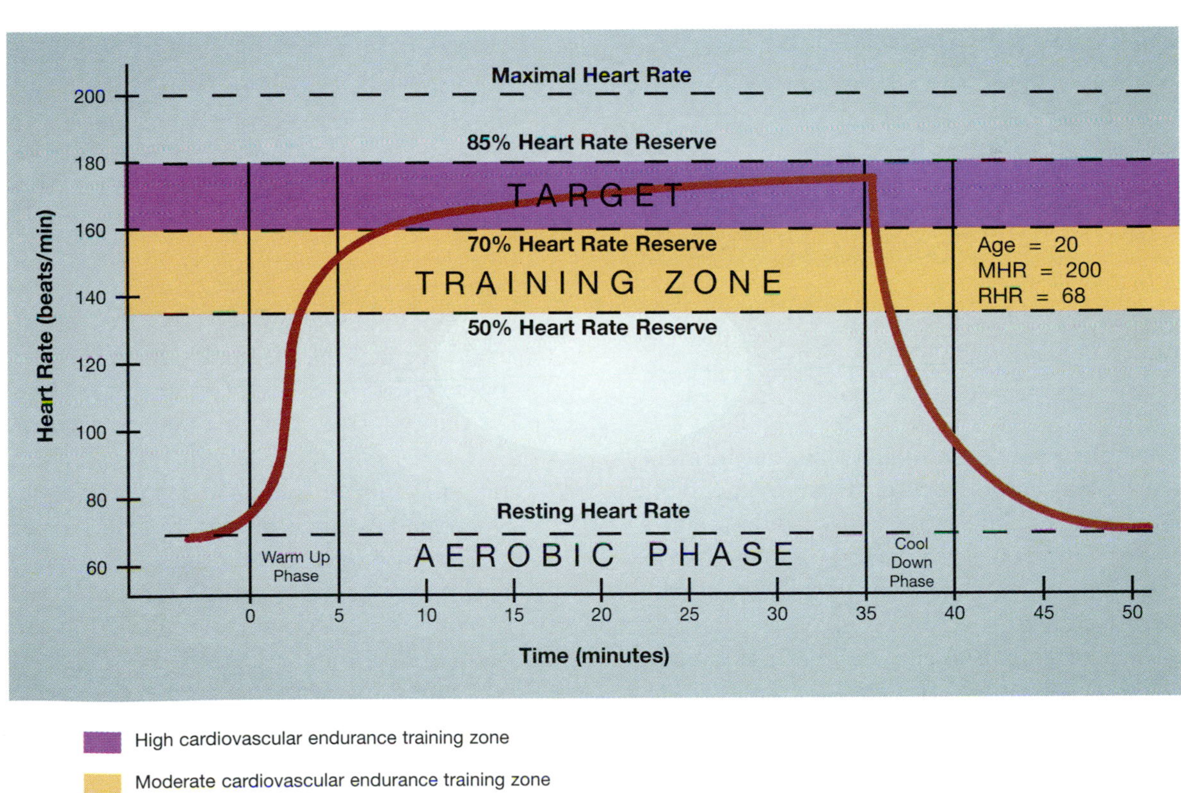


**FIGURE 3.2** ◆ Typical cardiovascular or aerobic training pattern.

Although three training sessions per week will maintain cardiovascular fitness, the importance of regular physical activity in preventing disease and enhancing quality of life was pointed out clearly in July 1993 at a news briefing held at the National Press Club in Washington, DC. At this briefing the American College of Sports Medicine and the U.S. Centers for Disease Control and Prevention, in conjunction with the President's Council on Physical Fitness and Sports, provided the American public with a set of recommendations on the types of physical activity needed for maintaining and promoting health.

In this summary statement every American is encouraged to accumulate at least 30 minutes of moderate-intensity physical activity almost daily. This daily routine has been promoted as an effective way to improve health. The entire contents of this statement on the benefits of physical activity are given in Figure 3.4.

Ideally, a person should engage in aerobic activities six to seven times per week. Based on the above discussion, to reap both the high-fitness and health-fitness benefits of exercise, a person needs to exercise a minimum of three times per week in the appropriate target zone (for high fitness maintenance) and three to four additional times per week in moderate-intensity activities (to enjoy the full benefits of health fitness). All exercise/activity sessions should last about 30 minutes.

## SPECIFIC EXERCISE CONSIDERATIONS

In addition to many of the exercise-related issues discussed to this point, other concerns require clarification or are somewhat controversial. Let's examine some of these issues.

1. **Does aerobic exercise make a person immune to heart and blood vessel disease?** Although aerobically fit individuals as a whole have a lower incidence of cardiovascular disease, a regular aerobic exercise program by itself does not offer an absolute guarantee against cardiovascular disease. Overall risk factor management is the best way to minimize the risk for cardiovascular disease (see Chapter 9). Many factors, including genetic predisposition, can increase the person's risk. Experts believe, however, that a regular aerobic exercise program not only will delay the onset of cardiovascular problems but that the chances of surviving a heart attack are much better for those who exercise regularly.

   Even moderate increases in aerobic fitness significantly lower the incidence of premature cardiovascular deaths. Data from the Aerobics Research Institute in Dallas, Texas (see Figure 1.7, Chapter 1) indicate that the decrease in cardiovascular mortality is greatest between the unfit (Group 1) and the moderately fit (2 and 3) groups. A further decrease in cardiovascular mortality is observed between the moderate and the highly fit groups (4 and 5), but the difference is not as much as that between the unfit and moderate fitness groups.

2. **How much aerobic exercise is required to decrease the risk for cardiovascular disease?** Although research has not yet indicated the exact amount of aerobic exercise required to lower the risk for cardiovascular disease, some general recommendations have been set forth. Dr. Ralph Paffenbarger and co-researchers showed that 2,000 calories expended per week as a result of physical activity yielded the lowest risk for cardiovascular disease in the group tested[4] (see Chapter 1, Figure 1.6). Two thousand calories per week represents about 300 calories per daily exercise session.

3. **Is it safe to exercise during pregnancy?** Women should not forsake exercise during pregnancy. If anything, they should exercise to strengthen the body and prepare for delivery. Moderate exercise during pregnancy helps to prevent excessive weight gain and speed up recovery following birth.

   Pregnant women in Indian tribes continue to do all of their difficult work chores up to the very day of delivery, and a few hours after the baby's birth they resume their normal activities. Several women athletes have competed in sports during the early stages of pregnancy. Nevertheless, the woman and her personal physician should make the final decision regarding her exercise program.

   Stretching exercises are to be performed very gently because hormonal changes during pregnancy increase the laxity of muscles and connective tissue. These changes facilitate delivery but they also make women more susceptible to injuries during exercise.

   In 1994, the American College of Obstetricians and Gynecologists released an update of

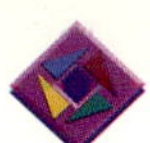

# — SUMMARY STATEMENT —
## Workshop On
## Physical Activity and Public Health

**Sponsored By:**
**U. S. Centers for Disease Control and Prevention**
**and**
**American College of Sports Medicine**

*In Cooperation with the President's Council on Physical Fitness and Sports*

Regular physical activity is an important component of a healthy lifestyle — preventing disease and enhancing health and quality of life. A persuasive body of scientific evidence, which has accumulated over the past several decades, indicates that regular, moderate-intensity physical activity confers substantial health benefits. Because of this evidence, the U.S. Public Health Service has identified increased physical activity as a priority in Healthy People 2000, our national health objectives for the year 2000.

A primary benefit of regular physical activity is protection against coronary heart disease. In addition, physical activity appears to provide some protection against several other chronic diseases such as adult-onset diabetes, hypertension, certain cancers, osteoporosis, and depression. Furthermore, on average, physically active people outlive inactive people, even if they start their activity late in life. It is estimated that more than 250,000 deaths per year in the U.S. can be attributed to lack of regular physical activity, a number comparable to the deaths attributed to other chronic disease risk factors such as obesity, high blood pressure, and elevated blood cholesterol.

Despite the recognized value of physical activity, few Americans are regularly active. Only 22% of adults engage in leisure time physical activity at the level recommended for health benefits in Healthy People 2000. Fully 24% of adult Americans are completely sedentary and are badly in need of more physical activity. The remaining 54% are inadequately active and they too would benefit from more physical activity. Participation in regular physical activity appears to have gradually increased during the 1960s, 1970s, and early 1980s, but has plateaued in recent years. Among ethnic minority populations, older persons, and those with lower incomes or levels of education, participation in regular physical activity has remained consistently low.

Why are so few Americans physically active? Perhaps one answer is that previous public health efforts to promote physical activity have overemphasized the importance of high-intensity exercise. The current low rate of participation may be explained, in part, by the perception of many people that they must engage in vigorous, continuous exercise to reap health benefits. Actually the scientific evidence clearly demonstrates that regular, moderate-intensity physical activity provides substantial health benefits. A group of experts brought together by the U.S. Centers for Disease Control and Prevention (CDC) and the American College of Sports Medicine (ACSM) reviewed the pertinent scientific evidence and formulated the following recommendation:

**Every American adult should accumulate 30 minutes or more of moderate-intensity physical activity over the course of most days of the week.** Incorporating more activity into the daily routine is an effective way to improve health. Activities that can contribute to the 30-minute total include walking up stairs (instead of taking the elevator), gardening, raking leaves, dancing, and walking part or all of the way to or from work. The recommended 30 minutes of physical activity may also come from planned exercise or recreation such as jogging, playing tennis, swimming, and cycling. One specific way to meet the standard is to walk two miles briskly.

**Because most adult Americans fail to meet this recommended level of moderate-intensity physical activity, almost all should strive to increase their participation in moderate or vigorous physical activity.** Persons who currently do not engage in regular physical activity should begin by incorporating a few minutes of increased activity into their day, building up gradually to 30 minutes of additional physical activity. Those who are irregularly active should strive to adopt a more consistent pattern of activity. Regular participation in physical activities that develop and maintain muscular strength and joint flexibility is also recommended.

This recommendation has been developed to emphasize the important health benefits of moderate physical activity. But recognizing the benefits of physical activity is only part of the solution to this important public health problem. Today's high-tech society entices people to be inactive. Cars, television, and labor-saving devices have profoundly changed the way many people perform their jobs, take care of their homes, and use their leisure time. Furthermore, our surroundings often present significant barriers to participation in physical activity. Walking to the corner store proves difficult if there are no sidewalks; riding a bicycle to work is not an option unless safe bike lanes or paths are available.

Many Americans will not change their lifestyles until the environmental and social barriers to physical activity are reduced or eliminated. Individuals can help to overcome these barriers by modifying their own lifestyles and by encouraging family members and friends to become more active. In addition, local, state, and federal public health agencies; recreation boards; school groups; professional organizations; and fitness and sports organizations should work together to disseminate this critical public health message and to promote national, community, worksite, and school programs that help Americans become more physically active.

*The American College of Sports Medicine and the U.S. Centers for Disease Control and Prevention, in cooperation with the President's Council on Physical Fitness and Sports, released this statement July 29, 1993, at the National Press Club in Washington, D.C.*



**FIGURE 3.4** ◆ Summary Statement: Workshop On Physical Activity and Public Health.

its guidelines for exercise during pregnancy.[5] Among the recommendations for pregnant women with no additional risk factors are:

- Continue to exercise at a mild-to-moderate pace throughout the pregnancy but decrease exercise intensity by about 25% from the pre-pregnancy program.)
- Exercise regularly a minimum of three times a week instead of doing occasional bouts of exercise.
- Attention must be paid to the body's signals of discomfort and distress. Stop exercise when tired. Never exercise to exhaustion. Stop if unusual symptoms arise. These include pain of any kind, cramping, nausea, bleeding or leaking amniotic fluid, faintness, dizziness, palpitations, numbness in any part of the body, or decreased fetal activity.
- Avoid exercises that require you to lie on your back after the first trimester. This position can block blood flow to the uterus and the baby.
- Do non-weight-bearing activities such as cycling, swimming, or water aerobics, which minimize the risk of injury and may allow the continuation of exercise throughout the pregnancy.
- Activities that could lead to a loss of balance or cause even mild trauma to the abdomen should be avoided.
- Care must be taken to get proper nourishment. Pregnancy also requires approximately 300 extra calories per day.
- During the first three months in particular, exercise in the heat is to be avoided. Clothing that allows for proper heat dissipation and drinking plenty of water are encouraged.

4. **Does participating in exercise hinder menstruation?** In some instances highly trained athletes may develop amenorrhea (stopping of menstruation) during training and competition. This condition is seen most often in extremely lean women who also engage in sports that require strenuous physical effort over a sustained time, but it is by no means irreversible. At present we do not know whether the condition is caused by physical stress or emotional stress related to high-intensity training, excessively low body fat, or other factors.

   Although women on the average have a lower physical capacity during menstruation, women have broken Olympic and world records at all stages of the menstrual cycle. Menstruation should not keep a woman from participating in athletics, and it will not necessarily have a negative impact on performance.

5. **Does exercise help relieve dysmenorrhea (painful menstruation)?** Exercise has not been shown to either cure or aggravate painful menstruation, but it has been shown to help relieve menstrual cramps because it improves circulation to the uterus. Particularly, stretching exercises of the muscles in the pelvic region seem to reduce and prevent painful menstruation that is not the result of a disease.[6]

6. **Does exercise offset the detrimental effects of cigarette smoking?** Physical exercise often motivates toward stopping smoking, but it does not offset any ill effects of smoking. If anything, smoking greatly diminishes the ability of the blood to transport oxygen to working muscles. Oxygen is carried in the circulatory system by hemoglobin, the iron-containing pigment of the red blood cells. Carbon monoxide, a byproduct of cigarette smoke, has 210 to 250 times greater affinity for hemoglobin than for oxygen. Consequently, carbon monoxide combines much faster with hemoglobin, decreasing the oxygen-carrying capacity of the blood.

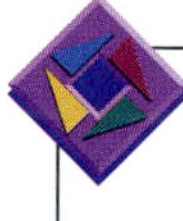

*A mild-to-moderate exercise program during pregnancy strengthens the body in preparation for delivery.*

Chronic smoking also increases airway resistance, requiring the respiratory muscles to work much harder and consume more oxygen just to ventilate a given amount of air. If a person quits smoking, exercise does help increase the functional capacity of the pulmonary system.

A regular exercise program does seem to be a powerful incentive to quit smoking. A random survey of 1,250 runners conducted at the 6.2-mile Peachtree Road Race in Atlanta provided impressive results. The results indicated that 81% and 75% of the men and women who smoked cigarettes when they started

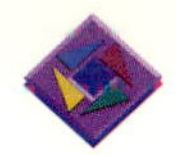

running had quit before the race date. (A comprehensive smoking cessation program is provided in Chapter 12 of this book.)

7. **Is exercise safe during a smog alert?** People who have respiratory or cardiovascular conditions should not exercise outdoors when air quality is poor. Everyone should refrain from outdoor exercise during periods of smog alert or "very poor" air quality. Exercising indoors is a safe alternative to outdoor activity in smoggy cities. If you have to exercise outdoors, air quality usually is best during the early morning and late evening hours.

8. **What type of clothing should a person wear during exercise?** The type of clothing you wear during exercise is important. Clothing should fit comfortably and allow free movement. Clothes should be geared to air temperature and humidity. Exercisers should avoid nylon and rubberized materials and tight clothes that will interfere with the cooling mechanism of the human body or obstruct normal blood flow.

   Properly fitting shoes, manufactured specifically for your choice of activity, are a *must* to help prevent lower limb injuries. Walking, running, aerobics, and court shoes all are manufactured differently to provide the most effective protection during each of these activities.

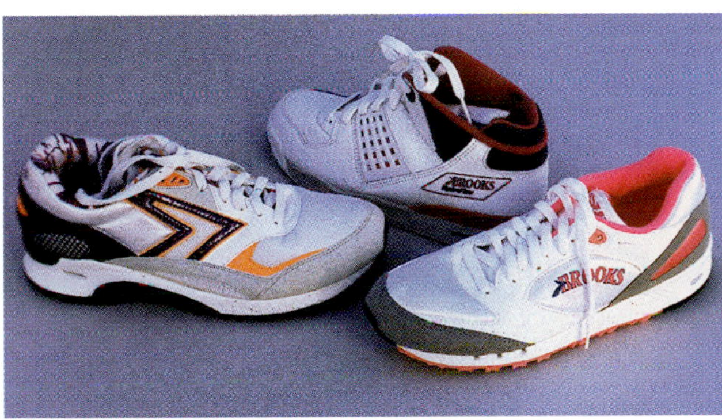


*Properly fitting shoes for specific activities are recommended to prevent exercise related injuries.*

9. **How long should a person wait after a meal before exercising strenuously?** The length of time to wait before exercising after a meal depends on the amount of food eaten. On the average, after a large meal you should wait about 2 hours before participating in strenuous physical activity. A walk or some other light physical activity is fine following a meal, though. If anything, it helps burn extra calories and may help the body metabolize fats more efficiently.

10. **What time of day is best for exercise?** You can do intense exercise almost any time of the day, with the exception of about 2 hours following a heavy meal, or the noon and early afternoon hours on hot and humid days. Moderate exercise seems to be beneficial shortly after a meal, because exercise enhances the *thermogenic response*, the amount of energy required to digest food. A walk after a meal burns more calories than a walk several hours after a meal.

    Many people enjoy exercising early in the morning because it gives them a boost to start the day. People who exercise in the morning also seem to stick with it more than others do. Some prefer the lunch hour for weight control reasons. By exercising at noon, they do not eat as big a lunch, which helps to keep down daily caloric intake. Highly stressed people seem to like the evening hours because of the relaxing effects of exercise.

11. **Why is exercising in hot and humid conditions unsafe?** When a person exercises, only 30% to 40% of the energy the body produces is used for mechanical work or movement. The rest of the energy (60% to 70%) is converted into heat. If this heat cannot be dissipated properly because the weather is too hot or the relative humidity is too high, body temperature increases and in extreme cases can result in death.

    The specific heat of body tissue (the heat required to raise the temperature of the body by 1°C) is .38 calories per pound of body weight per 1°C (.38 cal/lb/°C). This indicates that if no body heat is dissipated, a 150-pound person has to burn only 57 calories ($150 \times .38$) to increase total body temperature by 1°C. If this person were to conduct an exercise session requiring 300 calories (about 3 miles running) without any heat dissipation, the inner body temperature would increase by 5.3°C, the equivalent of going from 98.6°F to 108.1°F.

    This example clearly illustrates the need for caution when exercising in hot or humid weather. If the relative humidity is too high, body heat cannot be lost through evaporation because the atmosphere already is saturated with water vapor. In one instance a football casualty occurred at a temperature of only

64°F, but at a relative humidity of 100%. People must be cautious when air temperature is above 90°F and the relative humidity simultaneously is above 60%.

The American College of Sports Medicine recommends that individuals should not engage in strenuous physical activity when the readings of a wet bulb globe thermometer exceed 82.4°F. With this type of thermometer, the wet bulb is cooled by evaporation, and on dry days it shows a lower temperature than the regular (dry) thermometer. On humid days the cooling effect is less because of less evaporation; hence, the difference between the wet and dry readings is not as great.

The American Running and Fitness Association offers the following descriptions and first-aid measures for three signs of trouble when exercising in the heat:

- **Heat cramps.** Symptoms include cramps and spasms and muscle twitching in the legs, arms, and abdomen. To relieve heat cramps, stop exercising, get out of the heat, massage the painful area, slowly stretch, and drink plenty of fluids.
- **Heat exhaustion**. Symptoms include fainting; dizziness; profuse sweating; cold, clammy skin; weakness; headache; and a rapid, weak pulse. If you experience any of these symptoms, stop and find a cool place to rest. Drink plenty of cool fluids. Loosen or remove clothing, and rub your body with a cool, wet towel. Stay out of the heat for the rest of the day, and possibly for the next 2 or 3 days.
- **Heat stroke**. Symptoms include serious disorientation; warm, dry skin; no sweating; rapid, full pulse; vomiting; diarrhea; unconsciousness; and high body temperature. As the temperature climbs, unexplained anxiety sets in. When the body temperature reaches 104°F to 105°F, the individual may get goose bumps, feel a cold sensation in the trunk of the body, nauseous, throbbing in the temples, and numbness in the extremities. Most people become incoherent after this stage. When body temperature reaches 105°F to 106°F, disorientation, loss of fine-motor control, and muscular weakness set in. If the temperature exceeds 106°F, serious neurologic injury and death may be imminent.

  Heat stroke requires immediate emergency medical attention. Someone should request help (call 911) and get the person out of the sun. While you're waiting for the person to be taken to the hospital's emergency room, spray the person with cool water and rub the body with cool towels. Fan the person and give him or her plenty of cold liquids.

12. **What should a person do to replace fluids lost during prolonged aerobic exercise?** The main objective of fluid replacement during prolonged aerobic exercise is to maintain the blood volume so circulation and sweating can continue at normal levels. Adequate water replacement is the most important factor in preventing heat disorders. Drinking about 6 to 8 ounces of cool water every 15 to 20 minutes during exercise appears to be ideal to prevent dehydration. Cold fluids seem to be absorbed more rapidly from the stomach.

    Commercial fluid replacement solutions (e.g., Exceed, Gatorade) contain about 6 to 8% glucose, which seems to be optimal for fluid absorption and performance. Sugar does not become available to the muscles until about 30 minutes after drinking a glucose solution.

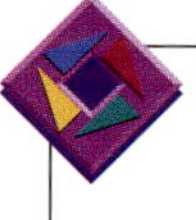

*Drinks with a glucose concentration above 8% slow down water absorption during exercise in the heat.*

Drinks high in fructose or with a glucose concentration above 8% will slow down water absorption when exercising in the heat.

Most soft drinks (cola, non-cola) contain between 10% and 12% glucose, an amount that is too high for proper rehydration during exercise in the heat (also see carbohydrate loading in Chapter 7).

Commercially prepared sports drinks are recommended when exercise will be strenuous and carried out for more than an hour. For exercise lasting less than an hour, water is just as effective in replacing fluid loss. The sports drinks that you select should be based on your personal preference. Try different drinks at 6% to 8% glucose concentration to see which drink you tolerate best and suits your tastes as well.

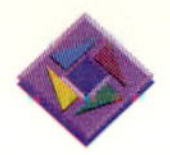

13. **What precautions should be taken when exercising in the cold?** In contrast to hot and humid conditions, exercising in the cold usually does not threaten one's health because clothing for heat conservation can be selected and exercise itself increases the production of body heat. The popular belief that exercising in cold temperatures (32°F and lower) freezes the lungs is totally false, because the air is warmed properly in the air passages before it ever reaches the lungs. Cold is not what poses a threat but, rather, wind velocity is what affects the chill factor greatly.

    For example, exercising at a temperature of 25°F with adequate clothing is not too cold, but if the wind is blowing at 25 miles per hour, the chill factor lowers the actual temperature to –5°F. This effect is even worse if a person is wet and exhausted.

    Even though the lungs are under no risk when exercising in the cold, the face, head, hands, and feet should be protected, as they are subject to frostbite. In cold temperatures, about 30% of the body's heat is lost through the head's surface area if it is unprotected. Wearing several layers of lightweight clothing is preferable to one single, thick layer because warm air is trapped between layers of clothes, enabling greater heat conservation.

## MANAGING EXERCISE-RELATED INJURIES

To enjoy and maintain physical fitness, preventing injury during a conditioning program is essential. Exercise-related injuries, nonetheless, are common in individuals who participate in exercise programs. Surveys indicate that more than half of all new participants incur injuries during the first 6 months of a conditioning program.

The three most common causes of injuries are: (a) rapid conditioning programs — doing too much too quickly, (b) improper shoes or training surfaces, and (c) anatomical predisposition (body propensity). A significant increase in quantity, intensity, and duration of activities is by far the most common cause of injuries. The body requires time to adapt to more intense activities. Most of these injuries can be prevented through a more gradual and moderate conditioning program.

Proper shoes for specific activities are essential. Shoes should be replaced when they show a lot of wear and tear. Softer training surfaces, such as grass and dirt, produce less trauma than asphalt and concrete do.

Few people have perfect body alignment, so injuries may occur eventually. These types of injuries often are associated with overtraining (working too hard and too long without sufficient rest for the body to recover from exhaustive exercise). In case of injury, proper treatment can avert a lengthy recovery process. A summary of common exercise-related injuries, and how to manage them, follows.

### Acute Sports Injuries

The best treatment always has been prevention itself. If an activity causes unusual discomfort or chronic irritation, the cause should be treated by decreasing the intensity of exercise, switching activities, substituting equipment, or upgrading clothing (such as proper-fitting shoes).

In cases of acute injury, the standard treatment is cold application, compression, or splinting (or both), and elevation of the affected body part. This commonly is referred to as ICE. I = ice application, C = compression, and E = elevation. Cold should be applied three to five times a day for 15 to 20 minutes at a time during the first 24 to 36 hours, by submerging the injured area in cold water, using an icebag, or applying ice massage to the affected part. An elastic bandage or wrap can be used for compression. Elevating the body part decreases blood flow to it.

The purpose of these three types of treatment is to minimize swelling in the area, which hastens recovery time. After the first 36 to 48 hours, heat can be applied if swelling or inflammation has not increased. If doubts remain regarding the nature or seriousness of the injury (such as suspected fracture), medical evaluation should be sought.

Obvious deformities (such as in fractures, dislocations, or partial dislocations) call for splinting, cold application with an icebag, and medical attention. Untrained individuals never should try to reset any of these conditions, as muscles, ligaments, and nerves could be damaged further. Treatment of these injuries always should be in the hands of specialized medical personnel. A quick reference guide for the signs or symptoms and treatment of exercise-related problems is provided in Table 3.1.

#### Muscle Soreness and Stiffness

Individuals who begin an exercise program or participate after a long layoff from exercise often

**TABLE 3.1**
**Reference Guide for Exercise Related Problems**

| Injury | Signs/Symptoms | Treatment* |
|---|---|---|
| Bruise (contusion) | Pain, swelling, discoloration | Cold application, compression, rest |
| Dislocations Fractures | Pain, swelling, deformity | Splinting, cold application, seek medical attention |
| Heat cramps | Cramps, spasms and muscle twitching in the legs, arms, and abdomen | Stop activity, get out of the heat, stretch, massage the painful area, drink plenty of fluids |
| Heat exhaustion | Fainting, profuse sweating, cold/clammy skin, weak/rapid pulse, weakness, headache | Stop activity, rest in a cool place, loosen clothing, rub body with cool/wet towel, drink plenty of fluids, stay out of heat for 2–3 days |
| Heat stroke | Hot/dry skin, no sweating, serious disorientation, rapid/full pulse, vomiting, diarrhea, unconsciousness, high body temperature | **Seek immediate medical attention**, request help and get out of the sun, bathe in cold water/spray with cold water/rub body with cold towels, drink plenty of cold fluids |
| Joint sprains | Pain, tenderness, swelling, loss of use, discoloration | Cold application, compression, elevation, rest, heat after 36 to 48 hours (if no further swelling) |
| Muscle cramps | Pain, spasms | Stretch muscle(s), use mild exercises for involved area |
| Muscle soreness and stiffness | Tenderness, pain | Mild stretching, low-intensity exercise, warm bath |
| Muscle strains | Pain, tenderness, swelling, loss of use | Cold application, compression, elevation, rest, heat after 36 to 48 hours (if no further swelling) |
| Shin splints | Pain, tenderness | Cold application prior to and following any physical activity, rest, heat (if no activity is carried out) |
| Side stitch | Pain on the side of the abdomen below the rib cage | Decrease level of physical activity or stop altogether, gradually increase level of fitness |
| Tendinitis | Pain, tenderness, loss of use | Rest, cold application, heat after 48 hours |

* Cold should be applied three to four times a day for 15 to 20 minutes. Heat can be applied three times a day for 15 to 20 minutes.

develop muscle soreness and stiffness. The acute soreness that sets in the first few hours after exercise is thought to be related to a lack of blood (oxygen) flow and general fatigue of the exercised muscles.

Delayed muscle soreness that appears several hours after exercise (usually about 12 hours later) and lasts for 2 to 4 days may be related to actual tiny tears in muscle tissue, muscle spasms that increase fluid retention, stimulating the pain nerve endings, and overstretching or tearing of connective tissue in and around muscles and joints.

Mild stretching before and adequately stretching after exercise helps to prevent soreness and stiffness. Gradually progressing into an exercise program is important, too. A person should not attempt to do too much too quickly. Mild stretching, low-intensity exercise to stimulate blood flow, and a warm bath might help to relieve pain.

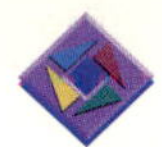

### Exercise Intolerance

When starting an exercise program, participants should stay within the safe limits. The best method to determine whether you are exercising too strenuously is to check your heart rate and make sure it does not exceed the limits of your target zone. Exercising above this target zone may not be safe for unconditioned or high-risk individuals. You do not have to exercise beyond your target zone to gain the desired cardiovascular benefits.

Several physical signs will tell you when you are exceeding your functional limitations. A rapid or irregular heart rate, difficult breathing, nausea, vomiting, lightheadedness, headaches, dizziness, pale skin, flushness, extreme weakness, lack of energy, shakiness, sore muscles, cramps, and tightness in the chest are all signs of intolerance to exercise. You should learn to listen to your body. If you notice any of these symptoms, you should seek medical attention before continuing your exercise program.

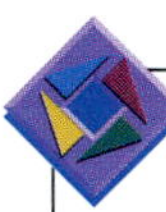

*Learn to listen to your body. Symptoms of exercise intolerance should be brought to the attention of medical personnel.*

Recovery heart rate is another indicator of overexertion. To a certain extent, recovery heart rate is related to fitness level. The higher your cardiovascular fitness level, the faster your heart rate will decrease following exercise. As a rule of thumb, heart rate should be below 120 beats per minute 5 minutes into recovery. If your heart rate is above 120, you most likely have overexerted yourself or possibly could have some other cardiac abnormality. If you lower the intensity or duration of exercise, or both, and still have a fast heart rate 5 minutes into recovery, you should consult your physician.

### Side Stitch

The exact cause of this sharp pain that sometimes occurs during exercise is unknown. Some experts suggest that it could be related to a lack of blood flow to the respiratory muscles during strenuous physical exertion. Side stitch seems to occur only in unconditioned beginners or trained individuals when they exercise at higher intensities than usual. This stitch is encountered primarily in the early stages of exercise participation. As you improve your physical condition, this problem will disappear unless you start training at a higher intensity. If it occurs, slow down, and if it persists, stop altogether.

### Shin Splints

The shin splint, one of the most common injuries to the lower limbs, is characterized by pain and irritation in the shin region of the leg. It usually results from one or more of the following: (a) lack of proper and gradual conditioning, (b) doing physical activities on hard surfaces (wooden floors, hard tracks, cement, and asphalt), (c) fallen arches in the feet, (d) chronic overuse, (e) muscle fatigue, (f) faulty posture, (g) improper shoes, and (h) participating in weight-bearing activities when excessively overweight.

Shin splints are managed by: (a) removing or reducing the cause (exercising on softer surfaces, wearing better shoes or arch supports, or both, completely stopping exercise until the shin splints heal); (b) doing mild stretching exercises before and after physical activity; (c) using ice massage for 10 to 20 minutes before and after physical exercise; and (d) applying active heat (whirlpool and hot baths) for 15 minutes, two to three times a day. In addition, supportive taping during physical activity is helpful (the proper taping technique can be learned readily from a qualified athletic trainer).

### Muscle Cramps

Muscle cramps are caused by the body's depletion of essential electrolytes or a breakdown in the coordination between opposing muscle groups. If you have a muscle cramp, you should first attempt to stretch the muscles involved. For example, in the case of the calf muscle, pull your toes up toward the knees. After stretching the muscles, gently rub them down, and finally do some mild exercises requiring the use of those muscles.

In pregnant and lactating women, muscle cramps often are related to a lack of calcium. If women get cramps during these times, calcium supplements may be the answer. Tight clothing also can cause cramps, by decreasing blood flow to active muscle tissue.

## AEROBIC ACTIVITY CHOICES

One of the fun aspects of aerobic exercise is the variety of activities that promote cardiovascular development. You may select one or a combination of activities for your program. This choice should be based on personal enjoyment, convenience, and availability.

Most people pick and adhere to a single mode of exercise, such as walking, swimming, or jogging. No single activity develops total fitness. Many activities contribute to cardiovascular development. The extent of their contribution to other fitness components is limited, though, and varies among the activities. For total fitness, aerobic activities should be supplemented with strength (resistance) and flexibility exercise programs. Selecting a combination of aerobic activities (cross-training) nonetheless can add enjoyment to the program and keep exercise from becoming monotonous.

As you learn about the various aerobic activities in this chapter, keep in mind that your exercise sessions must be convenient. So that you may enjoy exercise, select a time when you will not be rushed, and find a nearby location. People do not enjoy driving across town to get to the gym, health club, track, or pool. If parking is a problem, you may quickly get discouraged and use this as an excuse not to stick to your exercise program.

## Walking

The most natural, easiest, safest, and least expensive form of aerobic exercise is walking. For years many fitness practitioners believed that walking was not vigorous enough to improve cardiovascular functioning. Studies have established, however, that brisk walking at speeds of 4 miles per hour or faster does improve cardiovascular fitness.

From a health-fitness viewpoint, a regular walking program can prolong life significantly (also see Physical Inactivity, Chapter 9). Although walking takes longer than jogging, the caloric cost of brisk walking is only about 10% lower than jogging the same distance.

Walking is perhaps the best activity to start a conditioning program for the cardiovascular system. Inactive people should start with 1-mile walks four to five times per week. Walk times can be increased gradually by 5 minutes each week. Following 3 to 4 weeks of conditioning, people should be able to walk 2 miles at a 4-mile-per-hour pace, five times per week. For greater aerobic benefits, walk longer and swing the arms at a faster than normal pace. A backpack (4 to 6 pounds) or an Aero-belt* add to the intensity of walking. Because of the additional load to the cardiovascular system, extra weights are not recommended for people who have cardiovascular disease.

Walking in water (chest-deep level) is an excellent form of activity for people with leg and back problems. Because of water buoyancy, individuals submerged in water to armpit level weigh only about 10% to 20% of their weight outside the water. The resistance the water creates as a person walks in the pool makes the intensity quite high, providing an excellent cardiovascular workout.

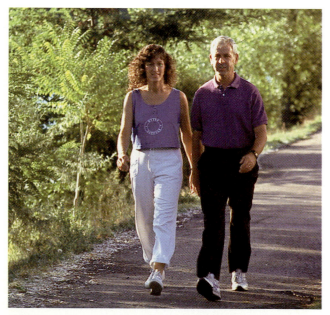

*Walking is the most natural aerobic exercise.*

## Hiking

Many people feel guilty if they are unable to continue their exercise routine during vacations. Hiking is an excellent activity for the entire family, especially during the summer and on summer vacations. The intensity of hiking over uneven terrain is greater than walking. An 8-hour hike can burn as many calories as a 20-mile walk or jog.

Another benefit of hiking is the relaxing effects of beautiful scenery. This is an ideal activity for highly stressed people who live near woods and hills. A rough day at the office can be forgotten quickly in the peacefulness and beauty of the outdoors.

*See Aero-belt exercise later in this chapter.

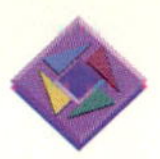

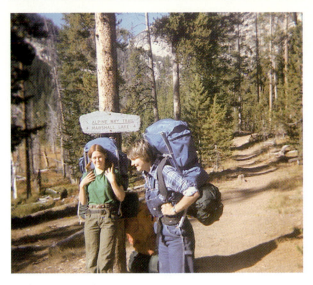


*An 8-hour hike can burn as many calories as a 20-mile walk or jog.*

## Jogging

Jogging is the most popular form of aerobic exercise. Next to walking, it is one of the most accessible and easiest forms of exercise. A person can find places to jog almost everywhere. The lone requirement to prevent injuries is a good pair of jogging shoes.

Jogging three to five times a week is one of the best ways to improve cardiovascular fitness. The risk of injury, however, is higher with jogging than walking, especially among beginners. For proper conditioning, jogging programs should start with 1 to 2 weeks of walking. As fitness improves, walking and jogging can be combined, gradually increasing the jogging segment until it comprises the full 20 to 30 minutes.

Unfortunately, too many people abuse this activity. People run too fast and too long. Many joggers think that if a little is good, more is better. Not so with cardiovascular endurance. As indicated under Frequency of Exercise, maximal oxygen uptake benefits of training more than five times per week are minimal. Furthermore, the risk of injury increases greatly as speed (running instead of jogging) and mileage go up.

Jogging approximately 15 miles per week near the 85% training intensity is enough to reach an excellent level of cardiovascular fitness. For those who want additional exercise, moderate-intensity activities (beyond the 15 miles) are recommended.

A good pair of shoes is a must for joggers. Many feet, knee, and leg problems originate from improperly fitting or worn-out shoes. A good pair of shoes should offer good lateral stability and not lean to either side when placed on a flat surface. The shoe also should bend at the ball of the foot, not at midfoot. Worn-out shoes should be replaced. After 500 miles of use, jogging shoes lose about a third of their shock absorption capabilities. If you suddenly have problems, check your shoes first. It may be time for a new pair. Guidelines for choosing the right jogging shoe are provided in Figure 3.5.

For safety reasons, joggers should stay away from high-speed roads, not wear headphones, and always run (or walk) against the traffic, so they will be able to see all oncoming traffic. At night, joggers should wear reflective clothing or fluorescent material on different parts of the body. Carrying a flashlight is even better because motorists can see the light from a greater distance than the reflective material.

An alternative form of jogging, especially for injured people, those with chronic back problems, and overweight individuals, is deep-water running (running in place while treading water). Deep-water running is almost as strenuous as jogging on land. In deep-water running, the land-running motions are accentuated by pumping the arms and legs hard through a full range of motion. The participant usually wears a floatation vest to help maintain the body in an upright position. Many elite athletes train frequently in water to lessen the wear and tear on the body caused by long-distance running. These athletes have been able to maintain high oxygen uptake values through rigorous water-running programs.

## Cross-Country Skiing

Many consider cross-country skiing as the ultimate aerobic exercise because it requires vigorous lower and upper body movements. The large amount of muscle mass involved in cross-country skiing makes the activity intense, yet it places little strain on muscles and joints.

Research has shown that, of all elite athletes, cross-country skiers have the greatest aerobic capacity. Some of the highest maximal oxygen uptakes ever measured have been found in elite cross-country skiers. Because more muscle mass is involved, more oxygen and energy (calories) are used during cross-country skiing than with most other aerobic activities.

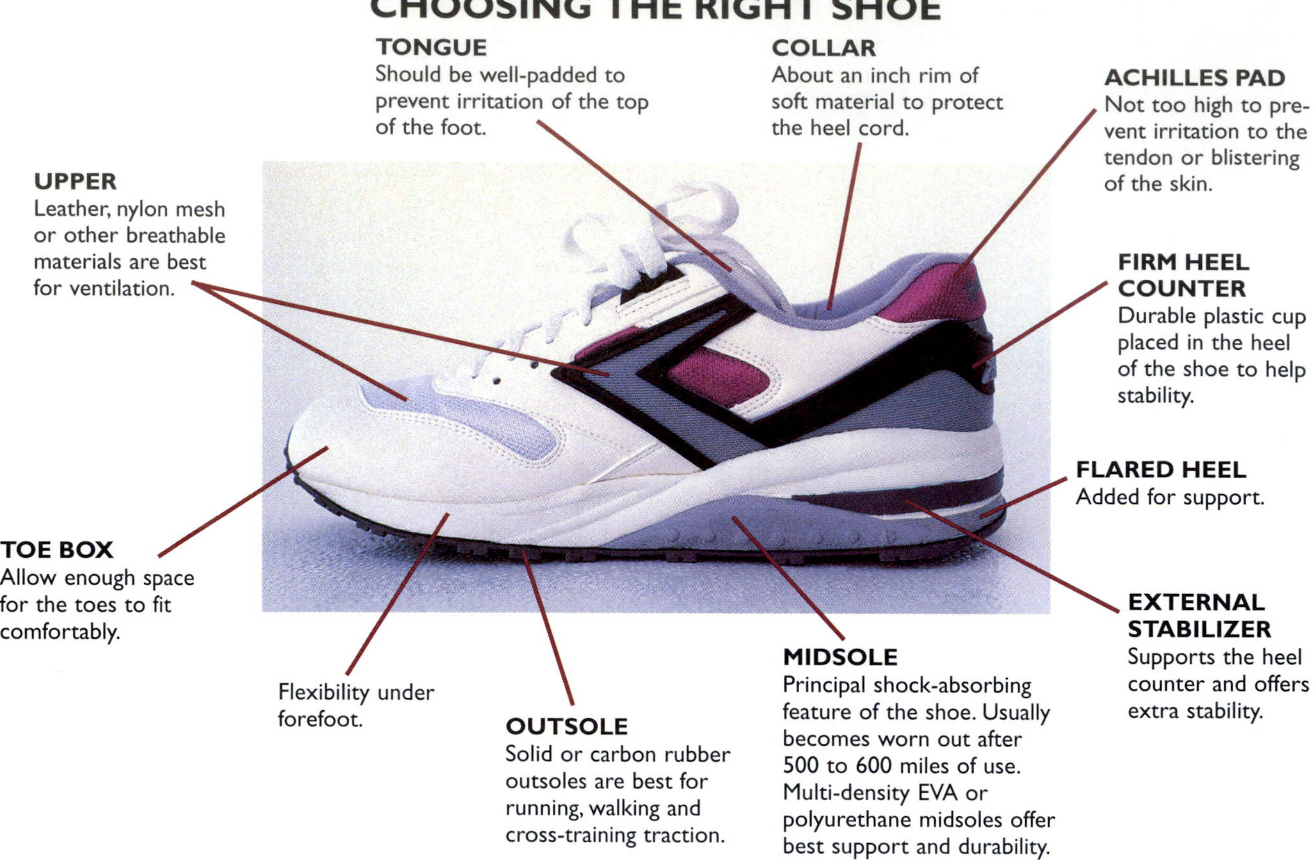
CHOOSING THE RIGHT SHOE
TONGUE
Should be well-padded to prevent irritation of the top of the foot.
COLLAR
About an inch rim of soft material to protect the heel cord.
ACHILLES PAD
Not too high to prevent irritation to the tendon or blistering of the skin.
UPPER
Leather, nylon mesh or other breathable materials are best for ventilation.
FIRM HEEL COUNTER
Durable plastic cup placed in the heel of the shoe to help stability.
FLARED HEEL
Added for support.
TOE BOX
Allow enough space for the toes to fit comfortably.
EXTERNAL STABILIZER
Supports the heel counter and offers extra stability.
MIDSOLE
Principal shock-absorbing feature of the shoe. Usually becomes worn out after 500 to 600 miles of use. Multi-density EVA or polyurethane midsoles offer best support and durability.
Flexibility under forefoot.
OUTSOLE
Solid or carbon rubber outsoles are best for running, walking and cross-training traction.

**FIGURE 3.5** ◆ What to look for in a good pair of jogging shoes.

In addition to being an excellent aerobic activity, cross-country skiing is soothing. Skiing through the beauty of the snow-covered countryside can be highly enjoyable. Although the need for snow is an obvious limitation, cross-country skiing simulating equipment for year-round training is available at many sporting goods stores.

Some skill is necessary for proficient cross-country skiing. Poorly skilled individuals are not able to elevate the heart rate enough to cause adequate aerobic development. Individuals contemplating this activity should seek out instruction to fully enjoy and reap the rewards of cross-country skiing.

## Aerobics

Aerobics, formerly known as aerobic dance, is thought to be the most common fitness activity for women in the United States. At first considered a fad, it now is a legitimate fitness activity with more than 20 million participants of all ages. Aerobics involves a series of exercise routines performed to music. Routines include a combination of stepping, walking, jogging, skipping, kicking, and arm-swinging movements. It is a fun way to exercise and promote cardiovascular development at the same time.

*High-impact-aerobics* (HIA), the traditional form of aerobics, involves actions in which both feet may be off the floor at the same time momentarily. These movements exert a great amount of vertical force on the feet as they contact the floor. Proper leg conditioning through other forms of weight-bearing aerobic exercises (brisk walking and jogging), as well as strength training, are recommended prior to participating in high-impact aerobics.

High-impact aerobics is an intense activity, and it also produces the highest rate of aerobics injuries. Shin splints, stress fractures, low back pain, and tendinitis are all too common among high-impact aerobics enthusiasts. These injuries are caused by the constant impact of the feet on firm surfaces. As a result, several alternative forms of aerobics have been developed.

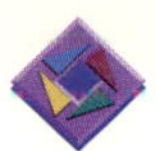

In *low-impact-aerobics* (LIA) at least one foot is in contact with the floor or ground at all times, reducing the impact as each foot contacts the surface. The recommended exercise intensity is more difficult to maintain with low-impact aerobics, though. To help elevate the exercise heart rate, all arm movements and weight-bearing actions that lower the center of gravity should be accentuated. Sustained movement throughout the program also is crucial to keep the heart rate in the target cardiovascular zone.

A relatively new form of aerobics is *step aerobics* (SA). Using a combination of stepping and arm movements, participants step up and down benches that range in height from 2 to 10 inches. Step aerobics adds another dimension to the aerobics movement and the exercise program. As noted previously, variety adds enjoyment to aerobic workouts.

Step aerobics is viewed as a high-intensity, but low-impact activity. The intensity of the activity can be controlled easily by changing the height of the steps. Aerobic benches or plates now are available commercially. The plates can be stacked together safely to adjust the height of the steps. Beginners are encouraged to use the lowest stepping height available and then advance gradually to a higher bench. This will lessen the risk of injury. Even though one foot is always in contact with the floor or bench during step aerobics, this activity is not recommended for individuals with ankle, knee, or hip problems.

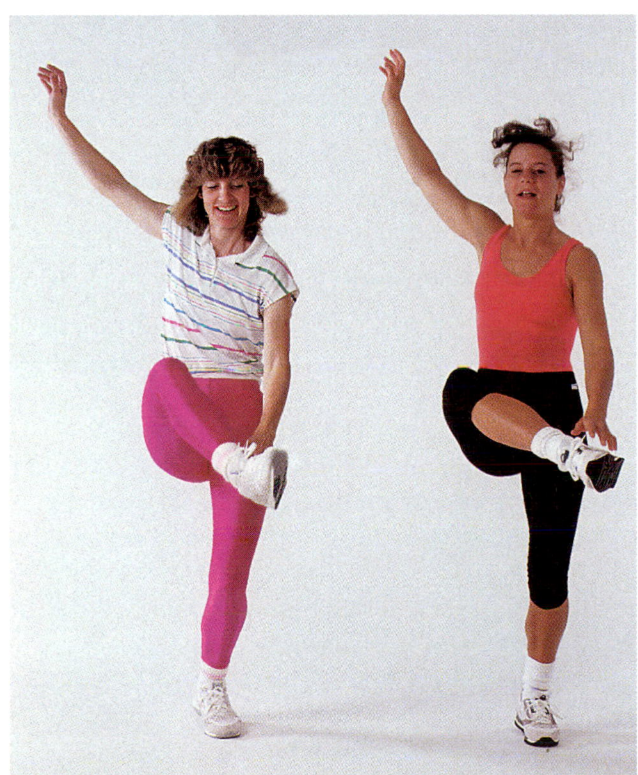

*Aerobics is the most popular fitness activity for women in the United States.*

Other forms of aerobics include a combination of HIA and LIA, as well as *moderate-impact aerobics* (MIA). The latter incorporates *plyometric training*. Plyometric aerobics requires forceful jumps or springing off the ground immediately after landing from a previous jump (also see Chapter 4). This type of training is used frequently by jumpers (high, long, and triple jumpers) and athletes in sports that require quick jumping ability, such as in basketball and gymnastics.

With moderate-impact aerobics, one foot is in contact with the ground most of the time. Participants, however, continually try to recover from all lower body flexion actions. This is done by quickly extending the hip, knee, and ankle joints without allowing the foot (or feet) to leave the ground. These quick movements make the exercise intensity of moderate-impact aerobics quite high.

## Aero-Belt Exercise

A new mode of aerobic activity is Aero-belt exercise. The Aero-belt™ (Aerobic Endurance Resistance Overloader) consists of a belt with an elastic band that slides freely through the belt and attaches to the wrists.* The objective of using the Aero-belt is to provide resistance to the arms during lower body physical activity, thereby increasing the person's oxygen consumption, energy expenditure, and development of upper body strength and endurance during aerobic exercise. As in cross-country skiing, the Aero-belt provides resistance to the arms while walking, jogging, bounding, stair stepping, riding a stationary bicycle, or doing aerobics.

Using the Aero-belt actually can provide more upper body conditioning benefits than cross-country skiing. Depending on individual strength and fitness levels, three different tension grades for the elastic cord are available. Medium and high tension are mainly for strength conditioning, and low tension is for developing endurance.

The physiologic responses to Aero-belt walking (4.0 and 4.2 mph), jogging (6 mph) and step

* Aero-belt is a registered trademark of Nurge Fitness Systems, P.O. Box 889, Ketchum, ID 83340 Phone: 1-800-TRY-TO-XL.

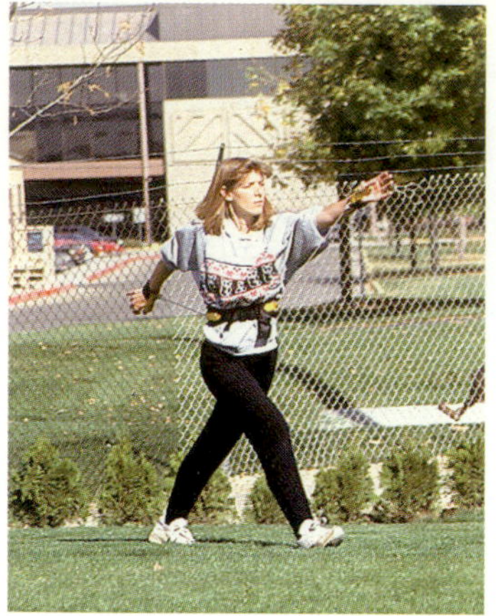

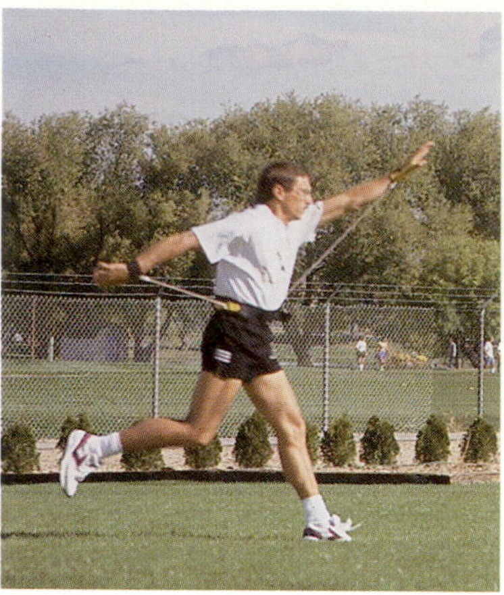

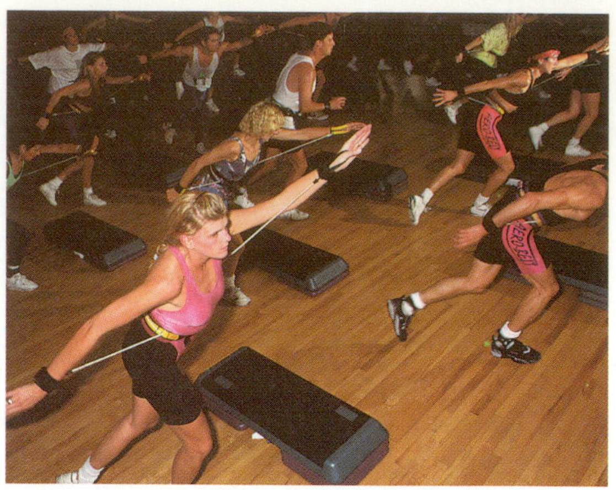

*Aero-belt Exercise is a new exercise modality designed to provide resistance to the arms during lower body physical activity; thereby increasing the person's oxygen consumption, energy expenditure, and upper body strength and endurance development during aerobic exercise.*

aerobics were investigated recently at Boise State University.[7,8,9] Increases in heart rate, oxygen uptake, and caloric expenditure ranged from 32% to 54% from regular walking and step-aerobics to walking and step-aerobics with an Aero-belt.

## Swimming

Swimming is another excellent form of aerobic exercise. It calls into play almost all major muscle groups in the body, providing a good training stimulus for the heart and lungs. Swimming is an excellent exercise option for individuals who cannot jog or walk for extended periods. Compared to other activities, the risk of injuries from swimming is low. The aquatic medium helps to support the body, taking pressure off bones and joints in the lower extremities and the back.

Maximal heart rates during swimming are approximately 13 beats per minute (bpm) lower than during running. The horizontal position of the body is thought to aid blood flow distribution throughout the body, decreasing the demand on the cardiovascular system. Cool water temperatures and direct contact with the water seem to help dissipate body heat more efficiently, further decreasing the strain on the heart.

Fitness experts recommend that this difference in maximal heart rate (13 bpm) be subtracted before determining cardiovascular training intensities. For example, the estimated maximal swimming heart rate for a 20-year old would be 187 bpm (220 – 20 – 13).

To produce better training benefits, gliding periods such as those in the breast stoke and side stroke should be minimized. Achieving proper training intensities with these strokes is difficult. The forward crawl is recommended for better aerobic results.

Overweight individuals need to swim fast enough to achieve an adequate training intensity. Excessive body fat makes the body more buoyant, and often the tendency is to just float along. This may be good for lowering stress and relaxing, but it does not increase caloric expenditure to aid with weight loss. Walking or jogging in waist- or armpit-deep water are better choices for overweight individuals who cannot walk or jog on land for a long time.

With reference to the principle of specificity of training, swimming participants need to realize that cardiovascular improvements cannot be measured adequately with a walk/jog test. Most of the work with swimming is done by the upper body musculature. Although the heart's ability to pump a greater amount of oxygenated blood improves significantly with any type of aerobic activity, the major increase in the ability of cells to utilize oxygen with swimming occurs in the upper body and not the lower extremities. Therefore, fitness improvements with swimming are best attained by comparing changes in distances swum using the swim test.

## Water Aerobics

Simple words best describe this relatively new form of exercise: fitness, fun, and safety for people of all ages. Besides developing fitness, water aerobics

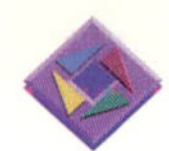

provides an opportunity for socialization and fun in a comfortable and refreshing setting.

Water aerobics incorporates a combination of rhythmic arm and leg actions performed in a vertical position while submerged in waist- to armpit-deep water. The vigorous limb movements against the water's resistance during water aerobics provide the training stimuli for cardiorespiratory development.

The popularity of water aerobics as an exercise modality to develop the cardiovascular system has been on the rise in recent years. This increase in popularity can be attributed to several factors:

1. Water buoyancy reduces weight-bearing stress on joints and therefore reduces the risk for injuries.
2. Water aerobics is a more feasible type of exercise for overweight individuals and those with arthritic conditions who may not be able to participate in weight-bearing activities such as walking, jogging, and aerobics.
3. Heat dissipation in water is beneficial to obese participants who seem to undergo a higher heat strain than individuals of average weight.
4. Water aerobics is available to swimmers and nonswimmers alike.

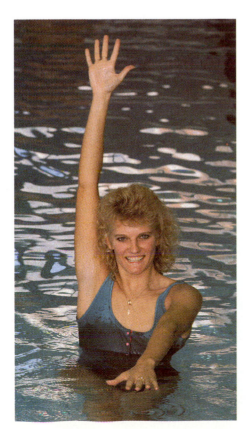

*Water aerobics represents fitness, fun, and safety for people of all ages.*

The exercises used during water aerobics are designed to elevate the heart rate, which contributes to cardiovascular development. In addition, the aquatic medium provides increased resistance for strength improvement with virtually no impact. Because of this resistance to movement, strength gains with water aerobics seem to be better than with most land-based aerobic activities.

Another benefit is that weight reduction can be facilitated without the pain and fear of injuries by many who initiate exercise programs. Water aerobics provides a relatively safe environment for participating in injury-free exercise. The cushioned environment of the water allows patients recovering from leg and back injuries, individuals with joint problems, injured athletes, pregnant women, and obese people to benefit from water aerobics. In water these people can exercise to develop and maintain cardiovascular endurance and yet limit or eliminate the potential for further injury.

Similar to swimming, maximal heart rates achieved during water aerobics are lower than during running. The difference between water aerobics and running, however, is only 10 bpm (as compared to 13 for swimming). The smaller difference is thought to be related to the upright position maintained during water aerobics, which may not facilitate blood flow distribution to the same extent as swimming. This difference of 10 bpm in maximal heart rate also should be considered when prescribing exercise intensities for water aerobics.

## Cycling

Cycling is an activity that most people learn in their youth. As a non-weight-bearing activity, it is a good exercise modality for people with lower body or lower back injuries. Cycling helps to develop the cardiovascular system, as well as muscular strength and endurance in the lower extremities. With the advent of stationary bicycles, this activity can be done year-round.

Raising the heart rate to the proper training intensity is more difficult with cycling. As the amount of muscle mass involved during aerobic exercise decreases, so does the demand placed on the cardiovascular system. In cycling the thigh muscles do most of the work, making a high cardiovascular training intensity harder to achieve and maintain.

Maintaining a continuous pedaling motion and eliminating coasting periods helps the participant achieve a higher heart rate. Exercising for longer periods also helps to compensate for the lower heart rate intensity during cycling. In comparing cycling to jogging, similar aerobic benefits take roughly three times the distance at twice the speed of jogging. Cycling, however, puts less stress on muscles and joints than jogging does, making the former a better exercise modality for people who cannot otherwise walk or jog.

To increase riding efficiency, the height of the bike seat should be adjusted so the legs are almost completely extended when the heels are placed on the pedals. The body should not sway from side to side as the person rides. The cycling cadence also is important for maximal efficiency. Bike tension or gears should be set at a moderate level to be able to ride at 70 to 90 revolutions per minute.

Skill is important in road cycling. Cyclists must be in control of the bicycle at all times. They have to be able to maneuver the bike in traffic, maintain balance at slow speeds, switch gears, apply the brakes, watch for pedestrians and stoplights, and ride through congested areas. Stationary cycling does not require special skills. Nearly everyone can do it.

Safety is a key issue in road cycling. More than a million bicycle injuries occur each year. Proper equipment and common sense are necessary. A well-designed and maintained bike is easier to maneuver. Toe clips are recommended to keep feet from sliding and to maintain equal upward and downward force on the pedals.

Bike riders must follow the same rules as motorists. Many accidents happen because cyclists run traffic lights and stop signs. Some further suggestions are:

- Use bike hand signals to let the traffic around you know of your actions.
- Don't ride side by side with another rider.
- Be aware of turning vehicles and cars backing out of alleys and parking lots; always yield to motorists in these situations.
- Watch out for storm drains. By not crossing them at the proper angle, front wheels can get caught and the rider thrown from the bike.
- Wear a good helmet, certified by the Snell Memorial Foundation or the American National Standards Institute. Many serious accidents and even deaths have been prevented by using helmets. Do not allow fashion, aesthetics, comfort, or price to be a factor when selecting and using a helmet for road cycling. Health and life are too precious to give up because of vanity and thriftiness.
- Wear appropriate clothes and shoes. Special clothing for cycling is not required. Clothing should be lightweight and not restrict movement. Shorts should be long enough to keep the skin from rubbing against the seat. For greater comfort, cycling shorts have extra padding sewn into the seat and crotch areas. Experienced cyclists often wear special shoes with a cleat that snaps directly onto the pedal.

The stationary bike is the most popular piece of equipment sold by sporting good stores. Before buying a stationary bike, though, be sure to try the activity a few days. If you enjoy it, you may want to purchase one. Invest with caution. If you opt to buy a lower-priced model, you may be disappointed. Good stationary bikes have comfortable

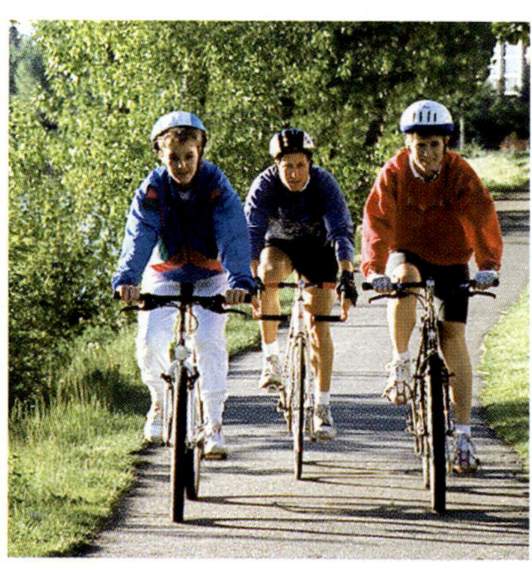

*Skill is an important factor for safety and enjoyment of road cycling.*

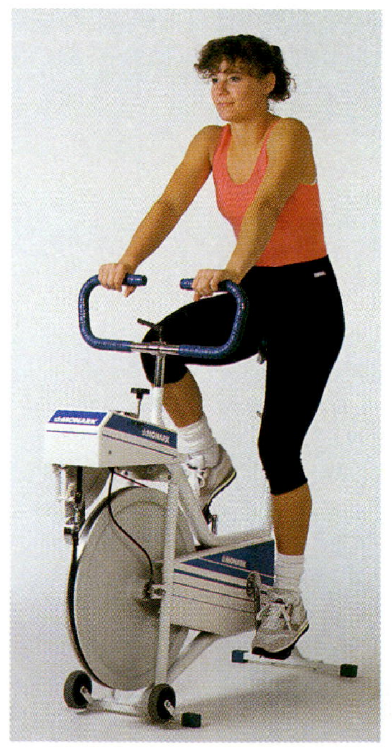

*Exercising on a stationary bicycle adds variety to aerobic workouts.*

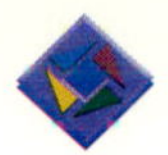

seats, are stable, and provide a smooth and uniform pedaling motion. A sticky bike that is hard to pedal only leads to discouragement and, along with many others, ends up stored in the corner of a basement.

## Cross-Training

An exercise program that combines two or more activities is referred to as cross-training. This type of training is designed to enhance fitness, decrease injuries, and eliminate the monotony of single-activity programs. Cross-training may combine aerobic and nonaerobic activities such as moderate jogging, speed training, and strength training.

Cross-training can produce better workouts than a single activity. For example, jogging develops the lower body and swimming builds the upper body. Rowing contributes to upper body development and cycling builds the legs. Combining activities such as these provides good overall conditioning and at the same time helps to improve or maintain fitness. Cross-training also offers an opportunity to develop skill and have fun with different activities.

Speed training often is coupled with cross-training. Faster performance times in aerobic activities (running, cycling) are generated with speed or interval training. People who want to improve their running times often run shorter intervals at faster speeds than the actual racing pace. For example, a person wanting to run a 6-minute mile may run four 440-yard intervals at a speed of 1 minute and 20 seconds per interval. A 440-yard walk/jog can become a recovery interval between fast runs.

Strength training is used frequently with cross-training. Strength training helps to condition muscles, tendons, and ligaments. In many activities improved strength enhances overall sports performance. For example, research has shown that, although road cyclists who trained with weights showed no improvement in aerobic capacity, the cyclists had a 33% improvement in riding time to exhaustion when exercising at 75% of their maximal capacity.[10]

## Rope Skipping

Rope skipping not only contributes to cardiovascular fitness, but it also helps to increase reaction time, coordination, agility, dynamic balance, and muscular strength in the lower extremities. At first, rope skipping may seem to be a highly strenuous form of aerobic exercise. Beginners often reach maximal heart rates after only 2 or 3 minutes of jumping. As skill improves, however, the energy demands decrease considerably.

Some people have claimed training benefits equal to a 30-minute jog in as few as 10 minutes of skipping. Although differences in strength and flexibility development are observed among various activities, 10 minutes at a certain heart rate provide similar cardiovascular benefits regardless of the nature of the activity. To obtain an adequate aerobic workout, the duration of exercise must be at least 20 minutes.

As with high-impact aerobics, a major concern of rope skipping is the stress placed on the lower extremities. Skipping with one foot at a time decreases the impact somewhat, but it does not eliminate the risk for injuries. Fitness experts recommend that skipping be used sparingly and primarily as a supplement to an aerobic exercise program.

## In-Line Skating

Frequently referred to as *blading*, in-line skating has become a highly popular fitness activity in recent years. Suddenly millions of children and adults are trying this activity. In the early 1990s stores could not keep up with the demand for in-line skates.

In-line skating has its origin in ice skating. Because warm-weather ice skating was not feasible, blades were replaced by wheels for summertime participation. Four-wheel roller skates were invented in the mid 1700s, but the activity did not really catch on until the late 1800s. The first in-line skate with five wheels in a row attached to the bottom of a shoe was developed in 1823. The in-line concept took hold in the United States in 1980, when hockey skates were adapted for this road-skating.

In-line skating is an excellent activity to develop cardiovascular fitness and lower body strength. The intensity of the activity is regulated by how hard you blade. The key to effective cardiovascular training is to maintain a constant and rhythmic pattern, using arms and legs and minimizing the gliding phase of blading. As a weight-bearing activity, in-line bladers also develop superior leg strength.

Instruction is necessary to achieve a minimum level of proficiency in this sport. Bladers commonly

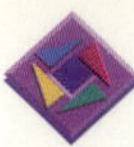



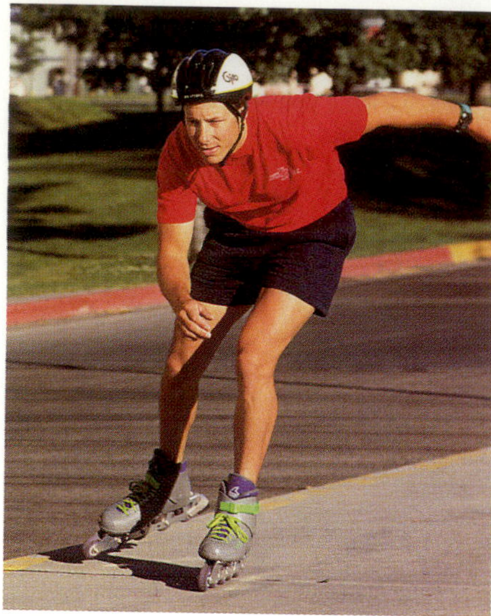

*In-line skating is a popular fitness activity in the 1990s.*

encounter hazards. Potholes, cracks, rocks, gravel, sticks, oil, street curbs, and driveways all pose challenges. Unskilled bladers are more prone to falls and injuries.

Good equipment will make the activity safer and more enjoyable. Blades range in price from $40 to $500. Recreational participants need not purchase the more costly competitive skates. An adequate blade should provide strong ankle support. Soft and flexible boots do not provide enough support. Small wheels offer more stability, and larger wheels enable greater speed. Blades should be purchased from stores that understand the sport and can provide sound advice according to skill level and needs.

Protective equipment is a *must* for in-line skating. Similar to road cycling, a good helmet that meets the safety standards set by the Snell Memorial Foundation or the American Standards Institute is important for protection in case of a fall. Wrist guards and knee and elbow pads also are recommended. The kneecap and the elbows are easily injured in any fall. Nighttime bladers should wear light-colored clothing and reflective tape.

## Rowing

Rowing is a low-impact activity that provides a complete body workout. It mobilizes most major muscle groups including the arms, legs, hips, abdominals, trunk, and shoulders. Rowing not only is a good form of aerobic exercise but, because of the nature of the activity (constant pushing and pulling against resistance), it also promotes total strength development. To accommodate different fitness levels, workloads can be regulated on most rowing machines.

Rowing is not among the most popular forms of aerobic exercise. Similar to stationary bicycles, a person should try the activity a few weeks before purchasing a unit.

## Stair Climbing

If sustained for at least 20 minutes, stair climbing is an extremely efficient form of aerobic exercise. Precisely because of the high intensity of stair climbing, many people in our society stay away from stairs and instead ride elevators! Many people dislike living in two-story homes because they have to climb the stairs frequently.

Not too many places have enough flights of stairs to climb continuously for 20 minutes. Stair-climbing machines offer an alternative. Stair climbing has become so popular that fitness enthusiasts often wait in line at health clubs to use the machines.

In terms of injuries, stair climbing seems to be relatively safe. Because the feet never leave the climbing surface, it is considered a low-impact activity. Joints and ligaments are not really strained during climbing. The intensity of exercise is controlled easily because most stair climbers can be programmed to regulate the workload.

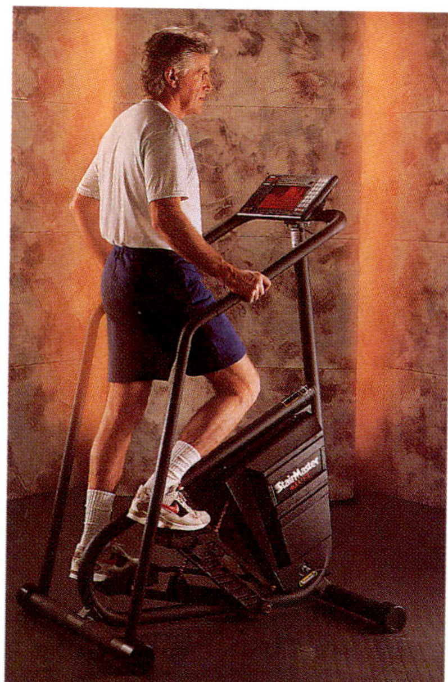


*Stair climbing provides a rigorous aerobic workout.*

## Racquet Sports

In racquet sports such as tennis, racquetball, squash, and badminton, the aerobic benefits are dictated by the individual's skill, intensity of the

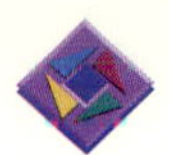

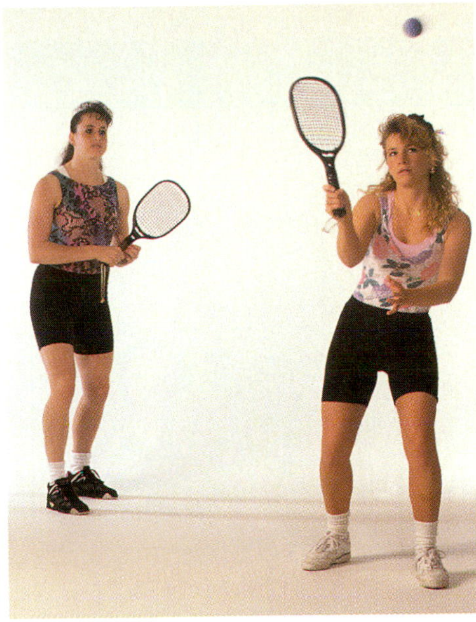

*Racquet sports require rhythmic and continuous activity to provide aerobic benefits.*

game, and how long the game is played. Skill is crucial to participate effectively in these sports and also to sustain continuous play. Frequent pauses during play do not allow people to maintain the heart rate in the appropriate target zone to stimulate cardiovascular development.

Many people who participate in racquet sports do so for enjoyment, social fulfillment, and relaxation. For developing cardiovascular fitness, these people supplement the sport with other forms of aerobic exercise such as jogging, cycling, or swimming.

If a racquet sport is the main form of aerobic exercise, participants need to try to run hard, fast, and as constantly as possible during play. They should not have to spend much time retrieving balls (bird or shuttlecock in badminton). Similar to low-impact aerobics, all movements should be accentuated by reaching out and bending more than usual, for better cardiovascular development.

## RATING THE FITNESS BENEFITS OF AEROBIC ACTIVITIES

The fitness contributions of different aerobic activities to the various health-related components of fitness vary. An accurate assessment of the contributions to each fitness component is difficult to establish, but a summary of likely benefits of several activities is provided in Table 3.2. Instead of a single rating or number, ranges are given for some of the categories. The benefits derived are based on the person's effort while participating in the activity.

The nature of the activity often dictates potential aerobic development. For example, jogging is much more strenuous than walking. The effort during exercise also has an impact on the amount of physiological development. The training benefits of going through the motions of a low-impact aerobics routine, as compared to accentuating all motions, are of a different magnitude.

Table 3.2 indicates a starting fitness level for each aerobic activity. Attempting to participate in high-intensity activities without proper conditioning often leads to injuries and discouragement. Beginners should start with low-intensity activities that carry a minimum risk for injuries.

In some cases, such as in high-impact aerobics and rope skipping, the risk for injuries remains high even if the participants have adequate conditioning. These activities should be supplemental only and are not recommended as the sole mode of exercise.

Physicians who work with cardiac patients frequently use METs, an alternative method of prescribing exercise intensity. The MET range for the various activities is included in Table 3.2. One MET represents the body's energy requirement at rest, or the equivalent of an oxygen uptake of 3.5 ml/kg/min. A 10-MET activity requires a tenfold increase in the resting energy requirement, or approximately 35 ml/kg/min. MET levels for a given activity vary according to the effort expended. The harder a person exercises, the higher is the MET level.

The effectiveness of various aerobic activities in weight management also is shown in Table 3.2. As a general rule, the greater the muscle mass involved in exercise, the better the results. Rhythmic and continuous activities that involve large amounts of muscle mass are most effective in burning calories.

Higher intensity activities increase caloric expenditure as well. Exercising longer, however, compensates for lower intensities. If carried out long enough (45 to 60 minutes five to six times per week), even walking can be an excellent exercise mode for weight loss. Additional information on a comprehensive weight management program is given in Chapter 8.

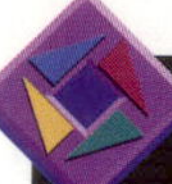

**TABLE 3.2**
**Ratings for Aerobic Activities**

| Activity | Recommended Starting Fitness Level[1] | Injury Risk[2] | Potential Cardiovascular Endurance Development ($VO_{2max}$)[3,5] | Upper Body Strength Development[3] | Lower Body Strength Development[3] | Upper Body Flexibility Development[3] | Lower Body Flexibility Development[3] | Weight Control[3] | MET Level[4,5,6] | Caloric Expenditure (cal/hour)[5,6] |
|---|---|---|---|---|---|---|---|---|---|---|
| Walking | B | L | 1–2 | 1 | 2 | 1 | 1 | 3 | 4–6 | 300–450 |
| Walking, Water—Chest-Deep | I | L | 2–4 | 2 | 3 | 1 | 1 | 3 | 6–10 | 450–750 |
| Hiking | B | L | 2–4 | 1 | 3 | 1 | 1 | 3 | 6–10 | 450–750 |
| Jogging | I | M | 3–5 | 1 | 3 | 1 | 1 | 5 | 6–15 | 450–1125 |
| Jogging, Deep Water | A | L | 3–5 | 2 | 2 | 1 | 1 | 5 | 8–15 | 600–1125 |
| High-Impact Aerobics | A | H | 3–4 | 2 | 4 | 3 | 2 | 4 | 6–12 | 450–900 |
| Low-Impact Aerobics | B | L | 2–4 | 2 | 3 | 3 | 2 | 3 | 5–10 | 375–750 |
| Step Aerobics | I | M | 2–4 | 2 | 3–4 | 3 | 2 | 3–4 | 5–12 | 375–900 |
| Moderate-Impact Aerobics | I | M | 2–4 | 2 | 3 | 3 | 2 | 3 | 6–12 | 450–900 |
| Swimming (front crawl) | B | L | 3–5 | 4 | 2 | 3 | 1 | 3 | 6–12 | 450–900 |
| Water Aerobics | B | L | 2–4 | 3 | 3 | 3 | 2 | 3 | 6–12 | 450–900 |
| Stationary Cycling | B | L | 2–4 | 1 | 4 | 1 | 1 | 3 | 6–10 | 450–750 |
| Road Cycling | I | M | 2–5 | 1 | 4 | 1 | 1 | 3 | 6–12 | 450–900 |
| Cross-Training | I | M | 3–5 | 2–3 | 3–4 | 2–3 | 1–2 | 3–5 | 6–15 | 450–1125 |
| Rope Skipping | I | H | 3–5 | 2 | 4 | 1 | 2 | 3–5 | 8–15 | 600–1125 |
| Cross-Country Skiing | B | M | 4–5 | 4 | 4 | 2 | 2 | 4–5 | 10–16 | 750–1200 |
| Aero-belt Exercise | B | M | 4–5 | 4 | 4 | 3 | 2 | 4–5 | 10–16 | 750–1200 |
| In-Line Skating | I | M | 2–4 | 2 | 4 | 2 | 2 | 3 | 6–10 | 450–750 |
| Rowing | B | L | 3–5 | 4 | 2 | 3 | 1 | 4 | 8–14 | 600–1050 |
| Stair Climbing | B | L | 3–5 | 1 | 4 | 1 | 1 | 4–5 | 8–15 | 600–1125 |
| Racquet Sports | I | M | 2–4 | 3 | 3 | 3 | 2 | 3 | 6–10 | 450–750 |

1 B = Beginner, I = Intermediate, A = Advanced
2 L = Low, M = Moderate, H = High
3 1 = Low, 2 = Fair, 3 = Average, 4 = Good, 5 = Excellent
4 One MET represents the rate of energy expenditure at rest (3.5 ml/kg/min). Each additional MET is a multiple of the resting value. For example, 5 METs represents an energy expenditure equivalent to five times the resting value or about 17.5 ml/kg/min.
5 Varies according to the person's effort (exercise intensity) during exercise.
6 Varies according to body weight.

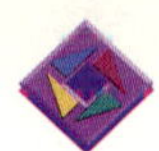

## GETTING STARTED AND ADHERING TO A LIFETIME EXERCISE PROGRAM

Having learned the basic principles of cardiovascular exercise prescription, you can proceed to Figure 3.6 and fill out your own prescription. This exercise prescription calls for a gradual increase in intensity, duration, and frequency.

If you have not been exercising regularly, you could go ahead and attempt to train five or six times a week for 30 minutes at a time. You may find this discouraging, however, and may drop out before getting too far because you probably will develop some muscle soreness and stiffness and possibly incur minor injuries. Muscle soreness and stiffness and the risk for injuries can be lessened or eliminated by increasing the intensity, duration, and frequency of exercise progressively as outlined in Figure 3.6. You can use Figure 3.7 to create and update a computer file regularly to keep a record of all your activities. This file is based on the EXLOG computer program available from Morton Publishing Company. You also can keep a daily log using the form provided in Figure 3.8.

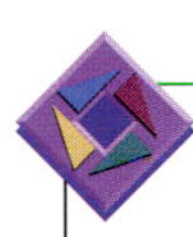

*Lifelong dedication to exercise and perseverance are necessary to reap and maintain good fitness.*

Once you have determined your exercise prescription, the difficult part begins: starting and sticking to a lifetime exercise program. Although you may be motivated after reading the benefits to be gained from physical activity, lifelong dedication and perseverance are necessary to reap and maintain good fitness.

The first few weeks are probably the most difficult, but where there's a will, there's a way. Once you begin to see positive changes, it won't be as hard. Soon you will develop a habit for exercise that will be deeply satisfying and will bring about a sense of self-accomplishment. People have utilized the following suggestions successfully:

1. **Select aerobic activities you enjoy.** If you pick an activity you don't enjoy, you will be less likely to keep exercising. Don't be afraid to try out a new activity, even if that means learning new skills.
2. **Combine different activities.** You can train by doing two or three different activities the same week. This cross-training may deter the monotony of repeating the same activity every day. Try lifetime sports. Many endurance sports, such as racquetball, basketball, soccer, badminton, roller skating, cross-country skiing, and surfing (paddling the board), provide a nice break from regular workouts.
3. **Set aside a regular time for exercise.** If you don't plan ahead, exercise is a lot easier to skip. Holding your exercise hour "sacred" helps you adhere to the program.
4. **Obtain the proper equipment for exercise.** A poor pair of shoes, for example, can make you more prone to injury, discouraging you right from the beginning.
5. **Find a friend or group of friends to exercise with.** Social interaction will make exercise more fulfilling. Besides, it's harder to skip if someone else is waiting for you.
6. **Set goals and share them with others.** Quitting is tougher when someone else knows what you are trying to accomplish. When you reach a targeted goal, reward yourself with a new pair of shoes or a jogging suit.
7. **Don't become a compulsive exerciser.** Learn to listen to your body. Overexercising can lead to chronic fatigue and injuries. Exercise should be enjoyable, and in the process you should stop and smell the roses.
8. **Exercise in different places and facilities.** This will add variety to your workouts.
9. **Keep a regular record of your activities.** Keeping a record allows you to monitor your progress and compare it against previous months and years.
10. **Conduct periodic assessments.** Improving to a higher fitness category is a reward in itself.
11. **If health problems arise, see a physician.** When in doubt, it's better to be safe than sorry.

## A LIFETIME COMMITMENT TO FITNESS

The benefits of fitness can be maintained only through a regular lifetime program. Exercise is not like putting money in the bank. Exercising several hours on Saturday and doing nothing else the rest of the week doesn't help. If anything, exercising only once a week is unsafe for unconditioned adults.

Even the greatest athletes on earth, if they were to stop exercising, would be at a similar risk for disease after just a few years as someone who has never done any physical activity. Staying with a physical fitness program long enough brings about positive physiological and psychological changes, and once you are there, you will not want to have it any other way.

The time involved in losing the benefits of exercise varies among the different components of physical fitness and also depends on the person's condition before the interruption. In regard to cardiovascular endurance, it has been estimated that 4 weeks of aerobic training are completely reversed in 2 consecutive weeks of physical inactivity. If you have been exercising regularly for months or years, however, 2 weeks of inactivity will not hurt you as much as it will someone who has exercised only a few weeks.

As a rule of thumb, after 48 to 62 hours of aerobic inactivity, the cardiovascular system starts to lose some of its capacity. Flexibility can be maintained with two or three stretching sessions per week. Strength is easily retained with just one maximal training session per week.

To maintain fitness, you should follow a regular exercise program, even during vacations. If you have to interrupt your program for reasons beyond your control, you should not attempt to resume training at the same level you left off but, rather, build up gradually again.

## NOTES

1. American College of Sports Medicine, *Guidelines for Exercise Testing and Prescription* (Philadelphia: Lea & Febiger, 1991).
2. American College of Sports Medicine, "The Recommended Quantity and Quality of Exercise for Developing and Maintaining Cardiorespiratory and Muscular Fitness in Healthy Adults," *Medicine and Science in Sports and Exercise,* 22 (1990), 265-274.
3. DeBusk, R. F., U. Stenestrand, M. Sheehan, and W. L. Haskell. "Training Effects of Long Versus Short Bouts of Exercise in Healthy Subjects." *American Journal of Cardiology,* 65 (1990), 1010-1013.
4. R. S. Paffenbarger, R. T. Hyde, A. L. Wing, and C. H. Steinmetz, in "Cause-Specific Death Rates per 10,000 Man-Years of Observation Among 16,936 Harvard Alumni, 1962 to 1968, by Physical Activity Index," *Journal of the American Medical Association*, 252 (1985), 491-495.
5. American College of Obstetricians and Gynecologists, "Guidelines for Exercise During Pregnancy," 1994.
6. University of California at Berkeley, *The Wellness Guide to Lifelong Fitness* (New York: Random House, 1993), p. 198.
7. Hopkins, D. R., W. W. K. Hoeger, D. E. Van Zee, and W. S. Nurge, "Physiologic Responses to Aero-Belt Walking," *Medicine and Science in Sports and Exercise*, 26 (1994), S43.
8. Hoeger, W. W. K., M. L. Chupurdia, W. S. Nurge, and D. E. Van Zee, " Physiologic Responses to Step-Aerobics and Aero-Belt Step-Aerobics," *Medicine and Science in Sports and Exercise*, 26 (1994), S43.
9. Nurge, W. J., D. E. Van Zee, and W. W. K. Hoeger, "Physiologic Responses to Aero-Belt Walking and Jogging," *Medicine and Science in Sports and Exercise*, 26 (1994), S43.
10. Marcinik, E. J., J. Potts, G. Schlabach, S. Will, P. Dawson, and B. F. Hurley, "Effects of Strength Training on Lactate Threshold and Endurance Performance," *Medicine and Science in Sports and Exercise*, 23 (1991), 739-743.

## SELECT BIBLIOGRAPHY

Arnheim, D. D. *Modern Principles of Athletic Training*. St. Louis: Times Mirror/Mosby College Publishing, 1988.

Borg, G. "Perceived Exertion: A Note on History and Methods." *Medicine and Science in Sports and Exercise* 5 (1973), 90-93.

Coleman, E. *Eating for Endurance.* Palo Alto, CA: Bull Publishing, 1992.

Cooper, K. H. *The Aerobics Program for Total Well-Being*. New York: Mount Evans and Co., 1982.

Karvonen, M. J., E. Kentala, and O. Mustala. "The Effects of Training on the Heart Rate, a Longitudinal Study." *Annales Medicinae Experimetalis et Biologiae Fenniae,* 35 (1957), 307-315.

McArdle, W. D., F. I. Katch, and V. L. Katch. *Essentials of Exercise Physiology.* Philadelphia: Lea & Febiger, 1994.

Pollock, M. L., J. H. Wilmore, and S. M. Fox III. *Health and Fitness Through Physical Activity*. New York: John Wiley & Sons, 1978.

Teitz, C. C. "Overuse Injuries." In *Scientific Foundations of Sports Medicine,* edited by C. C. Teitz. Philadelphia: B. C. Deckerm, 1989, pp. 299-328.

Wilmore, J. H., and D. L. Costill. *Training for Sport and Activity.* Dubuque, IA: Wm. C. Brown Publishers, 1988.

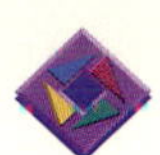

Name: ______________________________ Date: ______________________

**Intensity of Exercise**

1. Estimate your own maximal heart rate (MHR)

   MHR = 220 minus age (220 − age)

   MHR = 220 − 64 = 156 bpm

2. Resting Heart Rate (RHR) = 60 bpm

3. Heart Rate Reserve (HRR) = MHR − RHR

   HRR = 156 − 60 = 96 beats

4. Training Intensities (TI) = HRR × TI + RHR

   50 Percent TI = 96 × .50 + 60 = 108 bpm

   70 percent TI = 96 × .70 + 60 = 127 bpm ≈ 22 B IN 10 SECS

   85 Percent TI = 96 × .85 + 60 = 136 bpm

5. Cardiovascular Training Zone. The optimum cardiovascular training zone is found between the 70% and 85% training intensities. Individuals who have been physically inactive or are in the poor or fair cardiovascular fitness categories, however, should use a 50% training intensity during the first few weeks of the exercise program.

   Cardiovascular Training Zone: __________ (70% TI) to __________ (85% TI)

   Rate of Perceived Exertion (see Figure 3.1): ______________ to ______________

**Mode of Exercise**

Select any activity or combination of activities that you enjoy doing. The activity has to be continuous in nature and must get your heart rate up to the cardiovascular training zone and keep it there for as long as you exercise. Indicate your preferred mode(s) of exercise:

1. ____________________ 2. ____________________ 3. ____________________

4. ____________________ 5. ____________________ 6. ____________________

**Cardiovascular Exercise Program**

The following is your weekly program for developing cardiovascular endurance. If you are in the average, good, or excellent fitness category, you may start at week 5. After completing this 12-week program, for you to maintain your fitness level, you should exercise in the 70% to 85% training zone for about 20 to 30 minutes, a minimum of three times per week, on nonconsecutive days. You also should recompute your target zone periodically because you will experience a significant reduction in resting heart rate with aerobic training (approximately 10 to 20 beats in about 8 to 12 weeks).

| Week | Duration (min) | Frequency | Training Intensity | 10-Sec. Pulse Count* |
|---|---|---|---|---|
| 1 | 15 | 3 | Approximately 50% | |
| 2 | 15 | 4 | Approximately 50% | |
| 3 | 20 | 4 | Approximately 50% | _____ beats |
| 4 | 20 | 5 | Approximately 50% | |
| 5 | 20 | 4 | About 70% | |
| 6 | 20 | 5 | About 70% | |
| 7 | 30 | 4 | About 70% | _____ beats |
| 8 | 30 | 5 | About 70% | |
| 9 | 30 | 4 | Between 70% and 85% | |
| 10 | 30 | 5 | Between 70% and 85% | |
| 11 | 30–40 | 5 | Between 70% and 85% | _____ to _____ beats |
| 12 | 30–40 | 5 | Between 70% and 85% | |

*Fill out your own 10-second pulse count under this column.

**FIGURE 3.6** ◆ Cardiovascular exercise prescription form.

FITNESS & WELLNESS SERIES
By Werner W.K. Hoeger
Morton Publishing Company - Englewood, Colorado

MONTHLY EXERCISE LOG

Jim R. Davis
1234 Veterans Park
Los Escondidos, CA 99222

Month of January 1992

| Date | Body Weight | Type of Exercise | Exercise Heart Rate | Duration of Exercise | Distance (miles) | Calories Burned |
|---|---|---|---|---|---|---|
| 1 | 179.5 | Walking (4.5 mph) | 120 | 30 min. | 2.0 | 242 |
| | | Running 11 min/mile | 156 | 34 min. | 3.0 | 426 |
| | | Golf | 102 | 90 min. | | 483 |
| 4 | 179.0 | Running 11 min/mile | 156 | 33 min. | 3.0 | 413 |
| | | Tennis (moderate) | 126 | 60 min. | | 483 |
| 6 | 178.5 | Running 11 min/mile | 162 | 38 min. | 3.5 | 475 |
| 8 | 178.0 | Running 8.5 min/mile | 180 | 12 min. | 1.5 | 192 |
| | | Calisthenics | 96 | 30 min. | | 176 |
| 9 | 178.0 | Water Aerobics (vig) | 150 | 30 min. | | 534 |
| 11 | 177.5 | Running 8.5 min/mile | 174 | 28 min. | 3.0 | 439 |
| | | Racquetball | 144 | 60 min. | | 692 |
| 13 | 176.5 | Running 8.5 min/mile | 174 | 29 min. | 3.0 | 453 |
| 14 | 177.0 | Swimming 25 yrds/min | 138 | 25 min. | 0.5 | 177 |
| 16 | 177.5 | Running 8.5 min/mile | 174 | 26 min. | 3.0 | 415 |
| 17 | 176.5 | Dance (moderate) | 102 | 120 min. | | 635 |
| 18 | 176.0 | Basketball (mod) | 144 | 60 min. | | 486 |
| | | Skiing (downhill) | 96 | 60 min. | | 634 |
| 20 | 176.0 | Running 7 min/mile | 172 | 18 min. | 2.5 | 323 |
| 22 | 176.0 | Running 7 min/mile | 174 | 23 min. | 3.0 | 404 |
| 24 | 175.5 | Running 7 min/mile | 168 | 23 min. | 3.0 | 412 |
| 25 | 175.0 | Soccer | 150 | 90 min. | | 929 |
| 27 | 176.0 | Running 7 min/mile | 174 | 23 min. | 3.0 | 404 |
| 28 | 175.0 | Aerobic Dance (vig) | 156 | 30 min. | | 499 |
| | | Volleyball | 120 | 45 min. | | 236 |
| 30 | 175.0 | Strength Training | 108 | 60 min. | | 525 |
| 31 | 174.5 | Running 7 min/mile | 168 | 22 min. | 3.0 | 383 |
| | | Bowling | 102 | 90 min. | | 471 |

MONTHLY SUMMARY

| | |
|---|---|
| Average body weight: | 176.7 lbs. |
| Average exercise heart rate: | 144 bpm |
| Total number of days exercised: | 19 days |
| Average exercise time/day: | 62 min. |
| Total number of calories burned: | 11,943 |
| Average number of calories per day exercised: | 629 |
| Total number of miles run: | 35 |
| Total number of miles swum: | 1 |
| Total number of miles walked: | 2 |

**FIGURE 3.7** ◆ Computerized Exercise Log (EXLOG Software).

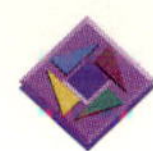

Month__________

| Date | Body Weight | Exercise Heart Rate | Type of Exercise | Distance In Miles | Time Hrs/Min | RPE* |
|---|---|---|---|---|---|---|
| 1 | | | | | | |
| 2 | | | | | | |
| 3 | | | | | | |
| 4 | | | | | | |
| 5 | | | | | | |
| 6 | | | | | | |
| 7 | | | | | | |
| 8 | | | | | | |
| 9 | | | | | | |
| 10 | | | | | | |
| 11 | | | | | | |
| 12 | | | | | | |
| 13 | | | | | | |
| 14 | | | | | | |
| 15 | | | | | | |
| 16 | | | | | | |
| 17 | | | | | | |
| 18 | | | | | | |
| 19 | | | | | | |
| 20 | | | | | | |
| 21 | | | | | | |
| 22 | | | | | | |
| 23 | | | | | | |
| 24 | | | | | | |
| 25 | | | | | | |
| 26 | | | | | | |
| 27 | | | | | | |
| 28 | | | | | | |
| 29 | | | | | | |
| 30 | | | | | | |
| 31 | | | | | | |
| | | | Total | | | |

*Rate of perceived exertion.

Month__________

| Date | Body Weight | Exercise Heart Rate | Type of Exercise | Distance In Miles | Time Hrs/Min | RPE* |
|---|---|---|---|---|---|---|
| 1 | | | | | | |
| 2 | | | | | | |
| 3 | | | | | | |
| 4 | | | | | | |
| 5 | | | | | | |
| 6 | | | | | | |
| 7 | | | | | | |
| 8 | | | | | | |
| 9 | | | | | | |
| 10 | | | | | | |
| 11 | | | | | | |
| 12 | | | | | | |
| 13 | | | | | | |
| 14 | | | | | | |
| 15 | | | | | | |
| 16 | | | | | | |
| 17 | | | | | | |
| 18 | | | | | | |
| 19 | | | | | | |
| 20 | | | | | | |
| 21 | | | | | | |
| 22 | | | | | | |
| 23 | | | | | | |
| 24 | | | | | | |
| 25 | | | | | | |
| 26 | | | | | | |
| 27 | | | | | | |
| 28 | | | | | | |
| 29 | | | | | | |
| 30 | | | | | | |
| 31 | | | | | | |
| | | | Total | | | |

*Rate of perceived exertion.

**FIGURE 3.8** ◆ Cardiovascular exercise record form.

Month________________

| Date | Body Weight | Exercise Heart Rate | Type of Exercise | Distance In Miles | Time Hrs/Min | RPE* |
|---|---|---|---|---|---|---|
| 1 | | | | | | |
| 2 | | | | | | |
| 3 | | | | | | |
| 4 | | | | | | |
| 5 | | | | | | |
| 6 | | | | | | |
| 7 | | | | | | |
| 8 | | | | | | |
| 9 | | | | | | |
| 10 | | | | | | |
| 11 | | | | | | |
| 12 | | | | | | |
| 13 | | | | | | |
| 14 | | | | | | |
| 15 | | | | | | |
| 16 | | | | | | |
| 17 | | | | | | |
| 18 | | | | | | |
| 19 | | | | | | |
| 20 | | | | | | |
| 21 | | | | | | |
| 22 | | | | | | |
| 23 | | | | | | |
| 24 | | | | | | |
| 25 | | | | | | |
| 26 | | | | | | |
| 27 | | | | | | |
| 28 | | | | | | |
| 29 | | | | | | |
| 30 | | | | | | |
| 31 | | | | | | |
| | | | Total | | | |

*Rate of perceived exertion.

Month________________

| Date | Body Weight | Exercise Heart Rate | Type of Exercise | Distance In Miles | Time Hrs/Min | RPE* |
|---|---|---|---|---|---|---|
| 1 | | | | | | |
| 2 | | | | | | |
| 3 | | | | | | |
| 4 | | | | | | |
| 5 | | | | | | |
| 6 | | | | | | |
| 7 | | | | | | |
| 8 | | | | | | |
| 9 | | | | | | |
| 10 | | | | | | |
| 11 | | | | | | |
| 12 | | | | | | |
| 13 | | | | | | |
| 14 | | | | | | |
| 15 | | | | | | |
| 16 | | | | | | |
| 17 | | | | | | |
| 18 | | | | | | |
| 19 | | | | | | |
| 20 | | | | | | |
| 21 | | | | | | |
| 22 | | | | | | |
| 23 | | | | | | |
| 24 | | | | | | |
| 25 | | | | | | |
| 26 | | | | | | |
| 27 | | | | | | |
| 28 | | | | | | |
| 29 | | | | | | |
| 30 | | | | | | |
| 31 | | | | | | |
| | | | Total | | | |

*Rate of perceived exertion.

**FIGURE 3.8** ◆ Cardiovascular exercise record form.

# Muscular Strength Assessment and Prescription

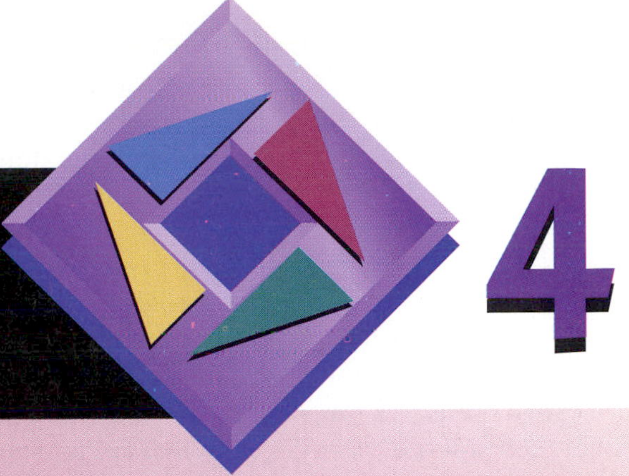


## Key Concepts

Muscular strength
Muscular endurance
Metabolism
Muscle hypertrophy
Anabolic steroids
1 RM
Hypertrophy
Atrophy
Red muscle fibers
White muscle fibers
Overload principle
Progressive resistance training
Specificity of training
Isometric training
Isotonic training
Fixed resistance
Variable resistance
Isokinetic training
Repetitions maximum
Resistance
Repetition
Set
Body building
Plyometrics

## Objectives

- Understand the importance of adequate strength levels in maintaining good health and well-being.
- Clarify misconceptions about women who engage in strength-training programs.
- Define muscular strength and muscular endurance.
- Be able to assess muscular strength and endurance through two different strength testing protocols.
- Learn to interpret strength testing results according to health fitness and physical fitness standards.
- Identify the factors that affect strength.
- Name the different types of muscle fibers.
- Understand the overload principle for strength development.
- Recognize the principles that govern muscular strength and muscular endurance development (mode, resistance, sets, and frequency).
- Become acquainted with three distinct strength-training programs.

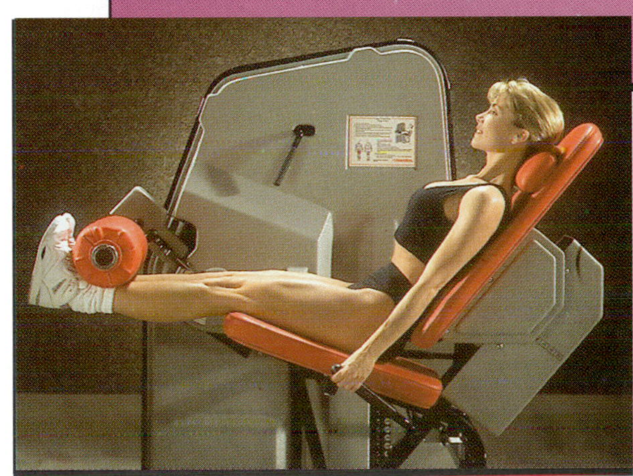

Evidence of the benefits of strength training in enhancing health and well-being is well-documented. Nevertheless, many people are still under the impression that strength is necessary only for highly trained athletes and other individuals who hold jobs that require heavy muscular work.

Strength is a basic component of fitness and wellness and is crucial for optimal performance in daily activities such as sitting, walking, running, lifting and carrying objects, doing housework, and even enjoying recreational activities. Strength also is of great value in improving posture, personal appearance and self-image, in developing sports skills, and in meeting certain emergencies in life in which strength is necessary to cope effectively. From a health standpoint, strength helps to maintain muscle tissue and a higher resting metabolism, lessens the risk for injury, helps to prevent and eliminate chronic low back pain, and is a key factor in childbearing.

Muscular strength also seems to be the most important health-related component of physical fitness in the older-adult population. While proper cardiovascular endurance helps maintain a healthy heart, good strength levels will do more toward independent living than any other fitness component. More than anything else, older adults want to enjoy good health and function independently. Many of them are, however, confined to nursing homes because they lack sufficient strength to move about. They cannot walk very far and many need to be helped in and out of beds, chairs, and tubs.

A strength training program can have a tremendous impact in enhancing quality of life. Research has shown leg strength improvements as high as 200% in previously inactive adults over the age of 90.[1] As strength improves, so does the ability to move about, the capacity for independent living, and enjoyment of life during the "golden years."

## Relationship Between Strength and Metabolism

Perhaps one of the most significant benefits of maintaining a good strength level is its relationship to human metabolism. *Metabolism* is defined as *all energy and material transformations within living cells*. A primary outcome of a strength training program is an increase in muscle mass or size (lean body mass), known as *muscle hypertrophy*.

Muscle tissue uses energy even at rest. In contrast, fatty tissue uses very little energy and may be considered metabolically inert from the point of view of caloric use. As muscle size increases, so does the resting metabolism or the amount of energy (calories) an individual requires during resting conditions to sustain proper cell function. Even small increases in muscle mass may affect resting metabolism.

Estimates indicate that each additional pound of muscle tissue increases resting metabolism by 30 to 50 calories per day. All other factors being equal, if two individuals both weigh 150 pounds but have different amounts of muscle mass, let's say 5 pounds, the one with more muscle mass will have a higher resting metabolic rate, allowing this person to ingest more calories to maintain the muscle tissue.

## Aging and Metabolic Rate

Loss of lean tissue also is thought to be the main reason for the decrease in metabolism as people grow older. Contrary to some beliefs, metabolism does not have to slow down significantly with aging. It is not so much that metabolism slows down. It's that we slow down.

Lean body mass decreases with sedentary living, which, in turn, slows down the resting metabolic rate. If people continue eating at the same rate, body fat increases. The average decrease in resting metabolism from age 26 to age 60 is about 360 calories per day. Hence, participating in a strength training program is important in preventing and reducing excess body fat.

# GENDER DIFFERENCES

One of the most common misconceptions about physical fitness is related to women and strength training. Because of the increase in muscle mass commonly seen in men, some women think a strength training program will be counterproductive because they, too, will develop large musculature. Even though the quality of muscle in men and women is the same, endocrinological differences do not allow women to achieve the same amount of muscle hypertrophy (size) as men. Men also have more muscle fibers, and because of the male sex-specific hormones, each individual fiber has more potential for hypertrophy.

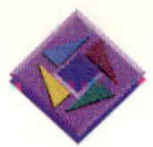

The idea that strength training allows women to develop muscle hypertrophy to the same extent as men do is as false as the notion that playing basketball will turn women into giants. *Masculinity and femininity are established by genetic inheritance*, not by the amount of physical activity. Variations in the extent of masculinity and femininity are determined by individual differences in hormonal secretions of androgen, testosterone, estrogen, and progesterone. Women with a bigger-than-average build often are inclined to participate in sports because of their natural physical advantage. As a result, many women have associated participation in sports and strength training with large muscle size.

As the number of women who participate in sports has increased steadily during the last few years, the myth that strength training in women leads to large increases in muscle size has been abated somewhat. For example, per pound of body weight, women gymnasts are considered to be among the strongest athletes in the world. These athletes engage regularly in serious strength training programs. Yet, female gymnasts have some of the most well-toned and graceful figures of all women. In recent years improved body appearance has become the rule rather than the exception for women who participate in strength training programs. Some of the most attractive women movie stars also train with weights to further improve their personal image. In his textbook *Weight Training for Life*, Dr. James Hesson points out that many beauty pageant participants engage in some sort of strength training program as they prepare for the pageant.[2] A survey at a recent state beauty pageant revealed that 86% of the participants (38 of 44 contestants) exercised with weights!

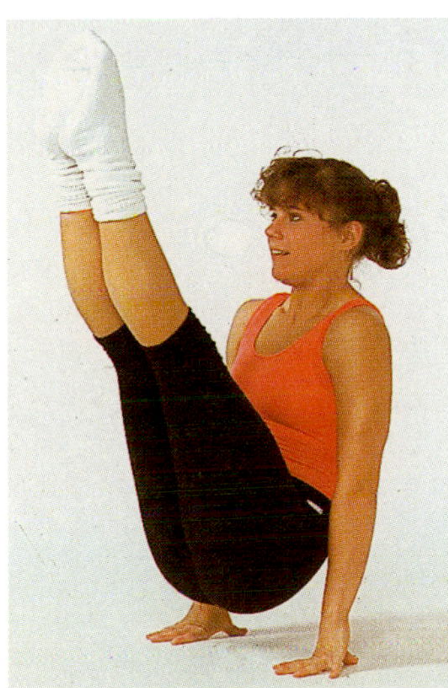

*Female gymnast performing a strength skill on the floor exercise event.*

At the same time, you may ask, "If weight training does not masculinize women, why do so many women body builders develop such heavy musculature?" In the sport of body building, the athletes follow intense training routines consisting of two or more hours of constant weight lifting with short rest intervals between sets. Many times body building training routines call for back-to-back exercises using the same muscle groups. The objective of this type of training is to "pump" extra blood into the muscles, which makes the muscles appear much bigger than they really are in a resting condition. Based on the intensity and the length of the training session, the muscles can remain filled with blood, appearing measurably larger for several hours after completing the training session. Therefore, in real life, these women are not as muscular as they seem when they are "pumped up" for a contest.

In the sport of body building, a big point of controversy is the use of anabolic steroids and human growth hormones, even among women participants. *Anabolic steroids* are synthetic versions of the male sex hormone testosterone, which promotes muscle development and hypertrophy. These hormones, however, produce detrimental and undesirable side effects, which some women deem tolerable (e.g., hypertension, fluid retention, decreased breast size, deepening of the voice, facial whiskers, and body hair growth). Anabolic steroid use in general, except for medical reasons and when carefully monitored by a physician, can lead to serious health consequences.

Anabolic steroid use among women body builders is widespread. According to several sports medicine physicians and women body builders, about 80% of women body builders have used steroids. Furthermore, according to several women's track-and-field coaches, as many as 95% of women athletes around the world in this sport had used anabolic steroids to remain competitive at the international level.

Women who take steroids undoubtedly will build heavy musculature, and, if the steroids are taken long enough, will produce masculinizing effects. As a result, the International Federation of Body Building instituted a mandatory steroid-testing program for women participating in the Miss Olympia contest. When drugs are not used to promote development, improved body image is the rule rather than the exception among women who participate in body building, strength training, or sports in general.

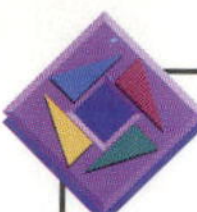

### SELECTED DETRIMENTAL EFFECTS OF ANABOLIC STEROID USE

- Liver tumors
- Hepatitis
- Hypertension
- Reduction of high density lipoprotein (HDL)
- Elevation of low density lipoprotein (LDL)
- Hyperinsulinism
- Impaired pituitary function
- Impaired thyroid function
- Mood swings
- Aggressive behavior
- Increased irritability
- Acne
- Fluid retention
- Decreased libido
- HIV infection (via injectable steroids)
- Prostate problems (men)
- Testicular atrophy (men)
- Reduced sperm count (men)
- Clitoral enlargement (women)
- Decreased breast size (women)
- Increased body and facial hair (nonreversible in women)
- Deepening of the voice (nonreversible in women)

## BODY COMPOSITION CHANGES

Another benefit of strength training, accentuated even more when combined with aerobic exercise, is a decrease in adipose or fatty tissue around muscle fibers themselves. The decrease in fatty tissue often is greater than the amount of muscle hypertrophy (see Figure 4.1). Therefore, losing inches but not body weight is common.

Because muscle tissue is more dense than fatty tissue, and despite the fact that inches are lost during a combined strength training and aerobic program, people, especially women, often become discouraged because they cannot see the results readily on the scale. They can offset this discouragement by determining body composition regularly to monitor changes in percent body fat rather than simply measure changes in total body weight.

## ASSESSMENT OF MUSCULAR STRENGTH AND ENDURANCE

Although muscular strength and endurance are interrelated, they differ in the following ways.

1. Strength is defined as the ability to exert maximum force against resistance.
2. Endurance is the ability of a muscle to exert submaximal force repeatedly over time.

Muscular endurance (also referred to as localized muscular endurance) depends to a large extent on muscular strength. Weak muscles cannot repeat an action several times or sustain it for a long time. Keeping these principles in mind, strength tests and training programs have been designed to measure and develop absolute muscular strength or muscular endurance, or a combination of the two.

*Muscular strength usually is determined by the maximal amount of resistance (one repetition maximum, or 1 RM) an individual is able to lift in a single effort.* This assessment yields a good measure of absolute strength, but it does require a considerable amount of time, as the 1 RM is determined through trial and error. For example, strength of

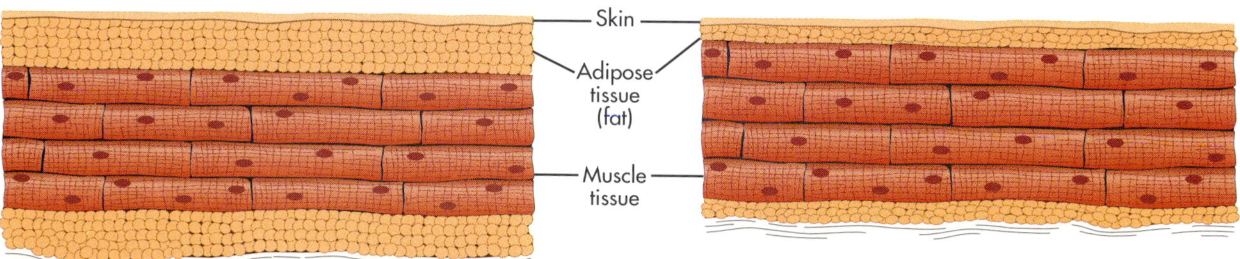

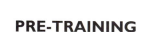

**FIGURE 4.1** ◆ Changes in body composition from combined aerobic and strength training program.

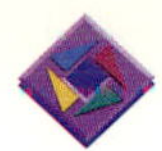

the chest muscles frequently is measured through the bench press exercise. If the individual has not trained with weights, he or she may try 100 pounds and lift this resistance quite easily. After adding 50 pounds, the person fails to lift the resistance. The resistance then is decreased by 10 or 20 pounds. Finally, after several trials the 1 RM is established.

A true 1 RM might be difficult to obtain the first time an individual is tested because fatigue becomes a factor. By the time the 1 RM is established, the person already has made several maximal or near-maximal attempts.

*Muscular endurance commonly is established by the number of repetitions an individual can perform against a submaximal resistance or by the length of time a given contraction can be sustained.* For example: How many push-ups can an individual do? Or how many times can he or she lift 50 pounds? Or how long can a person hold the chin above a bar while holding on to it?

In strength testing several body sites should be tested. Because different body parts have different strength levels, no single strength test provides a good assessment of overall body strength. As a minimum, a strength profile should include the upper body, the lower body, and the abdominal muscles.

If time is a factor and only one test item can be done, the Hand Grip Test commonly is used to assess strength. Even this test, though, provides only a weak correlation with overall body strength. (A description of this test is provided in Figure 4.8.)

As with cardiovascular endurance, you will have the opportunity to assess your own level of muscular strength or endurance, or both. Four tests are provided in this chapter. Your test selection should be based on the time and facilities available. Because individuals who have not been lifting regularly have a small increased risk for injury when attempting a maximal contraction, these individuals probably should avoid an absolute strength test (one that requires them to lift the greatest amount of weight in a single repetition).

After you have selected your test, go directly to the procedure that explains the respective test. For safety reasons, always take a friend or group of friends with you whenever you train with weights or conduct any type of strength assessment. Also, these are four different tests, so to make valid comparisons the same test should be used for pre-and post-assessments. The following are your options:

## Muscular Strength and Endurance Test

On this test you will lift a submaximal resistance as many times as possible on five different strength-training exercises, and you also will perform an abdominal crunch test. The resistance for each lift is determined according to selected percentages of body weight (see Figure 4.2). If you are not familiar with the different lifts, illustrations are provided at the end of this chapter.

A strength/endurance rating is determined according to the maximum number of repetitions you are able to do on each exercise. A 16-station, fixed-resistance, Universal Gym apparatus is necessary to administer all but the abdominal crunch exercise on this test (see Mode of Training, later in this chapter, for an explanation of fixed-resistance equipment).

For individuals who do only a few repetitions, the test will primarily measure absolute strength. For those who are able to do a lot of repetitions, the test will be an indicator of muscular endurance. A percentile rank for each exercise is given based on the number of repetitions performed (see Table 4.1), and an overall muscular strength/endurance rating can be determined by taking an average of the percentile ranks obtained for each exercise. A form to record your data for this test is provided in Figure 4.3.

If no fixed resistance Universal Gym equipment is available, you still can perform the test using different equipment. In that case, though, the percentile rankings and strength fitness categories may not be accurate because a certain resistance (for example, 50 pounds) is seldom the same on two different weight machines. The industry has no standard calibration procedure for strength equipment. Consequently, if you lift a certain weight on one machine, you may or may not be able to lift the same amount on a different piece of equipment.

Even though the percentile ranks may not be valid when using different equipment, test results still can be used to evaluate changes in fitness. For example, you may be able to do 7 repetitions on the equipment available to you (whereas you might have done 10 on Universal Gym fixed resistance), but if you can perform 14 repetitions after 12 weeks of training, that's a measure of improvement. When performing this test on different equipment, you should disregard the percentile ranks and use the test results to assess *changes* in fitness only.

## MUSCULAR STRENGTH AND ENDURANCE TEST

A 16-station, fixed resistance, Universal Gym apparatus is required to perform this test, along with a partner.

1. Familiarize yourself with the six lifts used for this test: lat pull-down, leg extension, bench press, abdominal crunch, leg curl, and arm curl. Graphic illustrations for each lift are given at the end of this chapter. For the leg curl exercise, the knees should be flexed to 90°. A description and illustration of the abdominal crunch exercise is provided in Figure 4.4. For the lateral pull-down exercise, use a sitting position and have your partner hold you down by the waist or shoulders. On the leg extension lift, maintain the trunk in an upright position.
2. Determine your body weight in pounds.
3. Determine the amount of resistance to be used on each lift. To obtain this number, multiply your body weight by the percent given below for each lift.

| Lift | Percent of Body Weight | |
|---|---|---|
| | Men | Women |
| Lat Pull-Down | .70 | .45 |
| Leg Extension | .65 | .50 |
| Bench Press | .75 | .45 |
| Abdominal Crunch | NA* | NA* |
| Leg Curl | .32 | .25 |
| Arm Curl | .35 | .18 |

*NA = not applicable — see Figure 4.4

4. Perform the maximum continuous number of repetitions possible and record this information in Figure 4.3.
5. Based on the number of repetitions performed, look up the percentile rank for each lift in the far left column of Table 4.1.
6. An overall strength fitness category can be obtained by determining an average percentile score for all six lifts. Determine your overall muscular endurance fitness category according to the following ratings:

| Average Score | Fitness Classification |
|---|---|
| ≥81 | Excellent |
| 61–80 | Good |
| 41–60 | Average |
| 21–40 | Fair |
| ≤20 | Poor |

**FIGURE 4.2** ◆ Procedure for the Muscular Strength and Endurance Test.

**TABLE 4.1**
**Muscular Strength and Endurance Scoring Table**

| Percentile Rank | Men: Lat Pull-Down | Men: Leg Extension | Men: Bench Press | Men: Abdominal Crunch | Men: Leg Curl | Men: Arm Curl | Women: Lat Pull-Down | Women: Leg Extension | Women: Bench Press | Women: Abdominal Crunch | Women: Leg Curl | Women: Arm Curl |
|---|---|---|---|---|---|---|---|---|---|---|---|---|
| 99 | 30 | 25 | 26 | 100 | 24 | 25 | 30 | 25 | 27 | 100 | 20 | 25 |
| 95 | 25 | 20 | 21 | 100 | 20 | 21 | 25 | 20 | 21 | 100 | 17 | 21 |
| 90 | 19 | 19 | 19 | 100 | 19 | 19 | 21 | 18 | 20 | 69 | 12 | 20 |
| 80 | 16 | 15 | 16 | 66 | 15 | 15 | 16 | 13 | 16 | 49 | 10 | 16 |
| 70 | 13 | 14 | 13 | 45 | 13 | 12 | 13 | 11 | 13 | 37 | 9 | 14 |
| 60 | 11 | 13 | 11 | 38 | 11 | 10 | 11 | 10 | 11 | 34 | 7 | 12 |
| 50 | 10 | 12 | 10 | 33 | 10 | 9 | 10 | 9 | 10 | 31 | 6 | 10 |
| 40 | 9 | 10 | 7 | 29 | 8 | 8 | 9 | 8 | 5 | 27 | 5 | 8 |
| 30 | 7 | 9 | 5 | 26 | 6 | 7 | 7 | 7 | 3 | 24 | 4 | 7 |
| 20 | 6 | 7 | 3 | 22 | 4 | 5 | 6 | 5 | 1 | 21 | 3 | 6 |
| 10 | 4 | 5 | 1 | 18 | 3 | 3 | 3 | 3 | 0 | 15 | 1 | 3 |
| 5 | 3 | 3 | 0 | 16 | 1 | 2 | 2 | 1 | 0 | 0 | 0 | 2 |

High physical fitness standard (rows 99–70)
Health fitness standard (rows 60–50)

Name: ______ Sex: ______ Date: ______

Body Weight: ______

| Lift | % Body Weight | | Resistance | Repetitions | % Rank |
|---|---|---|---|---|---|
| | Men | Women | | | |
| Lat Pull-Down | .70 | .45 | ______ | ______ | ______ |
| Leg Extension | .65 | .50 | ______ | ______ | ______ |
| Bench Press | .75 | .45 | ______ | ______ | ______ |
| Abdominal Crunch | NA* | NA* | ______ | ______ | ______ |
| Leg Curl | .32 | .25 | ______ | ______ | ______ |
| Arm Curl | .35 | .18 | ______ | ______ | ______ |

*NA = Not Applicable. See Figure 4.4.

Total: [ ]

Average Percentile Rank (divide total by 6): [ ] Overall Strength Category: ______

**FIGURE 4.3** ◆ Data form for Muscular Strength and Endurance test results.

## Muscular Endurance Test

Three exercises were selected to assess the endurance of the upper body, lower body, and mid-body muscle groups (see Figure 4.4). The advantage of this test is that it does not require strength training equipment.

For this test you will need a stopwatch, a metronome, a bench or gymnasium bleacher 16¼" high, a cardboard strip 3½" wide by 30" long, and a partner. As with the Muscular Strength and Endurance Test, a percentile rank is given for each exercise according to the number of repetitions performed (see Table 4.2). An overall endurance rating can be obtained through the average percentile rank for the three exercises. The data recording form for this test is given in Figure 4.5.

## MUSCULAR ENDURANCE TEST

Three exercises are conducted on this test: bench-jumps, modified dips (men) or modified push-ups (women), and abdominal crunches. All exercises should be conducted with the aid of a partner. The correct procedure for performing each exercise is as follows:

**Bench-jumps.** Using a bench or gymnasium bleacher 16¼" high, attempt to jump up and down the bench as many times as possible in 1-minute. If you cannot jump the full minute, you may step up and down. A repetition is counted each time both feet return to the floor.

**Modified dips.** Men only: Using a bench or gymnasium bleacher, place the hands on the bench with the fingers pointing forward. Have a partner hold your feet in front of you. Bend the hips at approximately 90° (you also may use three sturdy chairs, put your hands on two chairs placed by the sides of your body, and place your feet on the third chair in front of you). Lower your body by flexing the elbows until you reach a 90° angle at this joint, then return to the starting position (see Exercise 6 at the end of this chapter). Perform the repetitions to a two-step cadence (down-up) regulated with a metronome set at 56 beats per minute. Perform as many continuous repetitions as possible. Do not count any more repetitions if you fail to follow the metronome cadence.

**Modified push-ups.** Women: Lie down on the floor (face down), bend the knees (feet up in the air), and place the hands on the floor by the shoulders with the fingers pointing forward. The lower body will be supported at the knees (as opposed to the feet) throughout the test (see Exercise 3). The chest must touch the floor on each repetition. As with the modified-dip exercise, perform the repetitions (above) to a two-step cadence (up-down) regulated with a metronome set at 56 beats per minute. Perform as many continuous repetitions as possible. Do not count any more repetitions if you fail to follow the metronome cadence.

**Abdominal crunches.** Tape a 3½ x 30" strip of cardboard onto the floor. Lie down on the floor in a supine position (face up) with the knees bent at approximately 100° and the legs slightly apart. The feet should be on the floor and you must hold them in place yourself throughout the test. Straighten out your arms and place them on the floor alongside the trunk with the palms down and the fingers fully extended. The fingertips of both hands should barely touch the closest edge of the cardboard (see Figure 4.4a). Bring the head off the floor until the chin is 1" to 2" away from your chest. Keep the head in this position during the entire test (do not move the head by flexing or extending the neck). You are now ready to begin the test.

Perform the repetitions to a two-step cadence (up-down) regulated with a metronome set at 60 beats per minute. As you curl up, slide the fingers over the card-

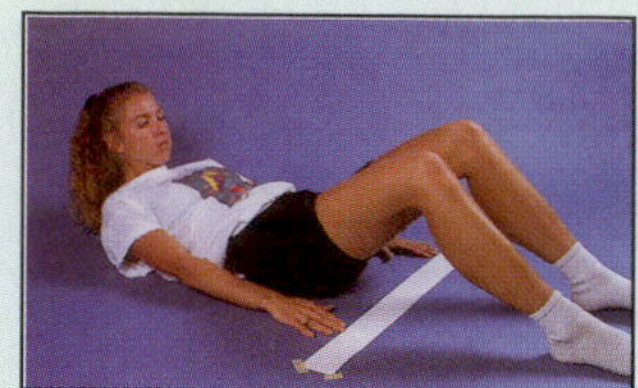

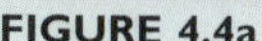

FIGURE 4.4a

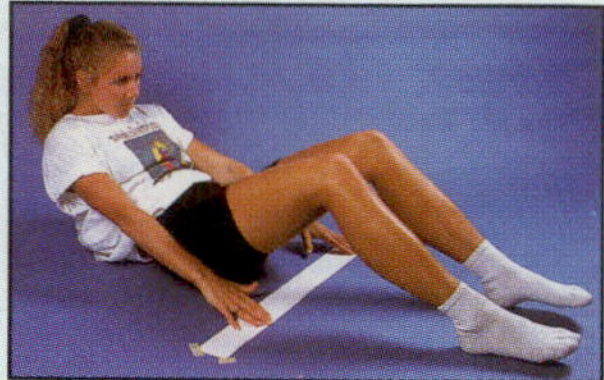

FIGURE 4.4b

board until the fingertips reach the far end (3½") of the board (see Figure 4.4b), then return to the starting position.

Allow a brief practice period of 5 to 10 seconds to familiarize yourself with the cadence. Initiate the up movement with the first beat and the down movement with the next beat. Accomplish one repetition every two beats of the metronome. Count as many repetitions as you are able to perform following the proper cadence. You may not count a repetition if the fingertips fail to reach the distant end of the cardboard.

Terminate the test if: (a) you fail to maintain the appropriate cadence, (b) the heels come off the floor, (c) the chin is not kept close to the chest, (d) you accomplish 100 repetitions, or (e) you no longer can perform the test. Have your partner check the angle at the knees throughout the test to make sure that the 100° angle is maintained as close as possible.

For this test you may also use a Crunch-Ster Curl-Up Tester, available from Novel Products.* An illustration of the test performed with this equipment is provided in Figures 4.4c and 4.4d.

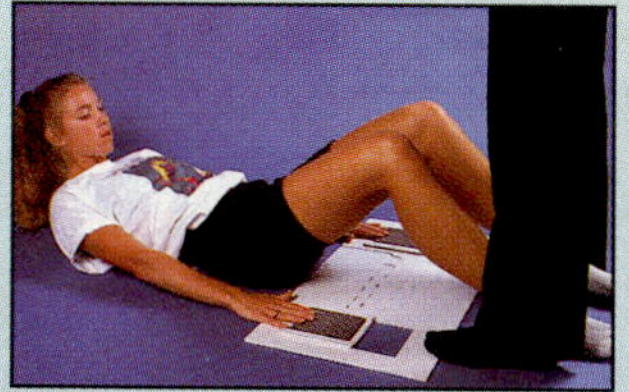

FIGURE 4.4c

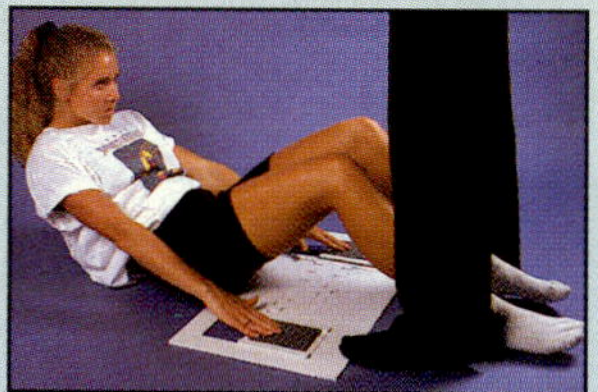

FIGURE 4.4d

You may record your test results in Figure 4.5. According to the results, look up your percentile rank for each exercise in the far left column of Table 4.2.

Total the percentile scores obtained for each exercise, and divide by 3 to obtain an average score. Determine your overall muscular endurance fitness category according to the following ratings:

| Average Score | Fitness Classification |
|---|---|
| >81 | Excellent |
| 61-80 | Good |
| 41-60 | Average |
| 21-40 | Fair |
| <20 | Poor |

*Novel Products, Inc. Figure Finder Collection. P.O. Box 408, Rockton, IL 61072-0408. 1-800-323-5143, FAX 815-624-4866.

**FIGURE 4.4** ◆ Procedure for the Muscular Endurance Test.

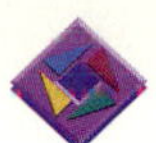

**TABLE 4.2**
**Muscular Endurance Scoring Table**

| | MEN | | | WOMEN | | |
|---|---|---|---|---|---|---|
| **Percentile Rank** | **Bench Jumps** | **Modified Dips** | **Abdominal Crunches** | **Bench Jumps** | **Modified Push-ups** | **Abdominal Crunches** |
| 99 | 66 | 54 | 100 | 58 | 95 | 100 |
| 95 | 63 | 50 | 100 | 54 | 70 | 100 |
| 90 | 62 | 38 | 100 | 52 | 50 | 69 |
| 80 | 58 | 32 | 66 | 48 | 41 | 49 |
| 70 | 57 | 30 | 45 | 44 | 38 | 37 |
| 60 | 56 | 27 | 38 | 42 | 33 | 34 |
| 50 | 54 | 26 | 33 | 39 | 30 | 31 |
| 40 | 51 | 23 | 29 | 38 | 28 | 27 |
| 30 | 48 | 20 | 26 | 36 | 25 | 24 |
| 20 | 47 | 17 | 22 | 32 | 21 | 21 |
| 10 | 40 | 11 | 18 | 28 | 18 | 15 |
| 5 | 34 | 7 | 16 | 26 | 15 | 0 |

High physical fitness standard
Health fitness standard

Name: ____________________ Sex: __________ Date: __________

| | Exercise | Metronome Cadence | Repetitions | % Rank |
|---|---|---|---|---|
| Men | Bench-Jumps | NA* | ______ | ______ |
| | Modified-Dips | 56 | ______ | ______ |
| | Abdominal Crunches | 60 | ______ | ______ |
| Women | Bench-Jumps | NA* | ______ | ______ |
| | Modified Push-Ups | 56 | ______ | ______ |
| | Abdominal Crunches | 60 | ______ | ______ |

*NA = No cadence required. Perform as many jumps as possible in one minute

Total: ______

Average Percentile Rank (divide total by 3): ______ Overall Endurance Category: ______

**FIGURE 4.5** ◆ Data form for Muscular Endurance test results.

## Strength-to-Body Weight Ratio Test

This is an absolute strength test that will require you to determine your 1 RM on six different lifts (see Figure 4.6). Each 1 RM is expressed as a percentage of your body weight (1 RM divided by body weight), and points are awarded based on the ratio obtained for each lift (see Table 4.3). The final strength score is obtained by totaling the points received for each lift (see Figure 4.7).

Because the 1 RM is determined through trial and error, individual assessments require about 20 to 30 minutes or longer. As with the Muscular Strength and Endurance Test (the first test), a 16-station, fixed-resistance, Universal Gym apparatus is necessary.

### STRENGTH-TO-BODY WEIGHT RATIO TEST

1. Familiarize yourself with the six lifts used for this test: bench press, arm curl, lat pull-down, leg press, leg extension, and leg curl (an illustration of each lift is given at the end of this chapter).
2. Determine your body weight in pounds.
3. Determine your one repetition maximum (1 RM) for each lift. This is done through trial and error. Estimate the amount of resistance (weight) that you think you will be able to lift. If the load is too light, increase the resistance by 5 to 10 pounds; if it is too heavy, decrease by the same amount. Allow 2 to 3 minutes between trials. Continue the process until you have determined the maximal amount of resistance you can lift in one single effort. Record this information under the 1 RM column in Figure 4.7.
4. Express each 1 RM as a percentage of your body weight. To obtain this number, divide the 1 RM for each lift by your weight. Enter this number under the ratio column in Figure 4.7. For example, the strength-to-body weight ratio for a 150-pound male who bench-presses 180 pounds is 1.20 (180 ÷ 150).
5. Using Table 4.3, look up on the far right column the number of points scored for the ratio obtained on each lift. In the previous example, a ratio of 1.2 on the bench press for a male would score seven points. Record this information in the appropriate points column in Figure 4.7.
6. Total the number of points obtained on each lift, and determine your overall strength fitness category according to the following ratings:

| Total Points | Strength Category |
|---|---|
| ≥48 | Excellent |
| 37–47 | Good |
| 25–36 | Average |
| 13–24 | Fair |
| ≤12 | Poor |

**FIGURE 4.6** ◆ Procedure for the Strength-to-Body Weight Ratio test.

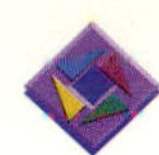

**TABLE 4.3**
**Strength-to-Body Weight Ratio Test Scoring Table**

| BENCH PRESS | ARM CURL | LAT PULL-DOWN | LEG PRESS | LEG EXTENSION* | LEG CURL | POINTS |
|---|---|---|---|---|---|---|
| **MEN** | | | | | | |
| 1.50 | 0.70 | 1.20 | 3.00 | 1.30 | 0.70 | 10 |
| 1.40 | 0.65 | 1.15 | 2.80 | 1.35 | 0.65 | 9 |
| 1.30 | 0.60 | 1.10 | 2.60 | 1.20 | 0.60 | 8 |
| 1.20 | 0.55 | 1.05 | 2.40 | 1.10 | 0.55 | 7 |
| 1.10 | 0.50 | 1.00 | 2.20 | 1.00 | 0.50 | 6 |
| 1.00 | 0.45 | 0.95 | 2.00 | 0.90 | 0.45 | 5 |
| 0.90 | 0.40 | 0.90 | 1.80 | 0.80 | 0.40 | 4 |
| 0.80 | 0.35 | 0.85 | 1.60 | 0.70 | 0.35 | 3 |
| 0.70 | 0.30 | 0.80 | 1.40 | 0.60 | 0.30 | 2 |
| 0.60 | 0.25 | 0.75 | 1.20 | 0.50 | 0.25 | 1 |
| **WOMEN** | | | | | | |
| 0.90 | 0.50 | 0.85 | 2.70 | 1.05 | 0.60 | 10 |
| 0.85 | 0.45 | 0.80 | 2.50 | 1.00 | 0.55 | 9 |
| 0.80 | 0.42 | 0.75 | 2.30 | 0.95 | 0.52 | 8 |
| 0.70 | 0.38 | 0.73 | 2.10 | 0.90 | 0.50 | 7 |
| 0.65 | 0.35 | 0.70 | 2.00 | 0.85 | 0.45 | 6 |
| 0.60 | 0.32 | 0.65 | 1.80 | 0.80 | 0.40 | 5 |
| 0.55 | 0.28 | 0.63 | 1.60 | 0.75 | 0.35 | 4 |
| 0.50 | 0.25 | 0.60 | 1.40 | 0.70 | 0.30 | 3 |
| 0.45 | 0.21 | 0.55 | 1.20 | 0.65 | 0.25 | 2 |
| 0.35 | 0.18 | 0.50 | 1.00 | 0.60 | 0.20 | 1 |

High physical fitness standard (points 10–7)
Health fitness standard (points 6–5)

*leg extension ratios adapted with permission by author.

From *Advanced Fitness and Exercise Prescription* (p. 108) by Vivian H. Heyward, 1991, Champaign, IL: Human Kinetics. Copyright © 1991 by Vivian H. Heyward. Reprinted by permission.

Name:______________________ Sex: ____________ Date: ____________

Body Weight: ____________ lbs.

| Lift | 1 RM | Ratio | Points | |
|---|---|---|---|---|
| Bench Press | ______ | ______ | ______ | |
| Leg Press | ______ | ______ | ______ | Overall Strength Category |
| Arm Curl | ______ | ______ | ______ | |
| Lat Pull-Down | ______ | ______ | ______ | ____________ |
| Leg Extension | ______ | ______ | ______ | |
| Leg Curl | ______ | ______ | ______ | |

Total Points: [ ]

**FIGURE 4.7** ◆ Data form for Strength-to-Body Weight Ratio test results.

## Hand Grip Test

As indicated earlier, when time is a factor, the Hand Grip Test can be used to provide a rough estimate of strength. Unlike the previous three tests, this is an isometric* (static contraction) test.

* A muscle contraction producing little or no movement. Also see Mode of Training later in this chapter.

If the proper grip is used, no finger or body movement is visible during the test. The test procedure is given in Figure 4.8 and you can record your test results in Figure 4.9.

Changes in strength may be more difficult to evaluate with this test. Most strength training programs are isotonic in nature, and this test provides an isometric assessment. Further, grip strength

### HAND GRIP STRENGTH TEST

1. Adjust the width of the dynamometer* so the middle bones (middle phalanges) of your fingers rest on the distant end of the dynamometer grip (see Figure 4.8a).

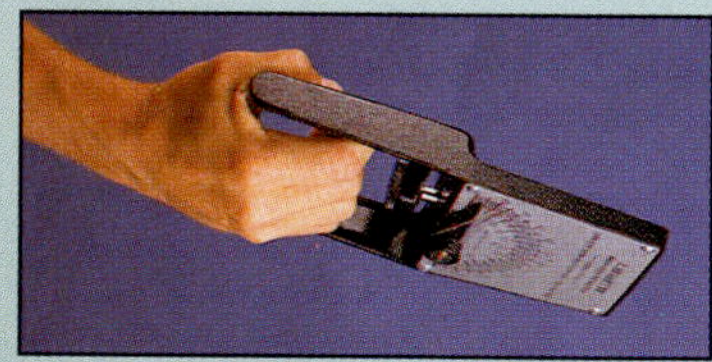

**FIGURE 4.8a** Proper grip size for the hand grip test.

2. Use your dominant hand for this test. Place your elbow at a 90° angle and about 2" away from the body (see page 85).
3. Now grip as hard as you can for a few seconds. Do not move any other body part as you perform the test (do not flex or extend the elbow, do not move the elbow away or toward the body, and do not lean forward or backward during the test).
4. Record the dynamometer reading in pounds (if reading is in kilograms, multiply by 2.2046).
5. Three trials are allowed for this test. Use the highest reading for your final test score. Record your test results in Figure 4.9 and look up your percentile rank in Table 4.4.
6. Obtain the hand grip strength fitness category according to the following guidelines:

| Percentile Rank | Fitness Classification |
|---|---|
| ≥81 | Excellent |
| 61–80 | Good |
| 41–60 | Average |
| 21–40 | Fair |
| ≤20 | Poor |

*A Lafayette model 78010 dynamometer is recommended for this test. Lafayette Instruments Co., Sagamore and North 9th Street, Lafayette, IN 47903.

**FIGURE 4.8** ◆ Procedure for the Hand Grip Strength Test.

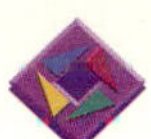

Name: ______ Sex: ______ Date: ______

Grip Strength Score: [ ] % Rank: ______ Strength Category: ______

**FIGURE 4.9** ◆ Data form for Hand Grip Strength test results.

**TABLE 4.4**
**Grip Strength Scoring Table**

| Percentile Rank | MEN | WOMEN |
|---|---|---|
| 99 | 153 | 101 |
| 95 | 145 | 94 |
| 90 | 141 | 91 |
| 80 | 139 | 86 |
| 70 | 132 | 80 |
| 60 | 124 | 78 |
| 50 | 122 | 74 |
| 40 | 114 | 71 |
| 30 | 110 | 66 |
| 20 | 100 | 64 |
| 10 | 91 | 60 |
| 5 | 76 | 58 |

High physical fitness standard (99–70)
Health fitness standard (60–50)

exercises seldom are used in strength training, and increases in strength are specific to the body parts exercised. This test also can be used to supplement the other three strength tests in this chapter.

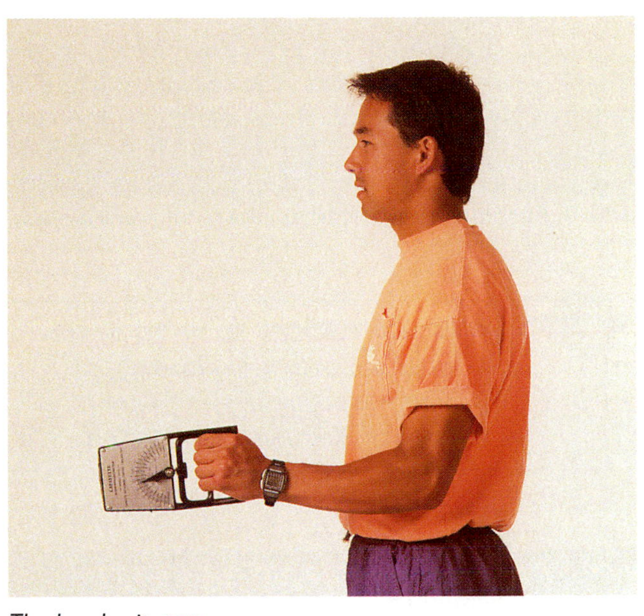

*The hand grip test.*

## Recording Your Strength Fitness Category

After you have established your own strength fitness category, record this information on Figure 4.10 and on your fitness and wellness profile in Appendix A. If you wish to conduct periodic strength assessments, extra blanks are included in Figure 4.10 for you to monitor your improvements.

Name: ______ Age: ______ Sex: ______

| Date | Test Used | Score | Fitness Classification |
|---|---|---|---|
| | | | |
| | | | |
| | | | |
| | | | |
| | | | |
| | | | |

**FIGURE 4.10** ◆ Muscular strength report.

## STRENGTH TRAINING PRESCRIPTION

Muscle cells increase and decrease their capacity to exert force according to the demands placed upon the muscular system. If muscle cells are overloaded beyond their normal use, such as in strength training programs, the cells increase in size (hypertrophy) and strength. If the demands placed on the muscle cells decrease, such as in sedentary living or required rest because of illness or injury, the cells decrease in size (atrophy) and lose strength. A good level of muscular strength is important to develop and maintain fitness, health, and total well-being.

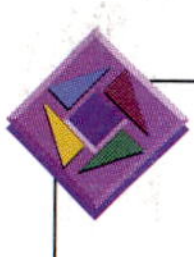

*Muscular strength seems to be the most important health-related component of physical fitness in the older-adult population.*

## FACTORS THAT AFFECT STRENGTH

Several physiological factors are related to muscle contraction and subsequent strength gains: neural stimulation, type of muscle fiber, the overload principle, and specificity of training. Basic knowledge of these concepts is important in understanding the principles involved in strength training.

### Neural Stimulation

Within the neuromuscular system single motor neurons (nerves traveling from the central nervous system to the muscle) branch and attach to multiple muscle fibers. The combination of the motor neuron and the fibers it innervates is called a *motor unit*. The number of fibers a motor neuron can innervate varies from just a few in muscles that require precise control (eye muscles, for example) to as many as 1,000 or more in large muscles that do not perform refined or precise movements.

Stimulation of a motor neuron causes the muscle fibers to contract maximally or not at all. Variations in the number of fibers innervated and the frequency of their stimulation determine the strength of the muscle contraction. As the number of fibers innervated and frequency of stimulation increases, so does the strength of the muscular contraction.

### Types of Fiber

Two basic types of muscle fibers determine muscle response: (a) slow-twitch or red fibers, and (b) fast-twitch or white fibers. Slow-twitch fibers have a greater capacity for aerobic work. Fast-twitch fibers have a greater capacity for anaerobic work and produce more overall force. The latter are important for quick and powerful movements commonly used in strength training activities.

The proportion of slow- and fast-twitch fibers is determined genetically, and consequently varies from one person to another. Nevertheless, training increases the functional capacity of both types of fiber, and more specifically, strength training increases their ability to exert force.

During muscular contraction slow-twitch fibers always are recruited first. As the force and speed of muscle contraction increase, the relative importance of the fast-twitch fibers also increases. To activate the fast-twitch fibers, an activity must be intense and powerful.

### Overload Principle

Strength gains are achieved in two ways:

1. Through increased ability of individual muscle fibers to generate a stronger contraction.
2. By recruiting a greater proportion of the total available fibers for each contraction.

These two factors combine in the overload principle. This principle states that for strength to improve, the demands placed on the muscle must be increased systematically and progressively over time, and the resistance must be of a magnitude significant enough to cause physiologic adaptation. In simpler terms, just like all other organs and systems of the human body, to increase in physical capacity, muscles have to be taxed beyond their accustomed loads. Because of this principle, strength training also is called *progressive resistance training*.

### Specificity of Training

The principle of specificity of training states that, for a muscle to increase in strength or endurance, the training program must be specific to obtain the

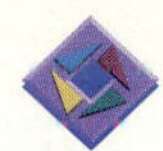

desired effects. In like manner, to increase static (isometric) versus dynamic (isotonic) strength, an individual must use static against dynamic training to achieve the desired results.

## PRINCIPLES INVOLVED IN STRENGTH TRAINING

Because muscular strength and endurance are important in developing and maintaining overall fitness and well-being, the principles necessary to develop a strength-training program have to be followed, as in the prescription of cardiovascular exercise. These principles are: mode, resistance, sets, and frequency of training.

### Mode of Training

Two basic types of training methods are used to improve strength: isometric (static) and isotonic (dynamic).

1. *Isometric training* refers to a muscle contraction that produces little or no movement, such as pushing or pulling against an immovable object.
2. *Isotonic training* refers to a muscle contraction with movement, such as extending the knees with resistance (weight) on the ankles (leg extension exercise).

Isometric training does not require much equipment. It was popular several years ago, but its popularity has waned. Because strength gains with isometric training are specific to the angle of muscle contraction, this type of training is beneficial in a sport such as gymnastics, which requires regular static contractions during routines.

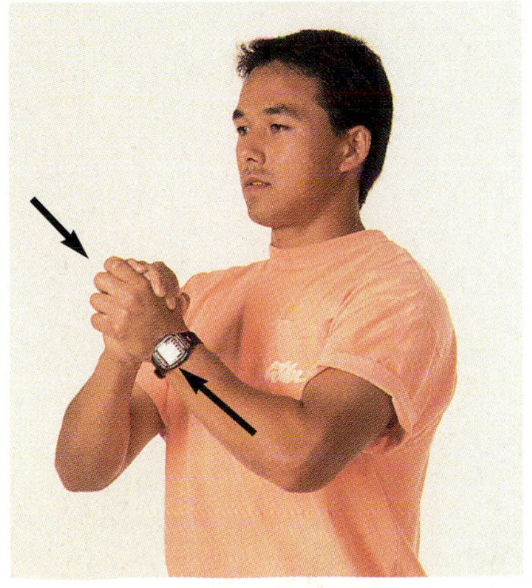

*Isometric training.*

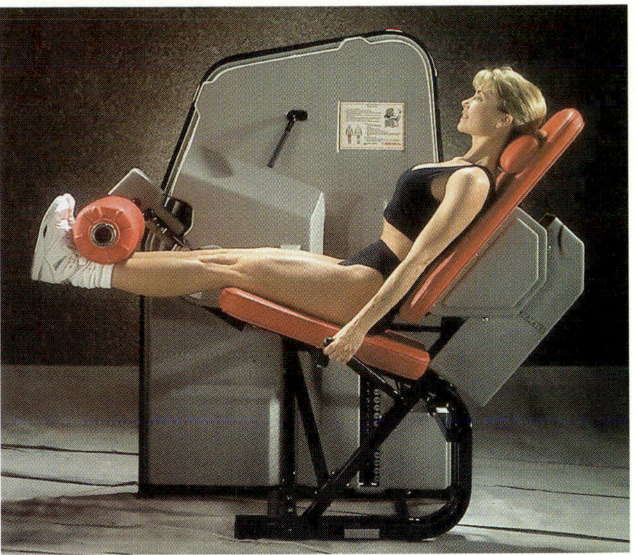

*Isotonic training.*

Isotonic training programs can be conducted without weights or with *free weights* (barbells and dumbbells), *fixed-resistance machines, variable-resistance machines*, and *isokinetic equipment*. When performing isotonic exercises without weights (for example, pull-ups, push-ups), with free weights, or with fixed-resistance machines, a constant resistance is moved through a joint's full range of motion. The greatest resistance that can be lifted equals the maximum weight that can be moved at the weakest angle of the joint. This is because of changes in muscle length and angle of pull as the joint moves through its range of motion.

As strength training became more popular, new strength training machines were developed. This technology brought about isokinetic and variable-resistance training programs which require special machines equipped with mechanical devices that provide differing amounts of resistance, with the intent of overloading the muscle group maximally through the entire range of motion. A distinction of isokinetic training is that the speed of the muscle contraction is kept constant because the machine provides resistance to match the user's force through the range of motion. The mode of training an individual selects depends mainly on the type of equipment available and the specific objective the training program is attempting to accomplish.

Isotonic training is the most popular mode for strength training. The primary advantage is that strength is gained through the full range of motion. Most daily activities are isotonic in nature. We are constantly lifting, pushing, and pulling objects, and strength is needed through a complete range of

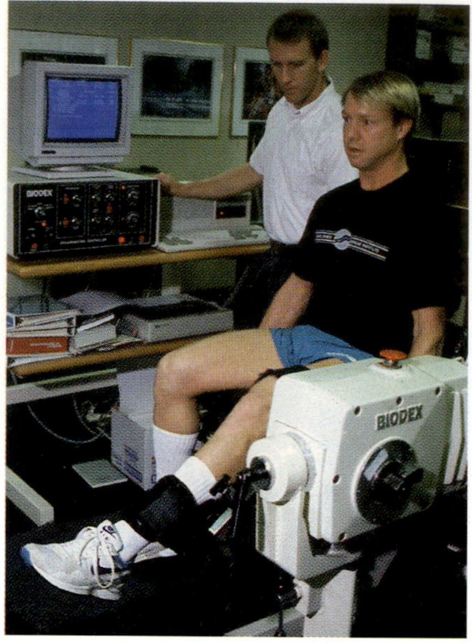


*Isokinetic training.*

motion. Another advantage is that improvements are measured easily by the amount lifted.

The benefits of isokinetic and variable-resistance training are similar to the other isotonic training methods. Theoretically, strength gains should be better because maximum resistance is applied at all angles. Research, however, has not shown this type of training to be more effective than other modes of isotonic training. A possible advantage, though, is that specific speeds used in various sport skills can be duplicated more closely with isokinetic strength training, which may enhance performance (specificity of training). A disadvantage is that the equipment is not readily available to many people.

## Resistance

Resistance in strength training is *the equivalent of intensity in cardiovascular exercise prescription.* The amount of resistance, or *weight lifted*, depends on whether the individual is trying to develop muscular strength or muscular endurance.

To stimulate strength development, a resistance of approximately 80% of the maximum capacity (1 RM) is recommended. For example, a person who can press 150 pounds should work with at least 120 pounds ($150 \times .80$). Less than 80% will help increase muscular endurance rather than strength.

Because of the time factor involved in constantly determining the 1 RM on each lift to ensure that the person is indeed working above 80%, a rule of thumb widely accepted by many authors and coaches is that individuals should perform between 3 and 12 repetitions maximum (3 to 12 RM) for adequate strength gains. For example, if a person is training with a resistance of 120 pounds and cannot lift it more than 12 times, the training stimulus is adequate for strength development.

Once the person can lift weight more than 12 times, the resistance should be increased by 5 to 10 pounds and the person again should build up to 12 repetitions. If training is conducted with more than 12 repetitions, primarily muscular endurance will be developed.

Strength research indicates that the closer a person trains to the 1 RM, the greater are the strength gains. A disadvantage of working constantly at or near the 1 RM is that it increases the risk for injury.

Highly trained athletes seeking maximum strength development often use 1 to 6 repetitions maximum. Working around 10 repetitions maximum seems to produce the best results in terms of muscular hypertrophy.

Body builders tend to work with moderate resistance levels (60% to 85% of the 1 RM) and perform 8 to 20 repetitions to near fatigue. A foremost objective of body building is to increase muscle size. Moderate resistance promotes blood flow to the muscles, "pumping up the muscles" (also known as "the pump") and making them look much larger than they are in a relaxed state.

From a health-fitness point of view, 8 to 12 repetitions maximum are ideal for adequate development. We live in an "isotonic world" in which muscular strength and endurance are both required to lead an enjoyable life. Therefore, working near a 10 repetition threshold seems best to improve overall performance.

## Sets

In strength training a set has been defined as *the number of repetitions performed for a given exercise.* For example, a person lifting 120 pounds eight times has performed one set of eight repetitions ($1 \times 8 \times 120$).

When working with 8 to 12 repetitions maximum, three sets per exercise are recommended. Because of the characteristics of muscle fiber, the number of sets that can be done is limited. As the number of sets increases, so does the amount of muscle fatigue and subsequent recovery time. Therefore, strength gains may be lessened by performing too many sets.

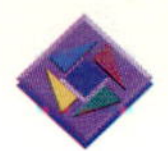

A recommended program for beginners in their first year of training is three heavy sets, up to the maximum number of repetitions, preceded by one or two light warm-up sets using about 50% of the 1 RM (no warm-up sets are necessary for subsequent exercises that use the same muscle group). Because of the lower resistances used in body building, four to eight sets can be done for each exercise.

To avoid muscle soreness and stiffness, new participants ought to build up gradually to the three sets of maximal repetitions. This can be done by performing only one set of each exercise with a lighter resistance on the first day, two sets of each exercise on the second day — one light and the second with the regular resistance — and three sets on the third day — one light and two heavy. After that, a person should be able to do all three heavy sets.

The time necessary to recover between sets depends mainly on the resistance used during each set. In strength training, the energy to lift heavy weights is derived primarily from the ATP-CP or phosphagen system (see Chapter 7 discussion on energy production). Ten seconds of maximal exercise pretty much depletes the CP stores in the exercised muscle(s). These stores are replenished in about 3 minutes of recovery.

Based on this principle, a rest period of about 3 minutes between sets is necessary for people who are trying to maximize their strength gains. Individuals training for health-fitness purposes might allow 2 minutes of rest between sets. Body builders should rest no more than a minute to maximize the "pumping" effect.

The exercise program will be more time-effective by alternating two or three exercises that require different muscle groups. In this way, an individual will not have to wait 2 to 3 minutes before proceeding to a new set on a different exercise. For example, bench press, leg extensions, and abdominal crunches may be combined so the person can go almost directly from one set to the next.

## Frequency of Training

Strength training should be done either through a total body workout three times a week, or more frequently if using a split body routine (upper body one day, lower body the next). After a maximum strength workout, the muscles should be rested for about 2 to 3 days to allow adequate recovery. If not completely recovered in 2 to 3 days, the person most likely is overtraining and therefore not reaping the full benefits of the program. In that case, the person should do fewer sets or exercises than in the previous workout. A summary of strength training guidelines for health-fitness purposes is provided in Figure 4.11.

To achieve significant strength gains, a minimum of 8 weeks of consecutive training is necessary. After achieving an ideal strength level, one training session per week will be sufficient to maintain the new strength level.

Frequency of strength training for body builders varies from person to person. Because they use moderate resistances, daily or even two-a-day workouts are common. The frequency depends on the amount of resistance, number of sets performed per session, and the person's ability to recover from the previous exercise bout (see Table 4.5). The latter often is dictated by level of conditioning.

| | |
|---|---|
| **Mode:** | 8 to 10 isotonic strength-training exercises involving the body's major muscle groups. |
| **Resistance:** | Enough resistance to perform 8 to 12 repetitions to near fatigue. |
| **Sets:** | A minimum of one set. |
| **Frequency:** | At least two times per week. |

Source: The recommended quantity and quality of exercise for developing and maintaining cardiorespiratory and muscular fitness in healthy adults by the American College of Sports Medicine, *Medicine Science in Sports and Exercise*, 22 (1990), 265–274.

**FIGURE 4.11** ◆ Strength training guidelines.

**TABLE 4.5**
**Guidelines for Various Strength Training Programs**

| Strength Training Program | Resistance | Sets | Rest Between Sets* | Frequency (workouts per week)** |
|---|---|---|---|---|
| Health fitness | 8–12 reps max | 3 | 2 min | 2–3 |
| Maximal strength | 1–6 reps max | 3–6 | 3 min | 2–3 |
| Muscular endurance | 10–30 reps | 3–6 | 2 min | 3–6 |
| Body building | 8–20 reps near max | 3–8 | 0–1 min | 4–12 |

* Recovery between sets can be decreased by alternating exercises that use different muscle groups.

** Weekly training sessions can be increased by using a split body routine.

## PLYOMETRICS

Strength, speed, and explosiveness are all crucial for success in athletics. All three of these factors are enhanced with a progressive resistance training program, but greater increases in speed and explosiveness are thought possible with plyometric training.

Plyometric exercise is defined best as *explosive jump training, incorporating speed and strength training to enhance explosiveness*. The objective is to generate the greatest amount of force in the shortest time. A sound strength base is necessary before attempting plyometric exercises.

Plyometric training is popular in sports that require powerful movements, such as basketball, volleyball, sprinting, jumping, and tumbling. A typical plyometric exercise involves jumping off and back onto a box, attempting to rebound as quickly as possible on each jump. Box heights are increased progressively from about 12" to 22".

The bounding action attempts to take advantage of the stretch-recoil and stretch reflex characteristics of muscle. The rapid stretch applied to the muscle during ground contact is thought to augment muscle contraction, leading to more explosiveness. Plyometrics can be used, too, for strengthening upper body muscles. An example is push-ups with a forceful extension of the arms to drive the hands (and body) completely off the floor during each repetition.

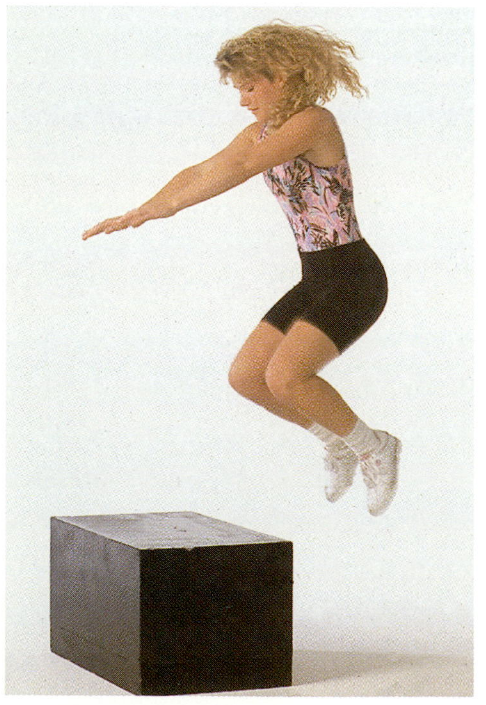

Plyometric training.

A drawback of plyometric training is the higher risk for injuries compared to conventional modes of progressive resistance training. The potential for injury escalates as the box height increases.

## STRENGTH TRAINING EXERCISES

The three strength training programs introduced next provide a complete body workout. The major muscles of the human body referred to in the exercises are pointed out in Figure 4.12.

Only a minimum of equipment is required for the first program, Strength Training Exercises Without Weights (Exercises 1 through 11). This program can be conducted within the walls of your own home. Your body weight is used as the primary resistance for most exercises. A few exercises call for a friend's help or some basic implements from around your house, to provide greater resistance.

The second program, Universal Gym Equipment Strength Training Exercises (Exercises 12 through 28), requires machines such as those shown in the accompanying photographs. These exercises can be conducted on either fixed-resistance or variable-resistance equipment. Many of these exercises also can be performed with free weights. The first eight exercises (12 to 19) are recommended to get a complete workout. The rest are optional. If one of the optional exercises involves the same body parts, however, the person may substitute the latter for one of the basic nine (Exercise 22 for 12, 20 or 21 for 13, 27 for 14, 24 or 25 for 15, 23 for 17, and 26 for 19).

Nautilus Strength-Training Exercises (Exercises 29 through 40) make up the third program. These also require machines, as illustrated in the photographs. All of these machines use variable resistance. In this last program, Exercises 29 through 38 are recommended for a complete body workout, and Exercise 40 may be substituted for Exercise 32.

## SETTING UP YOUR OWN STRENGTH TRAINING PROGRAM

Depending on the facilities available, you can choose one of the three training programs outlined in this chapter. Once you begin your strength

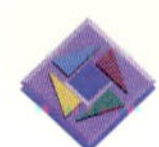

training program, you may use the form provided in Figure 4.13 to keep a record of your training sessions.

The resistance and the number of repetitions you use with your program should be based on whether you want to increase muscular strength or muscular endurance. Do up to 12 repetitions maximum for strength gains, and more than 12 for muscular endurance. For most people, three training sessions per week on nonconsecutive days is an ideal arrangement for proper development.

Because both strength and endurance are required in daily activities, three sets of about 12 repetitions maximum for each exercise are recommended. In doing this, you will obtain good strength gains and yet be close to the endurance threshold. If you are training for reasons other than health fitness, a summary of the guidelines is provided in Table 4.5.

Perhaps the only exercise that calls for more than 12 repetitions is the abdominal group of exercises. The abdominal muscles are considered primarily antigravity or postural muscles. Hence, a little more endurance may be required. When doing abdominal work, most people perform about 20 repetitions.

If time is a concern in completing a strength training exercise program, the American College of Sports Medicine[3] recommends as a minimum: (a) one set of 8 to 12 repetitions performed to near fatigue, and (b) 8 to 10 exercises involving the major muscle groups of the body, conducted twice a week. The recommendation is based on research showing that this training generates 70% to 80% of the improvements reported in other programs using three sets of about 10 RM.

## NOTES

1. W. J. Evans, "Exercise, Nutrition and Aging," *Journal of Nutrition*, 122 (1992), 796-801.
2. J. L. Hesson, *Weight Training for Life* (Englewood, CO: Morton Publishing, 1991).
3. American College of Sports Medicine, "The Recommended Quantity and Quality of Exercise for Developing and Maintaining Cardiorespiratory and Muscular Fitness in Healthy Adults," *Medicine and Science in Sports and Exercise*, 22 (1990), 265-274.

## SELECT BIBLIOGRAPHY


Allsen, P. E. *Strength Training: Beginners, Bodybuilders, and Athletes*. Glenview, IL: Scott, Foresman and Co., 1987.

Fox, E. L., R. W. Bowers, and M. L. Fossand. *The Physiological Basis for Exercise and Sport*. Philadelphia: Saunders College Publishing, 1993.

Getchell, B. *Physical Fitness: A Way of Life*. New York: Macmillan, 1992.

Hesson, J. L. *Weight Training for Life*. Englewood, CO: Morton Publishing, 1991.

Heyward, V. H. *Advanced Fitness Assessment & Exercise Prescription*. Champaign, IL: Human Kinetics, 1991.

Hoeger, W. W. K., and S. A. Hoeger. *Lifetime Physical Fitness and Wellness: A Personalized Program*. Englewood, CO: Morton Publishing, 1992.

Hoeger, W. W. K., D. R. Hopkins, S. L. Barette, and D. F. Hale. "Relationship Between Repetitions and Selected Percentages of One Repetition Maximum: A Comparison Between Untrained and Trained Males and Females." *Journal of Applied Sport Science Research*, 4:2 (1990), 47-51.

McArdle, W. D., F. I. Katch, and V. L. Katch. *Exercise Physiology: Energy, Nutrition and Human Performance*. Philadelphia: Lea and Febiger, 1991.

O'Shea, J. P. *Scientific Principles and Methods of Strength Fitness*. Reading, MA: Addison-Wesley, 1976.

Silvester, L. J. *Weight Training for Strength and Fitness*. Boston: Jones and Bartlett Publishers, 1992.

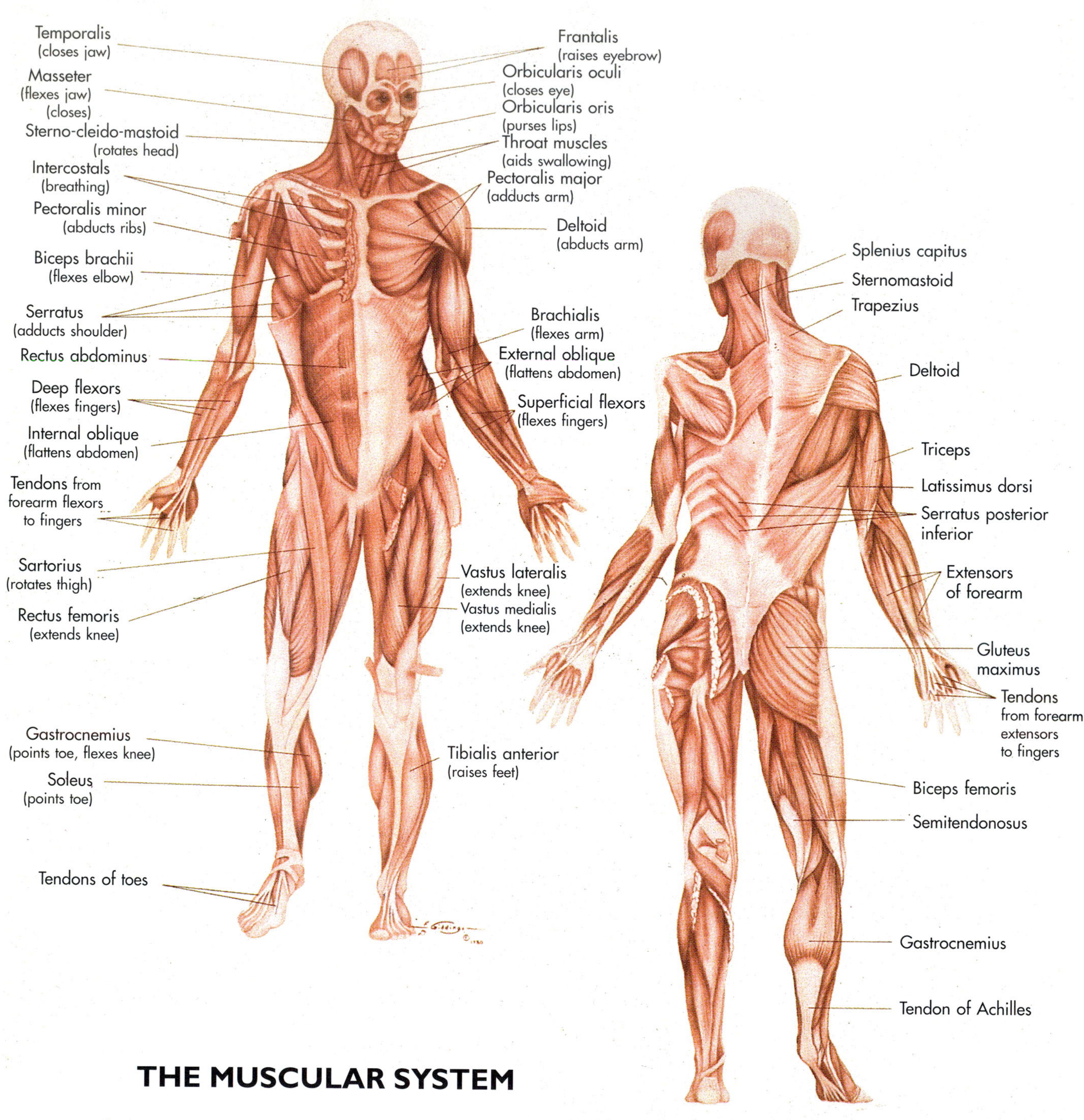


From *Basic Physiology and Anatomy* by E. Chaffee and F. Lytle (Philadelphia: Lippincott Co., 1980). Reproduced by permission.

**FIGURE 4.12** ♦ Major muscles of the human body.

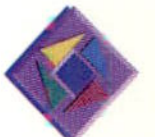

Name ______________________

| Date | | | | | | | | | | |
|---|---|---|---|---|---|---|---|---|---|---|
| Exercise | St/Reps/Res* | St/Reps/Res* | St/Reps/Res* | St/Reps/Res* | St/Reps/Res* | St/Reps/Res* | St/Reps/Res* | St/Reps/Res* | St/Reps/Res* | St/Reps/Res* |
| | | | | | | | | | | |
| | | | | | | | | | | |
| | | | | | | | | | | |
| | | | | | | | | | | |
| | | | | | | | | | | |
| | | | | | | | | | | |
| | | | | | | | | | | |
| | | | | | | | | | | |
| | | | | | | | | | | |
| | | | | | | | | | | |
| | | | | | | | | | | |
| | | | | | | | | | | |
| | | | | | | | | | | |
| | | | | | | | | | | |
| | | | | | | | | | | |
| | | | | | | | | | | |
| | | | | | | | | | | |
| | | | | | | | | | | |
| | | | | | | | | | | |
| | | | | | | | | | | |
| | | | | | | | | | | |
| | | | | | | | | | | |

*St/Reps/Res = Sets, Repetitions, and Resistance (e.g., 1/6/125 = 1 set of 6 repetitions with 125 pounds)

**FIGURE 4.13** ◆ Strength training record form.

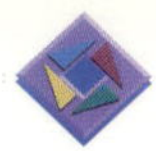



Name ______________________

| Date | | | | | | | | | | |
|---|---|---|---|---|---|---|---|---|---|---|
| Exercise | St/Reps/Res* | St/Reps/Res* | St/Reps/Res* | St/Reps/Res* | St/Reps/Res* | St/Reps/Res* | St/Reps/Res* | St/Reps/Res* | St/Reps/Res* | St/Reps/Res* |
| | | | | | | | | | | |
| | | | | | | | | | | |
| | | | | | | | | | | |
| | | | | | | | | | | |
| | | | | | | | | | | |
| | | | | | | | | | | |
| | | | | | | | | | | |
| | | | | | | | | | | |
| | | | | | | | | | | |
| | | | | | | | | | | |
| | | | | | | | | | | |
| | | | | | | | | | | |
| | | | | | | | | | | |
| | | | | | | | | | | |
| | | | | | | | | | | |
| | | | | | | | | | | |
| | | | | | | | | | | |
| | | | | | | | | | | |
| | | | | | | | | | | |
| | | | | | | | | | | |
| | | | | | | | | | | |
| | | | | | | | | | | |

*St/Reps/Res = Sets, Repetitions, and Resistance (e.g., 1/6/125 = 1 set of 6 repetitions with 125 pounds)

**FIGURE 4.13** ◆ Strength training record form.

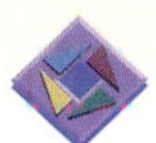

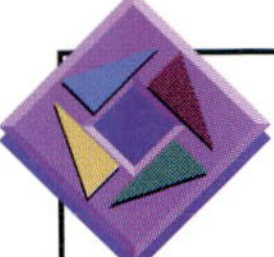

# 1
## Step-Up

**ACTION** Step up and down using a box or chair approximately 12" to 15" high. Conduct one set using the same leg each time you go up, and then conduct a second set using the other leg. You could also alternate legs on each step-up cycle. You may increase the resistance by holding a child or some other object in your arms (hold the child or object close to the body to avoid increased strain in the lower back).

**MUSCLES DEVELOPED**
Gluteal muscles, quadriceps, gastrocnemius, and soleus.

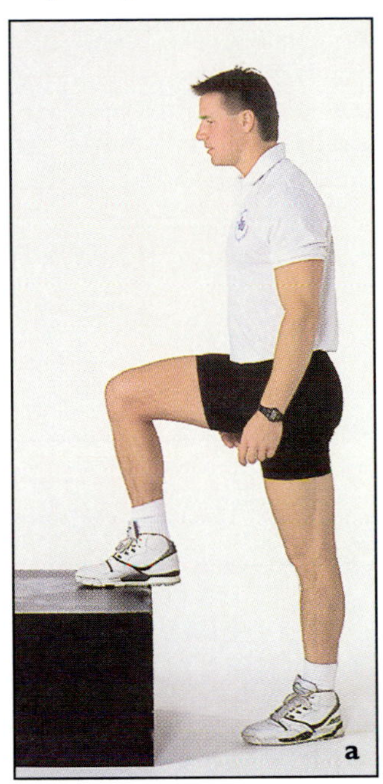
a

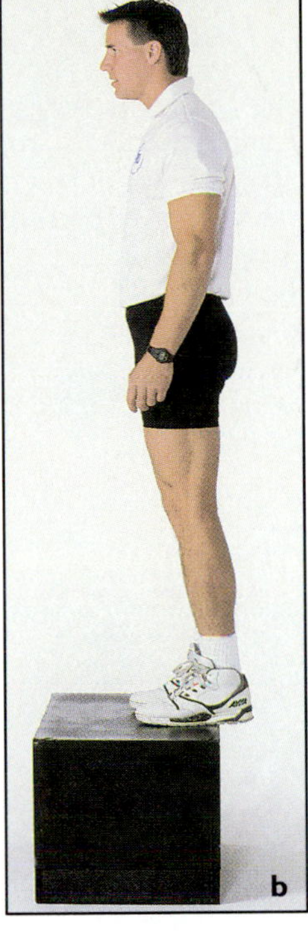
b

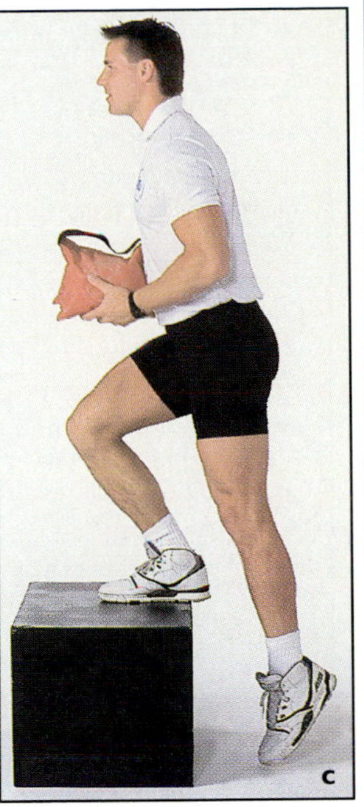
c

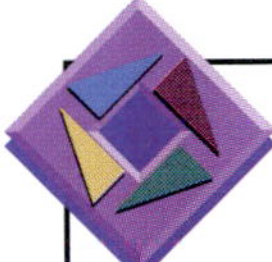

# 2
## High-Jumper

**ACTION** Start with the knees bent at approximately 150° and jump as high as you can, raising both arms simultaneously.

**MUSCLES DEVELOPED**
Gluteal muscles, quadriceps, gastrocnemius, and soleus.

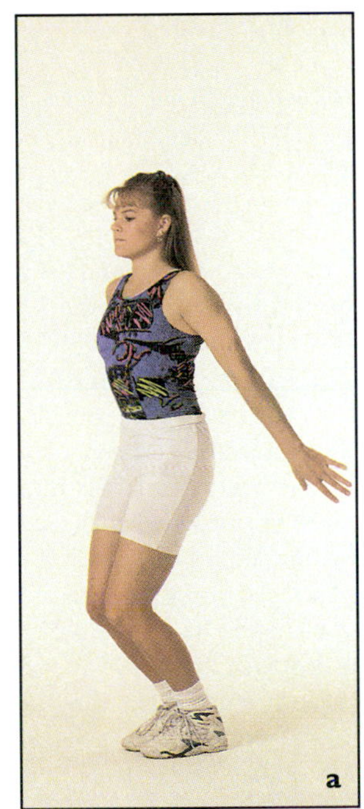
a

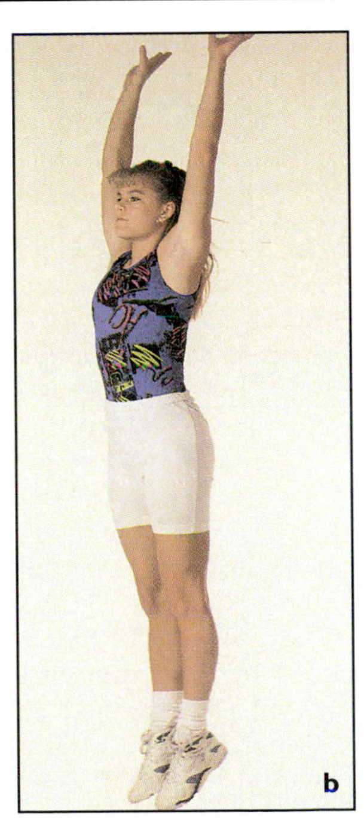
b

Photographs for Exercises 12, 13, and 15, through 28 are courtesy of Universal Gym® Equipment, Inc., 930 27th Avenue, S.W., Cedar Rapids, IA 52406. Photographs for Exercises 29 through 40 are courtesy of Nautilus®, a registered trademark of Nautilus® Sports/Medical Industries, Inc., 709 Powerhouse Road, Independence, Virginia 24348-0708.

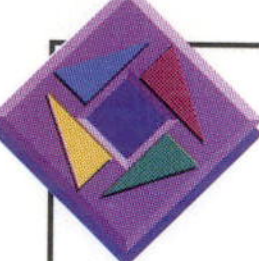

## 3
## Push-Up

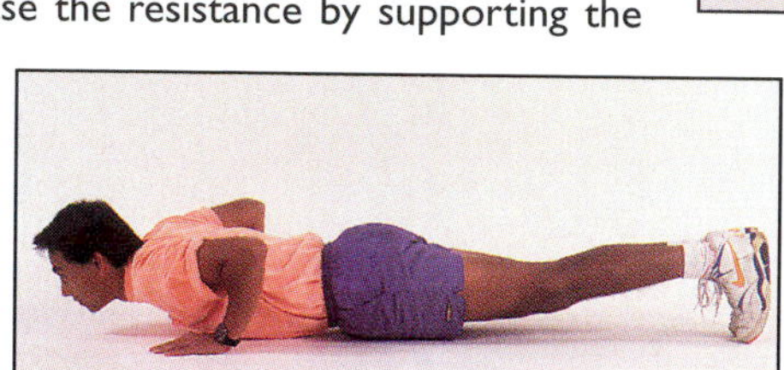

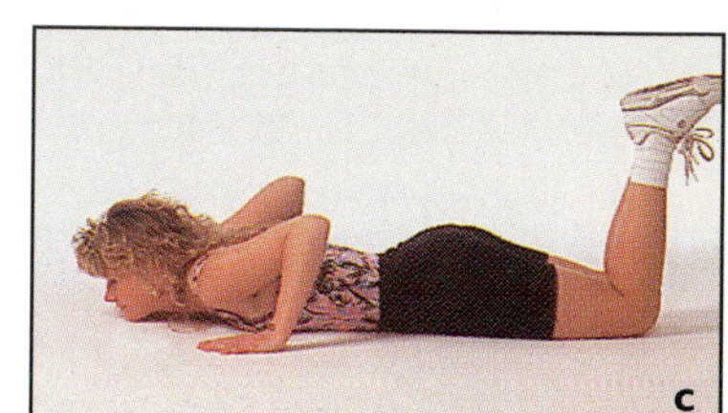

**ACTION** Maintaining your body as straight as possible, flex the elbows, lowering the body until you almost touch the floor, then raise yourself back up to the starting position. If you are unable to perform the push-up as indicated, you can decrease the resistance by supporting the lower body with the knees rather than the feet (see illustration c) or using an incline plane and supporting your hands at a higher point than the floor (see illustration d). If you wish to increase the resistance, have someone else add resistance to your shoulders as you are coming back up (see illustration e).

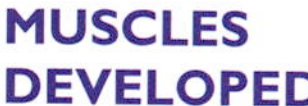

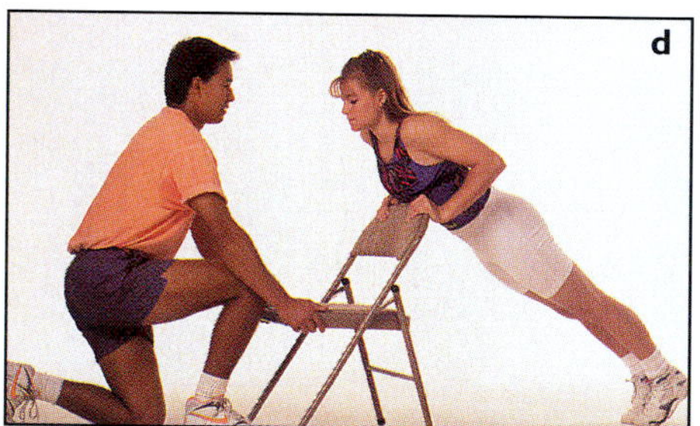

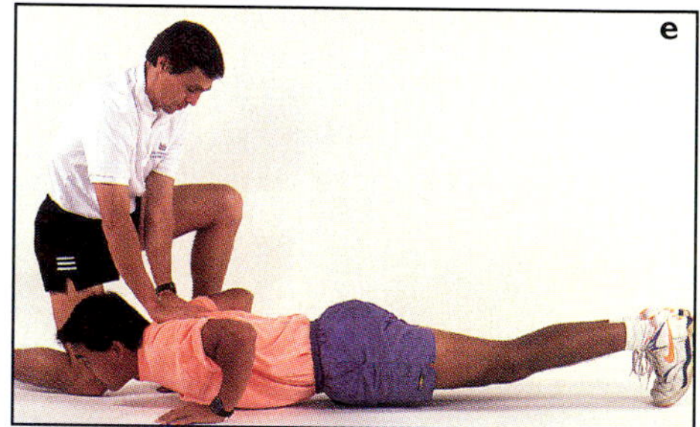

**MUSCLES DEVELOPED**
Triceps, deltoid, pectoralis major, erector spinae, and abdominals.

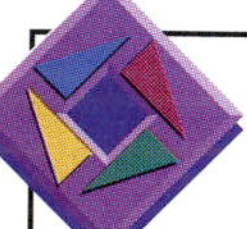

## 4
## Abdominal Crunch and Abdominal Curl-Up

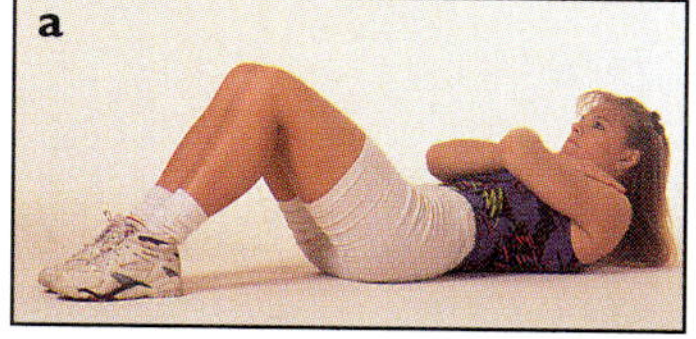

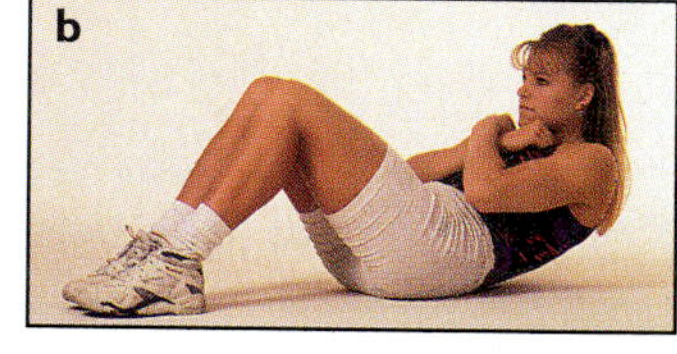

**ACTION** Start with your head and shoulders off the floor, arms crossed on your chest, and knees slightly bent (the greater the flexion of the knee, the more difficult the curl-up). Now curl up to about 30° (abdominal crunch — see illustration b) or curl all the way up (abdominal curl-up), then return to the starting position without letting the head or shoulders touch the floor, or allowing the hips to come off the floor. If you allow the hips to raise off the floor and the head and shoulders to touch the floor, you will most likely "swing up" on the next sit-up, which minimizes the work of the abdominal muscles. If you cannot curl up with the arms on the chest, place the hands by the side of the hips or even help yourself up by holding on to your thighs (illustrations d and e). Do not perform the sit-up exercise with your legs completely extended, as this will cause strain on the lower back.

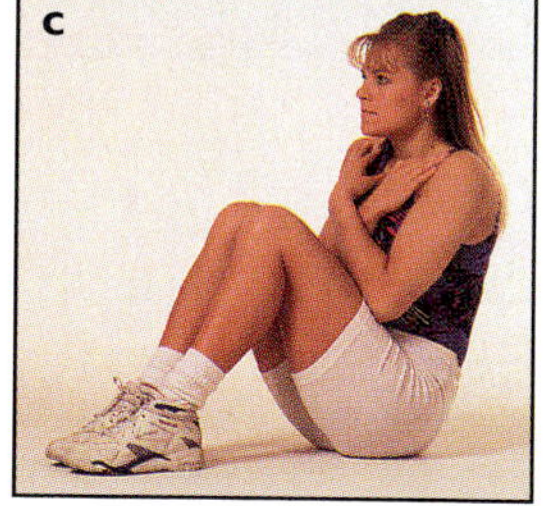

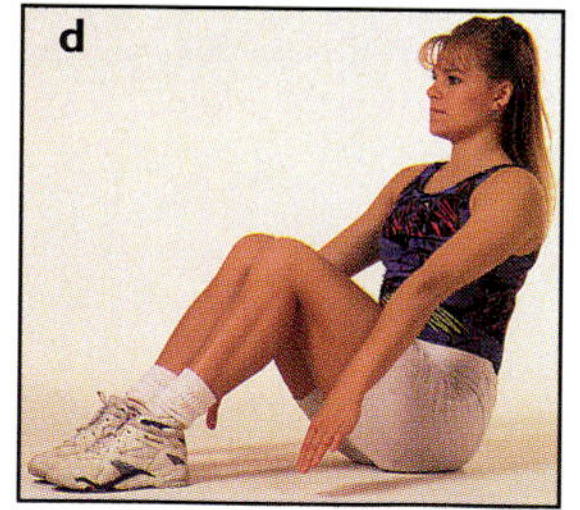

**MUSCLES DEVELOPED** Abdominal muscles (crunch) and hip flexors (complete curl-up).

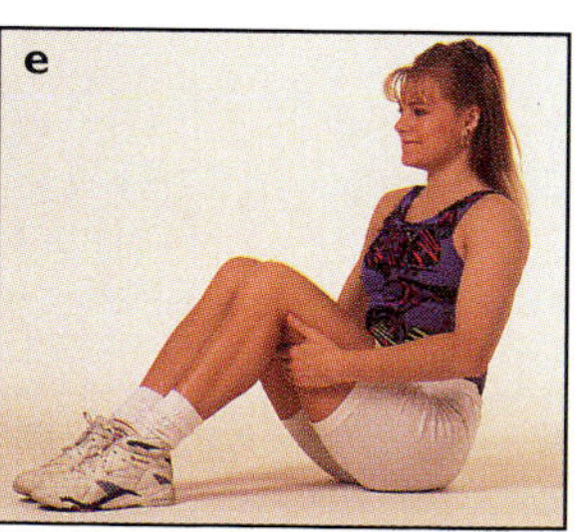

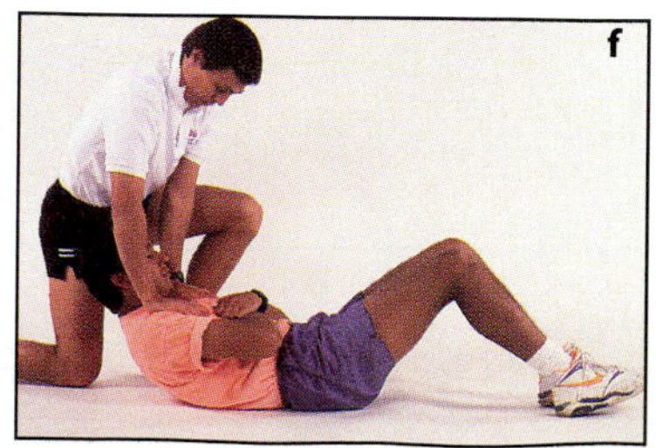

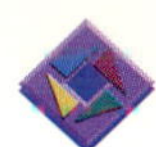

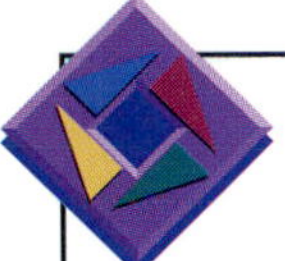

## 5
## Leg Curl

**ACTION** Lie on the floor face down. Cross the right ankle over the left heel. Apply resistance with your right foot, while you bring the left foot up to 90° at the knee joint. (Apply enough resistance so that the left foot can only be brought up slowly.) Repeat the exercise, crossing the left ankle over the right heel.

**MUSCLES DEVELOPED**
Hamstrings (and quadriceps).

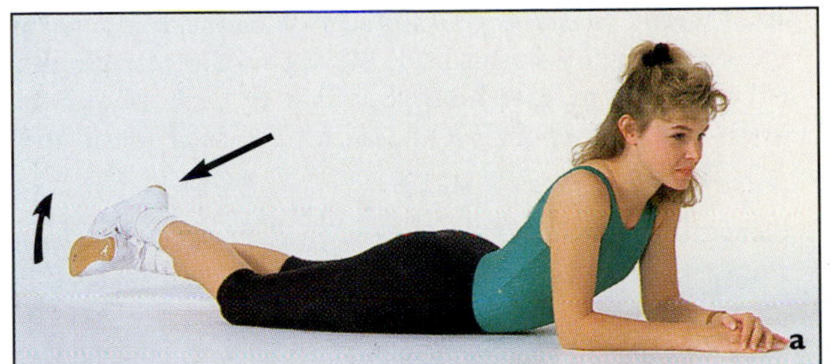
a

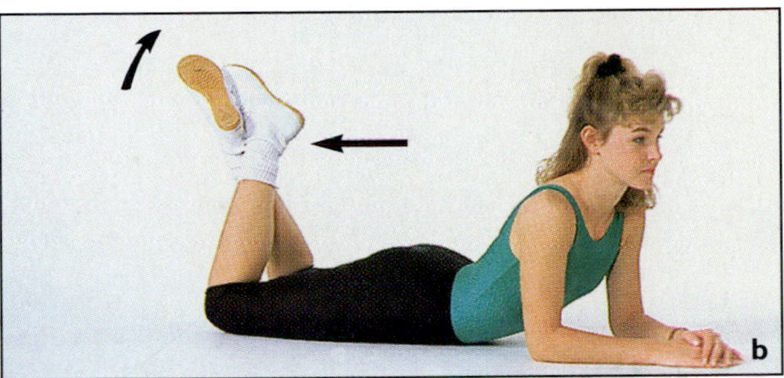
b

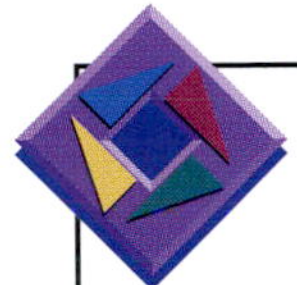

## 6
## Modified Dip

**ACTION** This upper-body exercise is performed by men only. Using a bench or gymnasium bleacher, place the hands on the bench with the fingers pointing forward. Have a partner hold your feet in front of you. The hips should be bent at approximately 90° (you also may use three sturdy chairs, put your hands on two chairs placed by the sides of your body, and the feet on the third chair in front of you). Lower your body by flexing the elbows until you reach a 90° angle at this joint, then return to the starting position.

**MUSCLES DEVELOPED**
Triceps, deltoid, and pectoralis major.

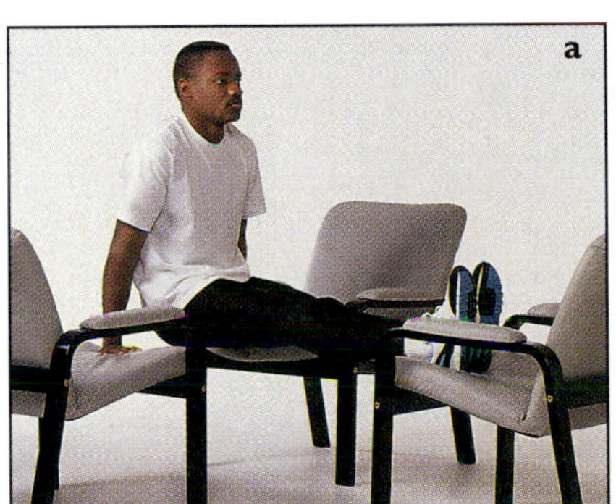
a

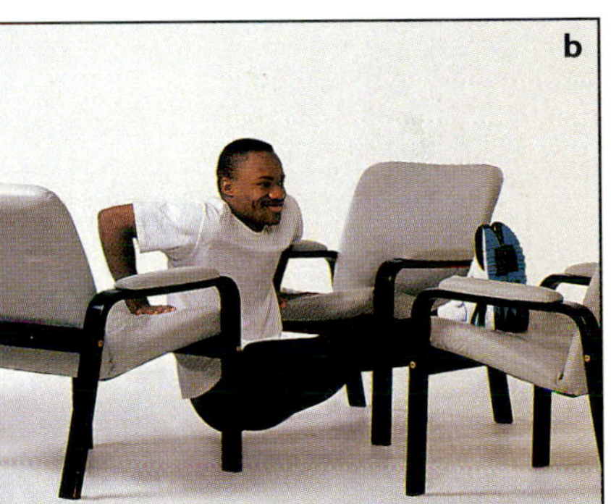
b

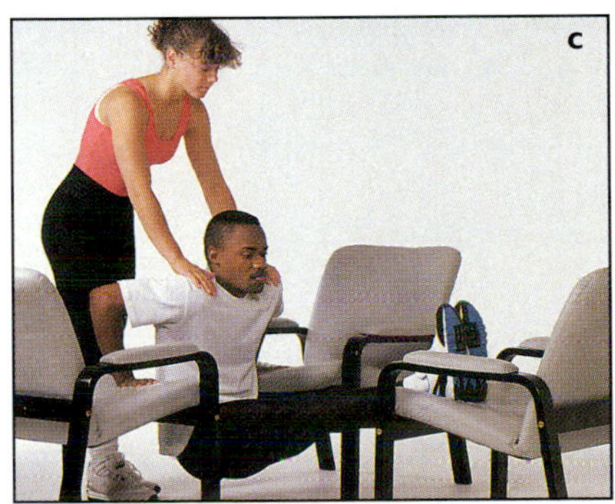
c

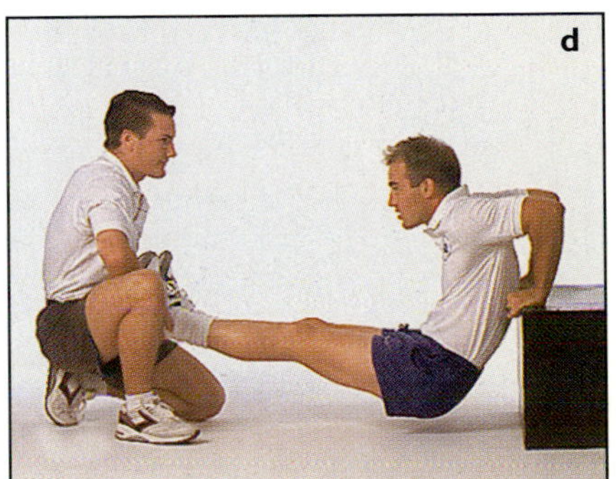
d

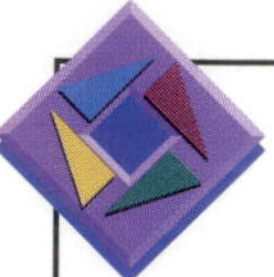

# 7
## Pull-Up

**ACTION** Suspend yourself from a bar with a pronated grip (thumbs in). Pull your body up until your chin is above the bar, then lower the body slowly to the starting position. If you are unable to perform the pull-up as described, either have a partner hold your feet to push off and facilitate the movement upward (illustrations c and d) or use a lower bar and support your feet on the floor (illustration e).

**MUSCLES DEVELOPED**
Biceps, brachioradialis, brachialis, trapezius, and latissimus dorsi.

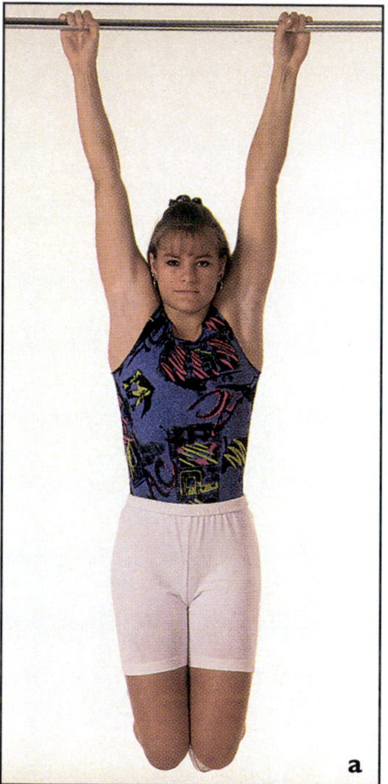
a

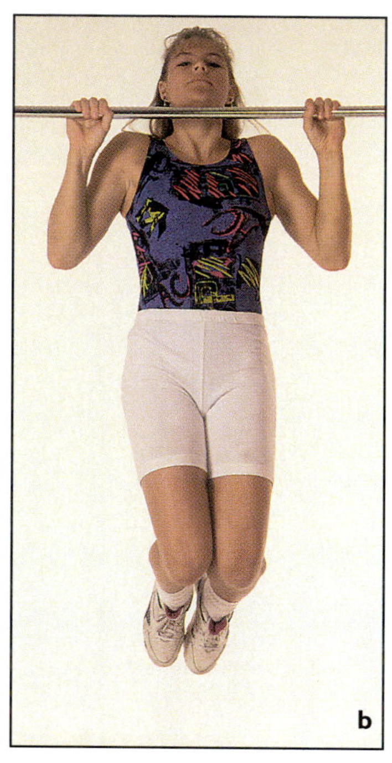
b

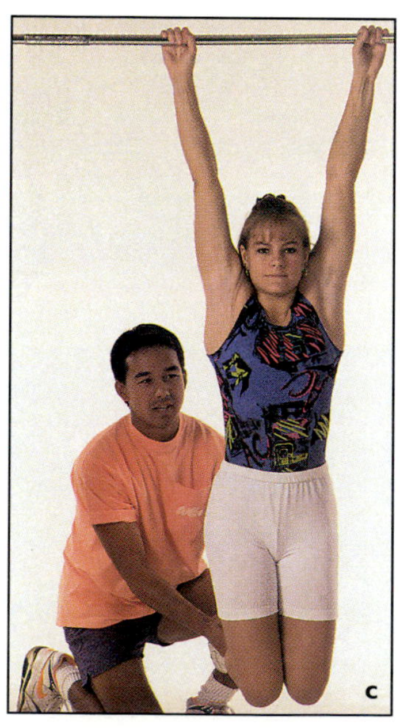
c

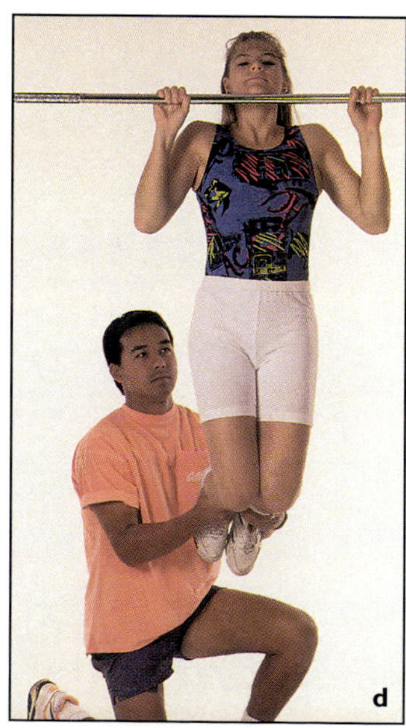
d

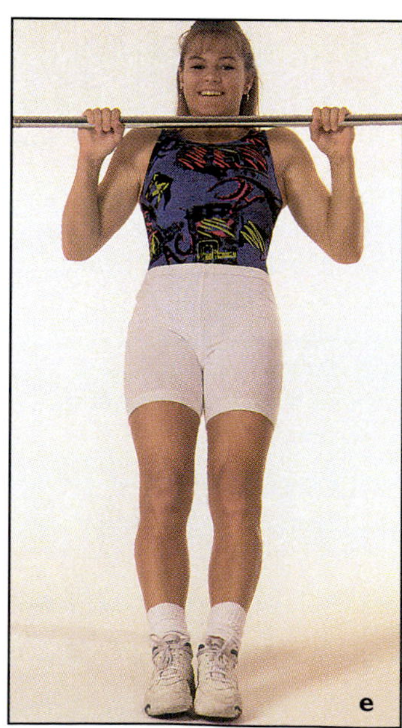
e

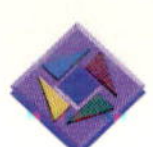

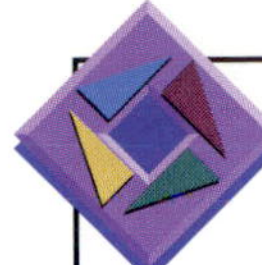

## 8
## Arm Curl

**ACTION** Using a palms-up grip, start with the arm completely extended, and with the aid of a sandbag or bucket filled (as needed) with sand or rocks, curl up as far as possible, then return to the initial position. Repeat the exercise with the other arm.

**MUSCLES DEVELOPED**
Biceps, brachioradialis, and brachialis.

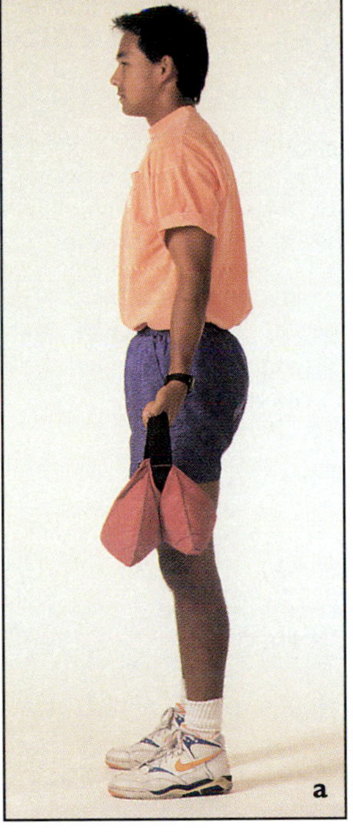
a

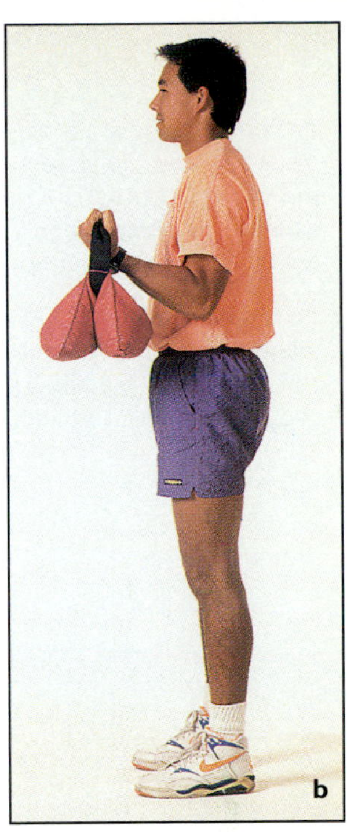
b

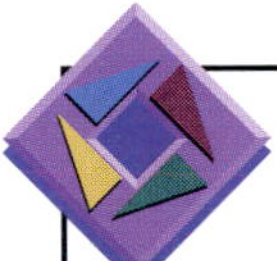

## 9
## Heel Raise

**ACTION** From a standing position with feet flat on the floor, raise and lower your body weight by moving at the ankle joint only (for added resistance, have someone else hold your shoulders down as you perform the exercise).

**MUSCLES DEVELOPED**
Gastrocnemius and soleus.

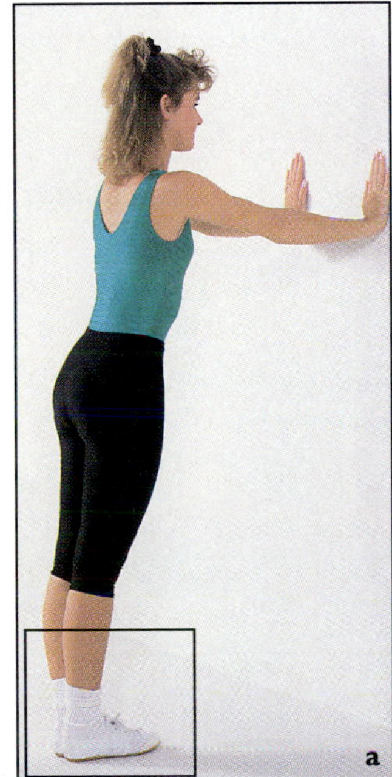
a

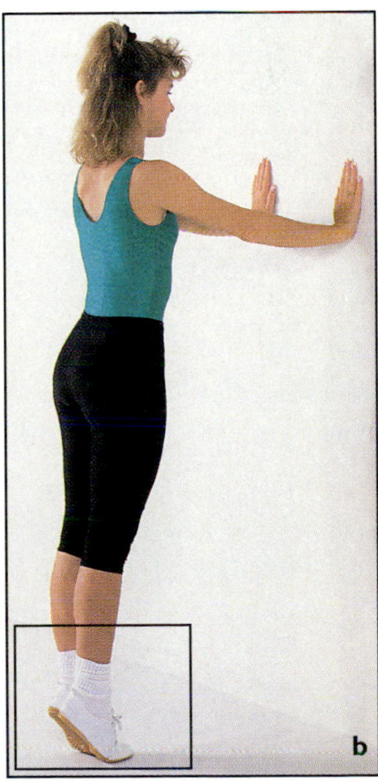
b

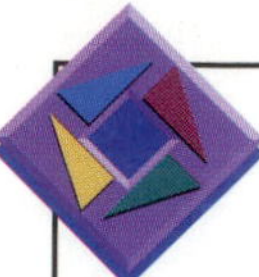

# 10

## Leg Abduction and Adduction

**ACTION** Both participants sit on the floor. The subject on the left places the feet on the inside of the other participant's feet. Simultaneously, the subject on the left presses the legs laterally (to the outside — abduction), while the subject on the right presses the legs medially (adduction). Hold the contraction for 5 to 10 seconds. Repeat the exercise at all three angles, and then reverse the pressing sequence. The subject on the left places the feet on the outside and presses inward, while the subject on the right presses outward.

**MUSCLES DEVELOPED** Hip abductors (rectus femoris, sartori, gluteus medius and minimus), and adductors (pectineus, gracilis, adductor magnus, adductor longus, and adductor brevis).

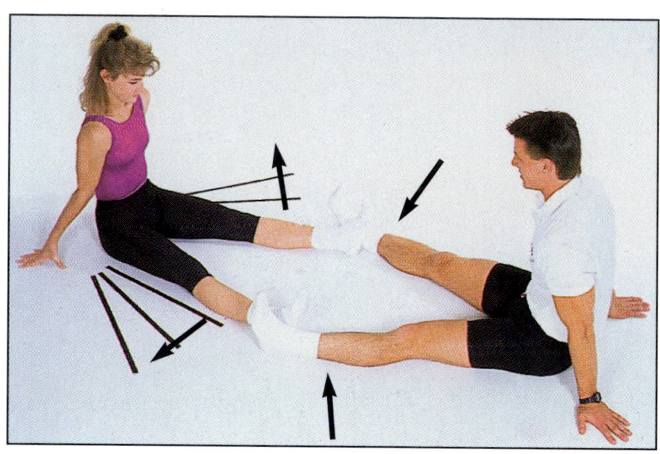

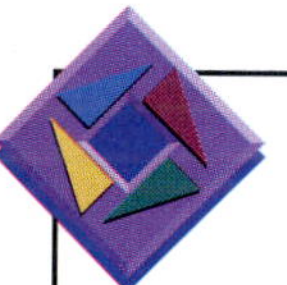

# 11

## Reverse Crunch

**ACTION** Lie on your back with arms crossed on your chest and knees and hips flexed at 90°. Now attempt to raise the pelvis off the floor by lifting vertically from the knees and lower legs. This is a challenging exercise that may be difficult to perform by beginners.

**MUSCLES DEVELOPED** Abdominals.

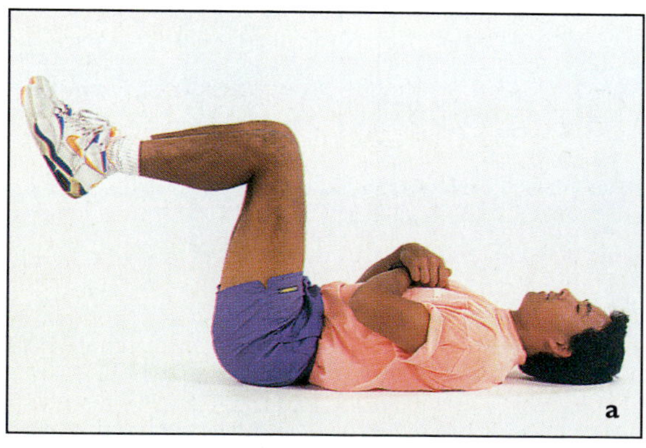

a

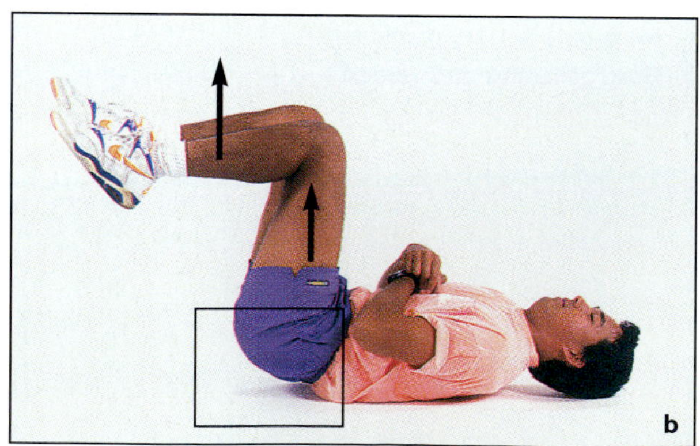

b

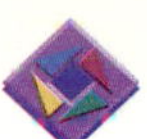

# Universal Gym® Equipment Strength-Training Exercises

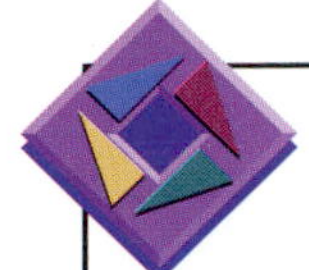

## 12

## Arm Curl

**ACTION** Use a supinated or palms-up grip, and start with the arms almost completely extended. Now curl up as far as possible, then return to the starting position.

**MUSCLES DEVELOPED** Biceps, brachioradialis, and brachialis.

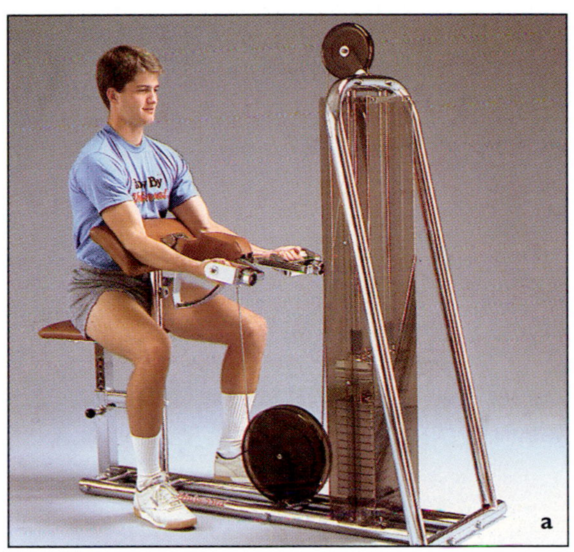

a

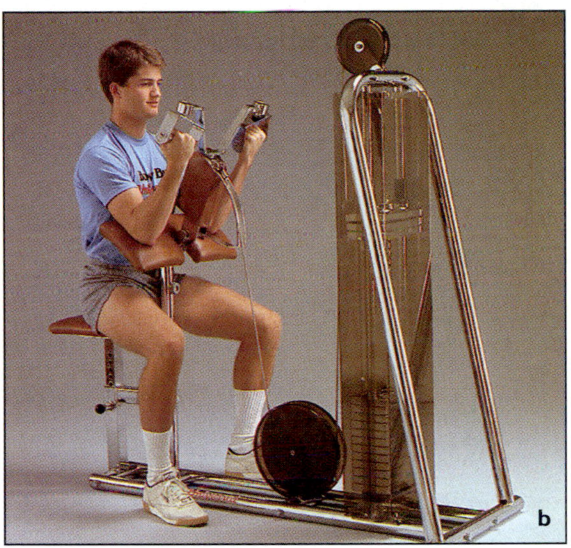

b

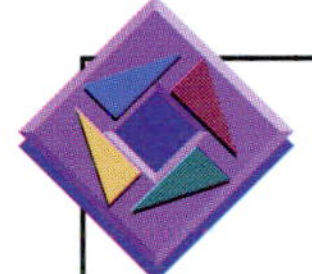

## 13

## Leg Press

**ACTION** From a sitting position with the knees flexed at about 90° and both feet on the footrest, fully extend the legs, then return slowly to the starting position.

**MUSCLES DEVELOPED** Quadriceps and gluteal muscles.

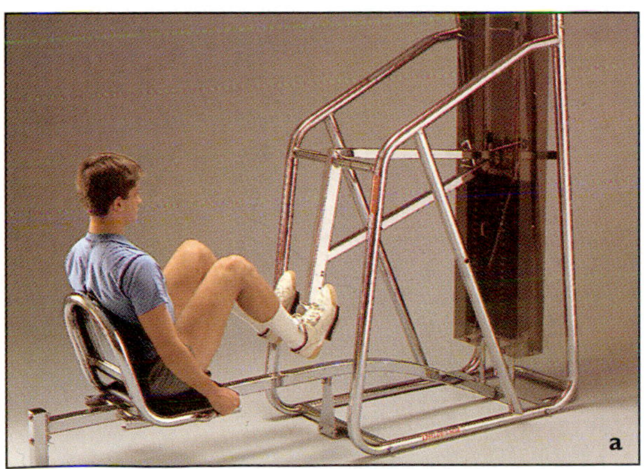

a

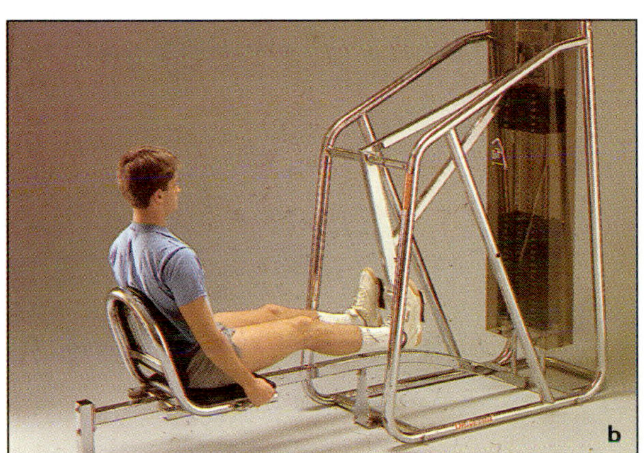

b

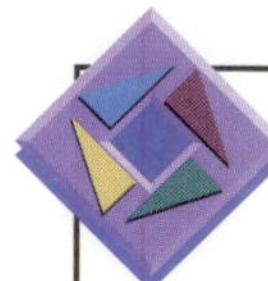

## 14
### Abdominal Curl-Up or Abdominal Crunch

SEE EXERCISE 4 IN THIS CHAPTER.

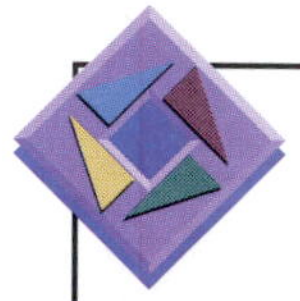

## 15
### Bench Press

**ACTION** Lie down on the bench with the head by the weight stack, the bench press bar above the chest, and keep the feet on the floor. Grasp the bar handles and press upward until the arms are completely extended, then return to the original position. Do not arch the back during this exercise. CAUTION: If you are susceptible to low back pain, place your feet on the bench.

**MUSCLES DEVELOPED** Pectoralis major, triceps, and deltoid.

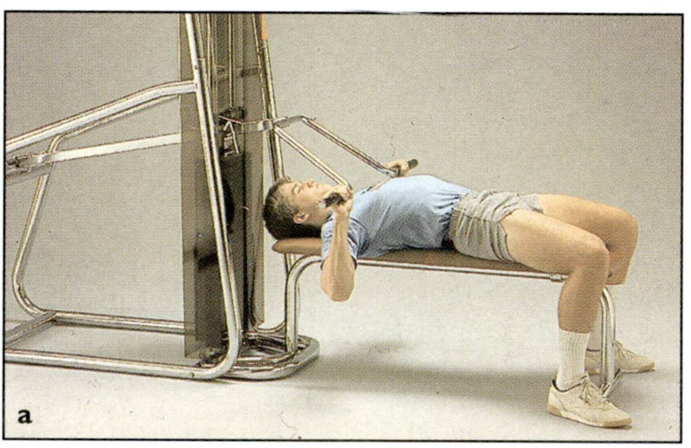
a

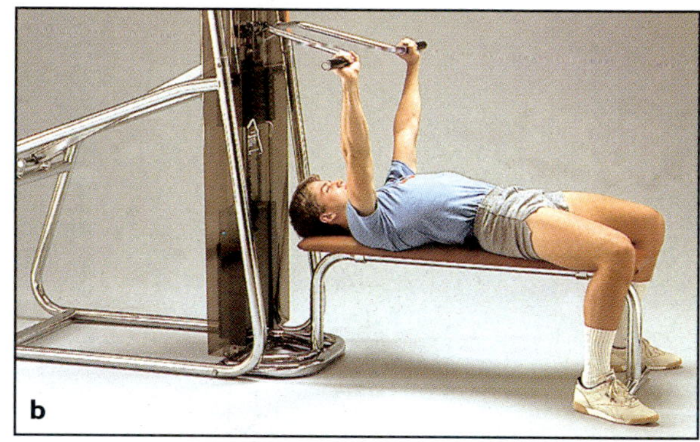
b

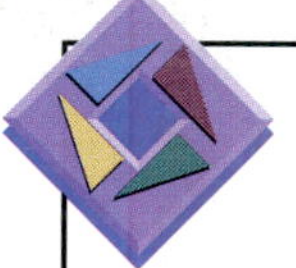

## 16
### Leg Curl

**ACTION** Lie with the face down on the bench, legs straight, and place the back of the feet under the padded bar. Curl up to at least 90°, and return to the original position.

**MUSCLES DEVELOPED** Hamstrings.

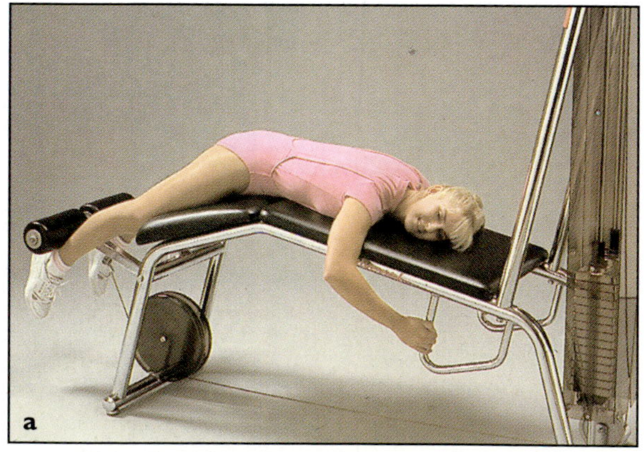
a

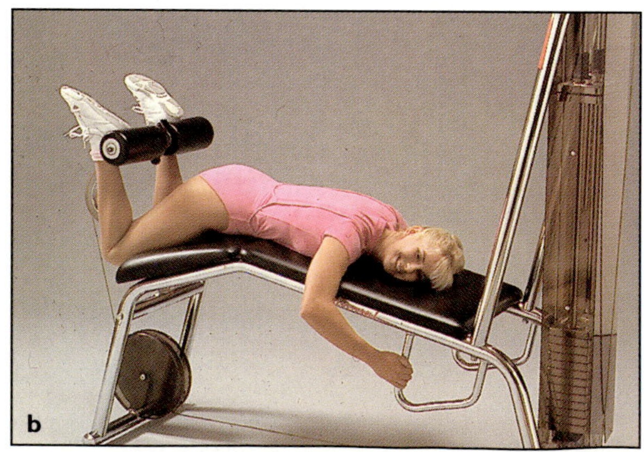
b

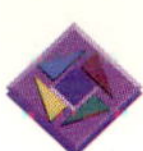

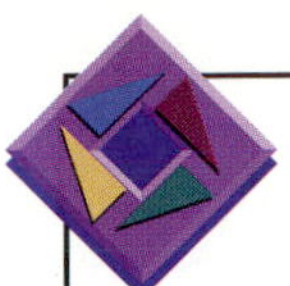

# 17

## Lat Pull-Down

**ACTION** Start from a sitting position, and hold the exercise bar with a wide grip. Pull the bar down until it touches the base of the neck, then return to the starting position (if a heavy resistance is used, stabilization of the body may be required by either using equipment as shown or by having someone else hold you down by the waist or shoulders).

**MUSCLES DEVELOPED** Latissimus dorsi, pectoralis major, and biceps.

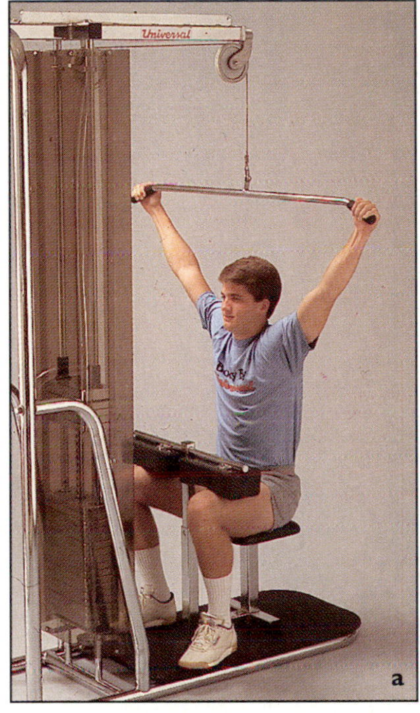
a

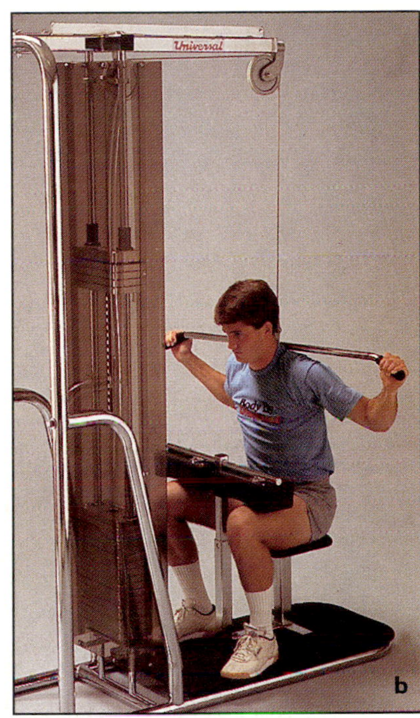
b

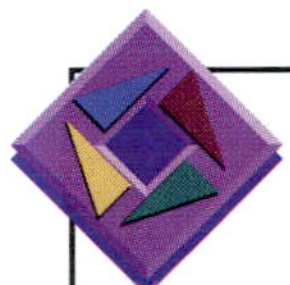

# 18

## Heel Raise

**ACTION** Start with your feet either flat on the floor or the front of the feet on an elevated block, then raise and lower yourself by moving at the ankle joint only. If additional resistance is needed, you can use a squat strength-training machine.

**MUSCLES DEVELOPED** Gastrocnemius and soleus.

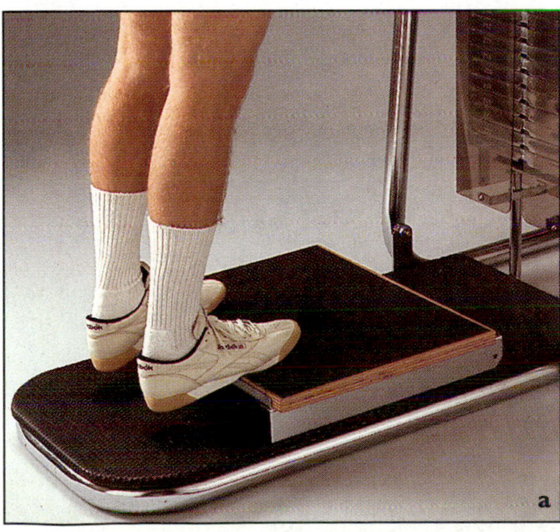
a

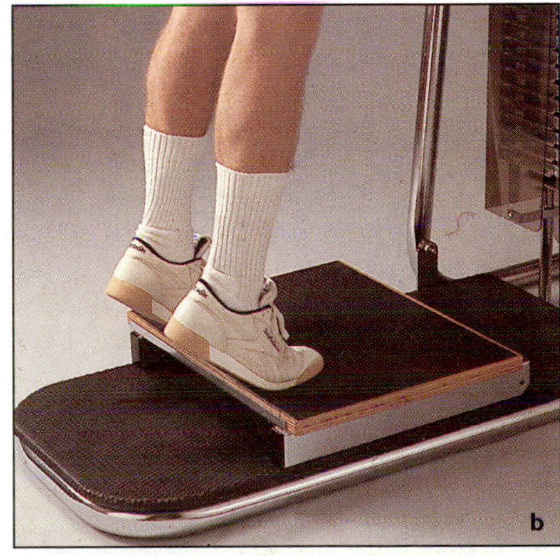
b

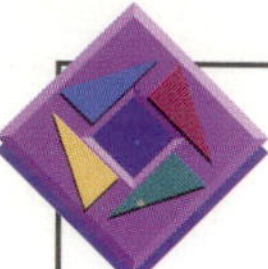

# 19
## Triceps Extension

**ACTION** Using a palms-down grip, grasp the bar slightly closer than shoulder width, and start wth the elbows almost completely bent. Fully extend the arms, then return to starting position.

**MUSCLES DEVELOPED**
Triceps.

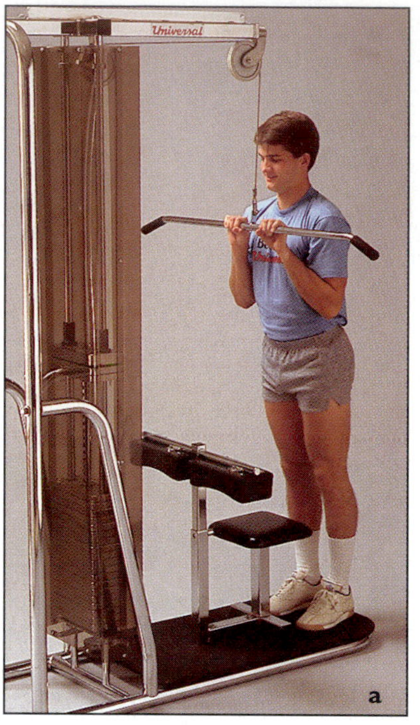

a

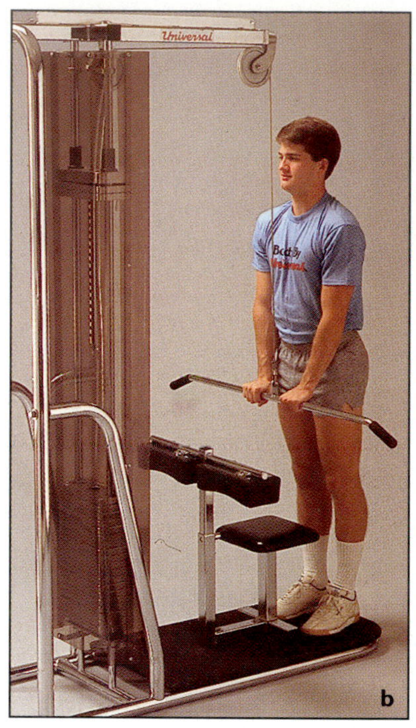

b

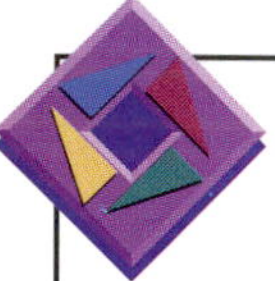

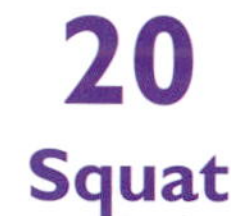

# 20
## Squat

**ACTION** Sit in an upright position with the feet under the padded bar and grasp the handles at the sides. Extend the legs until they are completely straight, then return to the starting position.

**MUSCLES DEVELOPED**
Quadriceps.

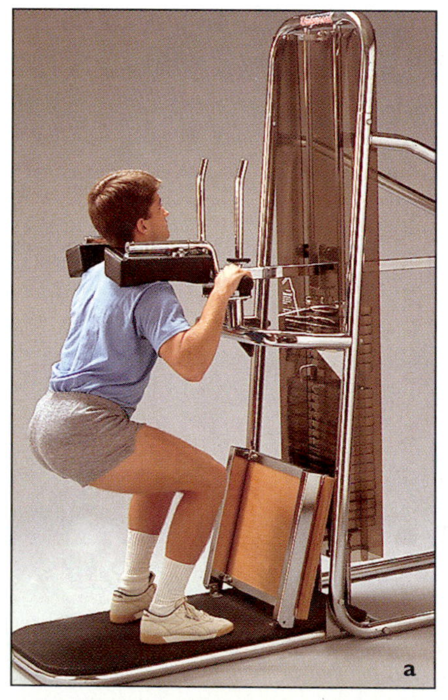
a

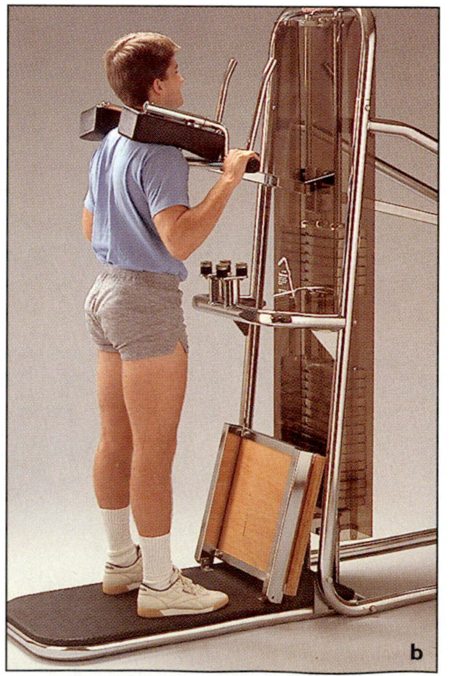
b

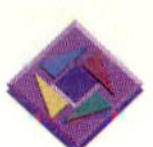

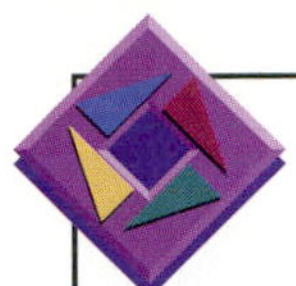

# 21
## Leg Extension

**ACTION** Sit in an upright position with the feet under the padded bar and grasp the handles at the sides. Extend the legs until they are completely straight, then return to the starting position.

**MUSCLES DEVELOPED** Quadriceps.

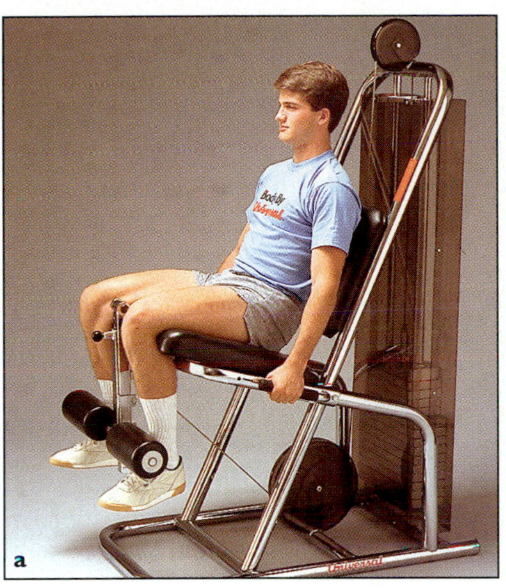
a

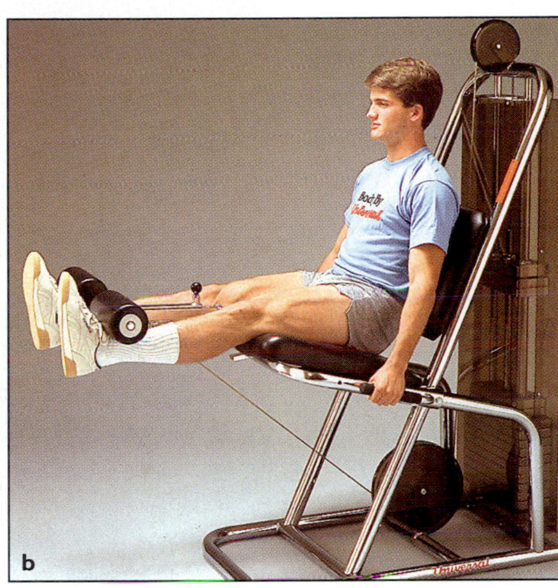
b

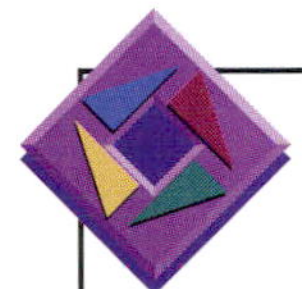

# 22
## Upright Rowing

**ACTION** Start with the arms extended and grip the handles with the palms down. Pull all the way up to the chin, then return to the starting position.

**MUSCLES DEVELOPED**
Biceps, brachioradialis, brachialis, deltoid, and trapezius.

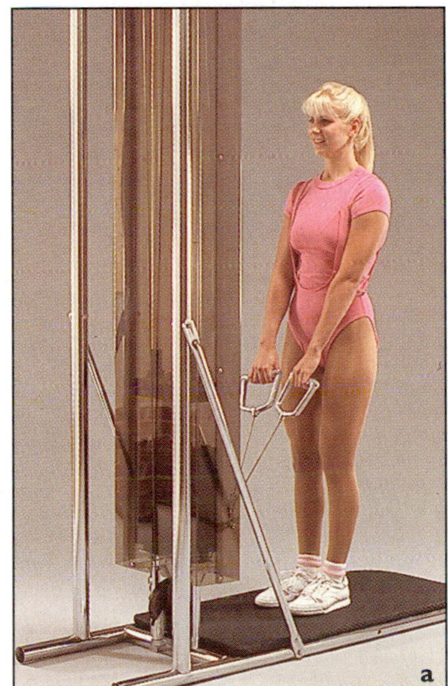
a

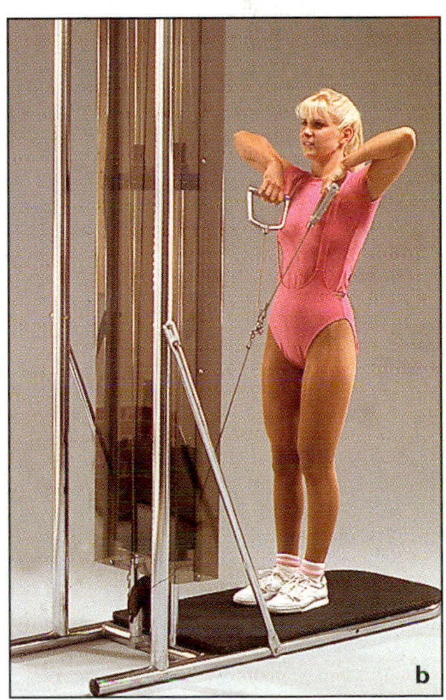
b

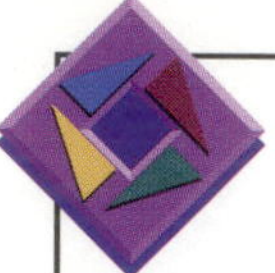

## 23

## Bent-arm Pullover

**ACTION** Sit back into the chair and grasp the bar behind your head. Pull the bar over your head all the way down to your abdomen and slowly return to the original position.

**MUSCLES DEVELOPED**
Latissimus dorsi, pectoral muscles, deltoid, and serratus anterior.

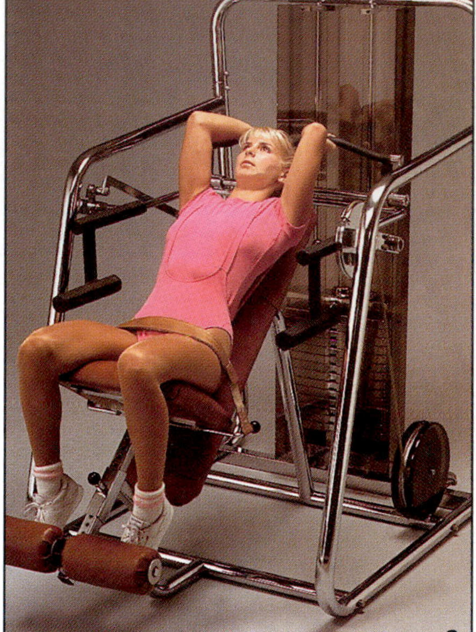

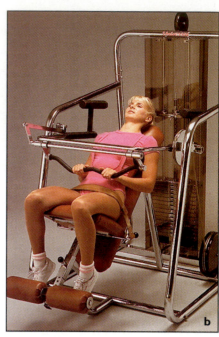


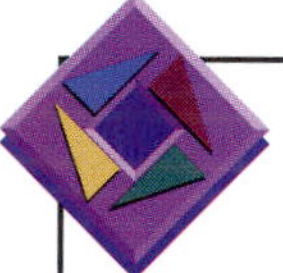

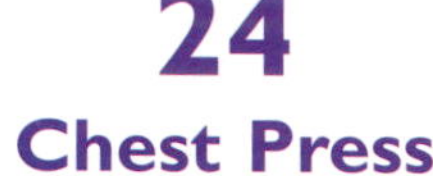

## 24

## Chest Press

**ACTION** Start with the arms to the side and elbows bent at 90°. Press your arms forward until the padded bars touch in front of your chest, then return to the starting position.

**MUSCLES DEVELOPED**
Pectoralis major and deltoid.

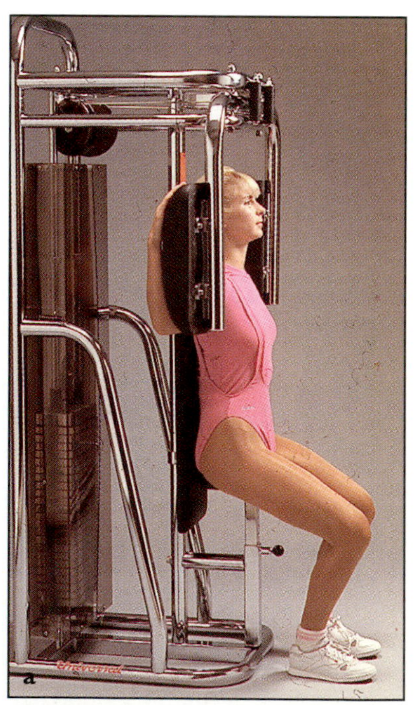


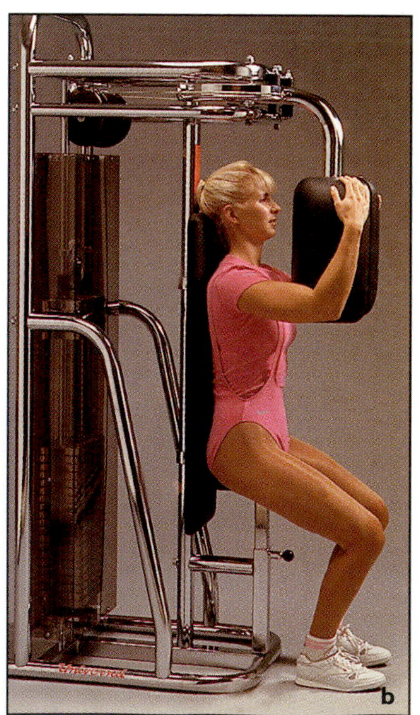

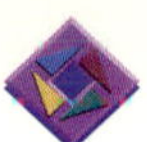

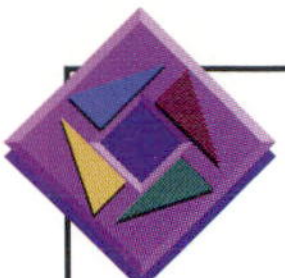

## 25
## Shoulder Press

**ACTION** Sit in an upright position and grasp the bar wider than the shoulder width. Press the bar all the way up until the arms are fully extended, then return to the initial position.

**MUSCLES DEVELOPED**
Triceps, deltoid, and pectoralis major.

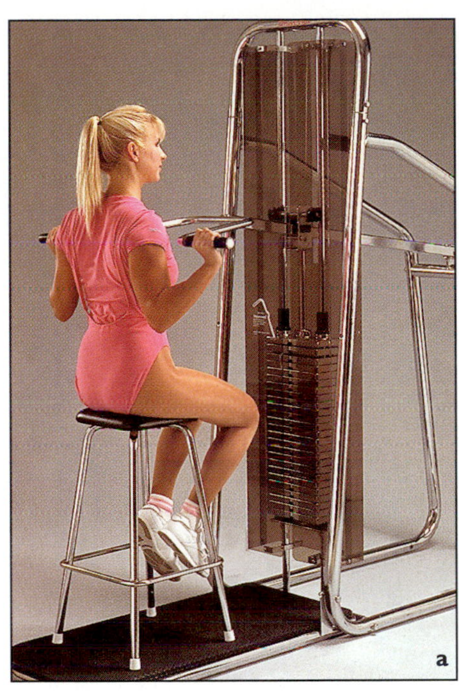
a

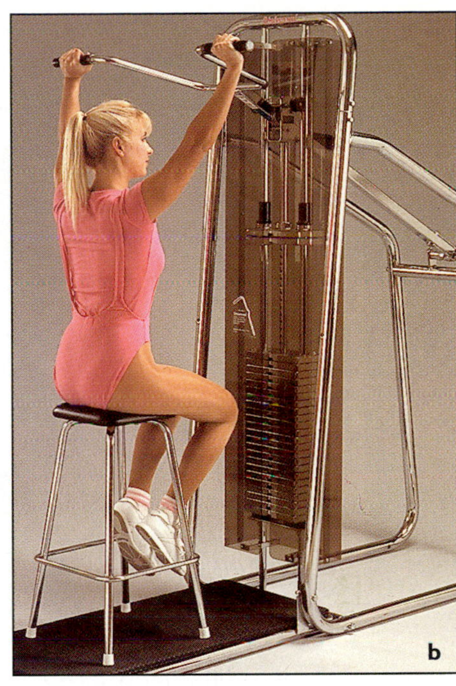
b

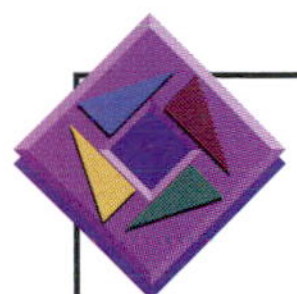

## 26
## Dip

**ACTION** Start with the elbows flexed, then fully extend the arms and slowly return to the initial position.

**MUSCLES DEVELOPED**
Triceps, deltoid, and pectoralis major.

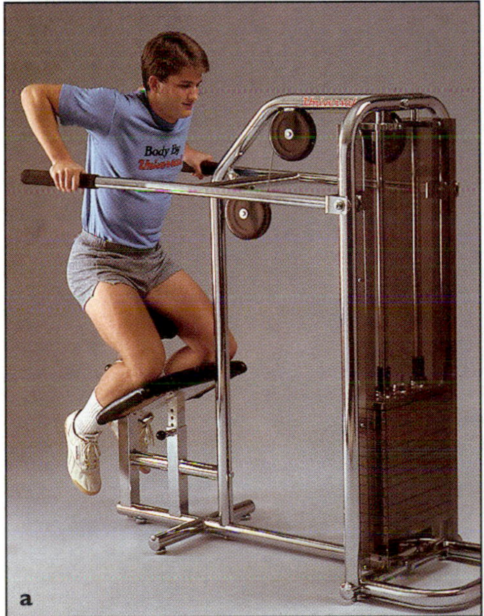

a

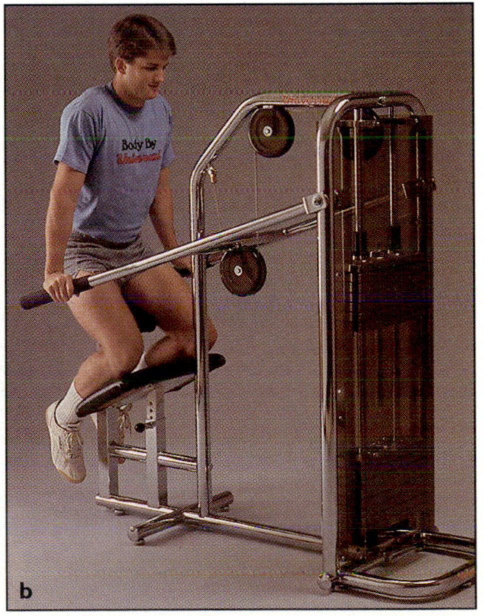

b

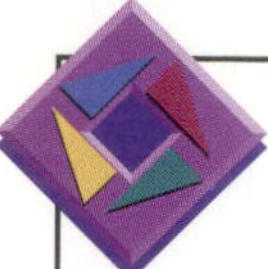

## 27
## Abdominal Crunch

**ACTION** Sit back into the machine and place the hands inside the straps as illustrated. Slowly crunch forward to a seated upright position, then return to the starting position.

**MUSCLES DEVELOPED** Abdominals.

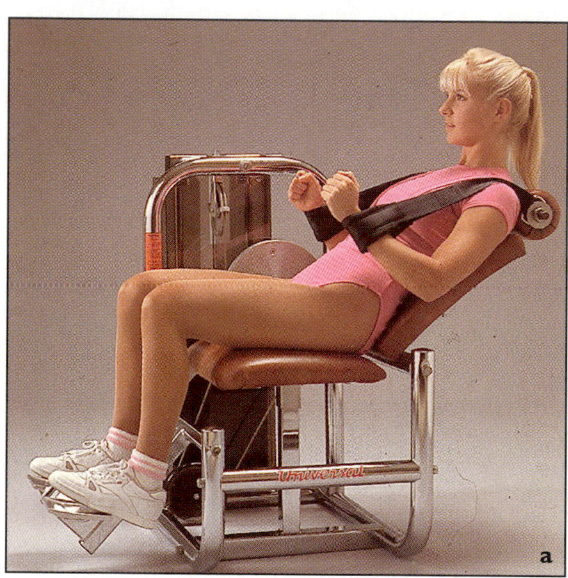
a

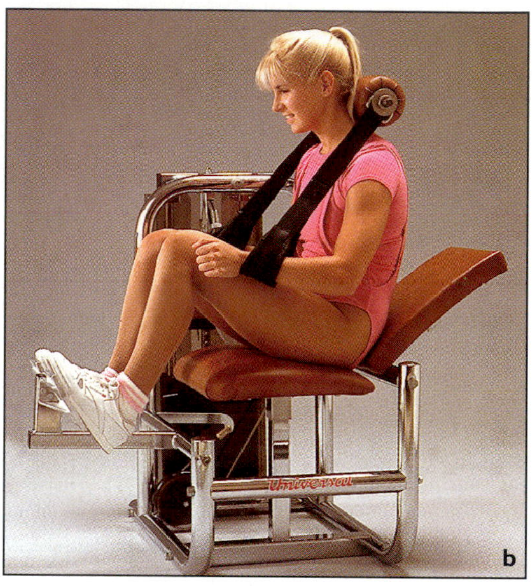
b

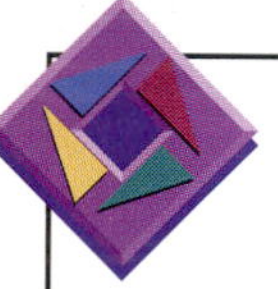

## 28
## Seated Back

**ACTION**
Sit in the machine with your trunk flexed and the upper back against the shoulder pad. Place the feet under the padded bar and hold on with your hands to the bars on the sides. Start the exercise by pressing backward, simultaneously extending the trunk and hip joints. Slowly return to the original position.

**MUSCLES DEVELOPED**
Erector spinae and gluteus maximus.

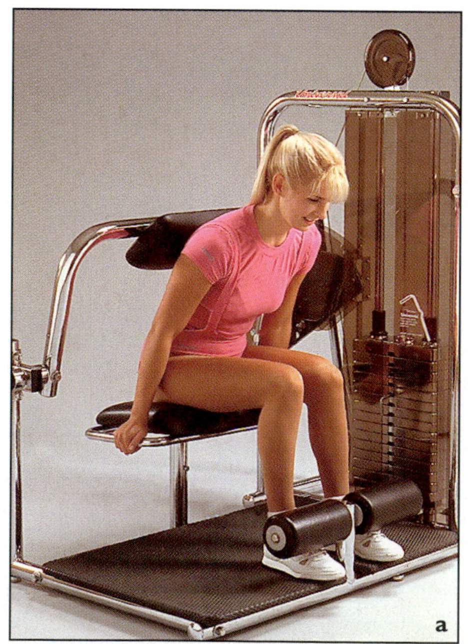
a

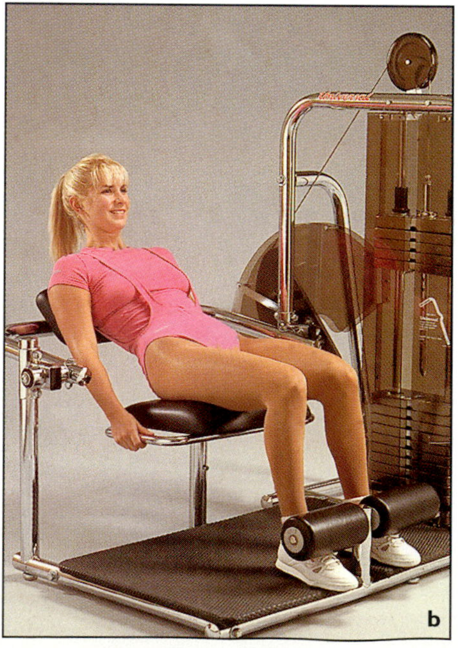
b

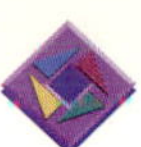

# Nautilus® Strength-Training Exercises

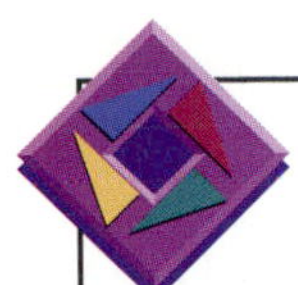

## 29

## Multi-Biceps (Arm Curl)

**ACTION** Sit into the machine and grasp the bar with the arms completely extended using a supinated or palms up grip. Curl up as far as possible and then return to the starting position.

**MUSCLES DEVELOPED**
Biceps, brachioradialis, and brachialis.

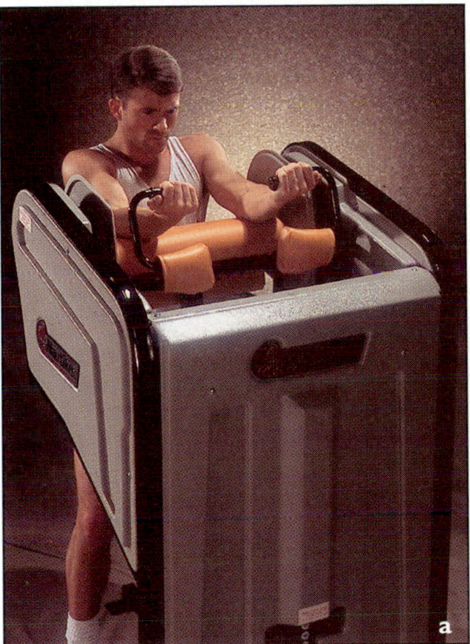

a

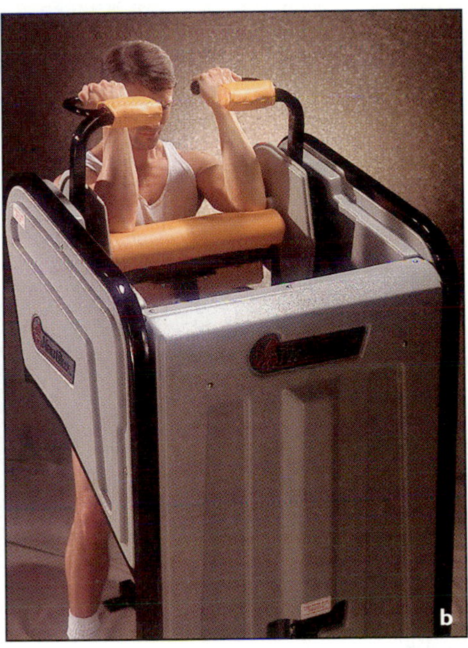

b

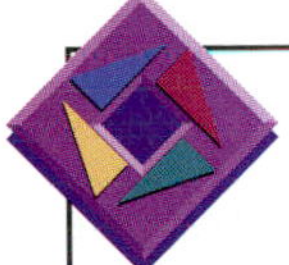

## 30

## Abdominal Crunch

**ACTION** Sit in an upright position and grasp the handles over your shoulders and crunch forward. Slowly return to the original position.

**MUSCLES DEVELOPED** Abdominals.

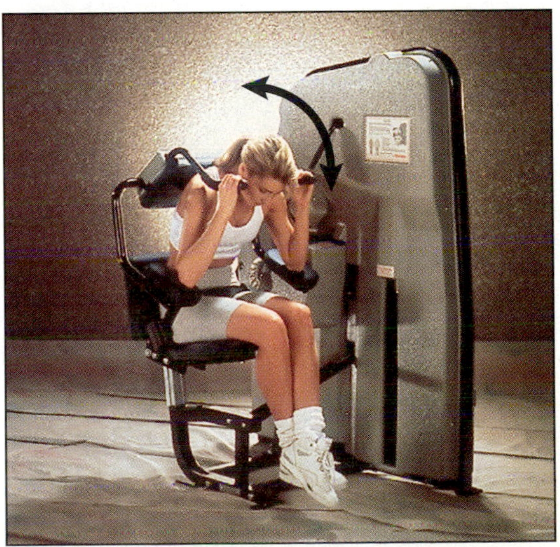

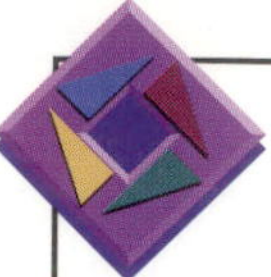

## 31

## Leg Extension

**ACTION** Sit in an upright position with the feet under the padded bar and grasp the handles at the sides. Extend the legs until they are completely straight, then return to the starting position.

**MUSCLES DEVELOPED** Quadriceps.

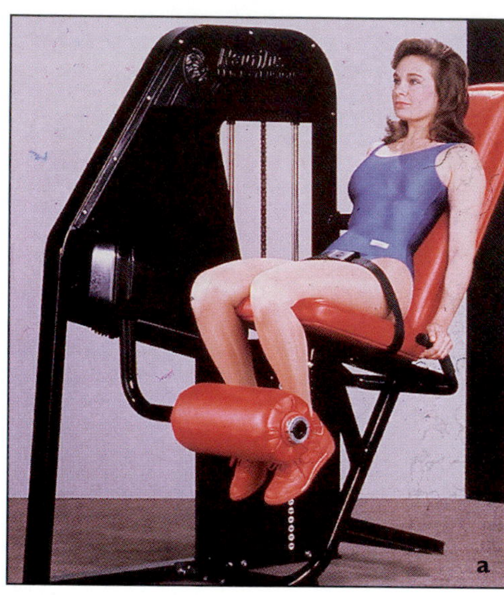
a

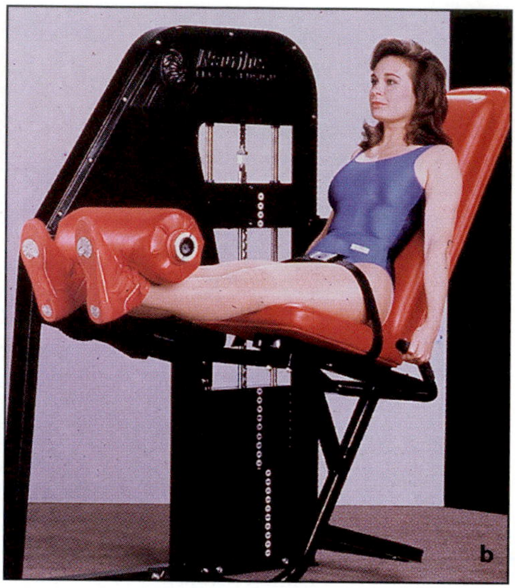
b

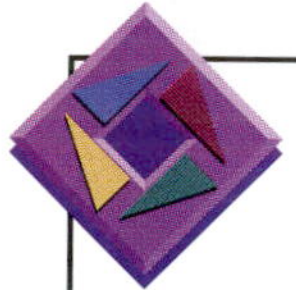

## 32

## Bench Press

**ACTION** Lie down on the bench with the head by the weight stack, the bench press bar above the chest, and the knees bent so the feet rest on the far end of the bench. Grasp the bar handles and press upward until the arms are completely extended, then return to the original position. Do not arch the back during this exercise.

**MUSCLES DEVELOPED** Pectoralis major, triceps, and deltoid.

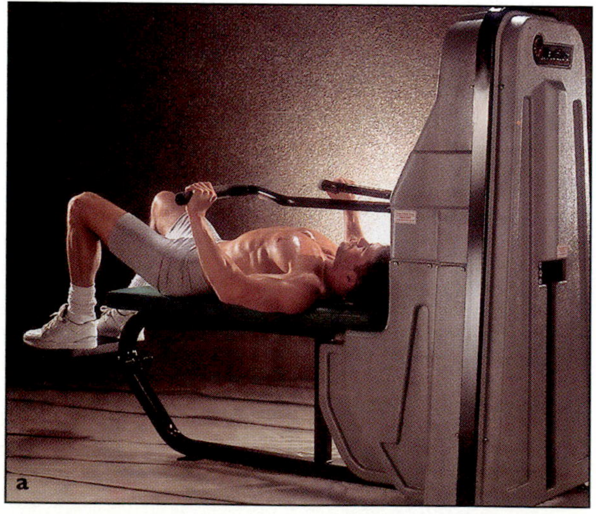
a

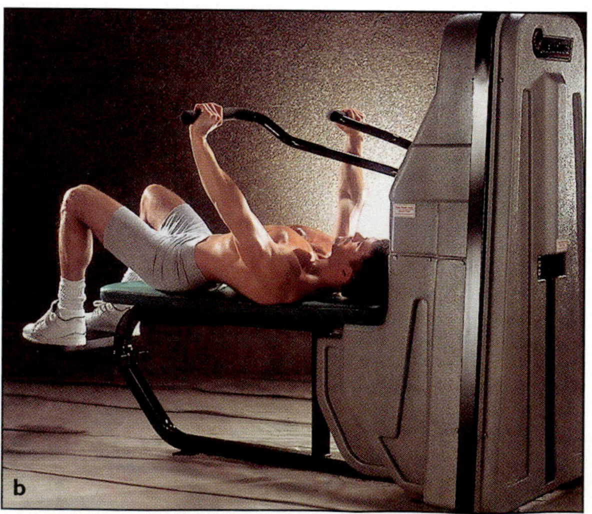
b

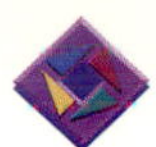

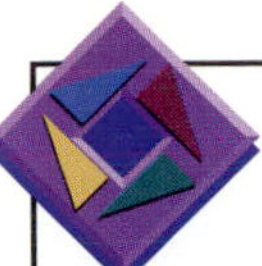

# 33

## Seated Leg Curl

**ACTION** Sit in the unit and place the strap over the upper thighs. With legs extended place the back of the feet over the padded rollers. Flex the knees until you reach a 90° to 100° angle. Slowly return to the starting position.

**MUSCLES DEVELOPED** Hamstrings.

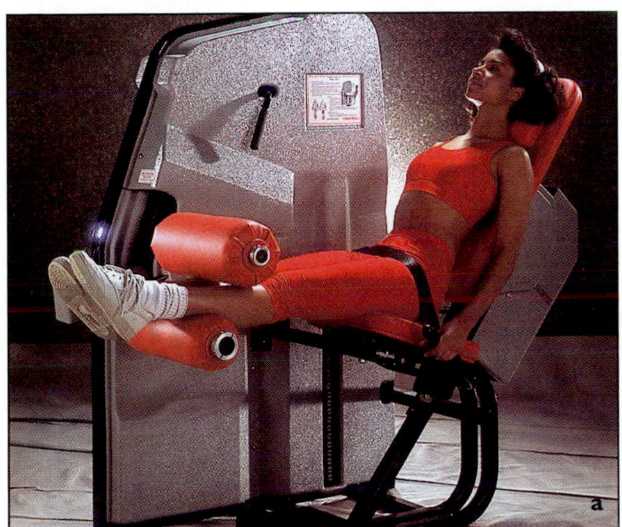
a

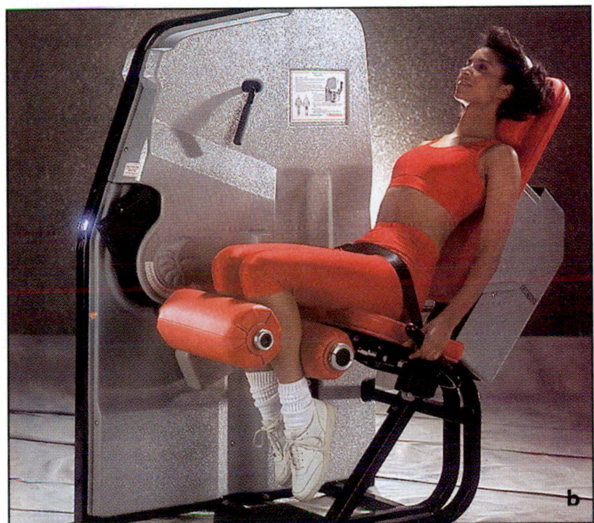
b

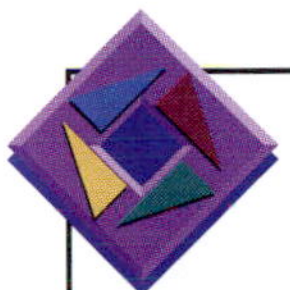

# 34

## Lower Back

**ACTION** Place yourself in the machine so that the front of the thigh and the upper back rest against the padded bars as illustrated. Slowly press backward against the padded bar until the back is fully extended. Slowly return to the original position.

**MUSCLES DEVELOPED** Erector spinae and gluteus maximus.

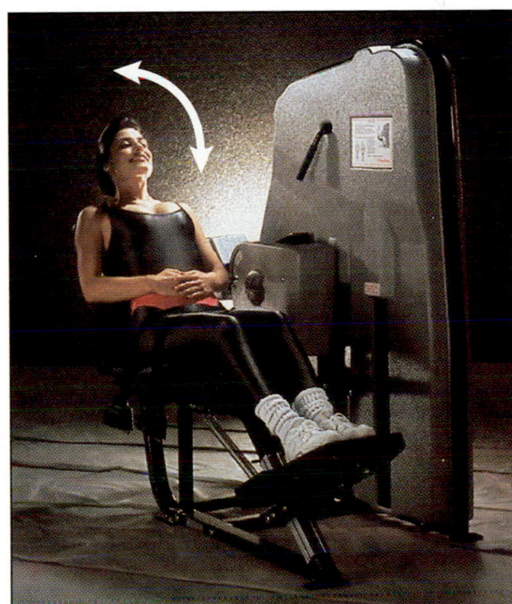

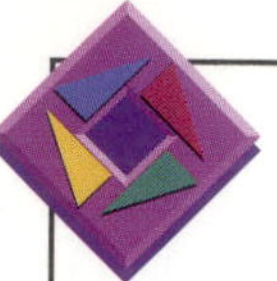

## 35
## Rowing Torso

**ACTION**
Sit in the machine with your arms in front of you, elbows bent and resting against the padded bars. Press back as far as possible, drawing the shoulder blades together. Return to the original position.

**MUSCLES DEVELOPED**
Posterior deltoid, rhomboids, and trapezius.

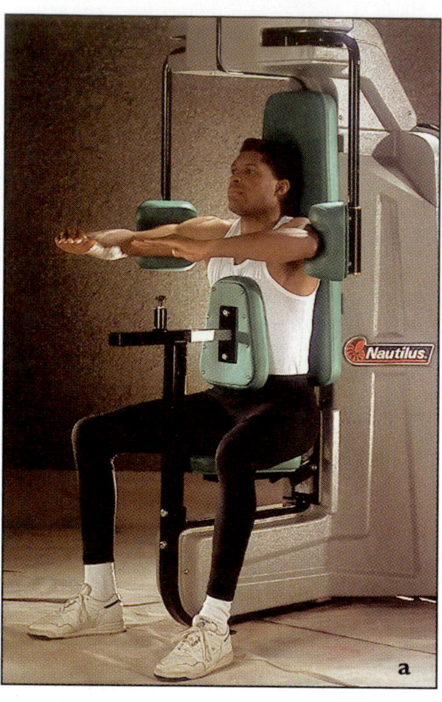


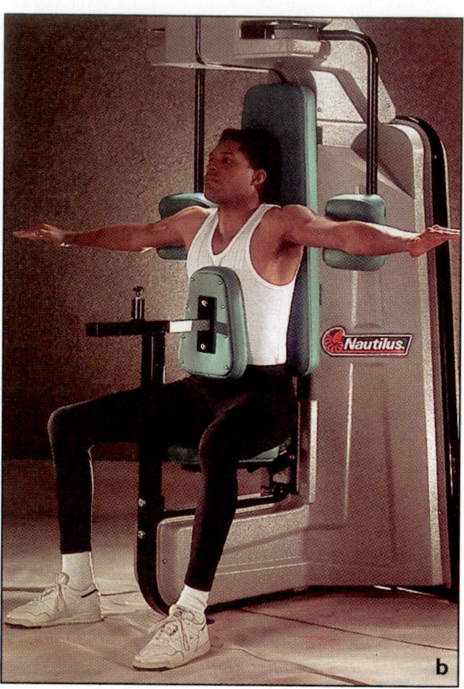


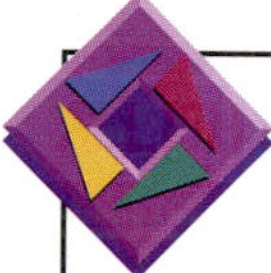

## 36
## Leg Press

**ACTION** From a sitting position with the knees flexed at about 90° and both feet on the footrest, fully extend the legs, then return slowly to the starting position.

**MUSCLES DEVELOPED**
Quadriceps and gluteal muscles.

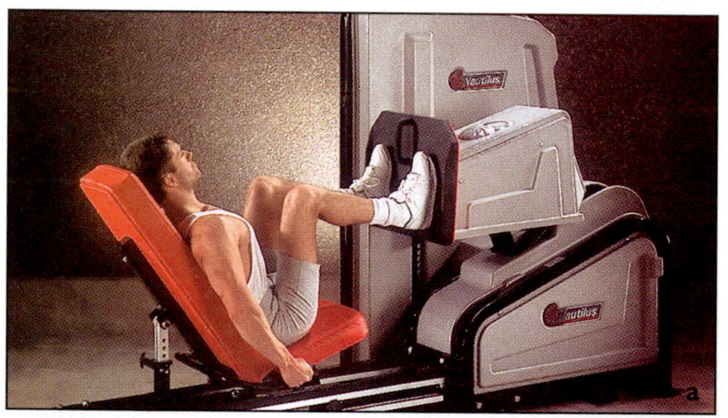


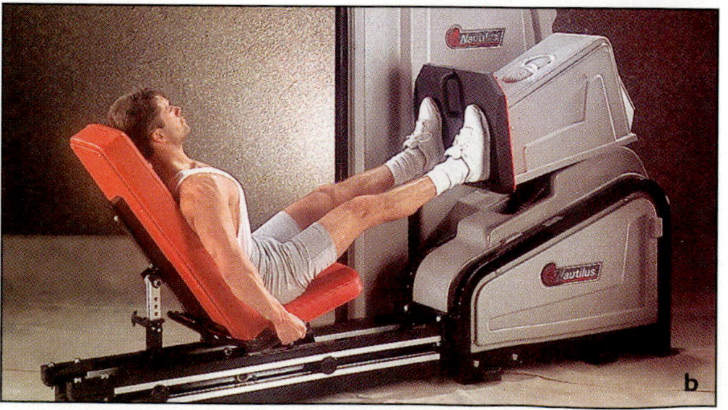

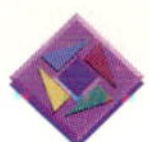

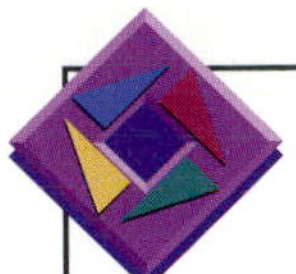

# 37
## Pullover

### ACTION
Sit back into the chair, arms bent, place the elbows against the padded end of the movement arm, and grasp the bar behind your head. Press forward and downward with your arms, pulling the bar over your head all the way down to your abdomen. Slowly return to the starting position.

### MUSCLES DEVELOPED
Latissimus dorsi, pectoral muscles, deltoid, and serratus anterior.

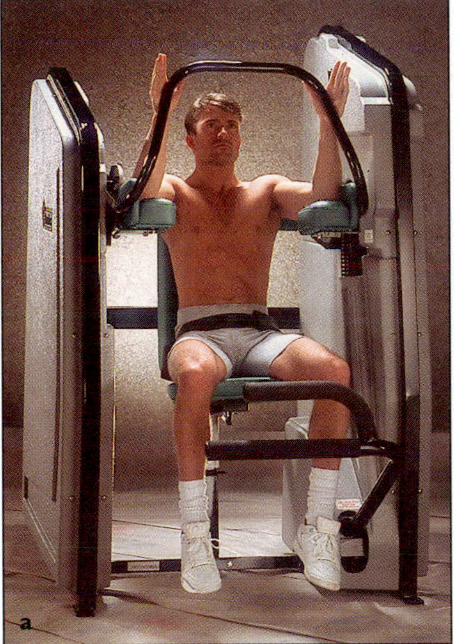
a

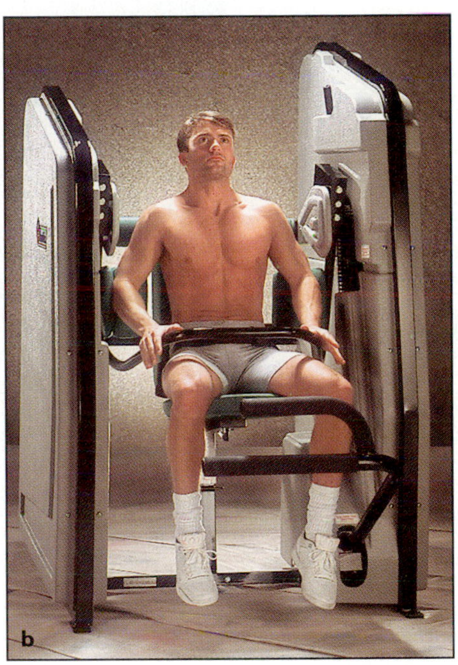
b

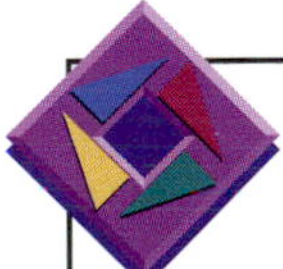

# 38
## Rotary Torso

### ACTION
Sit upright into the machine and place the elbows behind the padded bars. Rotate the torso as far as possible to one side and then slowly return to the starting position. Repeat the exercise to the opposite side.

### MUSCLES DEVELOPED
Internal and external obliques (abdominal muscles).

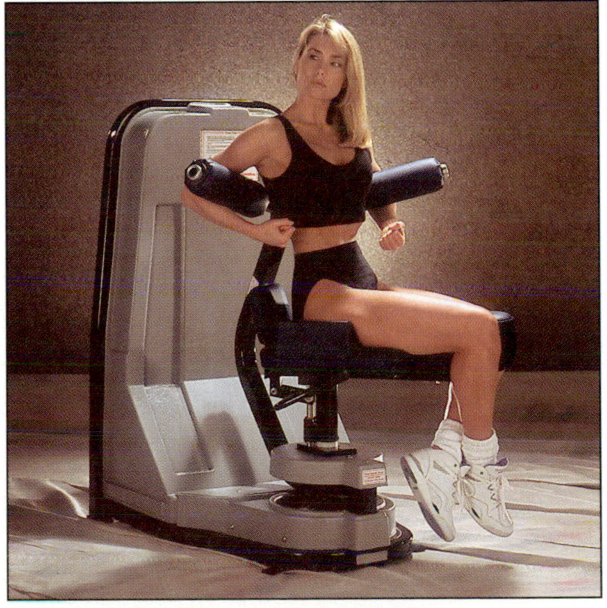

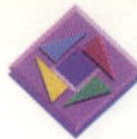



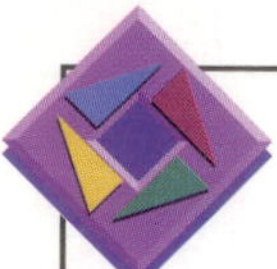

# 39
## Triceps Extension

**ACTION** Sit in an upright position, arms up, elbows bent, and place the little finger side of the hands and wrists against the pads (palms of the hands facing each other). Fully extend one arm at a time and then return to the original position. Repeat with the other arm.

**MUSCLES DEVELOPED**
Triceps.

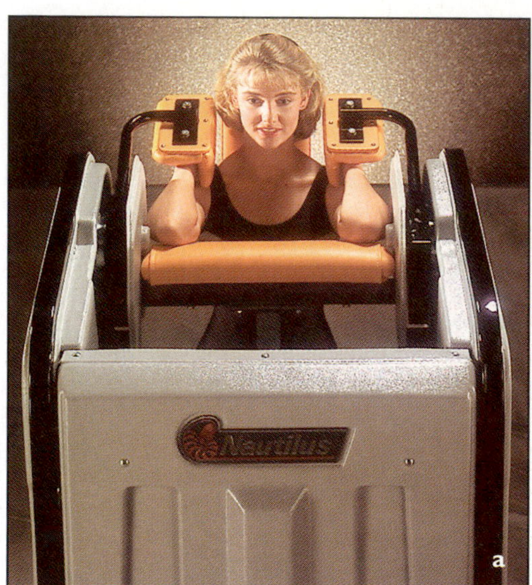


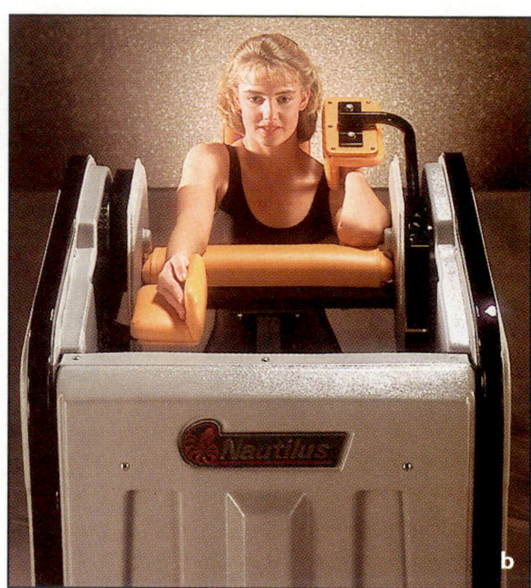


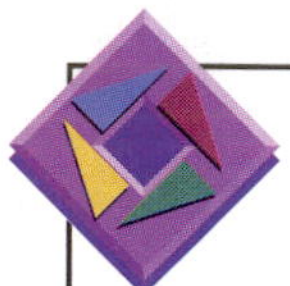

# 40
## Chest Press

**ACTION** Start with the arms up to the side, hands resting against the handle bars, and elbows bent at 90°. Press the movement arms forward as far as possible, leading with the elbows. Slowly return to the starting position.

**MUSCLES DEVELOPED** Pectoralis major and deltoid.

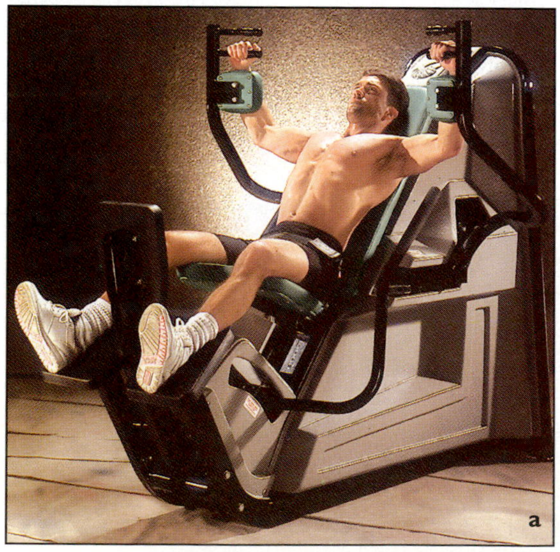


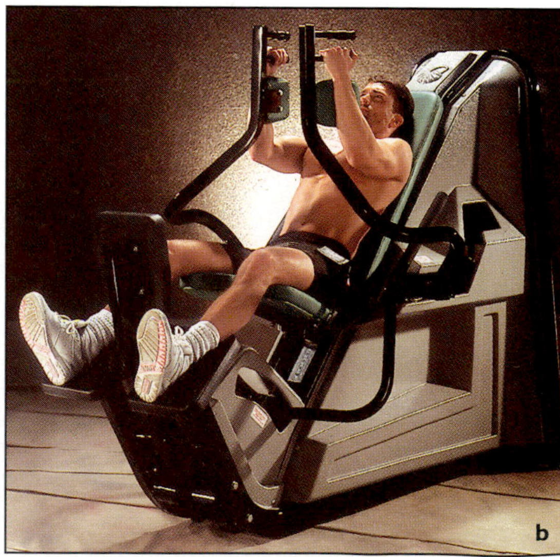

# Muscular Flexibility Assessment and Prescription

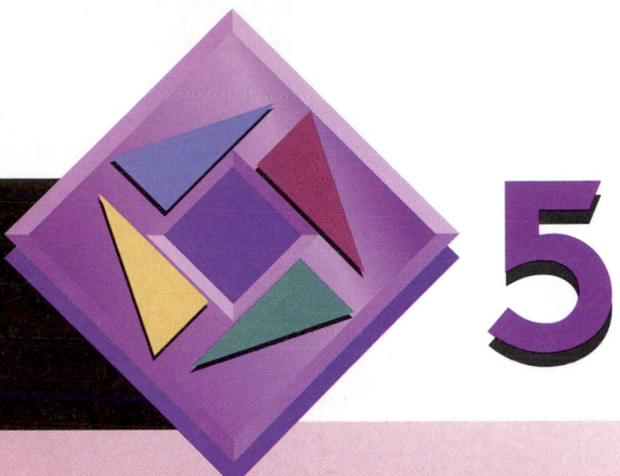


## Key Concepts

Flexibility
Range of motion
Specificity of flexibility
Plastic elongation
Elastic elongation
Modified Sit and Reach
Total Body Rotation
Shoulder Rotation
Ballistic stretching
Slow-sustained stretching
Proprioceptive neuromuscular facilitation (PNF)

## Objectives

- Understand the importance of muscular flexibility to adequate fitness and preventive health care.
- Identify the factors that affect muscular flexibility.
- Introduce a battery of muscular flexibility tests to assess overall body flexibility (Modified Sit and Reach Test, Body Rotation Test, Shoulder Rotation Test).
- Learn to interpret flexibility test results according to health fitness and physical fitness standards.
- Define ballistic stretching, slow-sustained stretching, and proprioceptive neuromuscular facilitation stretching.
- Understand the factors that contribute to the development of muscular flexibility.
- Become acquainted with a complete set of exercises for an overall body flexibility-development program.
- Be introduced to a program for the prevention and rehabilitation of low back pain.

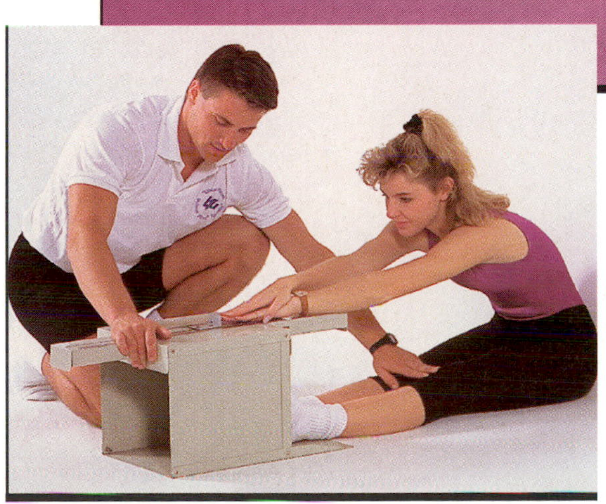

Flexibility is defined as *the ability of a joint to move freely through its full range of motion.* Health-care professionals and practitioners generally have underestimated and overlooked the contribution of good muscular flexibility to overall fitness and preventive health care.

In daily life we often have to make rapid or strenuous movements we are not accustomed to making, which may cause injury. Physical therapists have indicated that improper body mechanics often are the result of poor flexibility. Sports medicine specialists believe that many muscular/skeletal problems and injuries, especially in adults, may be related to a lack of flexibility.

Approximately 80% of all low back problems in the United States stems from improper alignment of the vertebral column and pelvic girdle, a direct result of inflexible and weak muscles. This backache syndrome costs American industry billions of dollars each year in lost productivity, health services, and worker's compensation.[1]

Improving and maintaining good range of motion in the joints is important to enhance the quality of life. Participating in a regular flexibility program will help a person maintain good joint mobility, increase resistance to muscle injury and soreness, prevent low-back and other spinal column problems, improve and maintain good postural alignment, promote proper and graceful body movement, improve personal appearance and self-image, and help to develop and maintain motor skills throughout life. In addition, flexibility exercises have been prescribed successfully to treat dysmenorrhea[2] (painful menstruation) and general neuromuscular tension (stress).

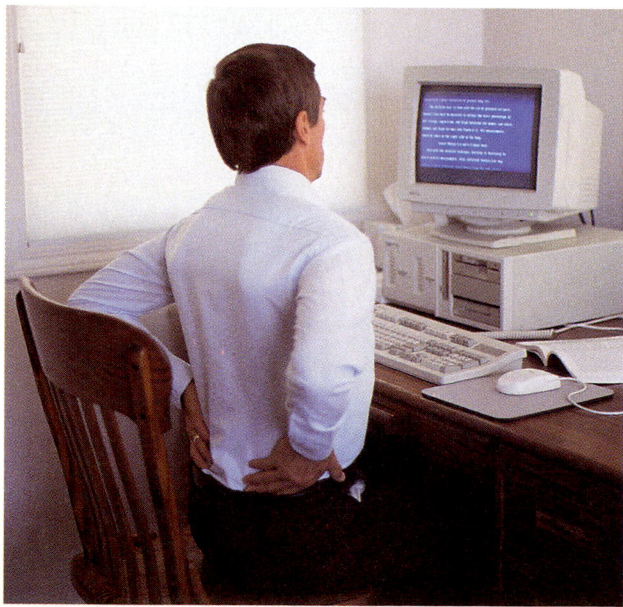

*Lack of physical conditioning frequently leads to chronic back pain.*

Further, stretching exercises, in conjunction with calisthenics, are helpful in warm-up routines to prepare the human body for more vigorous aerobic or strength training exercises, as well as cool-down routines following exercise to help the person return to a normal resting state. Fatigued muscles tend to contract to a shorter than average resting length, and stretching exercises help fatigued muscles reestablish their normal resting length.

Similar to muscular strength, good range of motion is critical in older life. Because of a lack of flexibility, some older adults are unable to perform simple daily tasks such as bending forward or turning. Many older adults do not turn their head or rotate their trunk to look over their shoulder but, rather, step around 90° to 180° to see behind them.

Physical activity and exercise also can be hampered severely by lack of good range of motion. Because of the pain involved with activity, older people who have tight hip flexors (muscles) cannot jog or walk very far. A vicious circle then ensues, because the condition usually worsens with further inactivity. A simple stretching program can alleviate or prevent this problem and help people return to an exercise program.

## FACTORS AFFECTING FLEXIBILITY

Total range of motion around a joint is highly specific and varies from one joint to another (hip, trunk, shoulder), as well as from one individual to the next. Muscular flexibility relates primarily to genetic factors and to physical activity. Beyond that, factors such as joint structure, ligaments, tendons, muscles, skin, tissue injury, adipose tissue (fat), body temperature, age, and sex influence range of motion about a joint. Because of the specificity of flexibility, indicating what constitutes an ideal level of flexibility is difficult. Nevertheless, flexibility is important to health and independent living.

The range of motion about a given joint depends mostly on the structure of that joint. Greater range of motion, however, can be attained through plastic and elastic elongation. *Plastic elongation is the permanent lengthening of soft tissue.* Even though joint capsules, ligaments, and tendons are

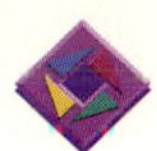

basically nonelastic, they can undergo plastic elongation. This permanent lengthening, accompanied by increases in range of motion, is best attained through slow-sustained stretching exercises.

*Elastic elongation is the temporary lengthening of soft tissue.* Muscle tissue has elastic properties and responds to stretching exercises by undergoing elastic or temporary lengthening. Elastic elongation increases the extensibility of the muscles.

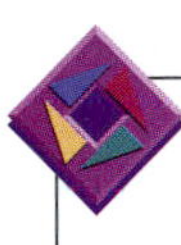

*Plastic elongation is permanent lengthening of soft tissue. Elastic elongation refers to temporary lengthening of soft tissue.*

Changes in muscle temperature can increase or decrease flexibility by as much as 20%. Properly warmed-up individuals have better flexibility than non-warmed-up people. Cool temperatures have the opposite effect, impeding joint range of motion. Because of the effects of temperature on muscular flexibility, many people prefer to do their stretching exercises after the aerobic phase of their workout. Aerobic activities raise body temperature, facilitating plastic elongation.

Another factor that influences flexibility is the amount of adipose (fat) tissue in and around joints and muscle tissue. A lot of adipose tissue not only increases resistance to movement but the added bulk also hampers joint mobility because of the contact between body surfaces.

On the average, women have more flexibility than men do, and they seem to retain this advantage throughout life. Aging does decrease the extensibility of soft tissue, though, resulting in less flexibility in both sexes.

The two most significant contributors to lower flexibility levels are sedentary living and lack of exercise. With less physical activity muscles lose their elasticity, and tendons and ligaments tighten and shorten. Inactivity also tends to be accompanied by an increase in adipose tissue, which further decreases joint range of motion. Finally, injury to muscle tissue, and tight skin from excessive scar tissue, has a negative effect on joint range of motion.

## ASSESSMENT OF FLEXIBILITY

Most of the flexibility tests developed over the years are specific to certain sports and are not practical for the general population. Their application in health and fitness programs is limited. For example, the Front-to-Rear Splits Test and the Bridge-Up Test may have applications in sports such as gymnastics and several track-and-field events, but they do not represent actions most people encounter in daily life.

Because of the lack of practical flexibility tests, most health/fitness centers have relied strictly on the Sit-and-Reach Test as an indicator of overall flexibility. This test measures flexibility of the hamstring muscles (back of the thigh) and, to a lesser extent, the lower back muscles.

Because flexibility is joint-specific and a lot of flexibility in one joint does not necessarily indicate the same is true in other joints, two additional tests — indicators of everyday movements such as reaching, bending, and turning — are included to determine your flexibility profile. These tests are the Total Body Rotation Test and the Shoulder Rotation Test.

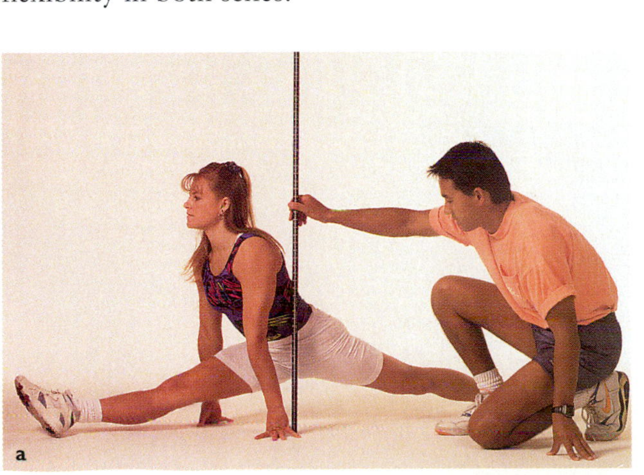


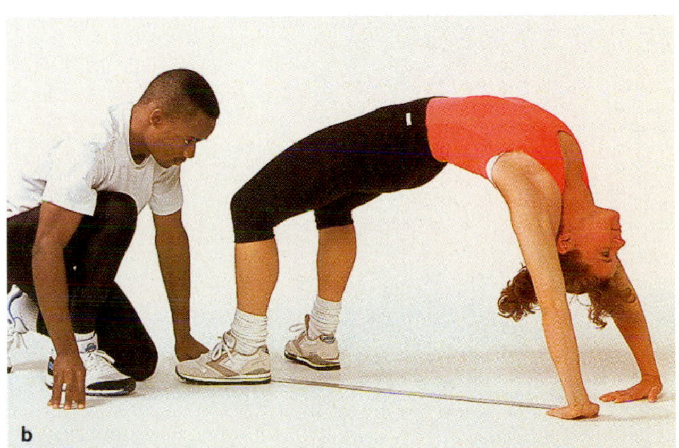


*Front-to-Rear Splits (A) and Bridge-Up (B) tests.*

The Sit-and-Reach Test has been modified from the traditional test. Unlike the traditional Sit-and-Reach Test, arm and leg lengths are taken into consideration to determine the score (see Figure 5.1a). In the original Sit-and-Reach Test, the 15" mark of the yardstick used to measure flexibility always is set at the edge of the box where the feet are placed. This does not take into consideration an individual with long arms and/or short legs or one with short arms and/or long legs, or both.[3,4,5] All other factors being equal, an individual with longer arms or shorter legs, or both, receives a better rating because of the structural advantage.

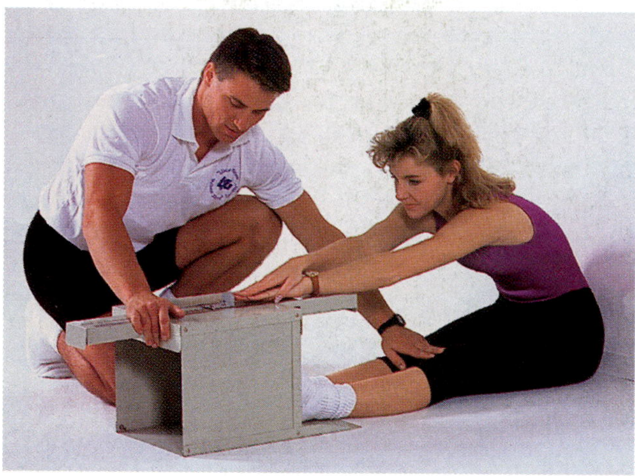

*Sit-and-Reach Test.*

The procedures and norms for the battery of flexibility tests are described in Figures 5.1 through 5.3 and Tables 5.1 through 5.3. For the flexibility profile, instead of a choice of tests, you should take all three tests. After obtaining your scores and percentile ranks for each test, you can determine the fitness category for each flexibility test using the guidelines given in Table 5.4.

## INTERPRETING FLEXIBILITY TEST RESULTS

After obtaining your scores and fitness ratings for each test, you can determine the fitness category for each flexibility test using the guidelines given in Table 5.4. You can use Figure 5.4 to record your flexibility fitness results. If you test your flexibility more than once, additional space is provided in this figure to record two separate sets of data. The overall flexibility fitness classification is obtained by computing an average percentile rank from all three tests and using the same guidelines given in Table 5.4. You also should record your overall flexibility results in the fitness and wellness profile given in Appendix A.

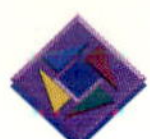

## MODIFIED SIT-AND-REACH TEST

To perform this test, you will need the Acuflex I* Sit-and-Reach Flexibility Tester, or you may simply place a yardstick on top of a box approximately 12" high.

1. Warm up properly before the first trial.
2. Remove your shoes for the test. Sit on the floor with the hips, back, and head against a wall; the legs fully extended; and the bottom of the feet against the Acuflex I or sit-and-reach box.
3. Place the hands one on top of the other, and reach forward as far as possible without letting the head and back come off the wall (the shoulders may be rounded as much as possible, but neither the head nor back should come off the wall at this time). The technician then can slide the reach indicator on the Acuflex I (or yardstick) along the top of the box until the end of the indicator touches the participant's fingers (see Figure 5.1a). The indicator then must be held firmly in place throughout the rest of the test.
4. Now your head and back can come off the wall. Gradually reach forward three times, the third time stretching forward as far as possible on the indicator (or yardstick) and holding the final position for at least 2 seconds. Be sure that during the test you keep the backs of the knees flat against the floor.
5. Record the final number of inches reached to the nearest one-half inch.

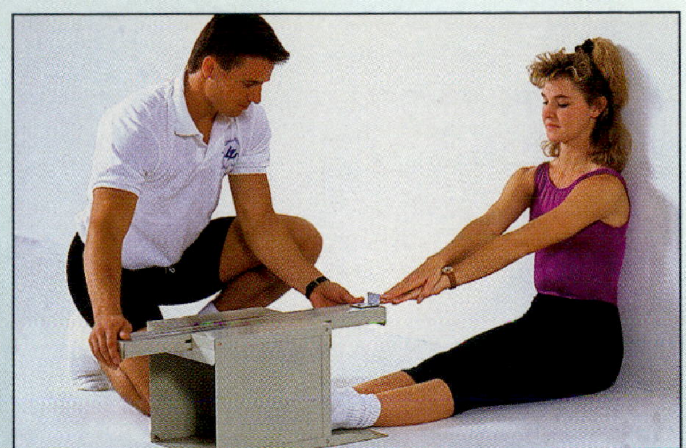

**FIGURE 5.1a** ◆ Determining the starting position for Sit-and-Reach Test.

You are allowed two trials, and an average of the two scores is used as the final test score. The respective percentile ranks and fitness categories for this test are given in Tables 5.1 and 5.4.

*The Acuflex I Flexibility Tester for the Modified Sit-and-Reach Test can be obtained from Figure Finder Collection, Novel Products, P. O. Box 408, Rockton, IL 61072-0480. Phone: 800-323-5143, FAX 815-624-4866.

**FIGURE 5.1** ◆ Procedure for the Modified Sit-and-Reach Test.

**TABLE 5.1**
**Percentile Ranks for Modified Sit-and-Reach Test**

| | Percentile Rank | Age Category ≤18 | 19–35 | 36–49 | ≥50 | | Percentile Rank | Age Category ≤18 | 19–35 | 36–49 | ≥50 |
|---|---|---|---|---|---|---|---|---|---|---|---|
| | 99 | 20.8 | 20.1 | 18.9 | 16.2 | | 99 | 22.6 | 21.0 | 19.8 | 17.2 |
| | 95 | 19.6 | 18.9 | 18.2 | 15.8 | | 95 | 19.5 | 19.3 | 19.2 | 15.7 |
| | 90 | 18.2 | 17.2 | 16.1 | 15.0 | | 90 | 18.7 | 17.9 | 17.4 | 15.0 |
| | 80 | 17.8 | 17.0 | 14.6 | 13.3 | | 80 | 17.8 | 16.7 | 16.2 | 14.2 |
| | 70 | 16.0 | 15.8 | 13.9 | 12.3 | | 70 | 16.5 | 16.2 | 15.2 | 13.6 |
| | 60 | 15.2 | 15.0 | 13.4 | 11.5 | | 60 | 16.0 | 15.8 | 14.5 | 12.3 |
| Men | 50 | 14.5 | 14.4 | 12.6 | 10.2 | Women | 50 | 15.2 | 14.8 | 13.5 | 11.1 |
| | 40 | 14.0 | 13.5 | 11.6 | 9.7 | | 40 | 14.5 | 14.5 | 12.8 | 10.1 |
| | 30 | 13.4 | 13.0 | 10.8 | 9.3 | | 30 | 13.7 | 13.7 | 12.2 | 9.2 |
| | 20 | 11.8 | 11.6 | 9.9 | 8.8 | | 20 | 12.6 | 12.6 | 11.0 | 8.3 |
| | 10 | 9.5 | 9.2 | 8.3 | 7.8 | | 10 | 11.4 | 10.1 | 9.7 | 7.5 |
| | 05 | 8.4 | 7.9 | 7.0 | 7.2 | | 05 | 9.4 | 8.1 | 8.5 | 3.7 |
| | 01 | 7.2 | 7.0 | 5.1 | 4.0 | | 01 | 6.5 | 2.6 | 2.0 | 1.5 |

High physical fitness standard (percentiles 70–99)
Health fitness standard (percentiles 50–60)

## TOTAL BODY ROTATION TEST

An Acuflex II* Total Body Rotation Flexibility Tester or a measuring scale with a sliding panel is needed to administer this test. The Acuflex II or scale is placed on the wall at shoulder height and should be adjustable to accommodate individual differences in height. If you need to build your own scale, use two measuring tapes and glue them above and below the sliding panel centered at the 15" mark. Each tape should be at least 30" long. If no sliding panel is available, simply tape the measuring tapes onto a wall. A line also must be drawn on the floor and centered with the 15" mark.

1. Warm up properly before beginning this test.
2. Stand sideways, an arm's length away from the wall, with the feet straight ahead, slightly separated, and the toes right up to the corresponding line drawn on the floor. Hold out the arm opposite to the wall horizontally from the body, making a fist with the hand. The Acuflex II, measuring scale, or tapes should be shoulder height at this time.
3. Rotate the trunk, the extended arm going backward (always maintaining a horizontal plane) and making contact with the panel, gradually sliding it forward as far as possible. If no panel is available, slide the fist alongside the tapes as far as possible. Hold the final position at least 2 seconds. Position the hand with the little finger side forward during the entire sliding movement as illustrated in Figure 5.2e. **Proper hand position is crucial. Many people attempt to open the hand, or push with extended fingers, or slide the panel with the knuckles — none of which is acceptable**. During the test the knees can be slightly bent, but **the feet cannot be moved, always pointing straight forward**. The body must be kept as straight (vertical) as possible.
4. Conduct the test on either the right or the left side of the body. Perform two trials on the selected side. Record the farthest point reached, measured to the nearest half inch and held for at least 2 seconds. Use the average of the two trials as the final test score. Referring to Tables 5.2 and 5.4, determine the percentile rank and flexibility fitness classification for this test.

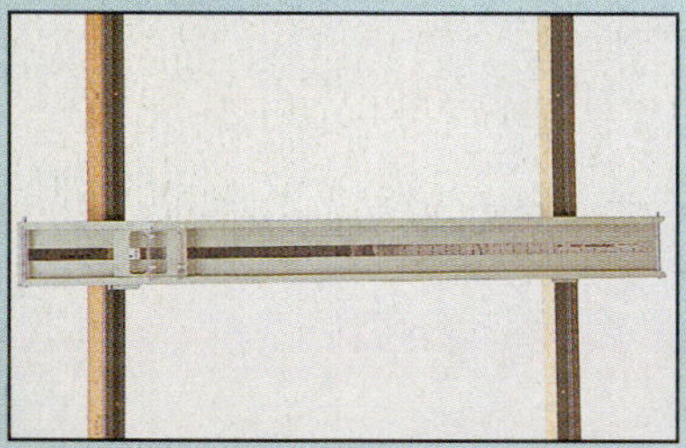

**FIGURE 5.2a** ◆ Acuflex II measuring device for the Total Body Rotation Test.

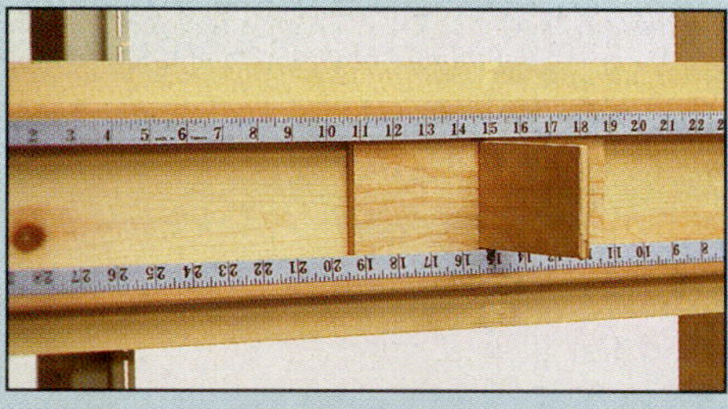

**FIGURE 5.2b** ◆ Homemade measuring device for the Total Body Rotation Test.

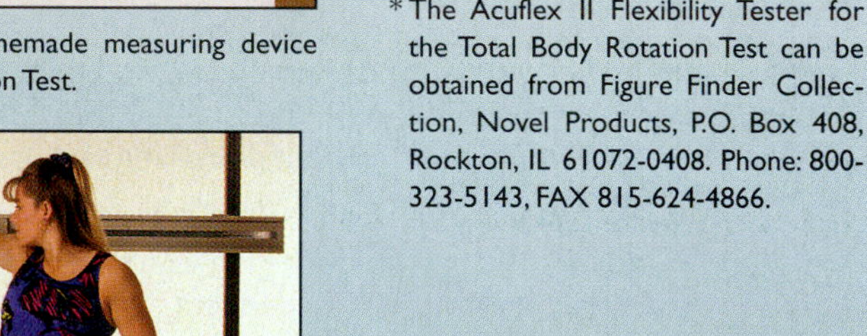

*The Acuflex II Flexibility Tester for the Total Body Rotation Test can be obtained from Figure Finder Collection, Novel Products, P.O. Box 408, Rockton, IL 61072-0408. Phone: 800-323-5143, FAX 815-624-4866.

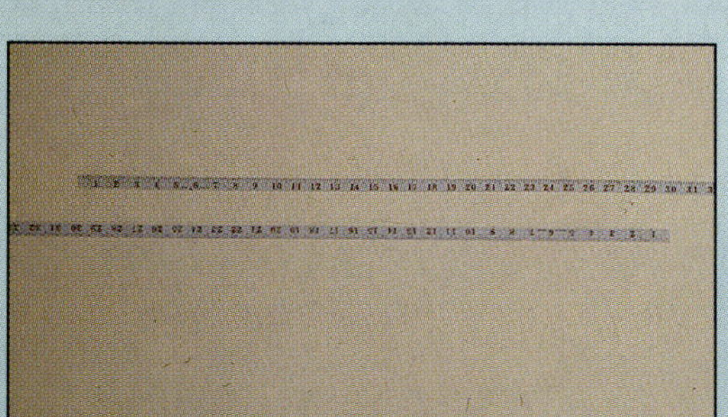

**FIGURE 5.2c** ◆ Measuring tapes for the Total Body Rotation Test.

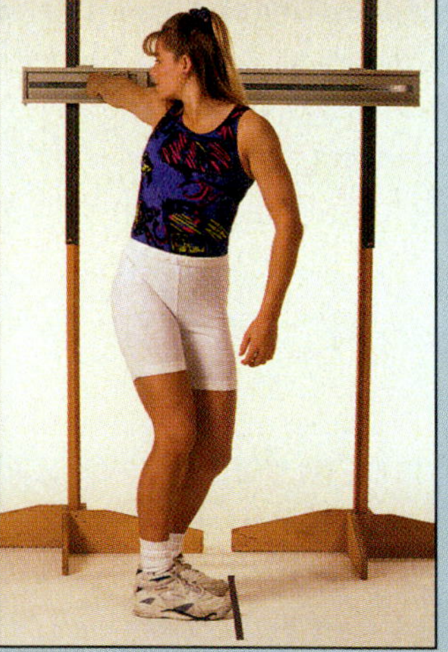

**FIGURE 5.2d** ◆ Total Body Rotation Test.

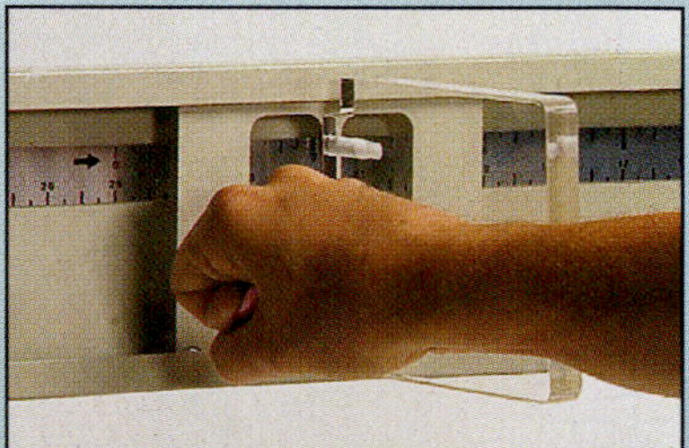

**FIGURE 5.2e** ◆ Proper hand position for the Total Body Rotation Test.

**FIGURE 5.2** ◆ Procedure for Total Body Rotation Test.

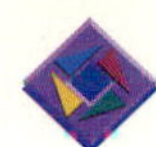

**TABLE 5.2**
**Percentile Ranks for Total Body Rotation Test**

| | Percentile Rank | Left Rotation ≤18 | Left Rotation 19–35 | Left Rotation 36–49 | Left Rotation ≥50 | Right Rotation ≤18 | Right Rotation 19–35 | Right Rotation 36–49 | Right Rotation ≥50 |
|---|---|---|---|---|---|---|---|---|---|
| Men | 99 | 29.1 | 28.0 | 26.6 | 21.0 | 28.2 | 27.8 | 25.2 | 22.2 |
| | 95 | 26.6 | 24.8 | 24.5 | 20.0 | 25.5 | 25.6 | 23.8 | 20.7 |
| | 90 | 25.0 | 23.6 | 23.0 | 17.7 | 24.3 | 24.1 | 22.5 | 19.3 |
| | 80 | 22.0 | 22.0 | 21.2 | 15.5 | 22.7 | 22.3 | 21.0 | 16.3 |
| | 70 | 20.9 | 20.3 | 20.4 | 14.7 | 21.3 | 20.7 | 18.7 | 15.7 |
| | 60 | 19.9 | 19.3 | 18.7 | 13.9 | 19.8 | 19.0 | 17.3 | 14.7 |
| | 50 | 18.6 | 18.0 | 16.7 | 12.7 | 19.0 | 17.2 | 16.3 | 12.3 |
| | 40 | 17.0 | 16.8 | 15.3 | 11.7 | 17.3 | 16.3 | 14.7 | 11.5 |
| | 30 | 14.9 | 15.0 | 14.8 | 10.3 | 15.1 | 15.0 | 13.3 | 10.7 |
| | 20 | 13.8 | 13.3 | 13.7 | 9.5 | 12.9 | 13.3 | 11.2 | 8.7 |
| | 10 | 10.8 | 10.5 | 10.8 | 4.3 | 10.8 | 11.3 | 8.0 | 2.7 |
| | 05 | 8.5 | 8.9 | 8.8 | 0.3 | 8.1 | 8.3 | 5.5 | 0.3 |
| | 01 | 3.4 | 1.7 | 5.1 | 0.0 | 6.6 | 2.9 | 2.0 | 0.0 |
| Women | 99 | 29.3 | 28.6 | 27.1 | 23.0 | 29.6 | 29.4 | 27.1 | 21.7 |
| | 95 | 26.8 | 24.8 | 25.3 | 21.4 | 27.6 | 25.3 | 25.9 | 19.7 |
| | 90 | 25.5 | 23.0 | 23.4 | 20.5 | 25.8 | 23.0 | 21.3 | 19.0 |
| | 80 | 23.8 | 21.5 | 20.2 | 19.1 | 23.7 | 20.8 | 19.6 | 17.9 |
| | 70 | 21.8 | 20.5 | 18.6 | 17.3 | 22.0 | 19.3 | 17.3 | 16.8 |
| | 60 | 20.5 | 19.3 | 17.7 | 16.0 | 20.8 | 18.0 | 16.5 | 15.6 |
| | 50 | 19.5 | 18.0 | 16.4 | 14.8 | 19.5 | 17.3 | 14.6 | 14.0 |
| | 40 | 18.5 | 17.2 | 14.8 | 13.7 | 18.3 | 16.0 | 13.1 | 12.8 |
| | 30 | 17.1 | 15.7 | 13.6 | 10.0 | 16.3 | 15.2 | 11.7 | 8.5 |
| | 20 | 16.0 | 15.2 | 11.6 | 6.3 | 14.5 | 14.0 | 9.8 | 3.9 |
| | 10 | 12.8 | 13.6 | 8.5 | 3.0 | 12.4 | 11.1 | 6.1 | 2.2 |
| | 05 | 11.1 | 7.3 | 6.8 | 0.7 | 10.2 | 8.8 | 4.0 | 1.1 |
| | 01 | 8.9 | 5.3 | 4.3 | 0.0 | 8.9 | 3.2 | 2.8 | 0.0 |

High physical fitness standard (percentile ranks 99–70)
Health fitness standard (percentile ranks 60–50)

## SHOULDER ROTATION TEST

This test can be done using the Acuflex III* Flexibility Tester, which consists of a shoulder caliper and a measuring device for shoulder rotation. If unavailable, you can construct your own device quite easily. The caliper can be built with three regular yardsticks. Nail and glue two of the yardsticks at one end at a 90° angle, and use the third one as the sliding end of the caliper. Construct the rotation device by placing a 60" measuring tape on an aluminum or wood stick, starting at about 6" or 7" from the end of the stick.

1. Warm up before the test.
2. Using the shoulder caliper, measure the biacromial width to the nearest fourth inch (use the top scale on the Acuflex III). Measure biacromial width between the lateral edges of the acromion processes of the shoulders, as shown in Figure 5.3a.

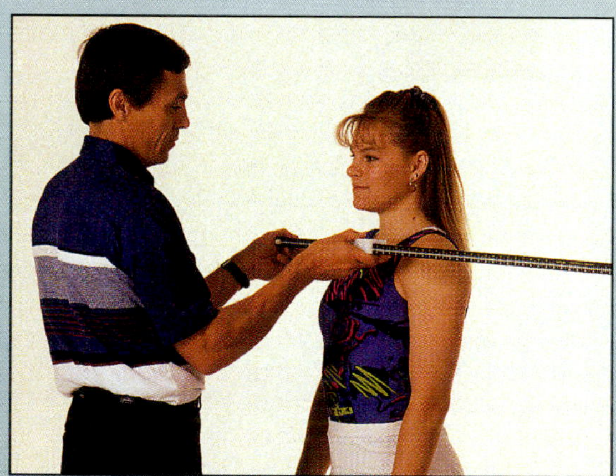

**FIGURE 5.3a** ◆ Measuring biacromial width.

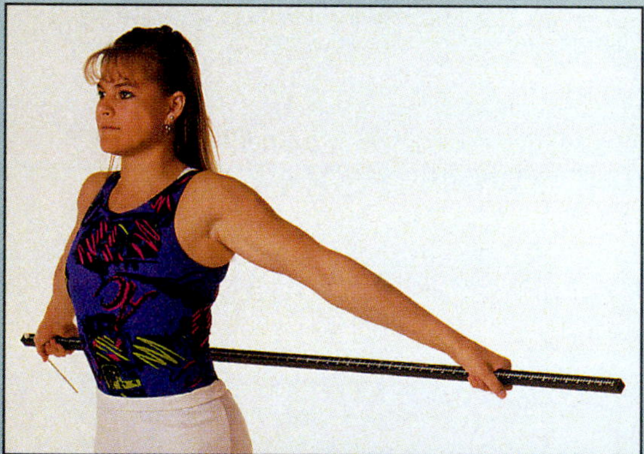

**FIGURE 5.3b** ◆ Starting position for the Shoulder Rotation Test (note the reverse grip used for this test).

3. Place the Acuflex III or homemade device behind the back and use a reverse grip (thumbs out) to hold on to the device (see Figure 5.3b). Place the right hand next to the zero point of the scale or tape (lower scale on the Acuflex III) and hold it firmly in place throughout the test. Place the left hand on the other end of the measuring device, as wide as needed.
4. Standing straight up and extending both arms to full length, with elbows locked, slowly bring the measuring device over the head until it reaches forehead level (Figure 5.3c). For subsequent trials, depending on the resistance encountered when rotating the shoulders, move the left grip in ½" to 1" at a time, and repeat the task until you no longer can rotate the shoulders without undue strain or start bending the elbows to do so. Always keep the right-hand grip against the zero point of the scale. Measure the last successful trial to the nearest half inch. Take this measurement right at the inner edge of the left hand on the side of the little finger.
6. Determine the final score for this test by subtracting the biacromial width from the best score (shortest distance) between both hands on the rotation test. For example, if the best score is 35" and the biacromial width is 15", the final score is 20" (35 – 15 = 20). Using Tables 5.3 and 5.4, determine the percentile rank and flexibility fitness classification for this test.

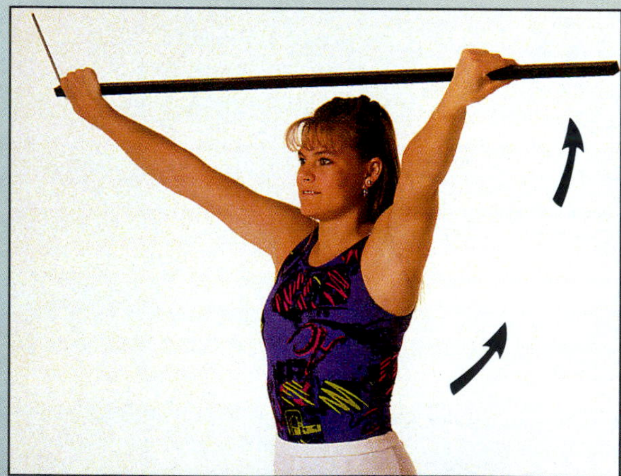

**FIGURE 5.3c** ◆ Shoulder Rotation Test.

* The Acuflex III Flexibility Tester for the Shoulder Rotation Test can be obtained from Figure Finder Collection, Novel Products, Inc., P. O. Box 408, Rockton, IL 61072-0408. Phone: (800) 323-5143, FAX 815-624-4866.

**FIGURE 5.3** ◆ Procedure for the Shoulder Rotation Test.

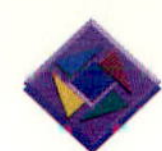

**TABLE 5.3**
**Percentile Ranks for the Shoulder Rotation Test**

| | Percentile Rank | Age Category ≤18 | 19–35 | 36–49 | ≥50 |
|---|---|---|---|---|---|
| Men | 99 | 2.2 | −1.0 | 18.1 | 21.5 |
| | 95 | 15.2 | 10.4 | 20.4 | 27.0 |
| | 90 | 18.5 | 15.5 | 20.8 | 27.9 |
| | 80 | 20.7 | 18.4 | 23.3 | 28.5 |
| | 70 | 23.0 | 20.5 | 24.7 | 29.4 |
| | 60 | 24.2 | 22.9 | 26.6 | 29.9 |
| | 50 | 25.4 | 24.4 | 28.0 | 30.5 |
| | 40 | 26.3 | 25.7 | 30.0 | 31.0 |
| | 30 | 28.2 | 27.3 | 31.9 | 31.7 |
| | 20 | 30.0 | 30.1 | 33.3 | 33.1 |
| | 10 | 33.5 | 31.8 | 36.1 | 37.2 |
| | 05 | 34.7 | 33.5 | 37.8 | 38.7 |
| | 01 | 40.8 | 42.6 | 43.0 | 44.1 |
| Women | 99 | 2.6 | −2.4 | 11.5 | 13.1 |
| | 95 | 8.0 | 6.2 | 15.4 | 16.5 |
| | 90 | 10.7 | 9.7 | 16.8 | 20.9 |
| | 80 | 14.5 | 14.5 | 19.2 | 22.5 |
| | 70 | 16.1 | 17.2 | 21.5 | 24.3 |
| | 60 | 19.2 | 18.7 | 23.1 | 25.1 |
| | 50 | 21.0 | 20.0 | 23.5 | 26.2 |
| | 40 | 22.2 | 21.4 | 24.4 | 28.1 |
| | 30 | 23.2 | 24.0 | 25.9 | 29.9 |
| | 20 | 25.0 | 25.9 | 29.8 | 31.5 |
| | 10 | 27.2 | 29.1 | 31.1 | 33.1 |
| | 05 | 28.0 | 31.3 | 33.4 | 34.1 |
| | 01 | 32.5 | 37.1 | 34.9 | 35.4 |

High physical fitness standard (percentiles 99–70)
Health fitness standard (percentiles 60–50)

**TABLE 5.4**
**Flexibility Fitness Categories**

| Percentile Rank | Fitness Category |
|---|---|
| ≥81 | Excellent |
| 61–80 | Good |
| 41–60 | Average |
| 21–40 | Fair |
| ≤20 | Poor |

## PRINCIPLES OF MUSCULAR FLEXIBILITY PRESCRIPTION

Even though genetics play a crucial role in body flexibility, range of joint mobility can be increased and maintained through a regular flexibility exercise program. Because range of motion is highly specific to each body part (ankle, trunk, shoulder), a comprehensive stretching program should include all body parts and follow the basic guidelines for flexibility development.

The overload and specificity of training principles discussed in conjunction with strength development in Chapter 4 apply as well to the development of muscular flexibility. To increase the total range of motion of a joint, the specific muscles surrounding that joint have to be stretched progressively beyond their accustomed length. The principles of mode, intensity, repetitions, and frequency of exercise also can be applied to flexibility programs.

### Mode of Training

Three modes of stretching exercises can increase flexibility:

1. Ballistic stretching.
2. Slow-sustained stretching.
3. Proprioceptive neuromuscular facilitation stretching.

Although research has indicated that all three types of stretching are effective in improving flexibility, each technique has certain advantages.

Ballistic or dynamic stretching exercises are done with jerky, rapid, and bouncy movements that provide the necessary force to lengthen the muscles. This type of stretching helps to develop flexibility, but the ballistic actions may cause muscle soreness and injury from small tears to the soft tissue.

Precautions must be taken not to overstretch ligaments, because they undergo plastic or permanent elongation. If the stretching force cannot be controlled, as in fast, jerky movements, ligaments easily can be overstretched. This, in turn, leads to excessively loose joints, increasing the risk for injuries, including joint dislocation and subluxation (partial dislocation). Most authorities, therefore, do not recommend ballistic exercises for development of flexibility.

Name: ______________________ Age: ________ Sex: ________

Date: ______________________

| Test | Score | % Rank | Classification |
|---|---|---|---|
| Modified Sit-and-Reach | | | |
| Total Body Rotation ___ Right ___ Left | | | |
| Shoulder Rotation | | | |

Total: [ ]

Average Percentile Rank (divide total by 3): [ ] Overall Flexibility Classification: ____________

Date: ______________________

| | | | |
|---|---|---|---|
| Modified Sit-and-Reach | | | |
| Total Body Rotation ___ Right ___ Left | | | |
| Shoulder Rotation | | | |

Total: [ ]

Average Percentile Rank (divide total by 3): [ ] Overall Flexibility Classification: ____________

**FIGURE 5.4** ◆ Muscular flexibility report.

With the slow-sustained stretching technique, muscles are lengthened gradually through a joint's complete range of motion, and the final position is held for a few seconds. A slow-sustained stretch causes the muscles to relax and thereby achieve greater length. This type of stretch causes little pain and has a low risk for injury. Slow-sustained stretching exercises are the most frequently used and recommended for flexibility development programs.

Proprioceptive neuromuscular facilitation (PNF) stretching has become more popular in the last few years. This technique, based on a "contract and relax" method, requires the assistance of another person. The procedure is as follows:

1. The person assisting with the exercise provides initial force by pushing slowly in the direction of the desired stretch. This first stretch does not cover the entire range of motion.
2. The person being stretched then applies force in the opposite direction of the stretch, against the assistant, who tries to hold the initial degree of stretch as close as possible. An isometric contraction is being performed at that angle.
3. After 4 or 5 seconds of isometric contraction, the muscle being stretched is relaxed completely. The assistant then increases the degree of stretch slowly to a greater angle.
4. The isometric contraction is repeated for another 4 or 5 seconds, following which the muscle is relaxed again. The assistant then can increase the degree of stretch slowly one more time. Steps 1 through 4 are repeated two to five

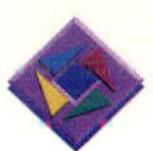

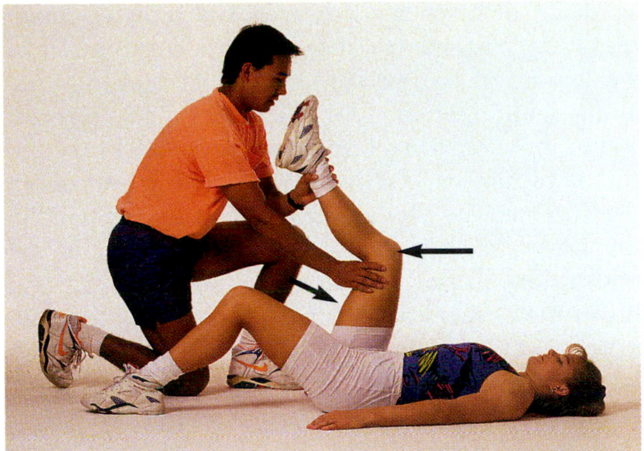

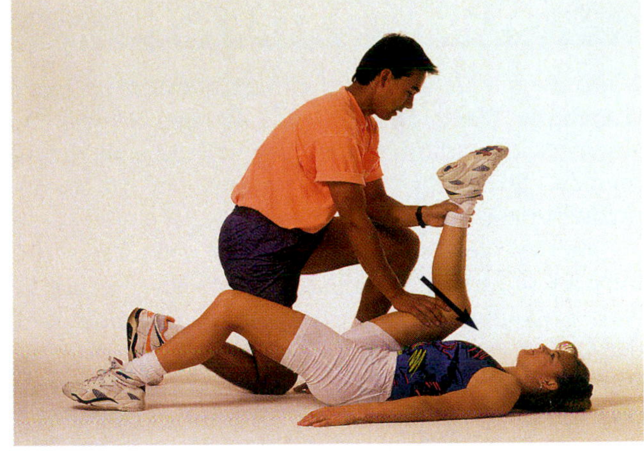

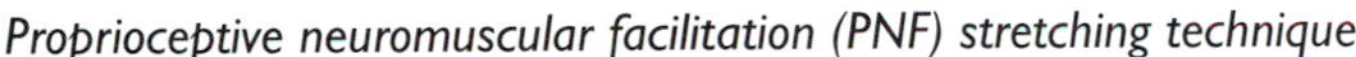

*Proprioceptive neuromuscular facilitation (PNF) stretching technique.*

times, until the exerciser feels mild discomfort. On the last trial the final stretched position should be held for several seconds.

Theoretically, with the PNF technique, the isometric contraction helps relax the muscle being stretched, which results in a longer muscle. Some fitness leaders believe PNF is more effective than slow-sustained stretching. Disadvantages, however, are that PNF is more painful, a second person is required to assist, and more time is necessary to conduct each session.

## Intensity of Exercise

The intensity, or degree of stretch, when doing flexibility exercises, should be only to a point of mild discomfort. Pain does not have to be part of the stretching routine. Excessive pain is an indication that the load is too high and may lead to injury.

All stretching should be done to slightly below the pain threshold. As participants reach this point, they should try to relax the muscle being stretched as much as possible. After completing the stretch, the body part is brought back gradually to the starting point.

## Repetitions

The time required for an exercise session for flexibility development is based on the number of repetitions and the length of time each repetition (final stretched position) is held. The general recommendation is that each exercise be done four or five times, holding the final position each time about 20 seconds.

As flexibility increases, a person can gradually increase the time each repetition is held, to a maximum of one minute. Individuals who are susceptible to flexibility injuries, however, should limit each stretch to 20 seconds.

## Frequency of Exercise

Flexibility exercises should be conducted five to six times a week in the early stages of the program. After a minimum of 6 to 8 weeks of almost daily stretching, flexibility levels can be maintained with only two or three sessions per week, doing about three repetitions of 10 to 15 seconds each. Figure 5.5 summarizes the flexibility development guidelines.

- **Mode**
  Static stretching or proprioceptive neuromuscular facilitation (PNF)
- **Intensity**
  Stretch to the point of mild discomfort
- **Repetitions**
  Repeat each exercise four to five times and hold the final stretched position for 10 to 60 seconds
- **Frequency**
  Two to six days per week

**FIGURE 5.5** ◆ Guidelines for flexibility development.

## WHEN TO STRETCH?

Many people do not differentiate a warm-up from stretching. Warming up means starting a workout slowly with walking, slow jogging, or light calisthenics. Stretching implies movement of joints through their range of motion.

Before performing flexibility exercises, the muscles should be warmed up properly. Failing to warm up increases the risk for muscle pulls and tears. Surveys have shown that individuals who stretch before workouts without an adequate warm-up actually have a higher rate of injuries than those who do not stretch at all.

A good time to do flexibility exercises is after aerobic workouts. Higher body temperature in itself helps to increase joint range of motion. Muscles also are fatigued following exercise. A fatigued muscle tends to shorten, which can lead to soreness and spasms. Stretching exercises help fatigued muscles reestablish their normal resting length and prevent unnecessary pain.

## FLEXIBILITY EXERCISES

To improve body flexibility, each major muscle group should be subjected to at least one stretching exercise. A complete set of exercises for developing muscular flexibility is presented at the end of this chapter.

You may not be able to hold a final stretched position with some of these exercises (examples: lateral head tilts and arm circles), but you still should perform the exercise through the joint's full range of motion. Depending on the number and length of repetitions, a complete workout will last between 15 and 30 minutes.

## PREVENTING AND REHABILITATING LOW BACK PAIN

Few people make it through life without having low back pain at some point. An estimated 75 million Americans currently suffer from chronic low back pain each year. About 80% of the time, backache syndrome is preventable and is caused by: (a) physical inactivity, (b) poor postural habits and body mechanics, and (c) excessive body weight.

Lack of physical activity is the most common reason for chronic low back pain. Deterioration or weakening of the abdominal and gluteal muscles, along with tightening of the lower back (erector spine) muscles, brings about an unnatural forward tilt of the pelvis (Figure 5.6). This tilt puts extra pressure on the spinal vertebrae, causing pain in the lower back. Accumulation of fat around the midsection of the body contributes to the forward tilt of the pelvis, which further aggravates the condition. Low back pain frequently is associated with faulty posture and improper body mechanics (body positions in all of life's daily activities, including sleeping, sitting, standing, walking, driving, working, and exercising). Incorrect posture and poor mechanics, as explained in Figure 5.7, increase strain not only on the lower back but on many other bones, joints, muscles, and ligaments as well.

Low back pain can be reduced greatly by including some specific stretching and strengthening exercises in the regular fitness program. In most cases back pain is present only with movement and physical activity. If the pain is severe and persists even at rest, the first step is to consult a physician, who can rule out any disc damage and most likely will prescribe proper bed rest using several pillows under the knees for leg support (see Figure 5.7). This position helps release muscle spasms by stretching the muscles involved. In addition, a

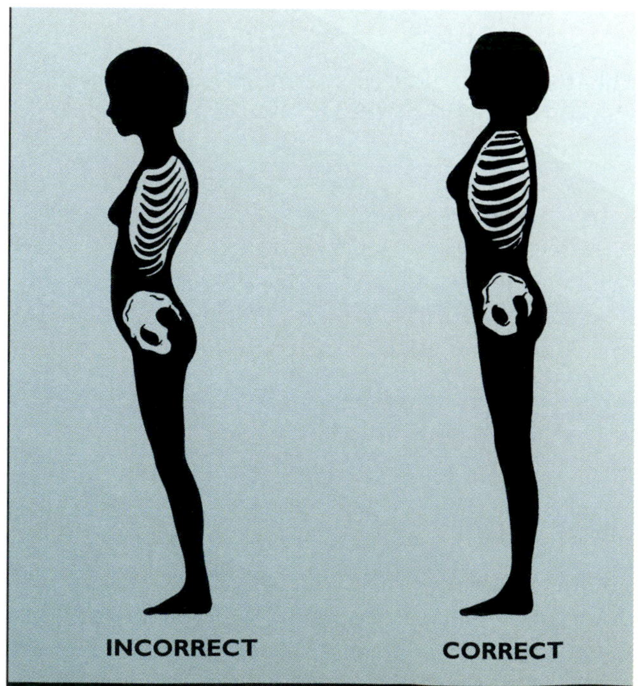


**FIGURE 5.6** ◆ Incorrect and correct pelvic alignment.

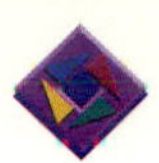

physician may prescribe a muscle relaxant or anti-inflammatory medication (or both) and some type of physical therapy.

Once a person is pain-free in the resting state, he or she needs to start correcting the muscular imbalance by stretching the tight muscles and strengthening the weak ones. Stretching exercises always are performed first.

Several exercises for preventing and rehabilitating the backache syndrome are given at the end of this chapter. These exercises can be done twice or more daily when a person has back pain. Under normal circumstances, doing these exercises three to four times a week is enough to prevent the syndrome.

## NOTES


1. S. A. Plowman, *Physical Fitness and Healthy Low Back Function,* President's Council on Physical Fitness and Sports: Physical Activity and Fitness Research Digest, Series 1 (3):3, 1993.
2. American College of Obstetricians and Gynecologists, "Guidelines for Exercise During Pregnancy," 1994.
3. W. W. K. Hoeger, and D. R. Hopkins, "A Comparison Between The Sit and Reach and The Modified Sit and Reach in the Measurement of Flexibility in Women," *Research Quarterly for Exercise and Sport*, 63:191-195.
4. W. W. K. Hoeger, D. R. Hopkins, S. Button, and T. A. Palmer, "Comparing the Sit and Reach with the Modified Sit and Reach in Measuring Flexibility in Adolescents," *Pediatric Exercise Science*, 2 (1990), 156-162.
5. D. R., Hopkins and W. W. K. Hoeger, "A Comparison of the Sit and Reach and the Modified Sit and Reach in the Measurement of Flexibility for Males," *Journal of Applied Sports Science Research*, 6 (1992), 7-10.


## SELECT BIBLIOGRAPHY


Billing, H., and E. Loewendahl. *Mobilization of the Human Body.* Palo Alto, CA: Stanford University Press, 1949.

Chapman, E. A., H. A. deVries, and R. Swezey. "Joint Stiffness: Effects of Exercise on Young and Old Men." *Journal of Gerontology* 27 (1972), 218-221.

Dickerson, R. V. "The Specificity of Flexibility." *Research Quarterly,* 33 (1962), 222-229.

Fleishman, E. A. *Examiners Manual for Basic Fitness Tests*. Englewood Cliffs, NJ: Prentice-Hall, 1964.

Heyward, V. H. *Advanced Methods for Physical Fitness Assessment and Exercise Prescription*. Champaign, IL: Human Kinetic Publishers, 1991.

Hoeger, W. W. K., S. Button, D. R. Hopkins, and T. A. Palmer. "Relationship Among Four Selected Flexibility Tests for High School-Age Students." *Northwest Journal for Health, Physical Education, Recreation and Dance*, 1:2 (1989), 6-10.

Hoeger, W. W. K., and D. R. Hopkins. "Assessing Muscular Flexibility." *Fitness Management*, 6:2 (1990), 34-36, 42.

Holt, L. E., T. M. Travis, and T. Okita. "Comparative Study of Three Stretching Techniques." *Perceptual and Motor Skills*, 31 (1970), 611-616.

Johnson, B. L., and J. K. Nelson. *Practical Measurements for Evaluation in Physical Education*. Minneapolis: Burgess Publishing, 1979.

Sapega, A. A., T. C. Quedenfeld, R. A. Moyer, and R. A. Butler. "Biophysical Factors in Range-of-Motion Exercise." *Physician and Sportsmedicine*, 9 (1981), 57-65.

Wright, V., and R. J. Johns. "Physical Factors Concerned with Stiffness of Normal and Diseased Joints." *Bulletin of Johns Hopkins Hospital,* 106 (1960), 215-231.

## Your back and how to care for it

Whatever the cause of low back pain, part of its treatment is the correction of faulty posture. But good posture is not simply a matter of "standing tall." It refers to correct use of the body at all times. In fact, for the body to function in the best of health it must be so used that no strain is put upon the muscles, joints, bones, and ligaments. To prevent low back pain, avoiding strain must become a way of life, practiced while lying, sitting, standing, walking, working, and exercising. When body position is correct, internal organs have enough room to function normally and blood circulates more freely.

With the help of this guide, you can begin to correct the positions and movements which bring on or aggravate backache. Particular attention should be paid to the positions recommended for resting, since it is possible to strain the muscles of the back and neck even while lying in bed. By learning to live with good posture, under all circumstances, you will gradually develop the proper carriage and stronger muscles needed to protect and support your hard-working back.

### HOW TO STAY ON YOUR FEET WITHOUT TIRING YOUR BACK

To prevent strain and pain in everyday activities, it is restful to change from one task to another before fatigue sets in. Housewives can lie down between chores; others should check body position frequently, drawing in the abdomen, flattening the back, bending the knees slightly.

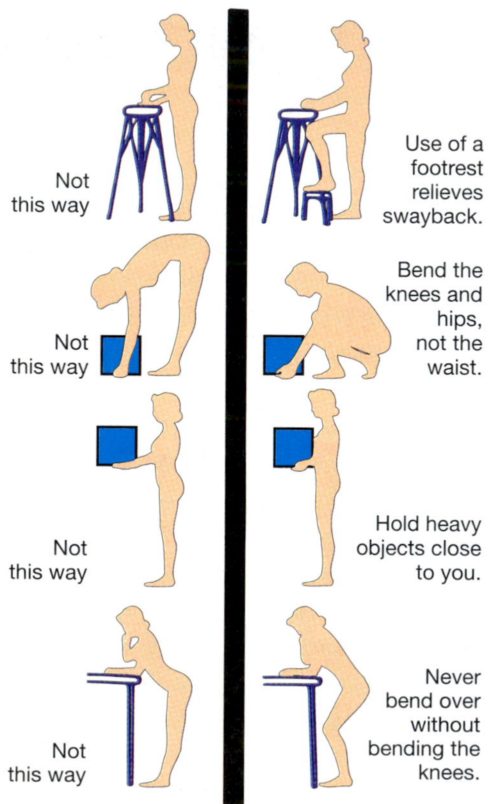
Not this way
Use of a footrest relieves swayback.
Not this way
Bend the knees and hips, not the waist.
Not this way
Hold heavy objects close to you.
Not this way
Never bend over without bending the knees.

### CHECK YOUR CARRIAGE HERE

In correct, fully erect posture, a line dropped from the ear will go through the tip of the shoulder, middle of hip, back of kneecap, and front of anklebone.

**Incorrect** Lower back is arched or hollow.

**Incorrect** Upper back is stooped, lower back is arched, abdomen sags.

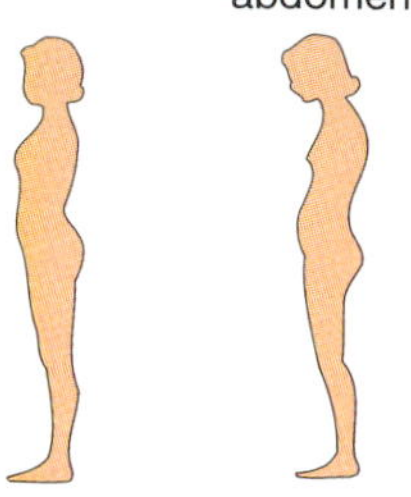

**Incorrect** Note how, in strained position pelvis tilts forward, chin is out, and ribs are down, crowding internal organs.

**Correct** In correct position, chin is in, head up back flattened, pelvis held straight.

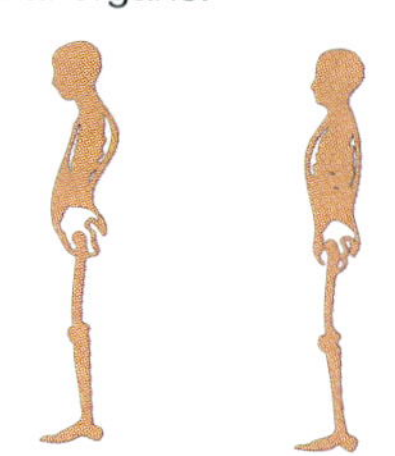

To find the correct standing position: Stand one foot away from wall. Now sit against wall, bending knees slightly. Tighten abdominal and buttock muscles. This will tilt the pelvis back and flatten the lower spine. Holding this position, inch up the wall to standing position, by straightening the legs. Now walk around the room, maintaining the same posture. Place back against wall again to see if you have held it.

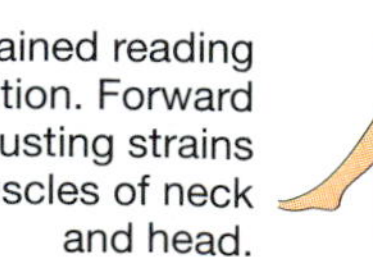

### HOW TO SIT CORRECTLY

A back's best friend is a straight, hard chair. If you can't get the chair you prefer, learn to sit properly on whatever chair you get. To correct sitting position from forward slump: Throw head well back, then bend it forward to pull in the chin. This will straighten the back. Now tighten abdominal muscles to raise the chest. Check position frequently.

Relieve strain by sitting well forward, flatten back by tightening abdominal muscles, and cross knees.

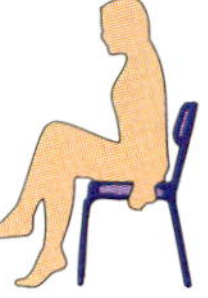

Use of footrest relieves swayback. Aim is to have knees higher than hips.

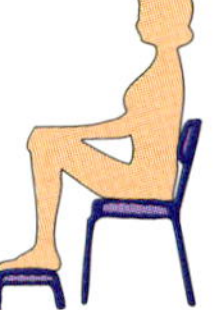

Correct way to sit while driving, close to pedals. Use seat belt or hard backrest, available commercially.

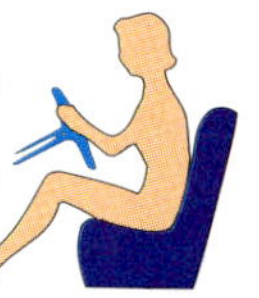

TV slump leads to "dowager's hump," strains neck and shoulders.

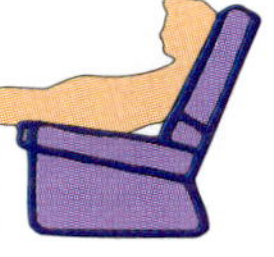

If chair is too high, swayback is increased.

Keep neck and back in as straight a line as possible with the spine. Bend forward from hips.

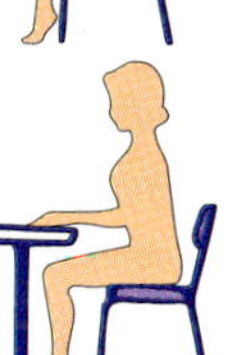

Driver's seat too far from pedals emphasizes curve in lower back.

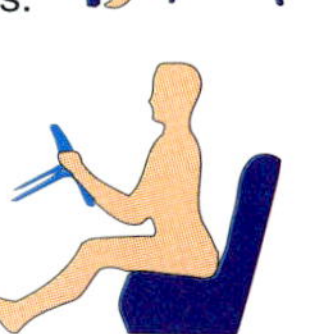

Strained reading position. Forward thrusting strains muscles of neck and head.

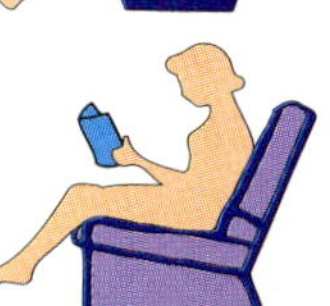

**FIGURE 5.7**

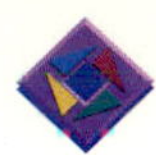

### HOW TO PUT YOUR BACK TO BED

For proper bed posture, a firm mattress is essential. Bedboards, sold commercially, or devised at home, may be used with soft mattresses. Bedboards, preferably, should be made of 3/4 inch plywood. Faulty sleeping positions intensify swayback and result not only in backache but in numbness, tingling, and pain in arms and legs.

**Incorrect:**
Lying flat on back makes swayback worse.

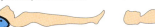

**Correct:**
Lying on side with knees bent effectively flattens the back. Flat pillow may be used to support neck, especially when shoulders are broad.

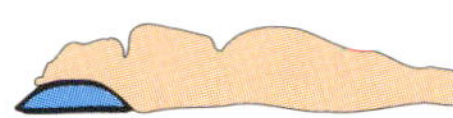

Use of high pillow strains neck, arms, shoulders.

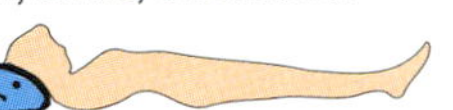

Sleeping on back is restful and correct when knees are properly supported.

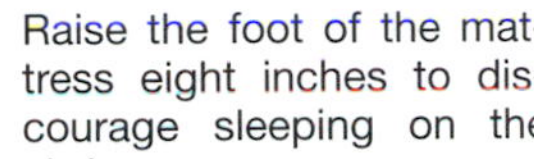

Sleeping face down exaggerates swayback, strains neck and shoulders.

Raise the foot of the mattress eight inches to discourage sleeping on the abdomen.

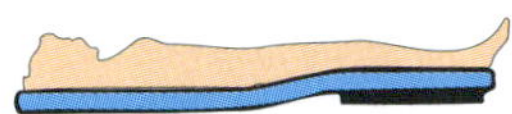

Bending one hip and knee does not relieve swayback.

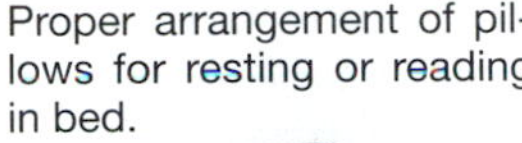

Proper arrangement of pillows for resting or reading in bed.

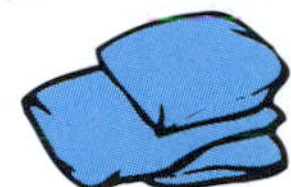

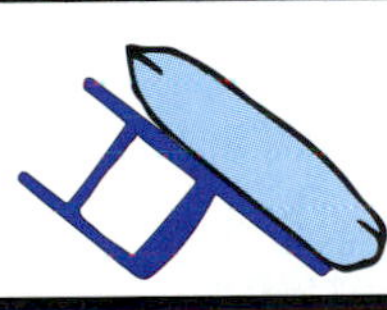

A straight-back chair used behind a pillow makes a serviceable backrest.

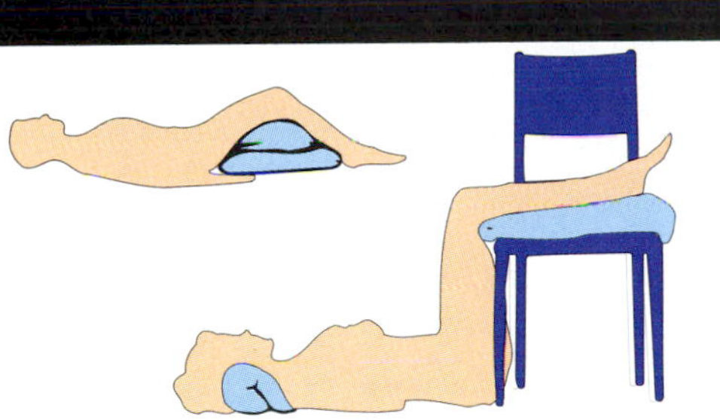

### WHEN DOING NOTHING, DO IT RIGHT

Rest is the first rule for the tired, painful back. The following positions relieve pain by taking all pressure and weight off the back and legs.

Note pillows under knees to relieve strain on spine.

For complete relief and relaxing effect, these positions should be maintained from 5 to 25 minutes.

**EXERCISE — WITHOUT GETTING OUT OF BED** Exercises to be performed while lying in bed are aimed not so much at strengthening muscles as at teaching correct positioning. But muscles used correctly become stronger and in time are able to support the body with the least amount of effort.

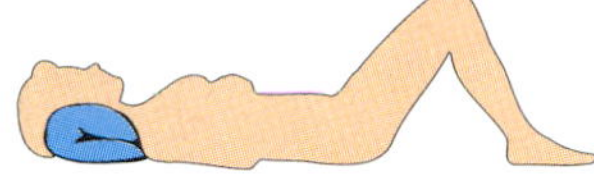

Do all exercises in this position. Legs should not be straightened.

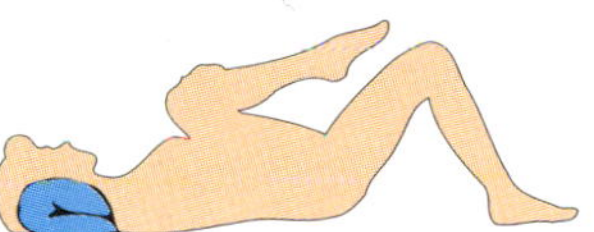

Bring knee up to chest. Lower slowly but do not straighten leg. Relax. Repeat with each leg 10 times.

**EXERCISE — WITHOUT ATTRACTING ATTENTION** Use these inconspicuous exercises whenever you have a spare moment during the day, both to relax tension and improve the tone of important muscle groups.

1. Rotate shoulders, forward and backward.
2. Turn head slowly side to side.
3. Watch an imaginary plane take off, just below the right shoulder. Stretch neck, follow it slowly as it moves up, around and down, disappearing below the other shoulder. Repeat, starting on left side.
4. Slowly, slowly, touch left ear to left shoulder, right ear to right shoulder. Raise both shoulders to touch ears, drop them as far down as possible.
5. At any pause in the day — waiting for an elevator to arrive, for a specific traffic light to change — pull in abdominal muscles, tighten, hold it for the count of eight without breathing. Relax slowly. Increase the count gradually after the first week, practice breathing normally with the abdomen flat and contracted. Do this sitting, standing, and walking.

Bring both knees slowly up to chest. Tighten muscles of abdomen, press back flat against bed. Hold knees to chest 20 seconds, then lower slowly. Relax. Repeat 5 times. This exercise gently stretches the shortened muscles of the lower back, while strengthening abdominal muscles. Clasp knees, bring them up to chest, at the same time coming to a sitting position. Rock back and forth.

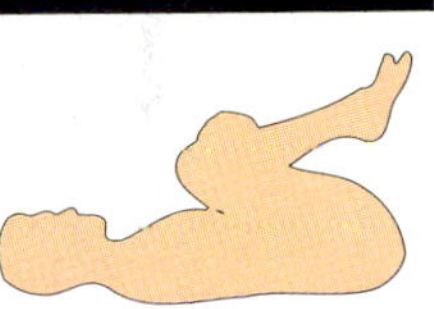

### RULES TO LIVE BY - FROM NOW ON

1. Never bend from the waist only; bend the hips and knees.
2. Never lift a heavy object higher than your waist.
3. Always turn and face the object you wish to lift.
4. Avoid carrying unbalanced loads; hold heavy objects close to your body.
5. Never carry anything heavier than you can manage with ease.
6. Never lift or move heavy furniture. Wait for someone to do it who knows the principles of leverage.
7. Avoid sudden movements, sudden "overloading" of muscles. Learn to move deliberately, swinging the legs from the hips.
8. Learn to keep the head in line with the spine, when standing, sitting, lying in bed.
9. Put soft chairs and deep couches on your "don't sit" list. During prolonged sitting, cross your legs to rest your back.
10. Your doctor is the only one who can determine when low back pain is due to faulty posture. He is the best judge of when you may do general exercises for physical fitness. when you do, omit any exercise which arches or overstrains the lower back: backward bends, or forward bends, touching the toes with the knees straight.
11. Wear shoes with moderate heels, all about the same height. Avoid changing from high to low heels.
12. Put a footrail under the desk, and a footrest under the crib.
13. Diaper the baby sitting next to him or her on the bed.
14. Don't stoop and stretch to hand the wash; raise the clothesbasket and lower the washline.
15. Beg or buy a rocking chair. Rocking rests the back by changing the muscle groups used.
16. Train yourself vigorously to use your abdominal muscles to flatten your lower abdomen. In time, this muscle contraction will become habitual, making you the envied possessor of a youthful body-profile!
17. Don't strain to open windows or doors.
18. For good posture, concentrate on strengthening "nature's corset" — the abdominal and buttock muscles. The pelvic roll exercise is especially recommended to correct the postural relation between the pelvis and the spine.



**FIGURE 5.7** ◆ *(Continued)*

# Flexibility Exercises

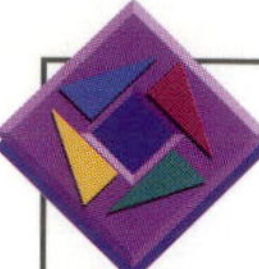

## 1 Lateral Head Tilt

**ACTION** Slowly and gently tilt the head laterally. Repeat several times to each side.

**AREAS STRETCHED** Neck flexors and extensors and ligaments of the cervical spine.

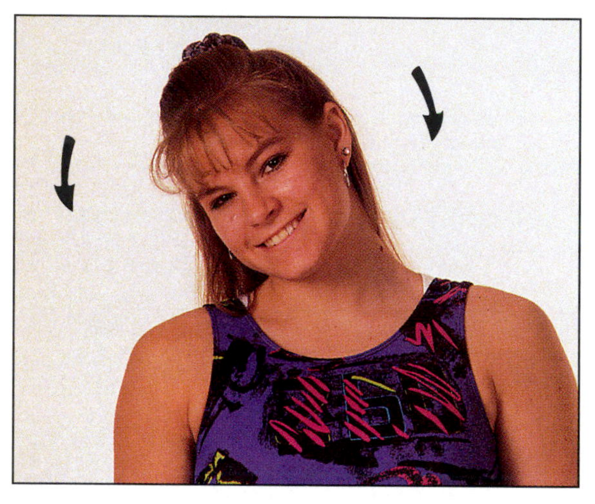

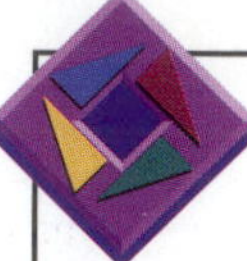

## 2 Arm Circles

**ACTION** Gently circle your arms all the way around. Conduct the exercise in both directions.

**AREAS STRETCHED** Shoulder muscles and ligaments.

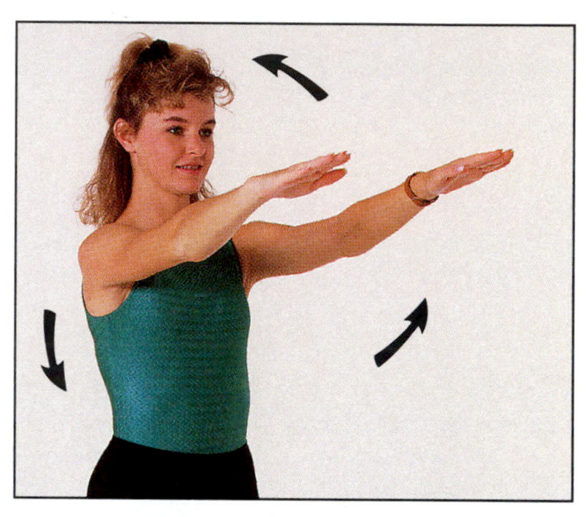

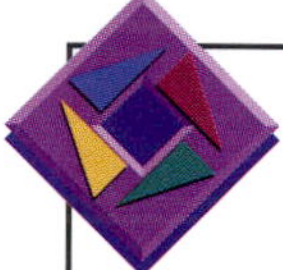

## 3 Side Stretch

**ACTION** Stand straight up, feet separated to shoulder width, and place your hands on your waist. Now move the upper body to one side and hold the final stretch for a few seconds. Repeat on the other side.

**AREAS STRETCHED**

Muscles and ligaments in the pelvic region.

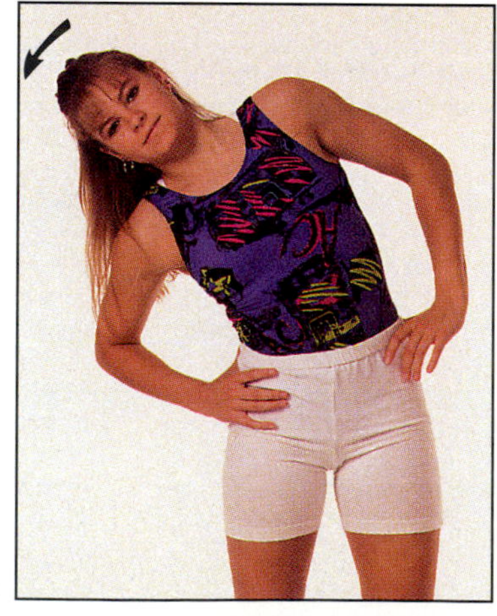

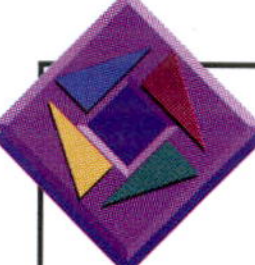

## 4 Body Rotation

**ACTION** Place your arms slightly away from your body and rotate the trunk as far as possible, holding the final position for several seconds. Conduct the exercise for both the right and left sides of the body. You can also perform this exercise by standing about two feet away from the wall (back toward the wall), and then rotate the trunk, placing the hands against the wall.

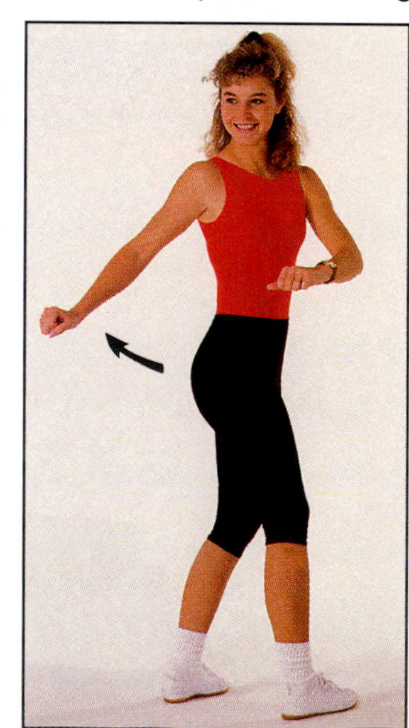

**AREAS STRETCHED**
Hip, abdominal, chest, back, neck, and shoulder muscles; hip and spinal ligaments.

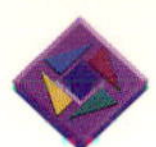

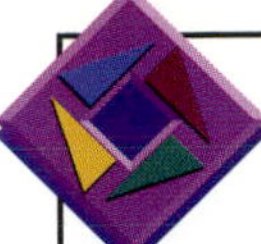

## 5
## Chest Stretch

**ACTION** Kneel down behind a chair and place both hands on the back of the chair. Gradually push your chest downward and hold for a few seconds.

**AREAS STRETCHED** Chest (pectoral) muscles and shoulder ligaments.

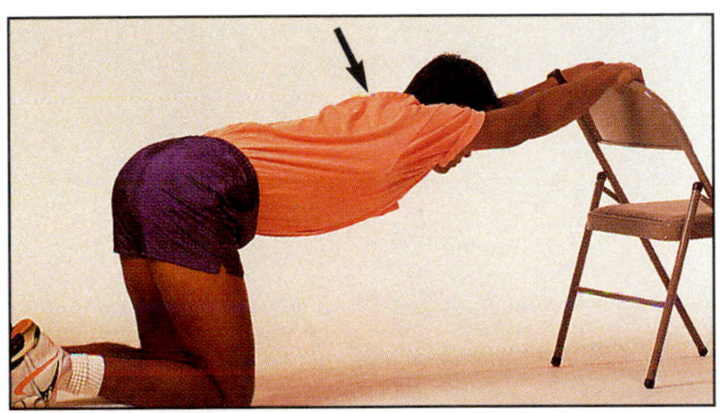

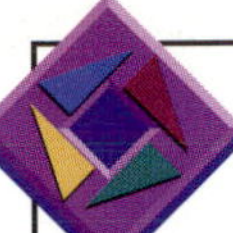

## 6
## Shoulder Hyperextension Stretch

**ACTION** Have a partner grasp your arms from behind by the wrists and slowly push them upward. Hold the final position for a few seconds.

**AREAS STRETCHED** Deltoid and pectoral muscles, and ligaments of the shoulder joint.

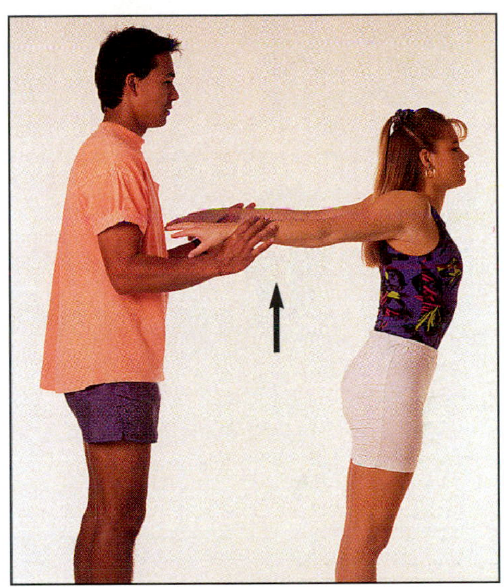

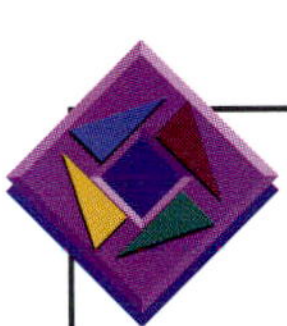

## 7
## Shoulder Rotation Stretch

**ACTION** With the aid of surgical tubing or an aluminum or wood stick, place the tubing or stick behind your back and grasp the two ends using a reverse (thumbs-out) grip. Slowly bring the tubing or stick over your head, keeping the elbows straight. Repeat several times (bring the hands closer together for additional stretch).

**AREAS STRETCHED** Deltoid, latissimus dorsi, and pectoral muscles; shoulder ligaments.

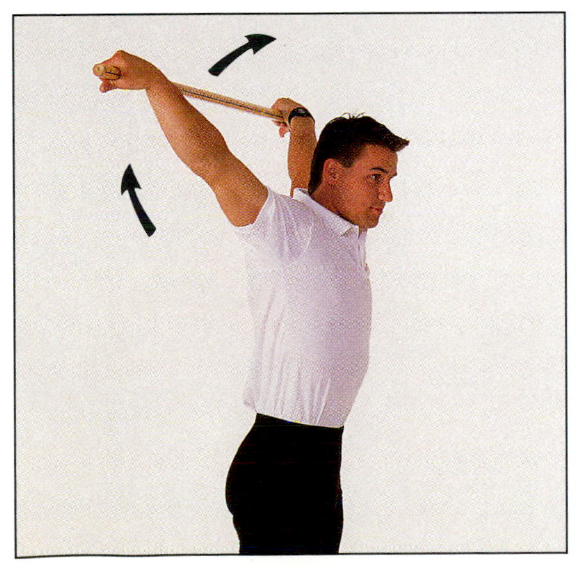

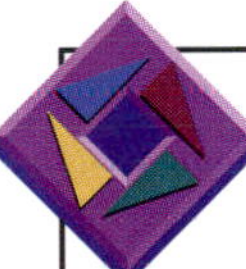

## 8
## Quad Stretch

**ACTION** Lie on your side and move one foot back by flexing the knee. Grasp the front of the ankle and pull the ankle toward the gluteal region. Hold for several seconds. Repeat with the other leg.

**AREAS STRETCHED** Quadriceps muscle, and knee and ankle ligaments.

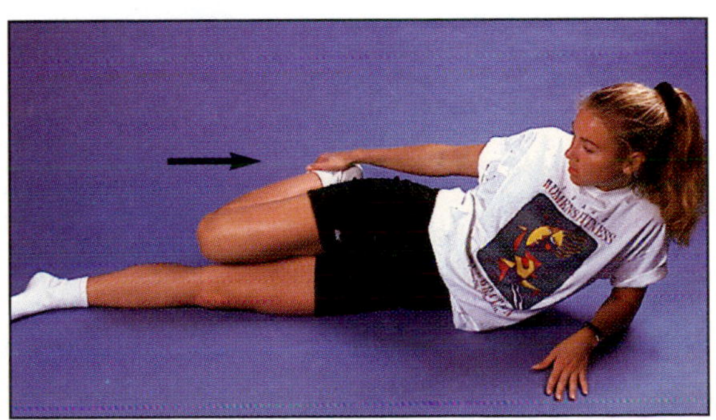

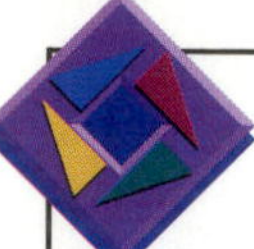

## 9

### Heel Cord Stretch

**ACTION** Stand against the wall or at the edge of a step and stretch the heel downward, alternating legs. Hold the stretched position for a few seconds.

**AREAS STRETCHED** Heel cord (Achilles tendon), gastrocnemius, and soleus muscles.

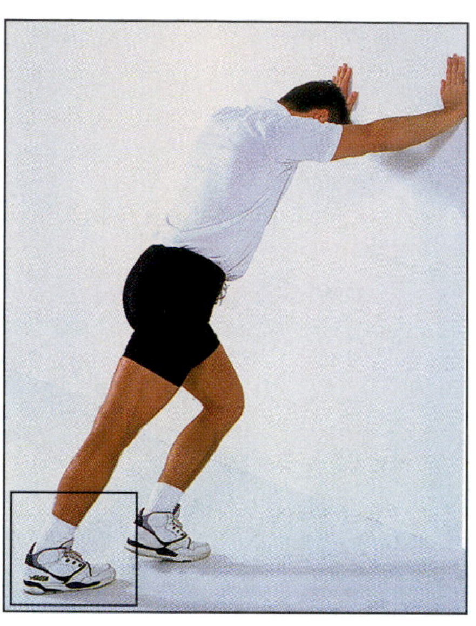

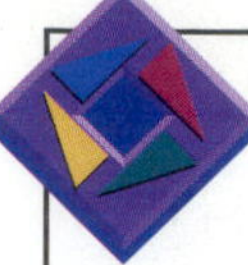

## 10

### Adductor Stretch

**ACTION** Stand with your feet about twice shoulder width and place your hands slightly above the knee. Flex one knee and slowly go down as far as possible, holding the final position for a few seconds. Repeat with the other leg.

**AREAS STRETCHED** Hip adductor muscles.

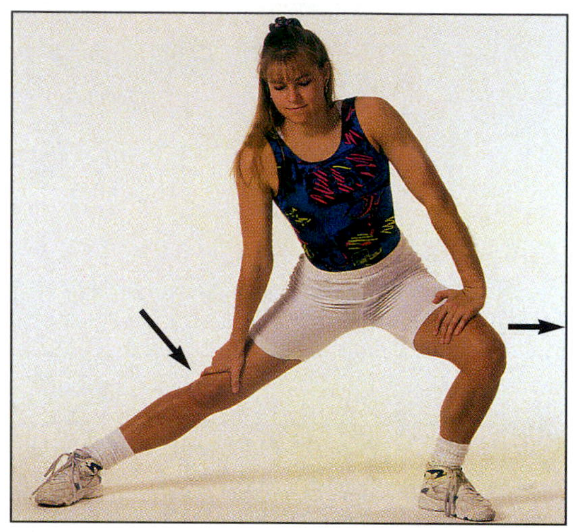

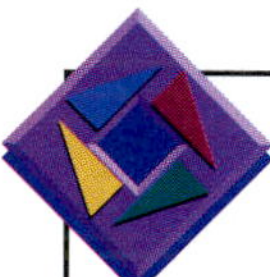

## 11

### Sitting Adductor Stretch

**ACTION** Sit on the floor and bring your feet in close to you, allowing the soles of the feet to touch each other. Now place your forearms (or elbows) on the inner part of the thigh and push the legs downward, holding the final stretch for several seconds.

**AREA STRETCHED** Hip adductor muscles.

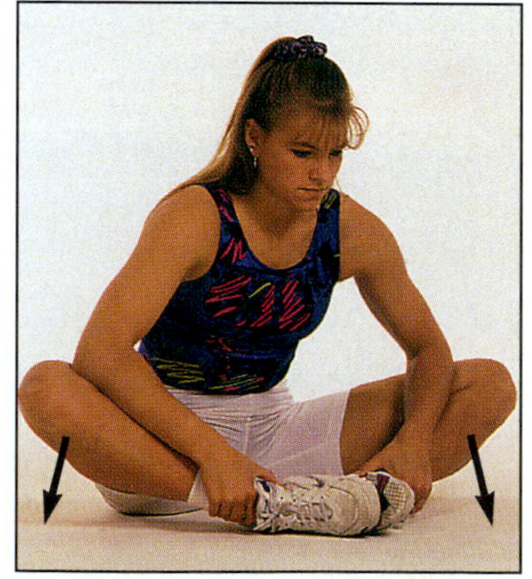

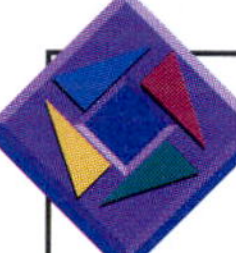

## 12

### Sit-and-Reach Stretch

**ACTION** Sit on the floor with legs together and gradually reach forward as far as possible. Hold the final position for a few seconds. This exercise may also be performed with the legs separated, reaching to each side as well as to the middle.

**AREAS STRETCHED** Hamstrings and lower back muscles, and lumbar spine ligaments.

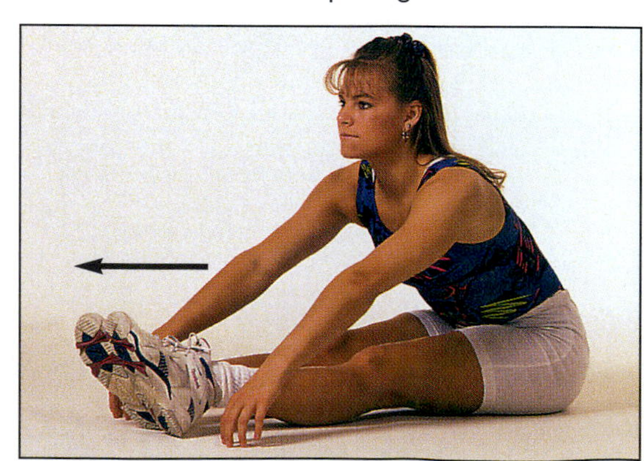

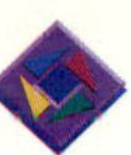

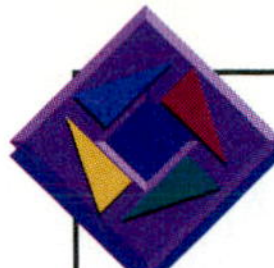

## 13
### Triceps Stretch

**ACTION** Place the right hand behind your neck. Grasp the right arm above the elbow with the left hand. Gently pull the elbow backward. Repeat the exercise with the opposite arm.

**AREAS STRETCHED** Back of upper arm (triceps muscle) and shoulder joint.

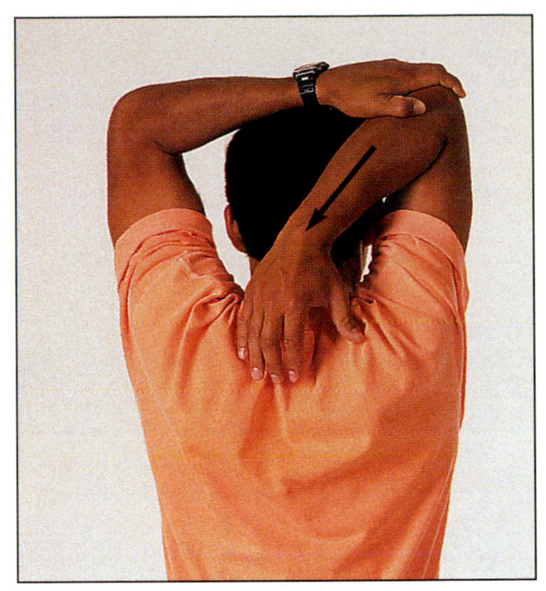

# Exercises for the Prevention and Rehabilitation of Low Back Pain

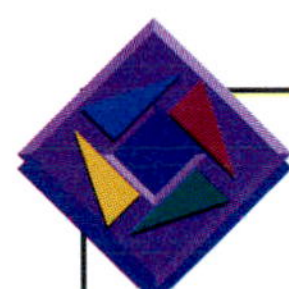

## 14
### Single-Knee to Chest Stretch

**ACTION** Lie down flat on the floor. Bend one leg at approximately 100° and gradually pull the opposite leg toward your chest. Hold the final stretch for a few seconds. Switch legs and repeat the exercise.

**AREAS STRETCHED** Lower back and hamstring muscles, and lumbar spine ligaments.

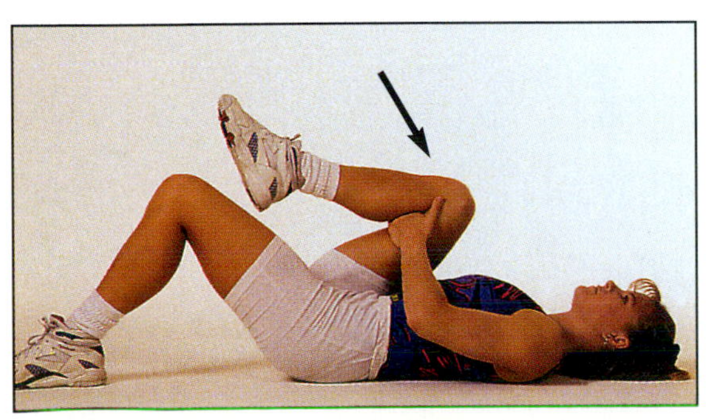

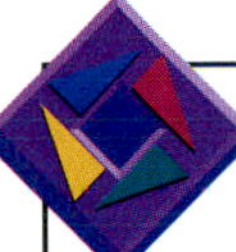

## 15
### Double-Knee to Chest Stretch

**ACTION** Lie flat on the floor and then slowly curl up into a fetal position. Hold for a few seconds.

**AREAS STRETCHED** Upper and lower back and hamstring muscles; spinal ligaments.

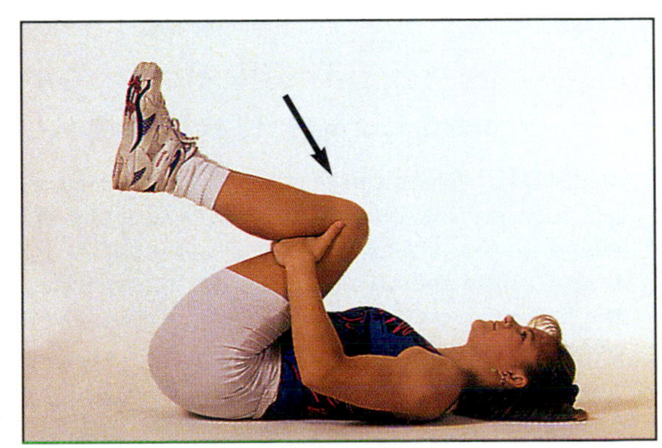

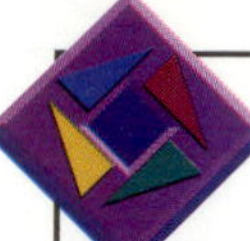

## 16
## Upper and Lower Back Stretch

**ACTION** Sit on the floor and bring your feet in close to you, allowing the soles of the feet to touch each other. Hold on to your feet and gently bring your head and upper chest toward your feet.

**AREAS STRETCHED** Upper and lower back muscles and ligaments.

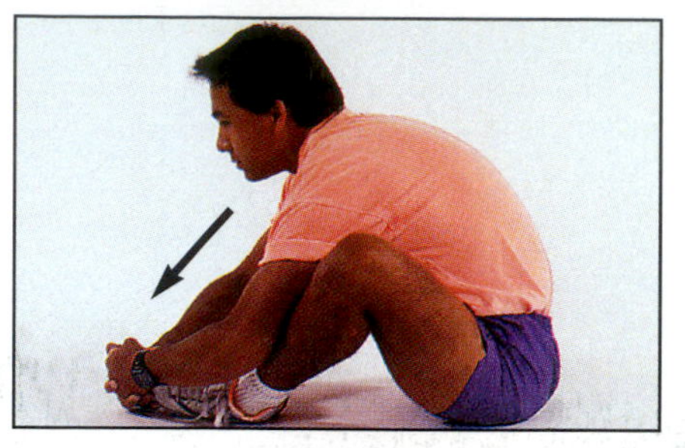

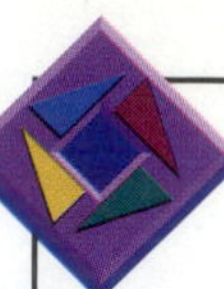

## 17
## Sit-and-Reach Stretch

(see Exercise 12 in this chapter)

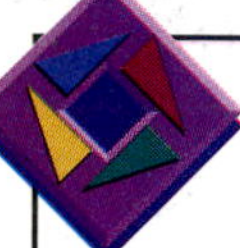

## 18
## Gluteal Stretch

**ACTION** Sit on the floor, bend the right leg and place your right ankle slightly above the left knee. Grasp the left thigh with both hands and gently pull the leg toward your chest. Repeat the exercise with the opposite leg.

**AREAS STRETCHED** Buttock area (gluteal muscles).

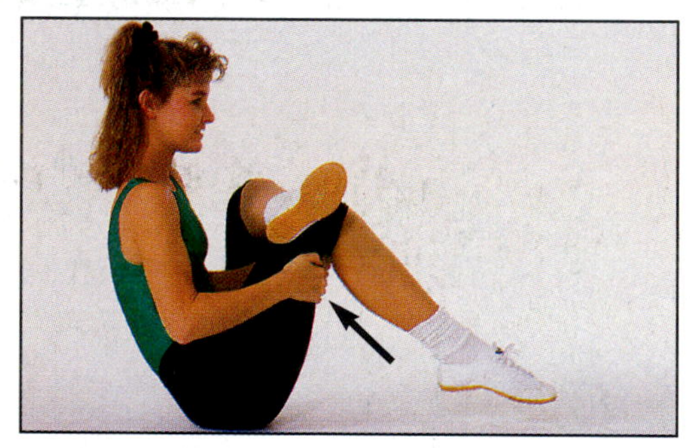

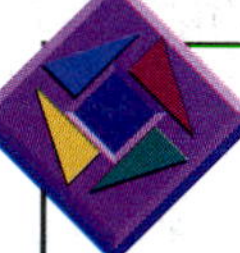

## 19
## Back Extension

**ACTION** Lie face down on the floor with the elbows by the chest, forearms on the floor, and the hands beneath the chin. Gently raise the trunk by extending the elbows until you reach an approximate 90° angle at the elbow joint. Be sure that the forearms remain in contact with the floor at all times. DO NOT extend the back beyond this point. Hyperextension of the lower back may lead to or aggravate an already existing back problem. Hold the stretched position for about ten seconds.

**AREA STRETCHED** Abdominal region.

**ADDITIONAL BENEFIT** Restore lower back curvature.

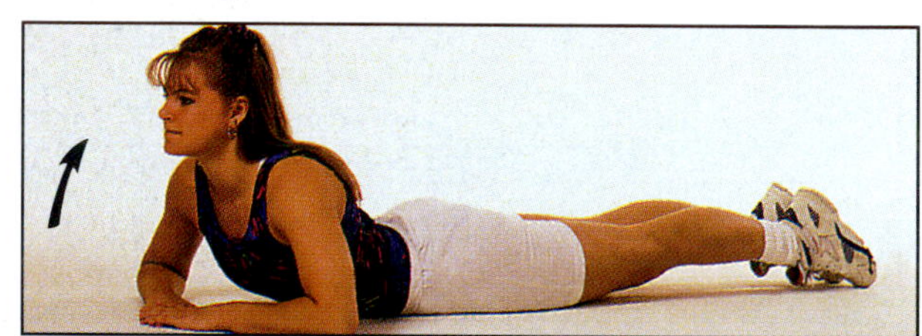

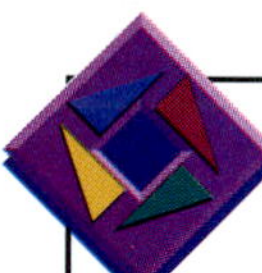

## 20
## Trunk Rotation and Lower Back Stretch

**ACTION** Sit on the floor and bend the left leg, placing the left foot on the outside of the right knee. Place the right elbow on the left knee and push against it. At the same time, try to rotate the trunk to the left (counterclockwise). Hold the final position for a few seconds. Repeat the exercise with the other side.

**AREAS STRETCHED** Lateral side of the hip and thigh; trunk, and lower back.

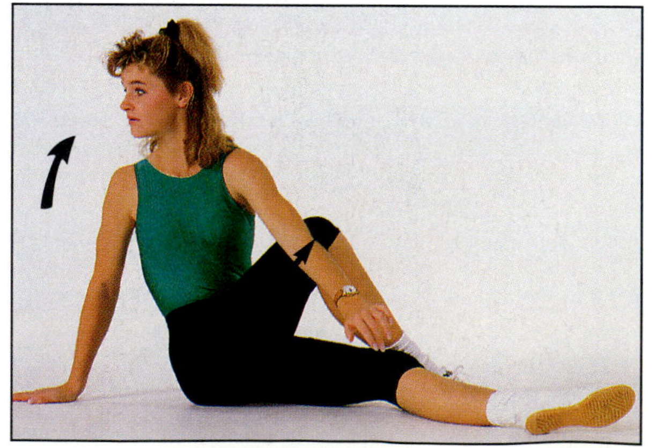

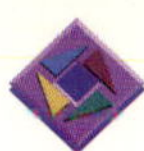

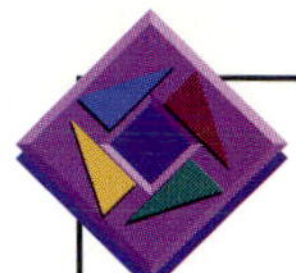

# 21

## Pelvic Tilt

**ACTION** Lie flat on the floor with the knees bent at about a 70° angle. Tilt the pelvis by tightening the abdominal muscles, flattening your back against the floor, and raising the lower gluteal area ever so slightly off the floor (see illustration b). Hold the final position for several seconds. The exercise can also be performed against a wall (as shown in illustration c). Repeat this exercise 4–5 times.

**AREAS STRETCHED** Low back muscles and ligaments.

**AREAS STRENGTHENED** Abdominal and gluteal muscles.

**NOTE:**

This is perhaps the most important exercise for the care of the lower back. It should be included as a part of the your daily exercise routine and should be performed several times throughout the day when pain in the lower back is present as a result of muscle imbalance.

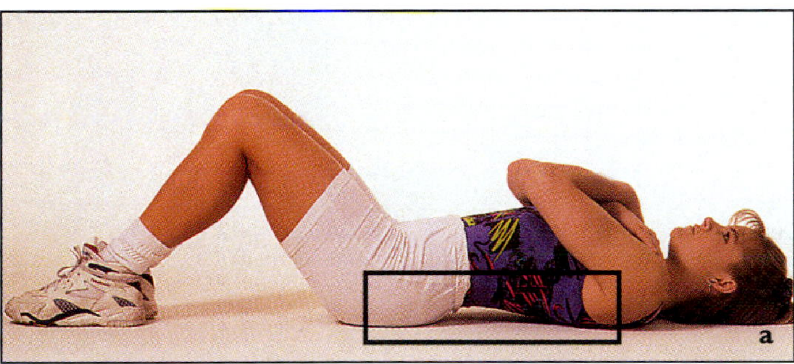

a

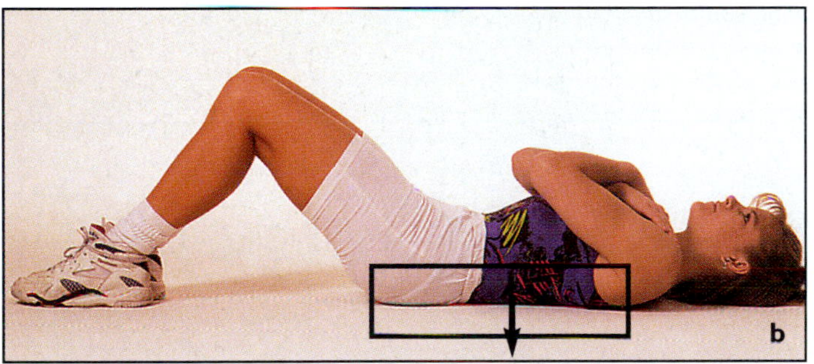

b

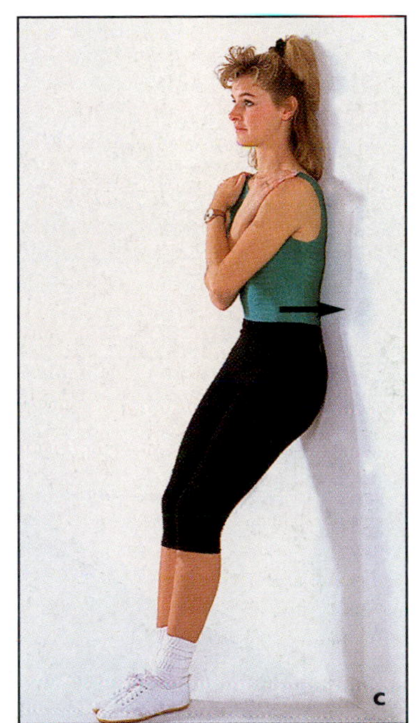

c

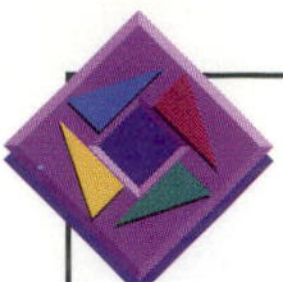

## 22

## The Cat

**ACTION** Kneel on the floor and place your hands in front of you (on the floor) about shoulder width apart. Relax your trunk and lower back (a). Now arch the spine and pull in your abdomen as far as you can and hold this position for 5–10 seconds (b). Repeat the exercise 4–5 times.

**AREAS STRETCHED** Low back muscles and ligaments.

**AREAS STRENGTHENED** Abdominal and gluteal muscles.

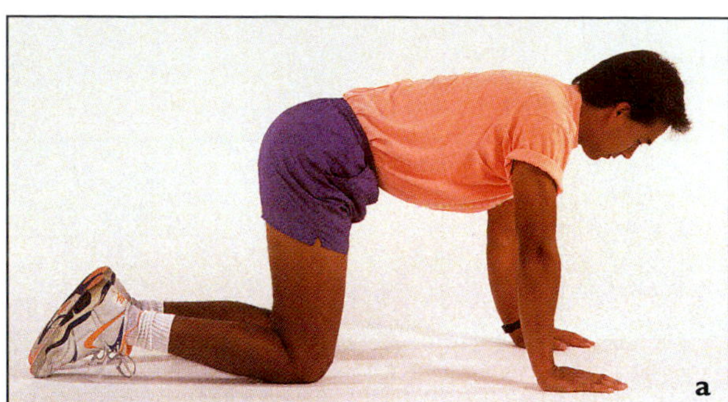
a

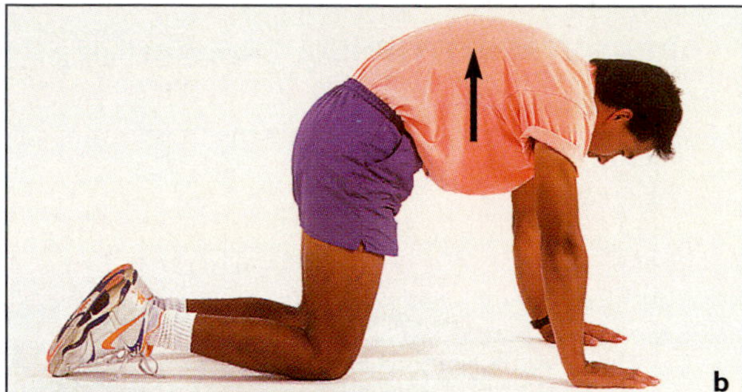
b

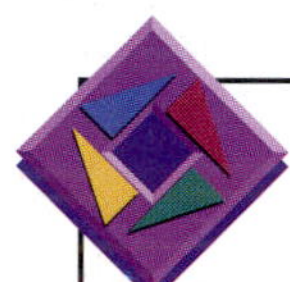

## 23

## Abdominal Crunch and Abdominal Curl-Up

**(see Exercise 4 in Chapter 8)**

It is important that you do not stabilize your feet when performing either of these exercises, because doing so decreases the work of the abdominal muscles. Also, remember not to "swing up" but rather to curl up as you perform these exercises.

# Body Composition Assessment

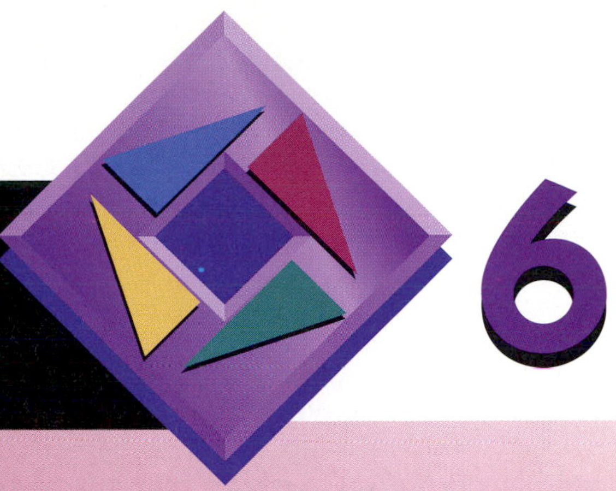


## Key Concepts

Body composition
Recommended body weight
Percent body fat
Lean body mass
Essential fat
Storage fat
Skinfold thickness
Girth measurements
Bioelectrical impedance
Waist-to-hip ratio
Body mass index

## Objectives

- Define body composition and its relationship to recommended body weight assessment.
- Learn the difference between essential and storage fat.
- Identify various techniques used in assessing body composition.
- Learn to assess body composition using the skinfold thickness technique.
- Be able to assess body composition using the girth measurements technique.
- Understand the importance of an adequate waist-to-hip ratio.
- Learn to calculate body mass index and be able to interpret the results.
- Be able to determine recommended weight according to recommended percent body fat values.

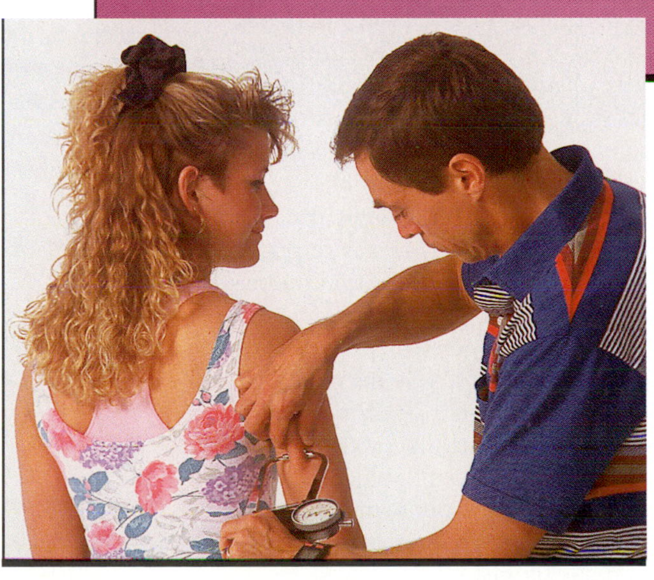

Obesity is a health hazard of epidemic proportions in most developed countries around the world. An estimated 35% of the adult population in industrialized nations is obese. According to 1993 estimates, 65% of adults in the United States was over recommended body weight. The prevalence continues to increase and seems to be getting worse.

When Yankee Stadium in New York was renovated several years ago, total seating capacity had to be reduced to accommodate the wider bodies of the spectators. During the last decade, the average weight of American adults increased by about 15 pounds. In 1991, 33% of adults were at least 10% above recommended body weight. In 1993, this figure grew to 40%.

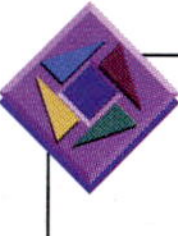

*During the last decade, the average weight of American adults increased by about 15 pounds.*

Obesity by itself has been associated with several serious health problems and accounts for 15% to 20% of the annual mortality rate in the United States. Obesity is a major risk factor for diseases of the cardiovascular system, including coronary heart disease, hypertension, congestive heart failure, high levels of blood lipids, atherosclerosis, strokes, thromboembolitic disease, diabetes, osteoarthritis, varicose veins, and intermittent claudication.

Other research points toward a possible link between obesity and cancer of the colon, rectum, prostate, gallbladder, breast, uterus, and ovaries. In addition, obesity has been associated with diabetes, ruptured intervertebral discs, gallstones, gout, respiratory insufficiency, and complications during pregnancy and delivery. Furthermore, it is implicated in psychological maladjustment and a higher accidental death rate.

The same is true for underweight people. Although the social pressure to be thin has retreated slightly in recent years, the pressure to attain model-like thinness is still with us and contributes to the gradual increase in the number of people who develop eating disorders (anorexia nervosa and bulimia, discussed in Chapter 8). Extreme weight loss can lead to medical conditions such as heart damage, gastrointestinal problems, shrinkage of internal organs, immune system abnormalities, disorders of the reproductive system, loss of muscle tissue, damage to the nervous system, and even death.

## WHAT DOES "BODY COMPOSITION" MEAN?

To understand body composition, we must recognize first that the human body consists of fat and nonfat components. The fat component usually is called *fat mass* or *percent body fat*. The nonfat component is termed *lean body mass*.

For many years people relied on height/ weight charts to determine recommended body weight. We now know, however, that these tables can be highly inaccurate and they fail to identify critical fat values associated with higher risk for disease. The proper way to determine recommended weight is by finding out what percent of total body weight is fat and what amount is lean tissue — determining body composition.

Once the fat percentage is known, recommended body weight can be calculated from recommended body fat. Recommended body weight, also called *healthy weight*, is defined as the body weight at which there seems to be no harm to human health. This assumes the absence of any medical condition that would improve with weight loss and a fat distribution pattern that is not associated with higher risk for illness.

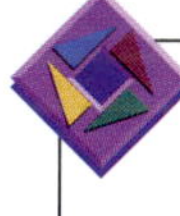

*Recommended body weight, also called healthy weight, is defined as the body weight at which there seems to be no harm to human health.*

Although various techniques for determining percent body fat were developed several years ago, many people still are unaware of these procedures and continue to depend on height/weight charts to find out their recommended body weight. The standard height/weight tables, first published in 1912, were based on average weights (including shoes and clothing) for men and women who obtained life insurance policies between 1888 and 1905. The recommended body weight on these tables is obtained according to sex, height, and frame size. Because no scientific guidelines are given to determine frame size, most people choose their frame size based on the column in which the weight comes closest to their own!

To determine whether people are truly obese or falsely at recommended body weight, body composition must be established. Obesity is related to

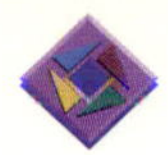

an excess of body fat. If body weight is the only criterion, an individual can easily be overweight, according to height/weight charts, yet not have too much body fat. Football players, body builders, weight lifters, and other athletes with large muscle size are typical examples. Some of these athletes who appear to be 20 or 30 pounds overweight really have little body fat.

The inaccuracy of height/weight charts was illustrated clearly when a young man who weighed about 225 pounds applied to join a city police force but was turned down without having been granted an interview. The reason? He was "too fat," according to the height/weight charts. When this young man's body composition later was assessed at a preventive medicine clinic, he was shocked to find out that only 5% of his total body weight was in the form of fat — considerably lower than the recommended standard. In the words of the technical director of the clinic, "The only way this fellow could come down to the chart's target weight would have been through surgical removal of a large amount of his muscle tissue."

At the other end of the spectrum, some people who weigh very little and may be viewed as skinny or underweight actually can be classified as obese because of their high body fat content. People who weigh as little as 100 pounds but are more than 30% fat (about one-third of their total body weight) are not uncommon. These cases are found more readily in the sedentary population and among people who are always dieting. Physical inactivity and constant negative caloric balance both lead to a loss in lean body mass (see Chapter 8). From these examples, body weight alone clearly does not always tell the true story.

## ESSENTIAL AND STORAGE FAT

Total fat in the human body is classified into two types: essential fat and storage fat. *Essential fat* is needed for normal physiological functions, and without it human health deteriorates. This type of fat is found in such tissues as muscles, nerve cells, bone marrow, intestines, heart, liver, and lungs. This essential fat constitutes about 3% of the total weight in men and 12% in women. The percentage is higher in women because it includes sex-specific fat, such as that found in the breast tissue, the uterus, and other sex-related fat deposits.

*Storage fat* is the fat stored in adipose tissue, mostly beneath the skin (subcutaneous fat) and around major organs in the body. This fat serves three basic functions:

1. As an insulator to retain body heat.
2. As energy substrate for metabolism.
3. As padding against physical trauma to the body.

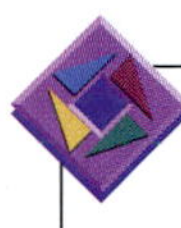

*Essential fat, needed for normal physiological functions, is about 3% of body weight in men and 12% in women.*

The amount of storage fat does not differ between men and women, except that men tend to store fat around the waist and women more so around the hips and thighs.

## TECHNIQUES FOR ASSESSING BODY COMPOSITION

Body composition can be assessed through several different procedures. The most common techniques are: (a) hydrostatic or underwater weighing, (b) skinfold thickness, (c) girth measurements, and (d) bioelectrical impedance. Because these procedures are used to estimate body fat, each technique may yield slightly different values. Therefore, when assessing body composition, the same technique should be used for pre- and post-test comparisons.

### Hydrostatic Weighing

Hydrostatic weighing has been called the "gold standard" of body composition. Almost all other techniques to determine body composition are validated against hydrostatic weighing. It is the most accurate technique if it is done properly and if the individual is able to perform the test adequately. The procedure requires a considerable amount of time, skill, space, and equipment and must be administered by a well-trained technician.

Because each individual assessment can take as long as 30 minutes, hydrostatic weighing is not feasible when testing a lot of people. Furthermore, the person's residual lung volume (amount of air left in the lungs following complete forceful exhalation) has to be measured before testing. If residual volume cannot be measured, as is the case in many laboratories and health/fitness centers, it can be estimated using the predicting equations, which

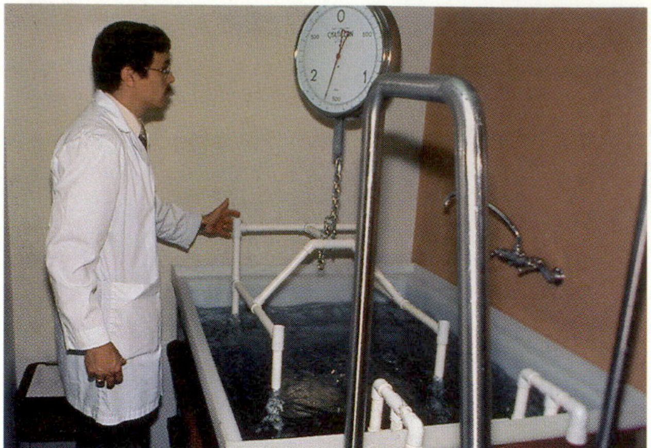

*Hydrostatic weighing technique for body composition assessment.*

may decrease the accuracy of hydrostatic weighing. Also, the psychological variables in being weighed while submerged underwater makes hydrostatic weighing difficult to administer to aquaphobic people (those with a fear of water).

Because of the cost, time, and complexity of hydrostatic weighing, most health and fitness programs prefer anthropometric measurement techniques, which correlate quite well with hydrostatic weighing. These techniques, primarily skinfold thickness and girth measurements, allow a quick, simple, and inexpensive estimate of body composition.

## Skinfold Thickness

Assessing body composition using skinfold thickness is based on the principle that approximately half of the body's fatty tissue is directly beneath the skin. Valid and reliable measurements of this tissue give a good indication of percent body fat.

The skinfold test is done with the aid of pressure calipers. Several sites must be measured to reflect the total percentage of fat: triceps, suprailium, and thigh skinfolds for women; and chest, abdomen, and thigh for men (see Figure 6.1). All measurements should be taken on the right side of the body.

Even with the skinfold technique, training is necessary to obtain accurate measurements. Also, different technicians may produce slightly different measurements from the same person. Therefore, the same technician should take pre- and post-measurements. And measurements should be done at the same time of the day, preferably in the

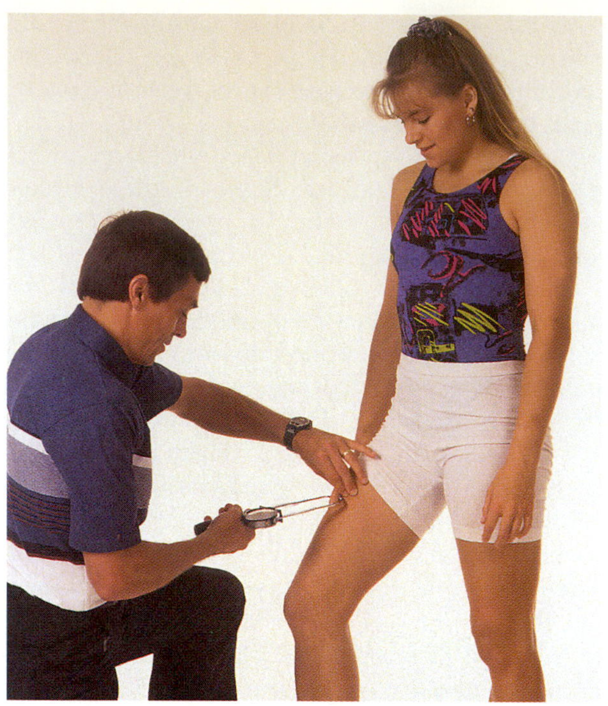

*Skinfold thickness technique for body composition assessment.*

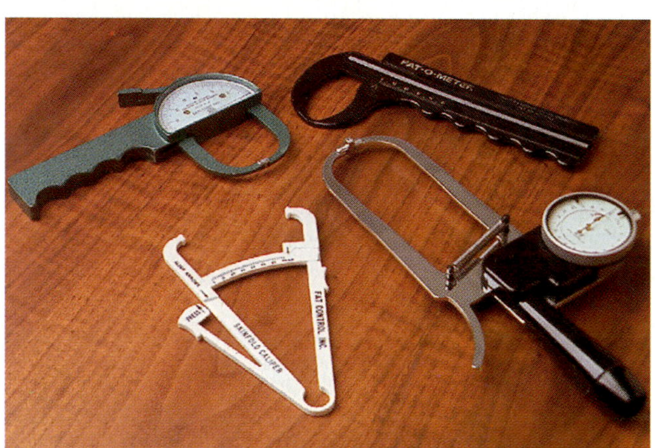


*Various types of skinfold calipers used to assess skinfold thickness.*

morning, as changes in water hydration from activity and exercise can affect skinfold girth. The procedure for assessing percent body fat using skinfold thickness is given in Figure 6.2. If skinfold calipers* are available to you, you may proceed to assess your percent body fat with the help of your instructor or an experienced technician.

*This instrument is available at most colleges and universities. If unavailable, you can purchase an inexpensive, yet reliable Skinfold Caliper from: Fat Control Inc., P. O. Box 10117, Towson, MD 21204, Phone (301) 296-1993

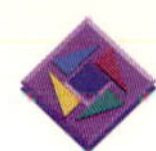

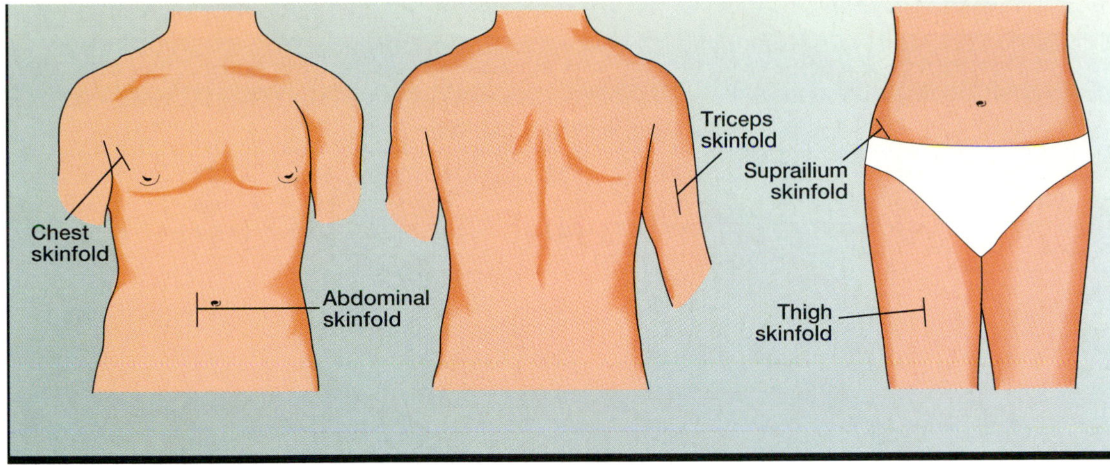


**FIGURE 6.1** ◆ Anatomical landmarks for skinfold measurements.

## BODY FAT ASSESSMENT ACCORDING TO SKINFOLD THICKNESS

1. Select the proper anatomical sites. For men: chest, abdomen, and thigh. For women: triceps, suprailium, and thigh (see Figure 6.1). Take all measurements on the right side of the body with the person standing. The correct anatomical landmarks for skinfolds are:

   Chest: a diagonal fold halfway between the shoulder crease and the nipple.

   Abdomen: a vertical fold taken about an inch to the right of the umbilicus.

   Triceps: a vertical fold on the back of the upper arm, halfway between the shoulder and the elbow.

   Thigh: a vertical fold on the front of the thigh, midway between the knee and hip.

   Suprailium: a diagonal fold above the crest of the ilium (on the side of the hip).

2. Measure each site by grasping a double thickness of skin firmly with the thumb and forefinger, pulling the fold slightly away from the muscular tissue. Hold the calipers perpendicular to the fold, and take the measurement ½" below the finger hold. Measure each site three times, and read the values to the nearest .1 to .5 mm. Record the average of the two closest readings as the final value. Take the readings without delay to avoid excessive compression of the skinfold. Releasing and refolding the skinfold is required between readings.

3. When doing pre- and post-assessments, conduct the measurement at the same time of day. The best time is early in the morning to avoid water hydration changes resulting from activity or exercise.

4. Obtain percent fat by adding the three skinfold measurements and looking up the respective values on Tables 6.1 for women, 6.2 for men under age 40, and 6.3 for men over 40.

   For example, if the skinfold measurements for an 18-year-old female are: (a) triceps = 16, (b) suprailium = 4, and (c) thigh = 30 (total = 50), the percent body fat is 20.6%

**FIGURE 6.2** ◆ Skinfold thickness procedure for body fat assessment.

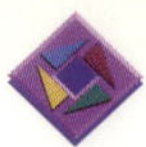



**TABLE 6.1**
**Percent Fat Estimates for Women Calculated from Triceps, Suprailium, and Thigh Skinfold Thickness**

| Sum of 3 Skinfolds | Age to the Last Year: Under 22 | 23 to 27 | 28 to 32 | 33 to 37 | 38 to 42 | 43 to 47 | 48 to 52 | 53 to 57 | Over 58 |
|---|---|---|---|---|---|---|---|---|---|
| 23- 25 | 9.7 | 9.9 | 10.2 | 10.4 | 10.7 | 10.9 | 11.2 | 11.4 | 11.7 |
| 26- 28 | 11.0 | 11.2 | 11.5 | 11.7 | 12.0 | 12.3 | 12.5 | 12.7 | 13.0 |
| 29- 31 | 12.3 | 12.5 | 12.8 | 13.0 | 13.3 | 13.5 | 13.8 | 14.0 | 14.3 |
| 32- 34 | 13.6 | 13.8 | 14.0 | 14.3 | 14.5 | 14.8 | 15.0 | 15.3 | 15.5 |
| 35- 37 | 14.8 | 15.0 | 15.3 | 15.5 | 15.8 | 16.0 | 16.3 | 16.5 | 16.8 |
| 38- 40 | 16.0 | 16.3 | 16.5 | 16.7 | 17.0 | 17.2 | 17.5 | 17.7 | 18.0 |
| 41- 43 | 17.2 | 17.4 | 17.7 | 17.9 | 18.2 | 18.4 | 18.7 | 18.9 | 19.2 |
| 44- 46 | 18.3 | 18.6 | 18.8 | 19.1 | 19.3 | 19.6 | 19.8 | 20.1 | 20.3 |
| 47- 49 | 19.5 | 19.7 | 20.0 | 20.2 | 20.5 | 20.7 | 21.0 | 21.2 | 21.5 |
| 50- 52 | 20.6 | 20.8 | 21.1 | 21.3 | 21.6 | 21.8 | 22.1 | 22.3 | 22.6 |
| 53- 55 | 21.7 | 21.9 | 22.1 | 22.4 | 22.6 | 22.9 | 23.1 | 23.4 | 23.6 |
| 56- 58 | 22.7 | 23.0 | 23.2 | 23.4 | 23.7 | 23.9 | 24.2 | 24.4 | 24.7 |
| 59- 61 | 23.7 | 24.0 | 24.2 | 24.5 | 24.7 | 25.0 | 25.2 | 25.5 | 25.7 |
| 62- 64 | 24.7 | 25.0 | 25.2 | 25.5 | 25.7 | 26.0 | 26.2 | 26.4 | 26.7 |
| 65- 67 | 25.7 | 25.9 | 26.2 | 26.4 | 26.7 | 26.9 | 27.2 | 27.4 | 27.7 |
| 68- 70 | 26.6 | 26.9 | 27.1 | 27.4 | 27.6 | 27.9 | 28.1 | 28.4 | 28.6 |
| 71- 73 | 27.5 | 27.8 | 28.0 | 28.3 | 28.5 | 28.8 | 29.0 | 29.3 | 29.5 |
| 74- 76 | 28.4 | 28.7 | 28.9 | 29.2 | 29.4 | 29.7 | 29.9 | 30.2 | 30.4 |
| 77- 79 | 29.3 | 29.5 | 29.8 | 30.0 | 30.3 | 30.5 | 30.8 | 31.0 | 31.3 |
| 80- 82 | 30.1 | 30.4 | 30.6 | 30.9 | 31.1 | 31.4 | 31.6 | 31.9 | 32.1 |
| 83- 85 | 30.9 | 31.2 | 31.4 | 31.7 | 31.9 | 32.2 | 32.4 | 32.7 | 32.9 |
| 86- 88 | 31.7 | 32.0 | 32.2 | 32.5 | 32.7 | 32.9 | 33.2 | 33.4 | 33.7 |
| 89- 91 | 32.5 | 32.7 | 33.0 | 33.2 | 33.5 | 33.7 | 33.9 | 34.2 | 34.4 |
| 92- 94 | 33.2 | 33.4 | 33.7 | 33.9 | 34.2 | 34.4 | 34.7 | 34.9 | 35.2 |
| 95- 97 | 33.9 | 34.1 | 34.4 | 34.6 | 34.9 | 35.1 | 35.4 | 35.6 | 35.9 |
| 98-100 | 34.6 | 34.8 | 35.1 | 35.3 | 35.5 | 35.8 | 36.0 | 36.3 | 36.5 |
| 101-103 | 35.2 | 35.4 | 35.7 | 35.9 | 36.2 | 36.4 | 36.7 | 36.9 | 37.2 |
| 104-106 | 35.8 | 36.1 | 36.3 | 36.6 | 36.8 | 37.1 | 37.3 | 37.5 | 37.8 |
| 107-109 | 36.4 | 36.7 | 36.9 | 37.1 | 37.4 | 37.6 | 37.9 | 38.1 | 38.4 |
| 110-112 | 37.0 | 37.2 | 37.5 | 37.7 | 38.0 | 38.2 | 38.5 | 38.7 | 38.9 |
| 113-115 | 37.5 | 37.8 | 38.0 | 38.2 | 38.5 | 38.7 | 39.0 | 39.2 | 39.5 |
| 116-118 | 38.0 | 38.3 | 38.5 | 38.8 | 39.0 | 39.3 | 39.5 | 39.7 | 40.0 |
| 119-121 | 38.5 | 38.7 | 39.0 | 39.2 | 39.5 | 39.7 | 40.0 | 40.2 | 40.5 |
| 122-124 | 39.0 | 39.2 | 39.4 | 39.7 | 39.9 | 40.2 | 40.4 | 40.7 | 40.9 |
| 125-127 | 39.4 | 39.6 | 39.9 | 40.1 | 40.4 | 40.6 | 40.9 | 41.1 | 41.4 |
| 128-130 | 39.8 | 40.0 | 40.3 | 40.5 | 40.8 | 41.0 | 41.3 | 41.5 | 41.8 |

Body density is calculated based on the generalized equation for predicting body density of women developed by A. S. Jackson, M. L. Pollock, and A. Ward. *Medicine and Science in Sports and Exercise* 12, (1980), 175–182. Percent body fat is determined from the calculated body density using the Siri formula.

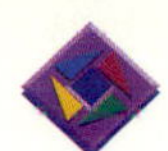

**TABLE 6.2**
**Percent Fat Estimates for Men Under Age 40 Calculated from Chest, Abdomen, and Thigh Skinfold Thickness**

| | Age to the Last Year | | | | | | | |
|---|---|---|---|---|---|---|---|---|
| Sum of 3 Skinfolds | Under 19 | 20 to 22 | 23 to 25 | 26 to 28 | 29 to 31 | 32 to 34 | 35 to 37 | 38 to 40 |
| 8- 10 | .9 | 1.3 | 1.6 | 2.0 | 2.3 | 2.7 | 3.0 | 3.3 |
| 11- 13 | 1.9 | 2.3 | 2.6 | 3.0 | 3.3 | 3.7 | 4.0 | 4.3 |
| 14- 16 | 2.9 | 3.3 | 3.6 | 3.9 | 4.3 | 4.6 | 5.0 | 5.3 |
| 17- 19 | 3.9 | 4.2 | 4.6 | 4.9 | 5.3 | 5.6 | 6.0 | 6.3 |
| 20- 22 | 4.8 | 5.2 | 5.5 | 5.9 | 6.2 | 6.6 | 6.9 | 7.3 |
| 23- 25 | 5.8 | 6.2 | 6.5 | 6.8 | 7.2 | 7.5 | 7.9 | 8.2 |
| 26- 28 | 6.8 | 7.1 | 7.5 | 7.8 | 8.1 | 8.5 | 8.8 | 9.2 |
| 29- 31 | 7.7 | 8.0 | 8.4 | 8.7 | 9.1 | 9.4 | 9.8 | 10.1 |
| 32- 34 | 8.6 | 9.0 | 9.3 | 9.7 | 10.0 | 10.4 | 10.7 | 11.1 |
| 35- 37 | 9.5 | 9.9 | 10.2 | 10.6 | 10.9 | 11.3 | 11.6 | 12.0 |
| 38- 40 | 10.5 | 10.8 | 11.2 | 11.5 | 11.8 | 12.2 | 12.5 | 12.9 |
| 41- 43 | 11.4 | 11.7 | 12.1 | 12.4 | 12.7 | 13.1 | 13.4 | 13.8 |
| 44- 46 | 12.2 | 12.6 | 12.9 | 13.3 | 13.6 | 14.0 | 14.3 | 14.7 |
| 47- 49 | 13.1 | 13.5 | 13.8 | 14.2 | 14.5 | 14.9 | 15.2 | 15.5 |
| 50- 52 | 14.0 | 14.3 | 14.7 | 15.0 | 15.4 | 15.7 | 16.1 | 16.4 |
| 53- 55 | 14.8 | 15.2 | 15.5 | 15.9 | 16.2 | 16.6 | 16.9 | 17.3 |
| 56- 58 | 15.7 | 16.0 | 16.4 | 16.7 | 17.1 | 17.4 | 17.8 | 18.1 |
| 59- 61 | 16.5 | 16.9 | 17.2 | 17.6 | 17.9 | 18.3 | 18.6 | 19.0 |
| 62- 64 | 17.4 | 17.7 | 18.1 | 18.4 | 18.8 | 19.1 | 19.4 | 19.8 |
| 65- 67 | 18.2 | 18.5 | 18.9 | 19.2 | 19.6 | 19.9 | 20.3 | 20.6 |
| 68- 70 | 19.0 | 19.3 | 19.7 | 20.0 | 20.4 | 20.7 | 21.1 | 21.4 |
| 71- 73 | 19.8 | 20.1 | 20.5 | 20.8 | 21.2 | 21.5 | 21.9 | 22.2 |
| 74- 76 | 20.6 | 20.9 | 21.3 | 21.6 | 22.0 | 22.2 | 22.7 | 23.0 |
| 77- 79 | 21.4 | 21.7 | 22.1 | 22.4 | 22.8 | 23.1 | 23.4 | 23.8 |
| 80- 82 | 22.1 | 22.5 | 22.8 | 23.2 | 23.5 | 23.9 | 24.2 | 24.6 |
| 83- 85 | 22.9 | 23.2 | 23.6 | 23.9 | 24.3 | 24.6 | 25.0 | 25.3 |
| 86- 88 | 23.6 | 24.0 | 24.3 | 24.7 | 25.0 | 25.4 | 25.7 | 26.1 |
| 89- 91 | 24.4 | 24.7 | 25.1 | 25.4 | 25.8 | 26.1 | 26.5 | 26.8 |
| 92- 94 | 25.1 | 25.5 | 25.8 | 26.2 | 26.5 | 26.9 | 27.2 | 27.5 |
| 95- 97 | 25.8 | 26.2 | 26.5 | 26.9 | 27.2 | 27.6 | 27.9 | 28.3 |
| 98-100 | 26.6 | 26.9 | 27.3 | 27.6 | 27.9 | 28.3 | 28.6 | 29.0 |
| 101-103 | 27.3 | 27.6 | 28.0 | 28.3 | 28.6 | 29.0 | 29.3 | 29.7 |
| 104-106 | 27.9 | 28.3 | 28.6 | 29.0 | 29.3 | 29.7 | 30.0 | 30.4 |
| 107-109 | 28.6 | 29.0 | 29.3 | 29.7 | 30.0 | 30.4 | 30.7 | 31.1 |
| 110-112 | 29.3 | 29.6 | 30.0 | 30.3 | 30.7 | 31.0 | 31.4 | 31.7 |
| 113-115 | 30.0 | 30.3 | 30.7 | 31.0 | 31.3 | 31.7 | 32.0 | 32.4 |
| 116-118 | 30.6 | 31.0 | 31.3 | 31.6 | 32.0 | 32.3 | 32.7 | 33.0 |
| 119-121 | 31.3 | 31.6 | 32.0 | 32.3 | 32.6 | 33.0 | 33.3 | 33.7 |
| 122-124 | 31.9 | 32.2 | 32.6 | 32.9 | 33.3 | 33.6 | 34.0 | 34.3 |
| 125-127 | 32.5 | 32.9 | 33.2 | 33.5 | 33.9 | 34.2 | 34.6 | 34.9 |
| 128-130 | 33.1 | 33.5 | 33.8 | 34.2 | 34.5 | 34.9 | 35.2 | 35.5 |

Body density is calculated based on the generalized equation for predicting body density of men developed by A. S. Jackson and M. L. Pollock, *British Journal of Nutrition* 40, (1978) 497–504. Percent body fat is determined from the calculated body density using the Siri formula.

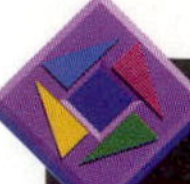

**TABLE 6.3**
**Percent Fat Estimates for Men Over Age 40 Calculated from Chest, Abdomen, and Thigh Skinfold Thickness**

| | Age to the Last Year | | | | | | | |
|---|---|---|---|---|---|---|---|---|
| Sum of 3 Skinfolds | 41 to 43 | 44 to 46 | 47 to 49 | 50 to 52 | 53 to 55 | 56 to 58 | 59 to 61 | Over 62 |
| 8- 10 | 3.7 | 4.0 | 4.4 | 4.7 | 5.1 | 5.4 | 5.8 | 6.1 |
| 11- 13 | 4.7 | 5.0 | 5.4 | 5.7 | 6.1 | 6.4 | 6.8 | 7.1 |
| 14- 16 | 5.7 | 6.0 | 6.4 | 6.7 | 7.1 | 7.4 | 7.8 | 8.1 |
| 17- 19 | 6.7 | 7.0 | 7.4 | 7.7 | 8.1 | 8.4 | 8.7 | 9.1 |
| 20- 22 | 7.6 | 8.0 | 8.3 | 8.7 | 9.0 | 9.4 | 9.7 | 10.1 |
| 23- 25 | 8.6 | 8.9 | 9.3 | 9.6 | 10.0 | 10.3 | 10.7 | 11.0 |
| 26- 28 | 9.5 | 9.9 | 10.2 | 10.6 | 10.9 | 11.3 | 11.6 | 12.0 |
| 29- 31 | 10.5 | 10.8 | 11.2 | 11.5 | 11.9 | 12.2 | 12.6 | 12.9 |
| 32- 34 | 11.4 | 11.8 | 12.1 | 12.4 | 12.8 | 13.1 | 13.5 | 13.8 |
| 35- 37 | 12.3 | 12.7 | 13.0 | 13.4 | 13.7 | 14.1 | 14.4 | 14.8 |
| 38- 40 | 13.2 | 13.6 | 13.9 | 14.3 | 14.6 | 15.0 | 15.3 | 15.7 |
| 41- 43 | 14.1 | 14.5 | 14.8 | 15.2 | 15.5 | 15.9 | 16.2 | 16.6 |
| 44- 46 | 15.0 | 15.4 | 15.7 | 16.1 | 16.4 | 16.8 | 17.1 | 17.5 |
| 47- 49 | 15.9 | 16.2 | 16.6 | 16.9 | 17.3 | 17.6 | 18.0 | 18.3 |
| 50- 52 | 16.8 | 17.1 | 17.5 | 17.8 | 18.2 | 18.5 | 18.8 | 19.2 |
| 53- 55 | 17.6 | 18.0 | 18.3 | 18.7 | 19.0 | 19.4 | 19.7 | 20.1 |
| 56- 58 | 18.5 | 18.8 | 19.2 | 19.5 | 19.9 | 20.2 | 20.6 | 20.9 |
| 59- 61 | 19.3 | 19.7 | 20.0 | 20.4 | 20.7 | 21.0 | 21.4 | 21.7 |
| 62- 64 | 20.1 | 20.5 | 20.8 | 21.2 | 21.5 | 21.9 | 22.2 | 22.6 |
| 65- 67 | 21.0 | 21.3 | 21.7 | 22.0 | 22.4 | 22.7 | 23.0 | 23.4 |
| 68- 70 | 21.8 | 22.1 | 22.5 | 22.8 | 23.2 | 23.5 | 23.9 | 24.2 |
| 71- 73 | 22.6 | 22.9 | 23.3 | 23.6 | 24.0 | 24.3 | 24.7 | 25.0 |
| 74- 76 | 23.4 | 23.7 | 24.1 | 24.4 | 24.8 | 25.1 | 25.4 | 25.8 |
| 77- 79 | 24.1 | 24.5 | 24.8 | 25.2 | 25.5 | 25.9 | 26.2 | 26.6 |
| 80- 82 | 24.9 | 25.3 | 25.6 | 26.0 | 26.3 | 26.6 | 27.0 | 27.3 |
| 83- 85 | 25.7 | 26.0 | 26.4 | 26.7 | 27.1 | 27.4 | 27.8 | 28.1 |
| 86- 88 | 26.4 | 26.8 | 27.1 | 27.5 | 27.8 | 28.2 | 28.5 | 28.9 |
| 89- 91 | 27.2 | 27.5 | 27.9 | 28.2 | 28.6 | 28.9 | 29.2 | 29.6 |
| 92- 94 | 27.9 | 28.2 | 28.6 | 28.9 | 29.3 | 29.6 | 30.0 | 30.3 |
| 95- 97 | 28.6 | 29.0 | 29.3 | 29.7 | 30.0 | 30.4 | 30.7 | 31.1 |
| 98-100 | 29.3 | 29.7 | 30.0 | 30.4 | 30.7 | 31.1 | 31.4 | 31.8 |
| 101-103 | 30.0 | 30.4 | 30.7 | 31.1 | 31.4 | 31.8 | 32.1 | 32.5 |
| 104-106 | 30.7 | 31.1 | 31.4 | 31.8 | 32.1 | 32.5 | 32.8 | 33.2 |
| 107-109 | 31.4 | 31.8 | 32.1 | 32.4 | 32.8 | 33.1 | 33.5 | 33.8 |
| 110-112 | 32.1 | 32.4 | 32.8 | 33.1 | 33.5 | 33.8 | 34.2 | 34.5 |
| 113-115 | 32.7 | 33.1 | 33.4 | 33.8 | 34.1 | 34.5 | 34.8 | 35.2 |
| 116-118 | 33.4 | 33.7 | 34.1 | 34.4 | 34.8 | 35.1 | 35.5 | 35.8 |
| 119-121 | 34.0 | 34.4 | 34.7 | 35.1 | 35.4 | 35.8 | 36.1 | 36.5 |
| 122-124 | 34.7 | 35.0 | 35.4 | 35.7 | 36.1 | 36.4 | 36.7 | 37.1 |
| 125-127 | 35.3 | 35.6 | 36.0 | 36.3 | 36.7 | 37.0 | 37.4 | 37.7 |
| 128-130 | 35.9 | 36.2 | 36.6 | 36.9 | 37.3 | 37.6 | 38.0 | 38.5 |

Body density is calculated based on the generalized equation for predicting body density of men developed by A. S. Jackson and M. L. Pollock, *British Journal of Nutrition* 40 (1978), 497–504. Percent body fat is determined from the calculated body density using the Siri formula.

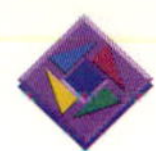

## Girth Measurements

A simpler method to determine body fat is by measuring circumferences at various body sites. This technique requires only a standard measuring tape. Good accuracy can be achieved with little practice. The limitation is that it may not be valid for athletic individuals (men or women) who participate actively in strenuous physical activity or for people who can be classified visually as thin or obese.

The required procedure for girth measurements is given in Figure 6.3. Measurements for women include the upper arm, hip, and wrist; for men, the waist and wrist.

### BODY FAT ASSESSMENT ACCORDING TO GIRTH MEASUREMENTS

**Girth Measurements for Women***

1. Using a regular tape measure, determine the following girth measurements in centimeters (cm):

   Upper Arm: take the measure halfway between the shoulder and the elbow.

   Hip: measure at the point of largest circumference.

   Wrist: take the girth in front of the bones where the wrist bends.

2. Obtain the person's age.
3. Using Table 6.4, find the girth measurement for each site and age in the lefthand columns. Look up the constant values in the righthand columns. These values will allow you to derive body density (BD) by substituting the constants in the following formula:

   BD = A – B – C + D

4. Using the derived body density, calculate percent body fat (%F) according to the following equation:

   %F = (495 ÷ BD) – 450**

   Example: Jane is 20 years old, and the following girth measurements were taken: biceps = 27 cm, hip = 99.5 cm, wrist = 15.4 cm.

| Data | Constant |
|---|---|
| Upper Arm = 27 cm | A = 1.0813 |
| Age = 20 | B = .0102 |
| Hip = 99.5 cm | C = .1206 |
| Wrist = 15.4 cm | D = .0971 |

BD = A – B – C + D
BD = 1.0813 – .0102 – .1206 + .0971 = 1.0476

%F = (495 ÷ BD) – 450
%F = (495 ÷ 1.0476) – 450 = 22.5

**Girth Measurements for Men*****

1. Using a regular tape measure, determine the following girth measurements in inches (the men's measurements are taken in inches as contrasted with centimeters for women):

   Waist: measure at the umbilicus (belly button)

   Wrist: measure in front of the bones where the wrist bends.

2. Subtract the wrist from the waist measurement.
3. Obtain the person's weight in pounds.
4. Look up the percent body fat (%F) in Table 6.5 by using the difference obtained in step 2 above and the person's body weight.

   Example: John weighs 160 pounds, and his waist and wrist girth measurements are 36.5 and 7.5 inches, respectively.

   Waist girth = 36.5 inches
   Wrist girth = 7.5 inches
   Difference = 29.0 inches
   Body weight = 160.0 lbs.
   %F = 22

* Reproduced by permission from R. B. Lambson, "Generalized Body Density Prediction Equations for Women Using Simple Anthropometric Measurements," unpublished doctoral dissertation, Brigham Young University, Provo, UT, August 1987.

** From W. E. Siri, *Body Composition From Fluid Spaces and Density* (Berkeley: University of California, Donner Laboratory of Medical Physics, 1956).

*** Table 3.5 reproduced by permission from A. G. Fisher, and P. E. Allsen, *Jogging* (Dubuque, IA: Wm. C. Brown, 1987). This table was developed according to the generalized body composition equation for men using simple measurement techniques by K. W. Penrouse, A. G Nelson, and A G. Fisher, *Medicine and Science in Sports and Exercise* 17(2):189, 1985. © American College of Sports Medicine 1985.

**FIGURE 6.3** ◆ Procedure for assessing body fat by girth measurements.

**TABLE 6.4**
**Conversion Constants from Girth Measurements (Centimeters) to Calculate Body Density for Women**

| Upper Arm (cm) | Constant A | Age | Constant B | Hip (cm) | Constant C | Hip (cm) | Constant C | Wrist (cm) | Constant D |
|---|---|---|---|---|---|---|---|---|---|
| 20.5 | 1.0966 | 17 | .0086 | 79 | .0957 | 114.5 | .1388 | 13.0 | .0819 |
| 21 | 1.0954 | 18 | .0091 | 79.5 | .0963 | 115 | .1394 | 13.2 | .0832 |
| 21.5 | 1.0942 | 19 | .0096 | 80 | .0970 | 115.5 | .1400 | 13.4 | .0845 |
| 22 | 1.0930 | 20 | .0102 | 80.5 | .0976 | 116 | .1406 | 13.6 | .0857 |
| 22.5 | 1.0919 | 21 | .0107 | 81 | .0982 | 116.5 | .1412 | 13.8 | .0807 |
| 23 | 1.0907 | 22 | .0112 | 81.5 | .0988 | 117 | .1418 | 14.0 | .0882 |
| 23.5 | 1.0895 | 23 | .0117 | 82 | .0994 | 117.5 | .1424 | 14.2 | .0895 |
| 24 | 1.0883 | 24 | .0122 | 82.5 | .1000 | 118 | .1430 | 14.4 | .0908 |
| 24.5 | 1.0871 | 25 | .0127 | 83 | .1006 | 118.5 | .1436 | 14.6 | .0920 |
| 25 | 1.0860 | 26 | .0132 | 83.5 | .1012 | 119 | .1442 | 14.8 | .0933 |
| 25.5 | 1.0848 | 27 | .0137 | 84 | .1018 | 119.5 | .1448 | 15.0 | .0946 |
| 26 | 1.0836 | 28 | .0142 | 84.5 | .1024 | 120 | .1454 | 15.2 | .0958 |
| 26.5 | 1.0824 | 29 | .0147 | 85 | .1030 | 120.5 | .1460 | 15.4 | .0971 |
| 27 | 1.0813 | 30 | .0152 | 85.5 | .1036 | 121 | .1466 | 15.6 | .0983 |
| 27.5 | 1.0801 | 31 | .0157 | 86 | .1042 | 121.5 | .1472 | 15.8 | .0996 |
| 28 | 1.0789 | 32 | .0162 | 86.5 | .1048 | 122 | .1479 | 16.0 | .1009 |
| 28.5 | 1.0777 | 33 | .0168 | 87 | .1054 | 122.5 | .1485 | 16.2 | .1021 |
| 29 | 1.0775 | 34 | .0173 | 87.5 | .1060 | 123 | .1491 | 16.4 | .1034 |
| 29.5 | 1.0754 | 35 | .0178 | 88 | .1066 | 123.5 | .1497 | 16.6 | .1046 |
| 30 | 1.0742 | 36 | .0183 | 88.5 | .1072 | 124 | .1503 | 16.8 | .1059 |
| 30.5 | 1.0730 | 37 | .0188 | 89 | .1079 | 124.5 | .1509 | 17.0 | .1072 |
| 31 | 1.0718 | 38 | .0193 | 89.5 | .1085 | 125 | .1515 | 17.2 | .1084 |
| 31.5 | 1.0707 | 39 | .0198 | 90 | .1091 | 125.5 | .1521 | 17.4 | .1097 |
| 32 | 1.0695 | 40 | ,0203 | 90.5 | .1097 | 126 | .1527 | 17.6 | .1109 |
| 32.5 | 1.0683 | 41 | .0208 | 91 | .1103 | 126.5 | .1533 | 17.8 | .1122 |
| 33 | 1.0671 | 42 | .0213 | 91.5 | .1109 | 127 | .1539 | 18.0 | .1135 |
| 33.5 | 1.0666 | 43 | .0218 | 92 | .1115 | 127.5 | .1545 | 18.2 | .1147 |
| 34 | 1.0648 | 44 | .0223 | 92.5 | .1121 | 128 | .1551 | 18.4 | .1160 |
| 34.5 | 1.0636 | 45 | .0228 | 93 | .1127 | 128.5 | .1558 | 18.6 | .1172 |
| 35 | 1.0624 | 46 | .0234 | 93.5 | .1133 | 129 | .1563 | | |
| 35.5 | 1.0612 | 47 | .0239 | 94 | .1139 | 129.5 | .1569 | | |
| 36 | 1.0601 | 48 | ,0244 | 94.5 | .1145 | 130 | .1575 | | |
| 36.5 | 1.0589 | 49 | .0249 | 95 | .1151 | 130.5 | .1581 | | |
| 37 | 1.0577 | 50 | .0254 | 95.5 | .1157 | 131 | .1587 | | |
| 37.5 | 1.0565 | 51 | .0259 | 96 | .1163 | 131.5 | .1593 | | |
| 38 | 1.0554 | 52 | .0264 | 96.5 | .1169 | 132 | .1600 | | |
| 38.5 | 1.0542 | 53 | .0269 | 97 | .1176 | 132.5 | .1606 | | |
| 39 | 1.0530 | 54 | .0274 | 97.5 | .1182 | 133 | .1612 | | |
| 39.5 | 1.0518 | 55 | .0279 | 98 | .1188 | 133.5 | .1618 | | |
| 40 | 1.0506 | 56 | .0284 | 98.5 | .1194 | 134 | .1624 | | |
| 40.5 | 1.0495 | 57 | .0289 | 99 | .1200 | 134.5 | .1630 | | |
| 41 | 1.0483 | 58 | .0294 | 99.5 | .1206 | 135 | .1636 | | |
| 41.5 | 1.0471 | 59 | .0300 | 100 | .1212 | 135.5 | .1642 | | |
| 42 | 1.0459 | 60 | .0305 | 100.5 | .1218 | 136 | .1648 | | |
| 42.5 | 1.0448 | 61 | .0310 | 101 | .1224 | 136.5 | .1654 | | |
| 43 | 1.0434 | 62 | .0315 | 101.5 | .1230 | 137 | .1660 | | |

*(Continued)*

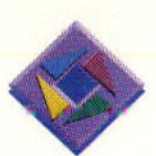

**TABLE 6.4** ***(continued)***
**Conversion Constants from Girth Measurements (Centimeters) to Calculate Body Density for Women**

| Upper Arm (cm) | Constant A | Age | Constant B | Hip (cm) | Constant C | Hip (cm) | Constant C | Wrist (cm) | Constant D |
|---|---|---|---|---|---|---|---|---|---|
| 43.5 | 1.0424 | 63 | .0320 | 102 | .1236 | 137.5 | .1666 | | |
| 44 | 1.0412 | 64 | .0325 | 102.5 | .1242 | 138 | .1672 | | |
| | | 65 | .0330 | 103 | .1248 | 138.5 | .1678 | | |
| | | 66 | .0335 | 103.5 | .1254 | 139 | .1685 | | |
| | | 67 | .0340 | 104 | .1260 | 139.5 | .1691 | | |
| | | 68 | .0345 | 104.5 | .1266 | 140 | .1697 | | |
| | | 69 | .0350 | 105 | .1272 | 140.5 | .1703 | | |
| | | 70 | .0355 | 105.5 | .1278 | 141 | .1709 | | |
| | | 71 | .0360 | 106 | .1285 | 141.5 | .1715 | | |
| | | 72 | .0366 | 106.5 | .1291 | 142 | .1721 | | |
| | | 73 | .0371 | 107 | .1297 | 142.5 | .1728 | | |
| | | 74 | .0376 | 107.5 | .1303 | 143 | .1733 | | |
| | | 75 | .0381 | 108 | .1309 | 143.5 | .1739 | | |
| | | | | 108.5 | .1315 | 144 | .1745 | | |
| | | | | 109 | .1321 | 144.5 | .1751 | | |
| | | | | 109.5 | .1327 | 145 | .1757 | | |
| | | | | 110 | .1333 | 145.5 | .1763 | | |
| | | | | 110.5 | .1339 | 146 | .1769 | | |
| | | | | 111 | .1345 | 146.5 | .1775 | | |
| | | | | 111.5 | .1351 | 147 | .1781 | | |
| | | | | 112 | .1357 | 147.5 | .1787 | | |
| | | | | 112.5 | .1363 | 148 | .1794 | | |
| | | | | 113 | .1369 | 148.5 | .1800 | | |
| | | | | 113.5 | .1375 | 149 | .1806 | | |
| | | | | 114 | .1382 | 149.5 | .1812 | | |
| | | | | | | 150 | .1818 | | |

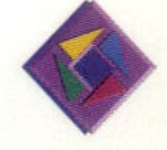

**TABLE 6.5**
**Estimated Percent Body Fat for Men Obtained from Waist Minus Wrist Girth Measurements (Inches) and Body Weight**

| | 22 | 22.5 | 23 | 23.5 | 24 | 24.5 | 25 | 25.5 | 26 | 26.5 | 27 | 27.5 | 28 | 28.5 | 29 | 29.5 | 30 | 30.5 | 31 | 31.5 | 32 | 32.5 | 33 | 33.5 | 34 | 34.5 | 35 | 35.5 | 36 |
|---|---|---|---|---|---|---|---|---|---|---|---|---|---|---|---|---|---|---|---|---|---|---|---|---|---|---|---|---|---|
| 120 | 4 | 6 | 8 | 10 | 12 | 14 | 16 | 18 | 20 | 21 | 23 | 25 | 27 | 29 | 31 | 33 | 35 | 37 | 39 | 41 | 43 | 45 | 47 | 49 | 50 | 52 | 54 | 56 | 58 |
| 125 | 4 | 6 | 7 | 9 | 11 | 13 | 15 | 17 | 19 | 20 | 22 | 24 | 26 | 28 | 30 | 32 | 33 | 35 | 37 | 39 | 41 | 43 | 45 | 46 | 48 | 50 | 52 | 54 | 56 |
| 130 | 3 | 5 | 7 | 9 | 11 | 12 | 14 | 16 | 18 | 20 | 21 | 23 | 25 | 27 | 28 | 30 | 32 | 34 | 36 | 37 | 39 | 41 | 43 | 44 | 46 | 48 | 50 | 52 | 53 |
| 135 | 3 | 5 | 7 | 8 | 10 | 12 | 13 | 15 | 17 | 19 | 20 | 22 | 24 | 26 | 27 | 29 | 31 | 32 | 34 | 36 | 38 | 39 | 41 | 43 | 44 | 46 | 48 | 50 | 51 |
| 140 | 3 | 5 | 6 | 8 | 10 | 11 | 13 | 15 | 16 | 18 | 19 | 21 | 23 | 24 | 26 | 28 | 29 | 31 | 33 | 34 | 36 | 38 | 39 | 41 | 43 | 44 | 46 | 48 | 49 |
| 145 | 3 | 4 | 6 | 7 | 9 | 11 | 12 | 14 | 15 | 17 | 19 | 20 | 22 | 23 | 25 | 27 | 28 | 30 | 31 | 33 | 35 | 36 | 38 | 39 | 41 | 43 | 44 | 46 | 47 |
| 150 | 2 | 4 | 6 | 7 | 9 | 10 | 12 | 13 | 15 | 16 | 18 | 19 | 21 | 23 | 24 | 26 | 27 | 29 | 30 | 32 | 33 | 35 | 36 | 38 | 40 | 41 | 43 | 44 | 46 |
| 155 | 2 | 4 | 5 | 7 | 8 | 10 | 11 | 13 | 14 | 16 | 17 | 19 | 20 | 22 | 23 | 25 | 26 | 28 | 29 | 31 | 32 | 34 | 35 | 37 | 38 | 40 | 41 | 43 | 44 |
| 160 | 2 | 4 | 5 | 6 | 8 | 9 | 11 | 12 | 14 | 15 | 17 | 18 | 19 | 21 | 22 | 24 | 25 | 27 | 28 | 30 | 31 | 33 | 34 | 35 | 37 | 38 | 40 | 41 | 43 |
| 165 | 2 | 3 | 5 | 6 | 8 | 9 | 10 | 12 | 13 | 15 | 16 | 17 | 19 | 20 | 22 | 23 | 24 | 26 | 27 | 29 | 30 | 31 | 33 | 34 | 36 | 37 | 38 | 40 | 41 |
| 170 | 2 | 3 | 4 | 6 | 7 | 9 | 10 | 11 | 13 | 14 | 15 | 17 | 18 | 19 | 21 | 22 | 24 | 25 | 26 | 28 | 29 | 30 | 32 | 33 | 34 | 36 | 37 | 39 | 40 |
| 175 | 2 | 3 | 4 | 6 | 7 | 8 | 10 | 11 | 12 | 13 | 15 | 16 | 17 | 19 | 20 | 21 | 23 | 24 | 25 | 27 | 28 | 29 | 31 | 32 | 33 | 35 | 36 | 37 | 39 |
| 180 | | 3 | 4 | 5 | 7 | 8 | 9 | 10 | 12 | 13 | 14 | 16 | 17 | 18 | 19 | 21 | 22 | 23 | 25 | 26 | 27 | 28 | 30 | 31 | 32 | 34 | 35 | 36 | 37 |
| 185 | | 3 | 4 | 5 | 6 | 8 | 9 | 10 | 11 | 13 | 14 | 15 | 16 | 18 | 19 | 20 | 21 | 23 | 24 | 25 | 26 | 28 | 29 | 30 | 31 | 33 | 34 | 35 | 36 |
| 190 | | 2 | 4 | 5 | 6 | 7 | 8 | 10 | 11 | 12 | 13 | 15 | 16 | 17 | 18 | 19 | 21 | 22 | 23 | 24 | 26 | 27 | 28 | 29 | 30 | 32 | 33 | 34 | 35 |
| 195 | | 2 | 3 | 5 | 6 | 7 | 8 | 9 | 11 | 12 | 13 | 14 | 15 | 16 | 18 | 19 | 20 | 21 | 22 | 24 | 25 | 26 | 27 | 28 | 30 | 31 | 32 | 33 | 34 |
| 200 | | 2 | 3 | 4 | 6 | 7 | 8 | 9 | 10 | 11 | 12 | 14 | 15 | 16 | 17 | 18 | 19 | 21 | 22 | 23 | 24 | 25 | 26 | 28 | 29 | 30 | 31 | 32 | 33 |
| 205 | | 2 | 3 | 4 | 5 | 6 | 8 | 9 | 10 | 11 | 12 | 13 | 14 | 15 | 17 | 18 | 19 | 20 | 21 | 22 | 23 | 25 | 26 | 27 | 28 | 29 | 30 | 31 | 32 |
| 210 | | 2 | 3 | 4 | 5 | 6 | 7 | 8 | 9 | 11 | 12 | 13 | 14 | 15 | 16 | 17 | 18 | 19 | 21 | 22 | 23 | 24 | 25 | 26 | 27 | 28 | 29 | 30 | 32 |
| 215 | | 2 | 3 | 4 | 5 | 6 | 7 | 8 | 9 | 10 | 11 | 12 | 13 | 15 | 16 | 17 | 18 | 19 | 20 | 21 | 22 | 23 | 24 | 25 | 26 | 28 | 29 | 30 | 31 |
| 220 | | | 2 | 3 | 4 | 6 | 7 | 8 | 9 | 10 | 11 | 12 | 13 | 14 | 15 | 16 | 17 | 18 | 19 | 20 | 22 | 23 | 24 | 25 | 26 | 27 | 28 | 29 | 30 |
| 225 | | | 2 | 3 | 4 | 6 | 7 | 8 | 9 | 10 | 11 | 12 | 13 | 14 | 15 | 16 | 17 | 18 | 19 | 20 | 21 | 22 | 23 | 24 | 25 | 26 | 27 | 28 | 29 |
| 230 | | | 2 | 3 | 4 | 5 | 6 | 7 | 8 | 9 | 10 | 11 | 12 | 13 | 14 | 15 | 16 | 17 | 18 | 19 | 20 | 21 | 22 | 23 | 24 | 25 | 26 | 27 | 28 |
| 235 | | | 2 | 3 | 4 | 5 | 6 | 7 | 8 | 9 | 10 | 11 | 12 | 13 | 14 | 15 | 16 | 17 | 18 | 19 | 20 | 21 | 22 | 23 | 24 | 25 | 26 | 27 | 28 |
| 240 | | | 2 | 3 | 4 | 5 | 6 | 7 | 8 | 9 | 10 | 11 | 12 | 13 | 14 | 15 | 16 | 17 | 17 | 18 | 19 | 20 | 21 | 22 | 23 | 24 | 25 | 26 | 27 |
| 245 | | | 2 | 3 | 4 | 5 | 6 | 7 | 8 | 9 | 9 | 10 | 11 | 12 | 13 | 14 | 15 | 16 | 17 | 18 | 19 | 20 | 21 | 22 | 23 | 24 | 25 | 26 | 27 |
| 250 | | | 2 | 3 | 4 | 5 | 6 | 6 | 7 | 8 | 9 | 10 | 11 | 12 | 13 | 14 | 15 | 16 | 17 | 18 | 18 | 19 | 20 | 21 | 22 | 23 | 24 | 25 | 26 |
| 255 | | | 2 | 3 | 3 | 4 | 5 | 6 | 7 | 8 | 9 | 10 | 11 | 12 | 13 | 14 | 14 | 15 | 16 | 17 | 18 | 19 | 20 | 21 | 22 | 23 | 24 | 24 | 25 |
| 260 | | | 2 | 2 | 3 | 4 | 5 | 6 | 7 | 8 | 9 | 10 | 10 | 11 | 12 | 13 | 14 | 15 | 16 | 17 | 18 | 19 | 19 | 20 | 21 | 22 | 23 | 24 | 25 |
| 265 | | | | 2 | 3 | 4 | 5 | 6 | 7 | 8 | 8 | 9 | 10 | 11 | 12 | 13 | 14 | 15 | 15 | 16 | 17 | 18 | 19 | 20 | 21 | 22 | 22 | 23 | 24 |
| 270 | | | | 2 | 3 | 4 | 5 | 6 | 7 | 7 | 8 | 9 | 10 | 11 | 12 | 13 | 13 | 14 | 15 | 16 | 17 | 18 | 19 | 19 | 20 | 21 | 22 | 23 | 24 |
| 275 | | | | 2 | 3 | 4 | 5 | 5 | 6 | 7 | 8 | 9 | 10 | 11 | 11 | 12 | 13 | 14 | 15 | 16 | 16 | 17 | 18 | 19 | 20 | 21 | 22 | 22 | 23 |
| 280 | | | | 2 | 3 | 4 | 4 | 5 | 6 | 7 | 8 | 9 | 9 | 10 | 11 | 12 | 13 | 14 | 14 | 15 | 16 | 17 | 18 | 19 | 19 | 20 | 21 | 22 | 23 |
| 285 | | | | 2 | 3 | 4 | 4 | 5 | 6 | 7 | 8 | 8 | 9 | 10 | 11 | 12 | 12 | 13 | 14 | 15 | 16 | 17 | 17 | 18 | 19 | 20 | 21 | 21 | 22 |
| 290 | | | | 2 | 3 | 3 | 4 | 5 | 6 | 7 | 7 | 8 | 9 | 10 | 11 | 11 | 12 | 13 | 14 | 15 | 15 | 16 | 17 | 18 | 19 | 19 | 20 | 21 | 22 |
| 295 | | | | 2 | 2 | 3 | 4 | 5 | 6 | 6 | 7 | 8 | 9 | 10 | 10 | 11 | 12 | 13 | 14 | 14 | 15 | 16 | 17 | 17 | 18 | 19 | 20 | 21 | 21 |
| 300 | | | | 2 | 2 | 3 | 4 | 5 | 5 | 6 | 7 | 8 | 9 | 9 | 10 | 11 | 12 | 12 | 13 | 14 | 15 | 16 | 16 | 17 | 18 | 19 | 19 | 20 | 21 |

| | 36.5 | 37 | 37.5 | 38 | 38.5 | 39 | 39.5 | 40 | 40.5 | 41 | 41.5 | 42 | 42.5 | 43 | 43.5 | 44 | 44.5 | 45 | 45.5 | 46 | 46.5 | 47 | 47.5 | 48 | 48.5 | 49 | 49.5 | 50 |
|---|---|---|---|---|---|---|---|---|---|---|---|---|---|---|---|---|---|---|---|---|---|---|---|---|---|---|---|---|
| 120 | | | | | | | | | | | | | | | | | | | | | | | | | | | | |
| 125 | 58 | | | | | | | | | | | | | | | | | | | | | | | | | | | |
| 130 | 55 | 57 | | | | | | | | | | | | | | | | | | | | | | | | | | |
| 135 | 53 | 55 | 56 | | | | | | | | | | | | | | | | | | | | | | | | | |
| 140 | 51 | 53 | 54 | 56 | | | | | | | | | | | | | | | | | | | | | | | | |
| 145 | 49 | 51 | 52 | 54 | 55 | | | | | | | | | | | | | | | | | | | | | | | |
| 150 | 47 | 49 | 50 | 52 | 53 | 55 | | | | | | | | | | | | | | | | | | | | | | |
| 155 | 46 | 47 | 49 | 50 | 52 | 53 | 55 | | | | | | | | | | | | | | | | | | | | | |
| 160 | 44 | 46 | 47 | 48 | 50 | 51 | 53 | 54 | | | | | | | | | | | | | | | | | | | | |
| 165 | 43 | 44 | 45 | 47 | 48 | 50 | 51 | 52 | 54 | | | | | | | | | | | | | | | | | | | |
| 170 | 41 | 43 | 44 | 45 | 47 | 48 | 49 | 51 | 52 | 54 | | | | | | | | | | | | | | | | | | |
| 175 | 40 | 41 | 43 | 44 | 45 | 47 | 48 | 49 | 51 | 52 | 53 | | | | | | | | | | | | | | | | | |
| 180 | 39 | 40 | 41 | 43 | 44 | 45 | 47 | 48 | 49 | 50 | 52 | 53 | | | | | | | | | | | | | | | | |
| 185 | 38 | 39 | 40 | 41 | 43 | 44 | 45 | 46 | 48 | 49 | 50 | 51 | 53 | | | | | | | | | | | | | | | |
| 190 | 37 | 38 | 39 | 40 | 41 | 43 | 44 | 45 | 46 | 48 | 49 | 50 | 51 | 52 | | | | | | | | | | | | | | |
| 195 | 35 | 37 | 38 | 39 | 40 | 41 | 43 | 44 | 45 | 46 | 47 | 49 | 50 | 51 | 52 | | | | | | | | | | | | | |
| 200 | 35 | 36 | 37 | 38 | 39 | 40 | 41 | 43 | 44 | 45 | 46 | 47 | 48 | 50 | 51 | 52 | | | | | | | | | | | | |
| 205 | 34 | 35 | 36 | 37 | 38 | 39 | 40 | 41 | 43 | 44 | 45 | 46 | 47 | 48 | 49 | 51 | 52 | | | | | | | | | | | |
| 210 | 33 | 34 | 35 | 36 | 37 | 38 | 39 | 40 | 42 | 43 | 44 | 45 | 46 | 47 | 48 | 49 | 50 | 51 | | | | | | | | | | |
| 215 | 32 | 33 | 34 | 35 | 36 | 37 | 38 | 39 | 40 | 42 | 43 | 44 | 45 | 46 | 47 | 48 | 49 | 50 | 51 | | | | | | | | | |
| 220 | 31 | 32 | 33 | 34 | 35 | 36 | 37 | 38 | 39 | 41 | 42 | 43 | 44 | 45 | 46 | 47 | 48 | 49 | 50 | 51 | | | | | | | | |
| 225 | 30 | 31 | 32 | 33 | 34 | 35 | 36 | 37 | 38 | 40 | 41 | 42 | 43 | 44 | 45 | 46 | 47 | 48 | 49 | 50 | 51 | | | | | | | |
| 230 | 30 | 31 | 32 | 33 | 34 | 35 | 36 | 37 | 38 | 39 | 40 | 41 | 42 | 43 | 44 | 45 | 46 | 47 | 48 | 49 | 50 | 51 | | | | | | |
| 235 | 29 | 30 | 31 | 32 | 33 | 34 | 35 | 36 | 37 | 38 | 39 | 40 | 41 | 42 | 43 | 44 | 45 | 46 | 47 | 48 | 49 | 50 | 51 | | | | | |
| 240 | 28 | 29 | 30 | 31 | 32 | 33 | 34 | 35 | 36 | 37 | 38 | 39 | 40 | 41 | 42 | 43 | 44 | 45 | 46 | 46 | 47 | 48 | 49 | 50 | | | | |
| 245 | 27 | 28 | 29 | 30 | 31 | 32 | 33 | 34 | 35 | 36 | 37 | 38 | 39 | 40 | 41 | 42 | 43 | 44 | 44 | 45 | 46 | 47 | 48 | 49 | 50 | | | |
| 250 | 27 | 28 | 29 | 30 | 31 | 31 | 32 | 33 | 34 | 35 | 36 | 37 | 38 | 39 | 40 | 41 | 42 | 43 | 44 | 44 | 45 | 46 | 47 | 48 | 49 | 50 | | |
| 255 | 26 | 27 | 28 | 29 | 30 | 31 | 32 | 33 | 34 | 34 | 35 | 36 | 37 | 38 | 39 | 40 | 41 | 42 | 43 | 44 | 44 | 45 | 46 | 47 | 48 | 49 | 50 | |
| 260 | 26 | 27 | 27 | 28 | 29 | 30 | 31 | 32 | 33 | 34 | 35 | 35 | 36 | 37 | 38 | 39 | 40 | 41 | 42 | 43 | 43 | 44 | 45 | 46 | 47 | 48 | 49 | 50 |
| 265 | 25 | 26 | 27 | 28 | 29 | 29 | 30 | 31 | 32 | 33 | 34 | 35 | 36 | 36 | 37 | 38 | 39 | 40 | 41 | 42 | 43 | 43 | 44 | 45 | 46 | 47 | 48 | 49 |
| 270 | 25 | 25 | 26 | 27 | 28 | 29 | 30 | 31 | 31 | 32 | 33 | 34 | 35 | 36 | 37 | 37 | 38 | 39 | 40 | 41 | 42 | 43 | 43 | 44 | 45 | 46 | 47 | 48 |
| 275 | 24 | 25 | 26 | 27 | 27 | 28 | 29 | 30 | 31 | 32 | 32 | 33 | 34 | 35 | 36 | 37 | 38 | 38 | 39 | 40 | 41 | 42 | 43 | 43 | 44 | 45 | 46 | 47 |
| 280 | 24 | 24 | 25 | 26 | 27 | 28 | 29 | 29 | 30 | 31 | 32 | 33 | 33 | 34 | 35 | 36 | 37 | 38 | 38 | 39 | 40 | 41 | 42 | 43 | 43 | 44 | 45 | 46 |
| 285 | 23 | 24 | 25 | 26 | 26 | 27 | 28 | 29 | 30 | 30 | 31 | 32 | 33 | 34 | 34 | 35 | 36 | 37 | 38 | 39 | 39 | 40 | 41 | 42 | 43 | 43 | 44 | 45 |
| 290 | 23 | 23 | 24 | 25 | 26 | 27 | 27 | 28 | 29 | 30 | 31 | 31 | 32 | 33 | 34 | 35 | 35 | 36 | 37 | 38 | 39 | 39 | 40 | 41 | 42 | 43 | 43 | 44 |
| 295 | 22 | 23 | 24 | 25 | 25 | 26 | 27 | 28 | 28 | 29 | 30 | 31 | 32 | 32 | 33 | 34 | 35 | 36 | 36 | 37 | 38 | 39 | 39 | 40 | 41 | 42 | 43 | 43 |
| 300 | 22 | 22 | 23 | 24 | 25 | 26 | 26 | 27 | 28 | 29 | 29 | 30 | 31 | 32 | 33 | 33 | 34 | 35 | 36 | 36 | 37 | 38 | 39 | 39 | 40 | 41 | 42 | 43 |

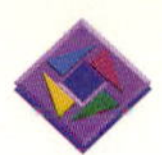

## Bioelectrical Impedance

The bioelectrical impedance technique is much simpler to administer, but it does require costly equipment. In this technique the individual is hooked up to a machine and a weak electrical current (totally painless) is run through the body to analyze body composition (body fat, lean body mass, and body water). The technique is based on the principle that fat tissue is not as good a conductor of an electrical current as lean tissue is. The easier the conductance, the leaner the individual.

The accuracy of current equations used to estimate percent body fat with this technique is still questionable. More research is required before the equations approach the accuracy of hydrostatic weighing, skinfolds, or girth measurements.

An advantage of bioelectrical impedance is that results are highly reproducible. Unlike other techniques, in which experienced technicians are necessary to obtain valid results, almost anyone can administer bioelectrical impedance. And, although the test results may not be completely accurate, this instrument is valuable in assessing body composition changes over time.

If this instrument or some other type of equipment for body composition assessment is available to you, you can use it to determine your percent body fat. You may want to compare the results with other techniques. Following all manufacturer's instructions will ensure the best possible result.

## Waist-to-Hip Ratio

Scientific evidence suggests that the way people store fat affects the risk for disease. Some individuals tend to store fat in the abdominal area (called the "apple" shape). Others store it mainly around the hips and thighs (gluteal femoral fat or "pear" shape).

Obese individuals with a lot of abdominal fat clearly are at higher risk for coronary heart disease, congestive heart failure, hypertension, Type II diabetes (adult-onset or non-insulin-dependent diabetes), and strokes than are obese people with similar amounts of total body fat stored primarily in the hips and thighs. Relatively new evidence also indicates that, among individuals with a lot of abdominal fat, those whose fat deposits are around internal organs (visceral fat) have an even greater risk for disease than those whose abdominal fat is mainly beneath the skin (subcutaneous fat).[1]

Because of the higher risk for disease in individuals who tend to store a lot of fat in the abdominal area, as contrasted with the hips and thighs, a waist-to-hip ratio test was designed by a panel of scientists appointed by the National Academy of Sciences and the Dietary Guidelines Advisory Council for the U.S. Departments of Agriculture and Health and Human Services. The waist measurement is taken at the point of smallest circumference, and the hip measurement is taken at the point of greatest circumference.

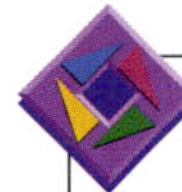

*Individuals with a lot of abdominal fat are at higher risk for coronary heart disease, congestive heart failure, hypertension, Type II diabetes, and strokes.*

The waist-to-hip ratio differentiates the "apples" from the "pears." Most men are apples, and most women are pears. The panel recommends that men need to lose weight if the waist-to-hip ratio is 1.0 or higher. Women need to lose weight if the ratio is .85 or higher (see Table 6.6). More conservative estimates indicate that the risk starts to increase when the ratio exceeds .95 and .80 for men and women, respectively. For example, the waist-to-hip ratio for a man with a 40-inch waist and a 38-inch hip would be 1.05 (40 ÷ 38). This ratio may indicate higher risk for disease.

## Body Mass Index

Another technique scientists use to determine thinness and excessive fatness is the Body Mass Index (BMI). This index incorporates height and weight to estimate critical fat values at which the risk for disease increases.

**TABLE 6.6**
**Disease Risk According to Waist-to-Hip Ratio**

| Waist-to-Hip Ratio | | |
|---|---|---|
| **Men** | **Women** | **Disease Risk** |
| ≤0.95 | ≤0.80 | Very Low |
| 0.96–0.99 | 0.81–0.84 | Low |
| ≥1.00 | ≥0.85 | High |

BMI is calculated by multiplying your weight in pounds by 705, dividing this figure by your height in inches, and then dividing by the same height again (or weight in kilograms divided by the square of the height in meters). For example, the BMI for an individual who weighs 172 pounds and is 67 inches tall would be 27 (172 × 705 ÷ 67 ÷ 67).

According to BMI, the lowest risk for chronic disease is in the 22 to 25 range (see Table 6.7). Individuals are classified as overweight between 25 and 30. BMIs above 30 are defined as obese and below 20 as underweight.

**TABLE 6.7**
**Disease Risk According to Body Mass Index (BMI)**

| BMI | Disease Risk |
|---|---|
| <20.00 | Moderate to Very High |
| 20.00 to 21.99 | Low |
| 22.00 to 24.99 | Very Low |
| 25.00 to 29.99 | Low |
| 30.00 to 34.99 | Moderate |
| 35.00 to 39.99 | High |
| ≥40.00 | Very High |

BMI is a useful tool to screen the general population, but, similar to height/weight charts, it fails to differentiate fat from lean body mass or where most of the fat is located (waist-to-hip ratio). Using BMI, athletes with a large amount of muscle mass (body builders, football players) easily can fall in the moderate or even high-risk categories. Therefore, body composition and waist-to-hip ratios are better procedures to determine health risk and recommended body weight.

## COMPUTING RECOMMENDED BODY WEIGHT

After finding out your percent body fat, you can determine your current body composition classification according to Table 6.8. In this table you will find the health fitness and the high physical fitness percent fat standards. For example, the recommended health fitness fat percentage for a 20-year-old female is 28% or less. The health fitness standard is established at the point at which there seems to be no harm to health in terms of percent body fat. A high physical fitness range for this same woman would be between 18% and 23%.

**TABLE 6.8**
**Body Composition Classification According to Percent Body Fat**

| | | MEN | | | |
|---|---|---|---|---|---|
| **Age** | **Excellent** | **Good** | **Moderate** | **Overweight** | **Significantly Overweight** |
| ≤19 | 12.0 | 12.1-17.0 | 17.1-22.0 | 22.1-27.0 | ≥27.1 |
| 20-29 | 13.0 | 13.1-18.0 | 18.1-23.0 | 23.1-28.0 | ≥28.1 |
| 30-39 | 14.0 | 14.1-19.0 | 19.1-24.0 | 24.1-29.0 | ≥29.1 |
| 40-49 | 15.0 | 15.1-20.0 | 20.1-25.0 | 25.1-30.0 | ≥30.1 |
| ≥50 | 16.0 | 16.1-21.5 | 21.1-26.0 | 26.1-31.0 | ≥31.1 |
| | | **WOMEN** | | | |
| **Age** | **Excellent** | **Good** | **Moderate** | **Overweight** | **Significantly Overweight** |
| ≤19 | 17.0 | 17.1-22.0 | 22.1-27.0 | 27.1-32.0 | ≥32.1 |
| 20-29 | 18.0 | 18.1-23.0 | 23.1-28.0 | 28.1-33.0 | ≥33.1 |
| 30-39 | 19.0 | 19.1-24.0 | 24.1-29.0 | 29.1-34.0 | ≥34.1 |
| 40-49 | 20.0 | 20.1-25.0 | 25.1-30.0 | 30.1-35.0 | ≥35.1 |
| ≥50 | 21.0 | 21.1-26.5 | 26.1-31.0 | 31.1-36.0 | ≥36.1 |

High physical fitness standard

Health fitness standard

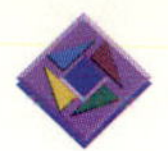

The high physical fitness standard does not mean you cannot be somewhat below this number. Many highly trained male athletes are as low as 3%, and some female distance runners have been measured at 6% body fat (which may not be healthy).

Although people generally agree that the mortality rate is higher for obese people, some evidence indicates that the same is true for underweight people. "Underweight" and "thin" do not necessarily mean the same thing. The body fat of a healthy thin person is around the high fitness percentage, whereas an underweight person has extremely low body fat, even to the point of compromising the essential fat.

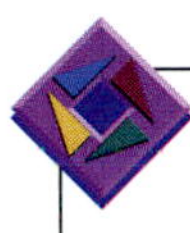

*A "desired" fat percentage should be based on your current percent body fat and your personal health/fitness objectives.*

The 3% essential fat for men and 12% for women seem to be the lower limits for people to maintain good health. Below these percentages normal physiologic functions can be seriously impaired. Some experts point out that a little storage fat (over the essential fat) is better than none at all. As a result, the health and high fitness standards for percent fat in Table 6.8 are set higher than the minimum essential fat requirements, at a point beneficial to optimal health and well-being. Finally, because lean tissue decreases with age, one extra percentage point is allowed for every additional decade of life.

Your recommended body weight is computed based on the selected health or high fitness fat percentage for your age and sex. Your decision to select a "desired" fat percentage should be based on your current percent body fat and your personal health/fitness objectives. To compute your own recommended body weight:

1. Determine the pounds of body weight in fat (FW). Multiply body weight (BW) by the current percent fat (%F) expressed in decimal form (FW = BW × %F).
2. Determine lean body mass (LBM) by subtracting the weight in fat from the total body weight (LBM = BW – FW). (Anything that is not fat must be part of the lean component.)
3. Select a desired body fat percentage (DFP) based on the health or high fitness standards given in Table 6.8.
4. Compute recommended body weight (RBW) according to the formula: RBW = LBM ÷ (1.0 – DFP).

As an example of these computations, a 19-year-old female who weighs 160 pounds and is 30% fat would like to know what her recommended body weight would be at 22%:

Sex: female
Age: 19
BW: 160 lbs
%F: 30% (.30 in decimal form)

1. FW = BW × %F
   FW = 160 × .30 = 48 lbs
2. LBM = BW – FW
   LBM = 160 – 48 = 112 lbs
3. DFP: 22% (.22 in decimal form)
4. RBW = LBM ÷ (1.0 – DFP)
   RBW = 112 ÷ (1.0 – .22)
   RBW = 112 ÷ (.78) = 143.6 lbs

In Figures 6.4 and 6.5 you will have the opportunity to determine your own body composition, recommended body weight, and disease risk according to waist-to-hip ratio and BMI.

Other than hydrostatic weighing, skinfold thickness seems to be the most practical and valid technique to estimate body fat. If skinfold calipers are available, use this technique to assess your percent body fat. If calipers are unavailable, estimate your percent fat according to the girth measurements technique or another technique available to you. (You may wish to use several techniques and compare the results.)

## I. Percent Body Fat According to Skinfold Thickness

**Men**

| | | |
|---|---|---|
| Date: | ________ | ________ |
| Chest (mm): | ________ | ________ |
| Abdomen (mm): | ________ | ________ |
| Thigh (mm): | ________ | ________ |
| Total (mm): | ________ | ________ |
| Percent Fat: | ________ | ________ |

**Women**

| | | |
|---|---|---|
| Date: | ________ | ________ |
| Triceps (mm): | ________ | ________ |
| Suprailium (mm): | ________ | ________ |
| Thigh (mm): | ________ | ________ |
| Total (mm): | ________ | ________ |
| Percent Fat: | ________ | ________ |

## II. Percent Body Fat According to Girth Measurements

**Men**

| | | |
|---|---|---|
| Date: | ________ | ________ |
| Waist (inches): | ________ | ________ |
| Wrist (inches): | ________ | ________ |
| Difference: | ________ | ________ |
| Body Weight: | ________ | ________ |
| Percent Fat: | ________ | ________ |

**Women**

| | | | | | |
|---|---|---|---|---|---|
| Date: | ________ | ________ | | | |
| Upper Arm (cm): | ________ | ________ | Constant A = | ________ | ________ |
| Age: | ________ | ________ | Constant B = | ________ | ________ |
| Hip (cm): | ________ | ________ | Constant C = | ________ | ________ |
| Wrist (cm): | ________ | ________ | Constant D = | ________ | ________ |
| BD:* | ________ | ________ | | | |
| Percent Fat:** | ________ | ________ | | | |

*Body density (BD) = A – B – C + D

**Percent Fat = (495 ÷ BD) – 450

## III. Recommended Body Weight Determination

| | | |
|---|---|---|
| Date: | ________ | ________ |
| Body Weight (BW): | ________ | ________ |
| Current Percent Fat (%F)*: | ________ | ________ |
| Fat Weight (FW) = BW × %F | | |
| FW = × = | ________ | ________ |
| Lean Body Mass (LBM) = BW – FW | | |
| LBM = – = | ________ | ________ |
| Desired Fat Percent (DFP – *see* Table 6.8): | ________ | ________ |
| Recommended Body Weight (RBW) = LBM ÷ (1.0 – DFP*) | | |
| RBW = ÷ (1.0 – ) = | ________ | ________ |

*Express percentages in decimal form (e.g., 25% = .25)

**FIGURE 6.4** ◆ Percent body fat and recommended body weight assessment (use second column for a retest or post-test).

**Waist-to-Hip Ratio**

| | | |
|---|---|---|
| Date: | ________ | ________ |
| Waist (inches): | ________ | ________ |
| Hip (inches): | ________ | ________ |
| Ratio (waist ÷ hip): | ________ | ________ |
| Disease risk: | ________ | ________ |

**Body Mass Index**

| | | |
|---|---|---|
| Date: | ________ | ________ |
| Weight (lbs): | ________ | ________ |
| Height (inches): | ________ | ________ |
| BMI:* | ________ | ________ |
| Disease risk: | ________ | ________ |

*BMI = Weight × 705 ÷ Height ÷ Height

**FIGURE 6.5** ◆ Waist-to-hip ratio and body mass index computation.

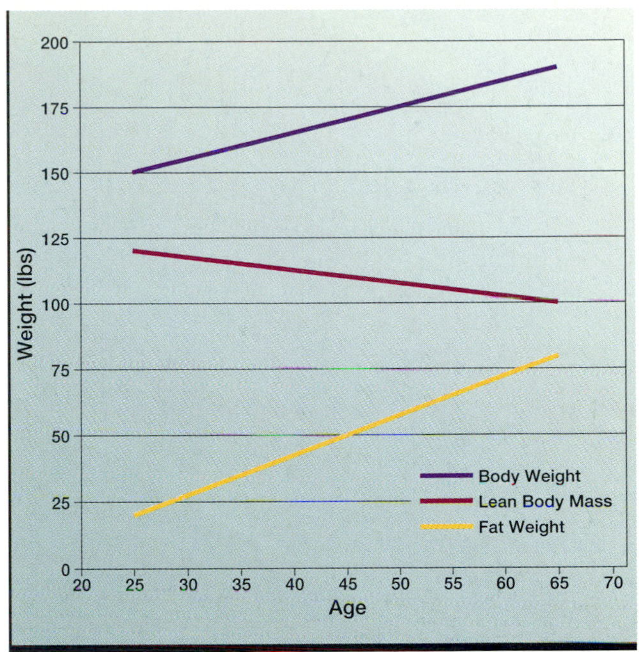


**FIGURE 6.6** ◆ Typical body composition changes for adults in the United States.

## IMPORTANCE OF REGULAR BODY COMPOSITION ASSESSMENT

Children in the United States do not start with a weight problem. Although a small group struggles with weight throughout life, most are not overweight when they reach age 20.

Current trends indicate that starting at age 25, the average man and woman in the United States gains 1 pound of weight per year. Thus, by age 65, the average American will have gained 40 pounds of weight. Because of the typical reduction in physical activity in our society, however, each year the average person also loses a half a pound of lean tissue. Therefore, over this span of 40 years there has been an actual fat gain of 60 pounds accompanied by a 20-pound loss of lean body mass (see Figure 6.6). These changes cannot be detected unless body composition is assessed periodically.

If you are on a diet/exercise program, you should repeat your percent body fat assessment and recommended weight computations about once a month. This is important because lean body mass is affected by weight reduction programs and amount of physical activity. As lean body mass changes, so will your recommended body weight. To make valid comparisons, the same technique should be used between pre- and post-assessments.

Changes in body composition resulting from a weight control/exercise program were illustrated in a co-ed aerobic dance course taught during a 6-week summer term. Students participated in aerobic dance routines four times a week, 60 minutes each time. On the first and last days of class, several physiological parameters, including body composition, were assessed. Students also were given information on diet and nutrition, and they basically followed their own dietary program.

At the end of the 6 weeks, the average weight loss for the entire class was 3 pounds (see Figure 6.7). But, because body composition was assessed, class members were surprised to find that the average fat loss was actually 6 pounds, accompanied by a 3-pound increase in lean body mass.

When dieting, body composition should be reassessed periodically because of the effects of negative caloric balance on lean body mass. As discussed in Chapter 8, dieting does decrease lean body mass. The loss of lean body mass can be offset or eliminated by combining a sensible diet with physical exercise.

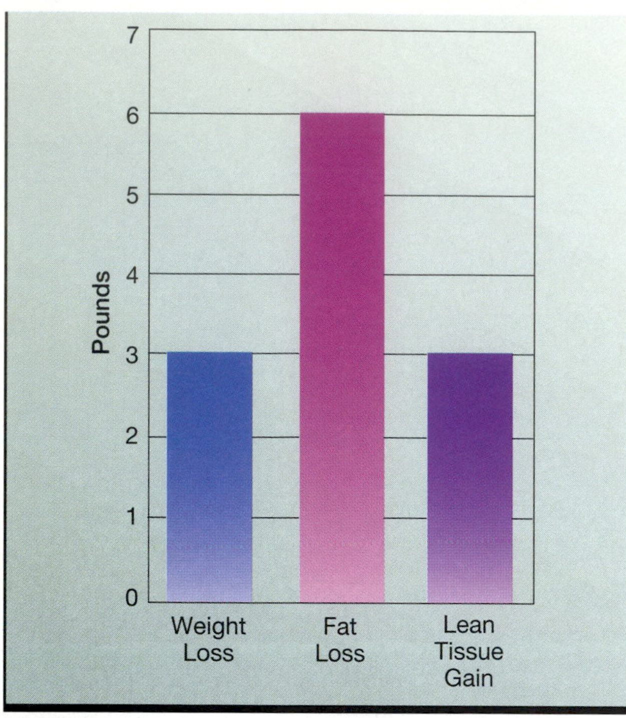


**FIGURE 6.7** ◆ Effects of a 6-week aerobics program on body composition.

## NOTES

1. C. Bouchard, G. A. Bray, and V. S. Hubbard. "Basic and Clinical Aspects of Regional Fat Distribution." *American Journal of Clinical Nutrition*, 52 (1990), 946-950.

## SELECT BIBLIOGRAPHY


Bouchard, C., and F. E. Johnson, Editors. *Fat Distribution During Growth and Later Health Outcomes*. New York: Alan R. Liss, 1988.

Bouchard, C., G. A. Bray, and V. S. Hubbard. "Basic and Clinical Aspects of Regional Fat Distribution." *American Journal of Clinical Nutrition*, 52 (1990), 946-950.

Bray, G. A. "Pathophysiology of Obesity." *American Journal of Clinical Nutrition*, 55 (1992), 488S-494S.

Fisher, A. G., and P. E. Allsen. *Jogging*. Dubuque, IA: Wm C. Brown, 1987.

Hoeger, W. W. K., and S. A. Hoeger. *Principles and Labs for Physical Fitness & Wellness*. Englewood, CO: Morton Publishing, 1994.

Jackson, A. S., and M. L. Pollock. "Generalized Equations for Predicting Body Density of Men." *British Journal of Nutrition*, 40 (1978), 497-504.

Jackson, A. S., M. L. Pollock, and A. Ward. "Generalized Equations for Predicting Body Density of Women." *Medicine and Science in Sports and Exercise*, 3 (1980), 175-182.

Lambson, R. B. *Generalized Body Density Prediction Equations for Women Using Simple Anthropometric Measurements*. Unpublished doctoral dissertation, Brigham Young University, Provo, UT, August 1987.

Penrouse, K. W., A. G. Nelson, and A. G. Fisher. "Generalized Body Composition Equation for Men Using Simple Measurement Techniques." *Medicine and Science in Sports and Exercise*, 17:2 (1985), 189.

Siri, W. E. "Body Composition from Fluid Spaces and Density." Berkeley, CA: Donner Laboratory of Medical Physics, University of California, 1956.

Stensland, S. H., and S. Margolis. "Simplifying the Calculation of Body Mass Index for Quick Reference." *Journal of the American Dietetic Association*, 90 (1990), 856.

# Principles of Nutrition for Wellness

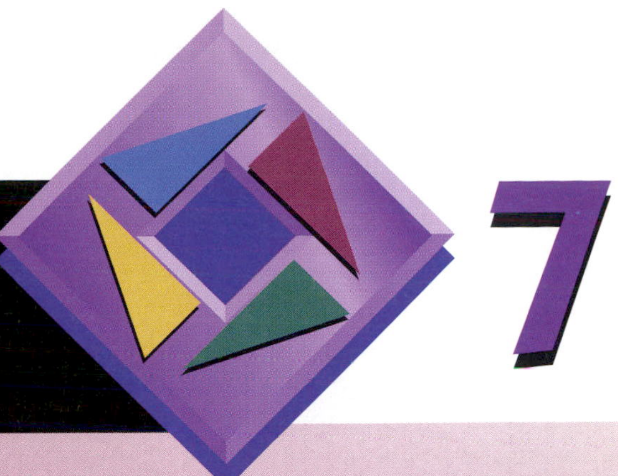


## Key Concepts

Nutrition
Carbohydrates
Simple carbohydrates
Complex carbohydrates
Dietary fiber
Fats
Saturated fat
Protein
Amino acid
Vitamins
Minerals
Eating disorders
Lipoproteins
RDA
Daily values
Phytochemicals
Glycogen
Osteoporosis

## Objectives

- Define nutrition and describe its relationship to health and well-being.
- Describe the functions of carbohydrates in the human body and be able to differentiate simple from complex carbohydrates.
- Describe the role and health benefits of adequate fiber in the diet.
- Describe the role of fats in the human body and be able to characterize saturated, monounsaturated, and polyunsaturated fats.
- Describe the functions of proteins in the human body.
- Describe the role of vitamins and minerals in the human body.
- Identify myths and fallacies regarding nutrition supplementation.
- Learn to conduct a comprehensive nutrient analysis, be capable of recognizing areas of deficiencies, and be able to implement changes to improve overall nutrition.
- Introduce the five food groups and learn how to achieve a balanced diet through the proper use of these groups.

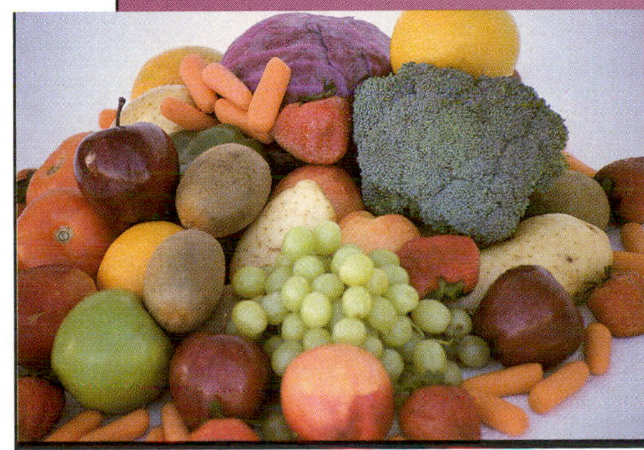

The science of nutrition studies the relationship of foods to optimal health and performance. Although all the answers are not in yet, scientific evidence has long linked good nutrition to overall health and well-being.

Proper nutrition means that a person's diet supplies all the essential nutrients to carry out normal tissue growth, repair, and maintenance. These nutrients should be obtained from a wide variety of sources. Figure 7.1 shows the basic food pyramid with the recommended number of servings from each food group for proper nutrition. The diet also should provide enough substrates to produce the energy necessary for work, physical activity, and relaxation.

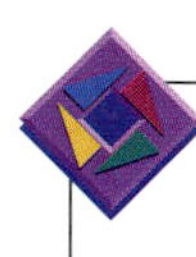

*Current dietary habits are leading many Americans to an early grave.*

Too much or too little of any nutrient can precipitate serious health problems. The typical American diet is too high in calories, sugar, fat, saturated fat, and sodium and not high enough in fiber — factors that undermine good health. Today's American diet has almost no deficiencies. Overconsumption is the major problem.

According to a 1988 report on nutrition and health issued by the U. S. Surgeon General — the first ever of its kind — diseases of dietary excess and imbalance are among the leading causes of death in the country. Of the total 2.1 million deaths in the United States in 1987, an estimated 1.5 million people died of diseases associated with faulty nutrition. In the report, based on more than 2,000 scientific studies, the U. S. Surgeon General said dietary changes can bring better health to all Americans. Other surveys reveal that on a given day nearly half of the American people eat no fruit and almost a fourth eat no vegetables.

Studies also indicate that diet and nutrition often play a crucial role in the development and progression of chronic diseases. A diet high in saturated fat and cholesterol increases the risk for atherosclerosis and coronary heart disease. In sodium-sensitive individuals, high salt intake has been linked to high blood pressure. Some researchers believe that 30% to 50% of all cancers are diet-related (see Chapter 10). Obesity, diabetes mellitus, and osteoporosis also have been associated with faulty nutrition.

An effective wellness program must incorporate current dietary recommendations to lower the risk for chronic disease. A summary of guidelines for a healthful diet include:

- Eating a variety of foods.

**Food Guide Pyramid**

**A Guide to Daily Food Choices**

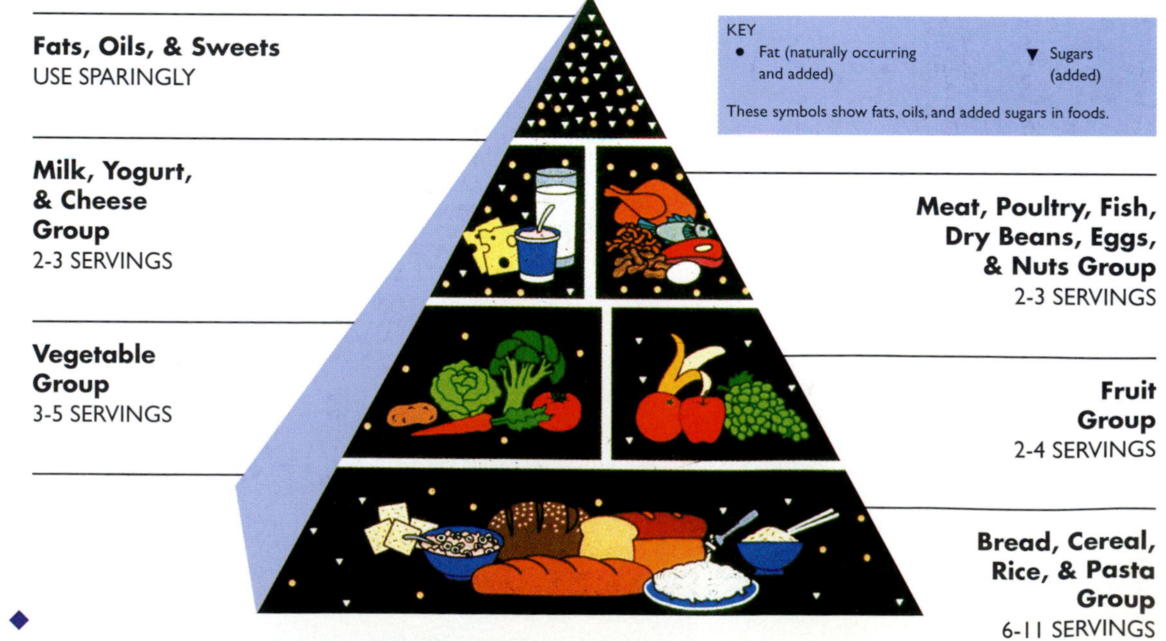


**FIGURE 7.1**

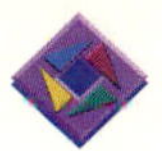

- Avoiding too much fat, saturated fat, and cholesterol.
- Eating foods with adequate starch and fiber.
- Avoiding too much sugar and sodium.
- Maintaining adequate calcium intake.
- Maintaining recommended body weight.
- Drinking alcoholic beverages in moderation, if at all.

These guidelines will be discussed throughout this chapter and in later Chapters (8, 9, and 10) of this book.

## NUTRIENTS

The essential nutrients the human body requires are carbohydrates, fat, protein, vitamins, minerals, and water. The first three are called *fuel nutrients* because they are the only substances the body uses to supply the energy (commonly measured in calories) needed for work and normal body functions. Vitamins, minerals, and water have no caloric value but still are necessary for a person to function normally and maintain good health. Many nutritionists add a seventh nutrient to this list, one that has received a great deal of attention recently: dietary fiber.

Carbohydrates, fats, proteins, and water are termed *macronutrients* because proportionately large amounts are needed daily. Vitamins and minerals are required only in small amounts. Therefore, nutritionists refer to them as *micronutrients*.

Depending on the amount of nutrients and calories, foods can be classified according to high nutrient density and low nutrient density. *High nutrient density* refers to foods that contain few or moderate calories but are packed with nutrients. Foods that have a lot of calories but few nutrients are of *low nutrient density* and commonly are called "junk food."

*Calorie is the unit of measure indicating the energy value of food and the cost of physical activity*. Technically, a kilocalorie (kcal) or large calorie is the amount of heat necessary to raise the temperature of 1 kilogram of water 1° Centigrade, but for simplification people call it a calorie rather than kcal. For example, if the caloric value of a food is 100 calories (kcal), the energy in this food would raise the temperature of 100 kilograms of water 1° Centigrade.

### Carbohydrates

Carbohydrates constitute the major source of calories the body uses to provide energy for work, maintain cells, and generate heat. They also help digest and regulate fat and metabolize protein. Each gram of carbohydrates provides the human body with four calories.

The major sources of carbohydrates are breads, cereals, fruits, vegetables, and milk and other dairy products. Carbohydrates are classified into simple carbohydrates and complex carbohydrates (Figure 7.2).

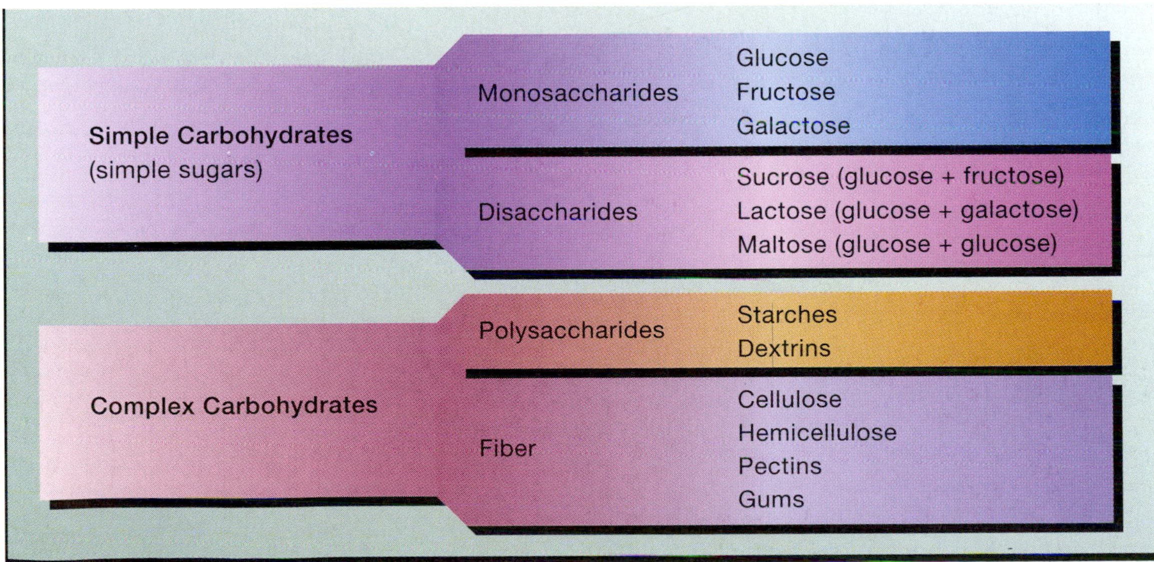


**FIGURE 7.2** ◆ Major types of carbohydrates.

## Simple Carbohydrates

Often called sugars, simple carbohydrates are formed by simple or double sugar units with little nutritive value (for example, candy, soda, cakes). Simple carbohydrates are divided into monosaccharides and disaccharides. These carbohydrates — with -ose endings — often take the place of more nutritive foods in the diet.

### Monosaccharides

The simplest sugars, monosaccharides are formed by five- or six-carbon skeletons. The three most common monosaccharides are glucose, fructose, and galactose.

1. *Glucose* is a natural sugar found in food, but it also is produced in the body from other simple and complex carbohydrates.
2. *Fructose*, or fruit sugar, occurs naturally in fruits and honey.
3. *Galactose* is produced from milk sugar in the mammary glands of lactating animals.

Both fructose and galactose are converted readily to glucose in the body. Glucose is used as a source of energy, or it may be stored in the muscles and liver in the form of glycogen (a long chain of glucose molecules hooked together). Excess glucose in the blood is converted to fat and stored in adipose (fat) tissue. Some of it is eliminated by the kidneys through the urine.

### Disaccharides

Formed by the linkage of two monosaccharide units, one of which is glucose, the three major disaccharides are:

1. *Sucrose* or table sugar (glucose + fructose).
2. *Lactose* (glucose + galactose).
3. *Maltose* (glucose + glucose).

## Complex Carbohydrates

Complex carbohydrates are formed when three or more simple sugar molecules bind together. Therefore, they also are called polysaccharides. Anywhere from about 10 to thousands of monosaccharide molecules can unite to form a single polysaccharide. Examples of complex carbohydrates are starches, dextrins, and glycogen.

1. **Starch** is the storage form of glucose in plants, needed to promote the earliest growth. Starch is found commonly in grains, seeds, corn, nuts, roots, potatoes, and legumes. Grains, the richest source of starch, should supply most of the energy in a healthful diet. Once eaten, starch is converted to glucose for the body's own energy use.
2. **Dextrins** are formed from the breakdown of large starch molecules exposed to dry heat, such as in baking bread or producing cold cereals. Complex carbohydrates of plant origin provide many valuable nutrients and can be an excellent source of fiber, or roughage.
3. **Glycogen** is the animal polysaccharide synthesized from glucose and found only in slight amounts in meats. Although it serves a function in humans similar to that of starch in plants, glycogen is not found in plants. Glycogen constitutes the body's reservoirs of glucose. Many hundreds to thousands of glucose molecules are linked together to be stored as glycogen in liver and muscle.

When a surge of energy is needed, enzymes in the muscle and the liver break down glycogen and thus make glucose readily available for energy transformation. This is discussed later in the chapter, under Nutrition for Athletes.

### Dietary Fiber

Dietary fiber is a type of complex carbohydrate made up of plant material the human body cannot digest. It is present mainly in leaves, skins, roots, and seeds. Processing and refining foods removes almost all of the natural fiber. In our daily diets the main sources of dietary fiber are whole-grain cereals and breads, fruits, and vegetables.

The most common types of fiber are:

1. *Cellulose* and *hemicellulose*, found in plant cell walls.
2. *Pectins*, found in fruits.
3. *Gums*, also found in small amounts in foods of plant origin.

Cellulose and hemicellulose are water-insoluble fibers. Pectins and gums are water-soluble fibers.

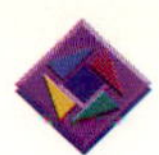

Fiber is important in the diet because it binds water, causing a softer and bulkier stool that increases peristalsis (involuntary muscle contraction of intestinal walls that force the stool onward) and allows food residues to pass through the intestinal tract more quickly. Many researchers believe that speeding up passage of food residues through the intestines lowers the risk for colon cancer, mainly because cancer-causing agents are not in contact as long with the intestinal wall. Fiber also is thought to bind with carcinogens (cancer-producing substances), and more water in the stool may dilute the cancer-causing agents, lessening their potency.

Increased fiber intake also may lower the risk for coronary heart disease because: (a) saturated fats often take the place of fiber in the diet, increasing cholesterol formation or absorption, and (b) specific water-soluble fibers such as pectin and guar gum, found in beans, oat bran, corn, and fruits, seem to bind cholesterol in the intestines, preventing its absorption. In addition to heart disease, several health disorders, including constipation, diverticulitis, hemorrhoids, gallbladder disease, and obesity have been linked to low fiber intake.

Determining the amount of fiber in your diet can be confusing at times because it can be measured either as crude fiber or as dietary fiber. *Crude fiber* is the smaller portion of the dietary fiber, which actually remains after chemical extraction in the digestive tract. The recommended amount of dietary fiber is 20 to 35 grams per day, the equivalent of 7 grams of crude fiber. Because most nutrition labels list the fiber content in terms of dietary fiber, the 20- to 35-gram guideline should be used (see Table 7.1).

This may be surprising, but *too much* fiber also can be detrimental to health. It can produce loss of calcium, phosphorus, and iron, not to mention gastrointestinal discomfort. When eating more fiber, a person also should drink more water, as too little fluid can cause constipation and even dehydration.

**TABLE 7.1**
**Dietary Fiber Content of Selected Foods**

| Food | Serving Size | Dietary Fiber (gm) |
|---|---|---|
| Almonds | 1 oz. | 3.0 |
| Apple | 1 medium | 4.3 |
| Banana | 1 medium | 3.3 |
| Beans — red, kidney | .5 cup | 10.2 |
| Blackberries | .5 cup | 4.9 |
| Beets (cooked) | .5 cup | 2.0 |
| Brazil nuts | 1 oz. | 2.5 |
| Broccoli (cooked) | .5 cup | 3.3 |
| Brown rice (cooked) | .5 cup | 2.0 |
| Carrots (cooked) | .5 cup | 2.9 |
| Cauliflower (cooked) | .5 cup | 1.7 |
| Cereal | | |
| All Bran | 1 oz. | 8.5 |
| Cheerios | 1 oz. | 1.1 |
| Cornflakes | 1 oz. | 0.5 |
| Fruit and Fibre | 1 oz. | 4.0 |
| Fruit Wheats | 1 oz. | 2.0 |
| Just Right | 1 oz. | 2.0 |
| Wheaties | 1 oz. | 2.0 |
| Corn (cooked) | .5 cup | 3.9 |
| Eggplant (cooked) | .5 cup | 3.0 |
| Lettuce (chopped) | .5 cup | 0.4 |
| Orange | 1 medium | 3.0 |
| Parsnips (cooked) | .5 cup | 2.1 |
| Pear | 1 medium | 5.0 |
| Peas (cooked) | .5 cup | 3.7 |
| Popcorn (plain) | 1 cup | 1.5 |
| Potato (baked) | 1 medium | 3.9 |
| Strawberries | .5 cup | 1.6 |
| Summer squash (cooked) | .5 cup | 1.6 |
| Watermelon | 1 cup | 0.8 |

## Fat

Fats, or lipids, are used by the human body as a source of energy. They are the most concentrated energy source. Each gram of fat supplies nine calories to the body. Fats are a part of the cell structure. They are used as stored energy and as an insulator to preserve body heat. They absorb shock, supply essential fatty acids, and carry the fat-soluble vitamins A, D, E, and K. Fats can be classified into three main groups: simple, compound, and derived (Figure 7.3). The basic sources of fat are milk and other dairy products, and meats and alternatives.

### Simple Fats

A simple fat consists of a glyceride molecule linked to one, two, or three units of fatty acids. According to the number of fatty acids attached, simple fats are divided into *monoglycerides* (one fatty acid), *diglycerides* (two fatty acids), and *triglycerides*

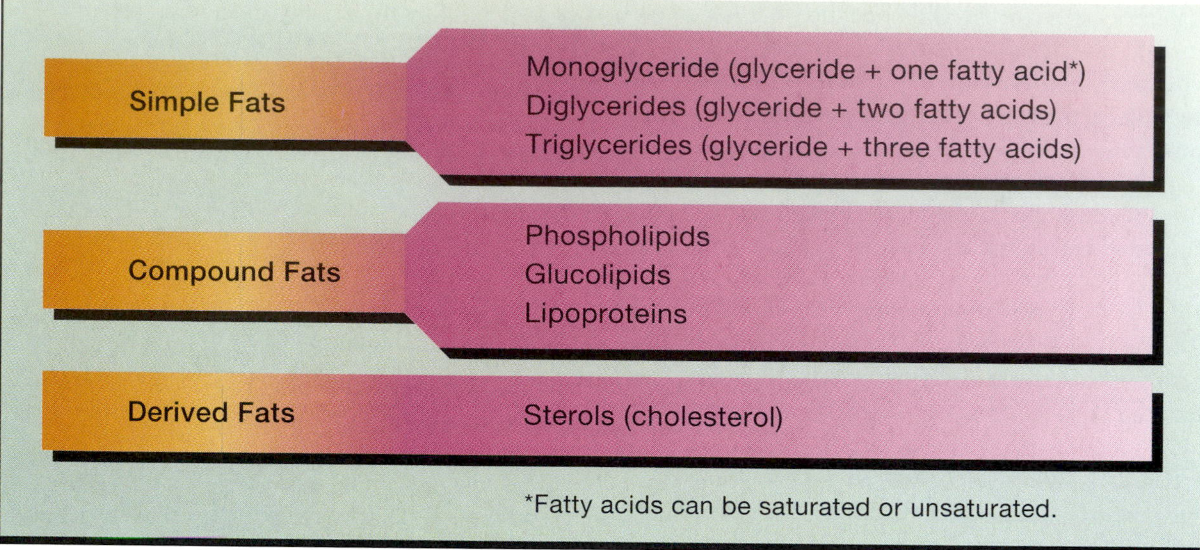

Simple Fats
Monoglyceride (glyceride + one fatty acid*)
Diglycerides (glyceride + two fatty acids)
Triglycerides (glyceride + three fatty acids)
Compound Fats
Phospholipids
Glucolipids
Lipoproteins
Derived Fats
Sterols (cholesterol)
*Fatty acids can be saturated or unsaturated.


**FIGURE 7.3** ◆ Major types of fats (lipids).

(three fatty acids). More than 90% of the weight of fat in foods and more than 95% of the stored fat in the human body are in the form of triglycerides.

The length of the carbon atom chain and the amount of hydrogen saturation in fatty acids vary. Based on the extent of saturation, fatty acids are said to be saturated or unsaturated. Unsaturated fatty acids are classified further into monounsaturated and polyunsaturated. Saturated fatty acids are mainly of animal origin. Unsaturated fats are found mostly in plant products.

In *saturated fatty acids* the carbon atoms are fully saturated with hydrogens; only single bonds link the carbon atoms on the chain (see Figure 7.4). These saturated fatty acids often are called saturated fats. Examples of foods high in saturated fatty acids are meats, meat fat, lard, whole milk, cream, butter, cheese, ice cream, hydrogenated oils (a process that makes oils saturated), coconut oil, and palm oils.

In *unsaturated fatty acids* (unsaturated fats), double bonds form between the unsaturated carbons. In *monounsaturated fatty acids* (MUFA) only one double bond is found along the chain. Olive, canola, rapeseed, peanut, and sesame oils are examples of monounsaturated fatty acids. *Polyunsaturated fatty acids* (PUFA) contain two or more double bonds between unsaturated carbon atoms along the chain. Corn, cottonseed, safflower, walnut, sunflower, and soybean oils are high in polyunsaturated fatty acids.

Saturated fats typically do not melt at room temperature. Unsaturated fats usually are liquid at room temperature. Coconut and palm oils are exceptions, as they are high in saturated fats. Shorter fatty acid chains also tend to be liquid at room temperature.

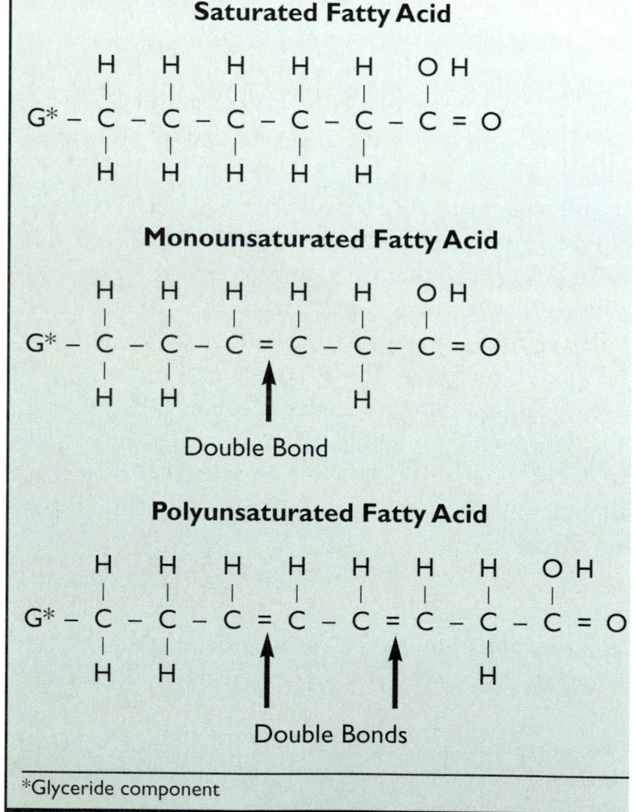


**FIGURE 7.4** ◆ Chemical structure of saturated and unsaturated fats.

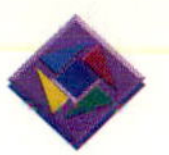

In general, saturated fats raise the blood cholesterol level, whereas polyunsaturated and monounsaturated fats tend to lower blood cholesterol (the role of cholesterol in health and disease is discussed in Chapter 9). Polyunsaturated fats, nonetheless, also seem to cause reduction of the "good" (HDL) cholesterol, which may not really improve the cholesterol profile (see compound fats, below, and also the discussion of cholesterol in Chapter 9). Monounsaturated fats, on the other hand, seem to lower only the "bad" (LDL) cholesterol and not the good (HDL) cholesterol.

Hydrogen often is added to monounsaturated and polyunsaturated fats to increase shelf life and to solidify them so they are more spreadable. During this process of partial hydrogenation, the position of hydrogen atoms may be changed along the chain, transforming the fat into a transfatty acid.

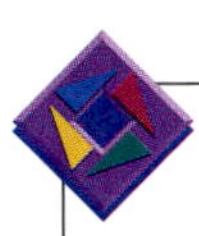

*Monounsaturated fats appear to lower only LDL (bad) cholesterol and not HDL (good) cholesterol.*

Margarine and spreads, crackers, cookies, and french fries often contain transfatty acids. Intake of these types of fats should be minimized. Studies suggest that diets rich in transfatty acids elevate LDL cholesterol and lower HDL cholesterol to the same extent as saturated fats.[1] Paying attention to food labels is important because the words "partially hydrogenated" or "transfatty acids" may indicate that the product carries as high a health risk as consuming saturated fat (eating margarine is still a better choice because its total transfatty acid and saturated fat is about half the saturated fat in butter).

One type of polyunsaturated fatty acids that has gained attention in recent years are *omega-3 fatty acids*. These fatty acids seem to be effective in lowering triglycerides (high blood triglyercides are a risk factor for coronary heart disease). Fish, especially fresh or frozen mackerel, herring, tuna, salmon, and lake trout, have omega-3 fatty acids. Canned fish is not recommended for this purpose because the canning process destroys most of the omega-3 oil. These fatty acids also are found, but to a lesser extent, in canola oil, walnuts, soybeans, and wheat germ.

Limited data suggest that eating one or two servings of fish weekly lessens the risk for coronary heart disease. People with diabetes, a history of hemorrhaging or strokes, on aspirin, blood-thinning therapy, and presurgical patients should not consume fish oil except under a physician's instruction.

### Compound Fats

Compound fats are a combination of simple fats and other chemicals. Examples are:

1. *Phospholipids*, similar to triglycerides except that phosphoric acid takes the place of one of the fatty acid units.
2. *Glucolipids*, a combination of carbohydrates, fatty acids, and nitrogen.
3. *Lipoproteins*, water-soluble aggregates of protein with triglycerides, phospholipids, or cholesterol.

Because lipids do not dissolve in water, lipoproteins transport fats in the blood. As the name indicates, lipoproteins are a combination of lipids covered by proteins (known as apoproteins).

The major forms of lipoproteins are *high density (HDL), low density (LDL), and very low density (VLDL) lipoproteins*. Lipoproteins play a large role in developing or in preventing heart disease. HDL is more than half protein and contains little cholesterol. High HDL levels have been associated with a lower risk for coronary heart disease. LDL is approximately a fourth protein and nearly half cholesterol. High LDL levels have been linked to increased risk for coronary heart disease. VLDL contains mostly (about half) triglycerides and only about 10% protein and 20% cholesterol. Chapter 9 provides more information on the role these lipoproteins play in coronary heart disease.

### Derived Fats

Derived fats combine simple and compound fats. Sterols are an example. Although sterols contain no fatty acids, they are considered fats because they do not dissolve in water. The most often mentioned sterol is cholesterol, which is found in many foods or can be manufactured from saturated fats in the body.

## Protein

Proteins are the main substances the body uses to build and repair tissues such as muscles, blood, internal organs, skin, hair, nails, and bones. They are a part of hormones, antibodies, and enzymes. Enzymes play a key role in all of the body's processes. Because all enzymes are formed by proteins, this nutrient is necessary for normal functioning. Proteins also help maintain the normal balance of body fluids.

Proteins can be used as a source of energy, too, but only if not enough carbohydrates are available. Each gram of protein yields four calories of energy. The main sources of protein are meats and alternatives, and milk and other dairy products. Excess proteins maybe converted to glucose or fat or even excreted in the urine.

The human body uses 20 *amino acids*, the basic building blocks to form different types of protein. Amino acids contain nitrogen, carbon, hydrogen, and oxygen. Nine of the 20 amino acids are called *essential amino acids* because the body cannot produce them. The other 11, termed *nonessential amino acids*, can be manufactured in the body if food proteins in the diet provide enough nitrogen (see Table 7.2). For normal body function all amino acids must be present at the same time.

Proteins that contain all the essential amino acids are known as *complete* or *higher-quality protein*. These types of proteins usually are of animal source. If one or more of the essential amino acids is missing, the proteins are termed incomplete or lower-quality protein. Individuals have to take in enough protein to ensure nitrogen for adequate amino acid production and also to get enough high-quality protein to obtain the essential amino acids.

**TABLE 7.2**
**Amino Acids**

| Essential Amino Acids* | Nonessential Amino Acids |
|---|---|
| Histidine | Alanine |
| Isoleucine | Arginine |
| Leucine | Asparagine |
| Lysine | Aspartic acid |
| Methionine | Cysteine |
| Phenylalanine | Glutamic acid |
| Threonine | Glutamine |
| Tryptophan | Glycine |
| Valine | Proline |
| | Serine |
| | Tyrosine |

*Must be provided in the diet as the body cannot manufacture them.

Protein deficiency is not a problem in the usual American diet. Two glasses of skim milk combined with about 4 ounces of poultry or fish meet the daily protein requirement. Protein deficiency, however, could be a concern in some vegetarian diets.Vegetarians rely primarily on foods from the bread and cereal and fruit and vegetable groups and avoid most foods from animal sources found in the milk and meat groups. The four basic types of vegetarians are:

1. *Vegans*, who eat no animal products at all.
2. *Ovovegetarians*, who allow eggs in the diet.
3. *Lactovegetarians*, who eat foods from the milk group.
4. *Ovolactovegetarians*, who include egg and milk products in the diet.

Vegans in particular must be careful to eat protein foods that provide a balanced distribution of essential amino acids, such as grain products and beans. Strict vegans also need a supplement of vitamin $B_{12}$. This vitamin is not found in plant foods, and its deficiency may lead to anemia.

Vegetarians who do not select their food combinations properly may develop nutritional deficiencies of protein, vitamins, minerals, and even calories. Vegetarian diets can be balanced, but this is a complicated issue that cannot be covered adequately in a few paragraphs. Those who are interested in vegetarian diets should consult other resources.

Too much animal protein can cause serious health problems as well. Many people eat twice as much protein as they need. Protein foods from animal sources often are high in fat, saturated fat, and cholesterol, which can lead to cardiovascular disease and cancer. Too much animal protein also decreases blood enzymes that prevent precancerous cells from developing into tumors.

As discussed later in this chapter, a well-balanced diet contains a variety of foods from all five basic food groups, including wise selection of foods from animal sources. Based on current nutrition data, meat (poultry and fish included) should be replaced by grains, legumes, vegetables, and fruits as main courses. Meats should be used more for flavoring than for substance. Daily consumption of beef, poultry, or fish should be limited to 3 to 6 ounces (about the size of a deck of cards).

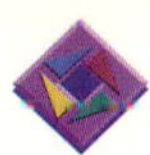

## Vitamins

Vitamins are organic substances necessary for normal bodily metabolism, growth, and development. Vitamins function as antioxidants, as coenzymes (primarily the B complex), which regulate the work of the enzymes; and vitamin D even functions as a hormone.

Vitamins C, E, beta-carotene (a precursor to vitamin A), and the mineral selenium serve as antioxidants, preventing oxygen from combining with other substances that it may damage. During metabolism oxygen changes carbohydrates and fats into energy. In this process oxygen is transformed into stable forms of water and carbon dioxide. A small amount of oxygen, however, ends up in an unstable form, referred to as *oxygen free radicals*. Solar radiation, cigarette smoke, radiation, and other environmental factors also seem to encourage the formation of free radicals.

A free radical molecule has a normal proton nucleus with a single unpaired electron. Having only one electron makes the free radical extremely reactive, and it constantly looks to pair the electron up with one from another molecule. When it steals the second electron from another molecule, that other molecule in turn becomes a free radical. This chain reaction goes on until two free radicals meet to form a stable molecule. Antioxidants help stabilize free radicals so they will not be as reactive until a match can be found.

Free radicals attack and damage proteins and lipids, in particular the cell membrane and DNA. This damage is thought to play a key role in the development of conditions such as heart disease, cancer, and emphysema (also see Chapters 9 and 10). The beneficial effects of antioxidants are given in Table 7.3.

Researchers believe that antioxidants offer protection by absorbing free radicals before they can cause damage and also by interrupting the sequence of reactions once damage has begun (Figure 7.5), thwarting certain chronic diseases.[2]

Vitamins are classified into two types based on their solubility: *fat-soluble vitamins* (A, D, E, and K), and *water-soluble vitamins* (B complex and C).

**TABLE 7.3**
**Antioxidant Nutrients, Sources, and Functions**

| Nutrient | Good Sources | Antioxidant Effect |
|---|---|---|
| **Vitamin C** | Citrus fruit, kiwi fruit, cantaloupe, strawberries, broccoli, green or red peppers, cauliflower, cabbage | Appears to inactivate oxygen-free radicals |
| **Vitamin E** | Vegetable oils, yellow and green leafy vegetables, margarine, wheatgerm, oatmeal, almonds, and whole grain breads, cereals | Protects lipids from oxidation. |
| **Beta-carotene** | Carrots, squash, pumpkin, sweet potatoes, broccoli, green leafy vegetables | Soaks up oxygen-free radicals |
| **Selenium** | Seafood, meat, whole grains | Helps prevent damage to cell structures |

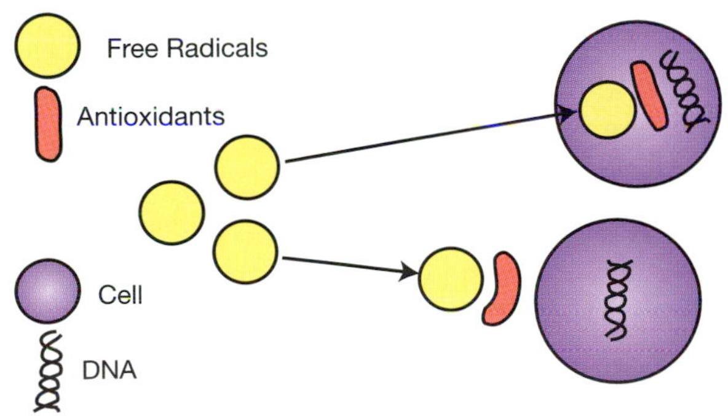

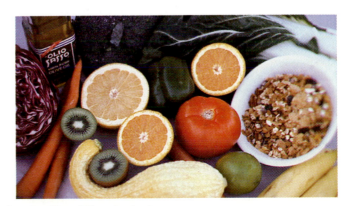


**FIGURE 7.5** ◆ The antioxidant effect of beta-carotene, vitamins C and E, and selenium.

In general, the body does not manufacture vitamins. Vitamins can be obtained only through a well-balanced diet. To decrease vitamin losses during cooking, natural foods should be microwaved or steamed rather than boiled in water that later is thrown out.

A few exceptions, such as A, D, and K, are formed in the body. Vitamin A is produced from beta-carotene, found in foods such as carrots, pumpkin, and sweet potatoes. Ultraviolet light from the sun changes a compound in the skin called 7-dehydrocholesterol into vitamin D. Vitamin K is created in the body by intestinal bacteria. The major functions of vitamins are outlined in Table 7.4.

## Minerals

Minerals are inorganic elements found in the body and in food. Approximately 25 minerals have important roles in body functioning. Minerals are contained in all cells, especially those in hard parts of the body (bones, nails, teeth).

Minerals are crucial in maintaining water balance and the acid-base balance. They are essential components of respiratory pigments, enzymes, and enzyme systems, and they regulate muscular and nervous tissue excitability, blood clotting, and normal heart rhythm.

The three minerals mentioned most commonly are calcium, iron, and sodium. As pointed out later in this chapter, calcium deficiency may result in osteoporosis, and low iron intake can induce iron-deficiency anemia. High sodium intake may lead to hypertension (also see blood pressure in Chapter 9). The specific functions of some of the most important minerals are given in Table 7.5.

## Water

Approximately 70% of total body weight is water. Water is the most important nutrient, involved in almost every vital body process: in digesting and absorbing food, in the circulatory process, in removing waste products, in building and rebuilding cells, and in transporting other nutrients.

Water is contained in almost all foods but primarily in liquid foods, fruits, and vegetables. Besides the natural content in foods, every person should drink about eight glasses of fluids a day.

# ENERGY (ATP) PRODUCTION

The energy derived from food is not used directly by the cells. It is transferred to form an energy-rich compound called adenosine triphosphate, or ATP. The subsequent breakdown of this compound provides the energy used by all energy-requiring processes of the body. ATP must be recycled continually to sustain life and work. ATP can be resynthesized in three ways (also see Figure 7.6):

1. **ATP and ATP-CP system.** The body stores small amounts of ATP and creatine phosphate (CP). These stores are used during all-out activities up to 10 seconds in duration, such as sprinting, long jumping, and power (weight) lifting. The amount of stored ATP provides energy for just a few seconds. With all-out efforts, ATP is resynthesized from CP, another high-energy phosphate compound. This is referred to as the ATP-CP or phosphagen system.

   Depending on the amount of physical training, the concentration of CP stored in cells is sufficient to allow maximum exertion for up to 10 seconds. Once the CP stores are depleted, the person is forced to slow down or rest to allow ATP to form through anaerobic and aerobic pathways.

2. **Anaerobic or lactic acid system.** During high-intensity (anaerobic) exercise that is sustained between 10 and 180 seconds maximum, ATP is replenished from the breakdown of glucose through a series of chemical reactions that do not require oxygen. In the process, though, lactic acid is produced, which causes muscular fatigue.

   Because of the accumulation of lactic acid with high-intensity exercise, the formation of ATP during anaerobic activities is limited to about 3 minutes. A recovery period then is necessary to allow for the elimination of lactic acid. Formation of ATP through the anaerobic system is possible from glucose (carbohydrates) only.

3. **Aerobic system.** The production of energy during slow-sustained exercise is derived primarily through aerobic metabolism. Both glucose (carbohydrates) and fatty acids (fat) are used in this process. Oxygen is required to form ATP, and under steady state exercise conditions lactic acid accumulation is minimal.

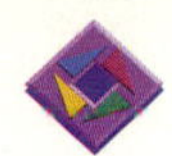

**TABLE 7.4**
**Major Functions of Vitamins**

| Nutrient | Good Sources | Major Functions | Deficiency Symptoms |
|---|---|---|---|
| Vitamin A | Milk, cheese, eggs, liver, and yellow/dark green fruits and vegetables | Required for healthy bones, teeth, skin, gums, and hair. Maintenance of inner mucous membranes, thus increasing resistance to infection. Adequate vision in dim light. | Night blindness, decreased growth, decreased resistance to infection, rough-dry skin. |
| Vitamin D | Fortified milk, cod liver oil, salmon, tuna, egg yolk | Necessary for bones and teeth. Needed for calcium and phosphorus absorption | Rickets (bone softening), fractures, and muscle spasms |
| Vitamin E | Vegetable oils, yellow and green leafy vegetables, margarine, wheat germ, whole-grain breads and cereals | Related to oxidation and normal muscle and red blood cell chemistry | Leg cramps, red blood cell breakdown |
| Vitamin K | Green leafy vegetables, cauliflower, cabbage, eggs, peas, and potatoes | Essential for normal blood clotting | Hemorrhaging |
| Vitamin $B_1$ (Thiamine) | Whole-grain or enriched bread, lean meats and poultry, organ fish, liver, pork, poultry, organ meats, legumes nuts, and dried yeast | Assists in proper use of carbohydrates. Normal functioning of nervous system. Maintenance of good appetite. | Loss of appetite, nausea, confusion, cardiac abnormalities, muscle spasms |
| Vitamin $B_2$ (Riboflavin) | Eggs, milk, leafy green vegetables, whole grains, lean meats, dried beans and peas | Contributes to energy release from carbohydrates, fats, and proteins. Needed for normal growth and development, good vision, and healthy skin | Cracking of the corners of the mouth, inflammation of the skin, impaired vision. |
| Vitamin $B_6$ (Pyridoxine) | Vegetables, meats, whole-grain cereals,soybeans, peanuts, and potatoes | Necessary for protein and fatty acids metabolism,and normal red blood cell formation | Depression, irritability, muscle spasms, nausea |
| Vitamin $B_{12}$ | Meat, poultry, fish, liver, organ meats, eggs, shellfish, milk, and cheese | Required for normal growth, red blood cell formation, nervous system and digestive tract | Impaired balance, weakness, drop in red blood cell count functioning |
| Niacin | Liver and organ meats, meat, fish, poultry, whole grains, enriched breads, nuts, green leafy vegetables, and dried beans and peas | Contributes to energy release from carbohydrates, fats, and proteins. Normal growth and development, and formation of hormones and nerve-regulating substances | Confusion, depression, weakness, weight loss |
| Biotin | Liver, kidney, eggs, yeast, legumes, milk, nuts, dark green vegetables | Essential for carbohydrate metabolism and fatty acid synthesis | Inflamed skin, muscle pain, depression, weight loss |
| Folic Acid | Leafy green vegetables, organ meats, whole grains and cereals, and dried beans | Needed for cell growth and reproduction and red blood cell formation | Decreased resistance to infection |
| Pantothenic Acid | All natural foods, especially liver, kidney, eggs, nuts, yeast, milk, dried peas and beans, and green leafy vegetables | Related to carbohydrate and fat metabolism | Depression, low blood sugar, leg cramps, nausea, headaches |
| Vitamin C (Ascorbic Acid) | Fruits and vegetables | Helps protect against infection; formation of collagenous tissue. Normal blood vessels, teeth, and bones | Slow-healing wounds, loose teeth, hemorrhaging, rough-scaly skin, irritability |

**TABLE 7.5**
**Major Functions of Minerals**

| Nutrient | Good Sources | Major Functions | Deficiency Symptoms |
|---|---|---|---|
| Calcium | Milk, yogurt, cheese, green leafy vegetables, dried beans, sardines, and salmon | Required for strong teeth and bone formation. Maintenance of good muscle tone, heart beat, and nerve function | Bone pain and fractures, periodontal disease, muscle cramps |
| Iron | Organ meats, lean meats, seafoods, eggs, dried peas and beans, nuts, whole and enriched grains, and green leafy vegetables | Major component of hemoglobin. Aids in utilization of energy | Nutritional anemia and overall weakness |
| Phosphorus | Meats, fish, milk, eggs, dried beans and peas, whole grains, and processed foods | Required for bone and teeth formation. Energy release regulation | Bone pain and fracture, weight loss, and weakness |
| Zinc | Milk, meat, seafood, whole grains, nuts, eggs, and dried beans | Essential component of hormones, insulin, and enzymes. Used in normal growth and development | Loss of appetite, slow-healing wounds, and skin problems |
| Magnesium | Green leafy vegetables, whole grains, nuts, soybeans, seafood, and legumes | Needed for bone growth and maintenance. Carbohydrate and protein utilization. Nerve function. Temperature regulation | Irregular heartbeat, weakness, muscle spasms, and sleeplessness |
| Sodium | Table salt, processed foods, and meat | Body fluid regulation. Transmission of nerve impulse. Heart action | Rarely seen |
| Potassium | Legumes, whole grains, bananas, orange juice, dried fruits, and potatoes | Heart action. Bone formation and maintenance. Regulation of energy release. Acid-base regulation | Irregular heartbeat, nausea, weakness |
| Selenium | Seafood, meat, whole grains | Component of enzyme; functions in close association with vitamin E | Muscle pain, possible heart muscle deterioration; possible hair and nail loss |

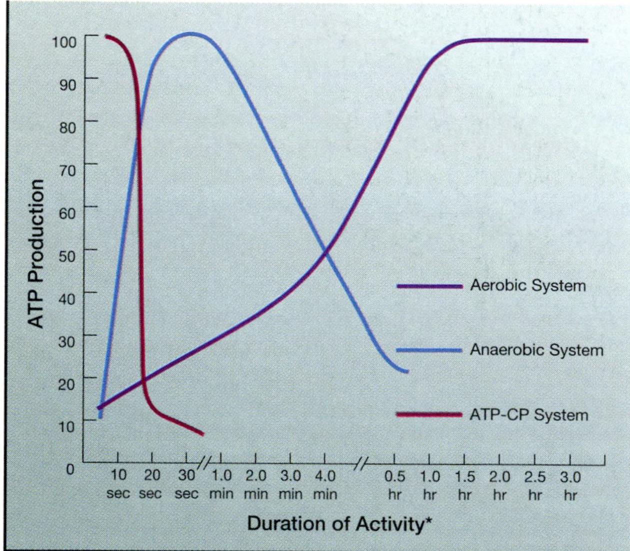


**FIGURE 7.6** ◆ Contributions of the energy formation mechanisms during various forms of physical activity.

Because oxygen is required, a person's capacity to utilize oxygen (maximal oxygen uptake, or Max $VO_2$ — see Chapter 2) is crucial for successful athletic performance in aerobic events. The higher the Max $VO_2$, the greater is the capacity to generate ATP through the aerobic system.

## BALANCING THE DIET

Most people would like to have good health and live life to its fullest. One of the fundamental ways to accomplish this is through a well-balanced diet. As illustrated in Figure 7.7, the recommended guidelines state that daily caloric intake should be distributed so about 58% of the total calories come from carbohydrates (48% complex carbohydrates

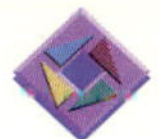

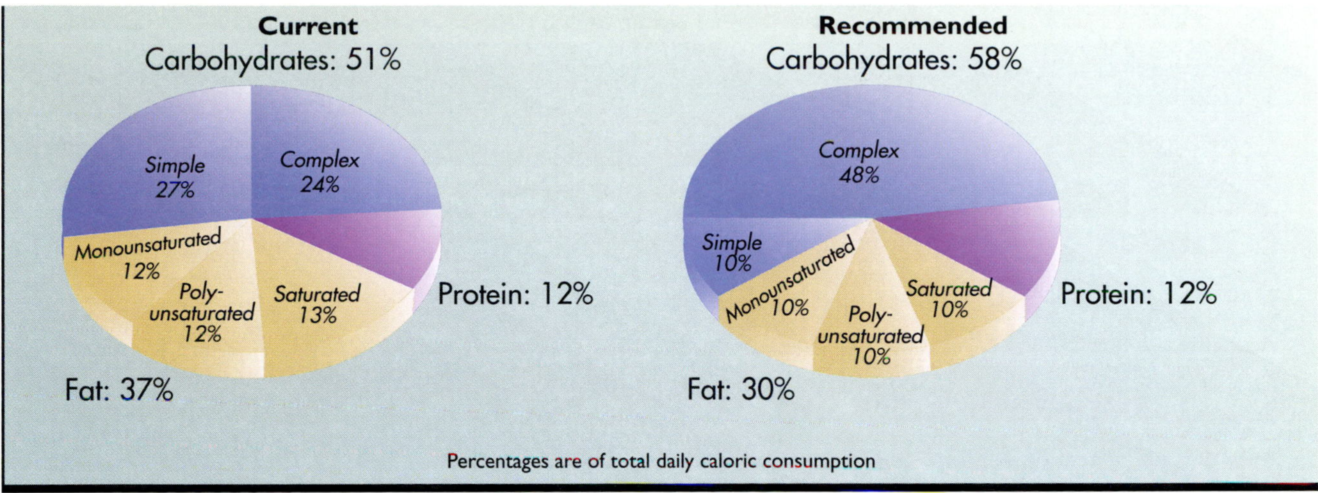


**FIGURE 7.7** ◆ Fat, carbohydrate, and protein intake.

and 10% sugar), less than 30% of the total calories from fat (equally divided [10% each] among saturated, monounsaturated, and polyunsaturated fats), and 12% of the total calories from protein (0.8 grams of protein per kilogram [2.2 pounds] of body weight). The diet also must include all of the essential vitamins, minerals, and water. To rate a diet accurately is difficult without a complete nutrient analysis.

The American diet has changed significantly since the turn of the century. People in the 1990s eat more fat, fewer carbohydrates, and about the same amount of protein, but fewer calories. At the same time, we weigh more than we did in 1900, an indication that we are not as physically active as our grandparents were.

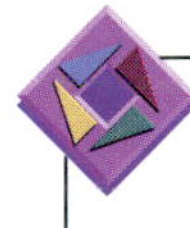

*People in the 1990s eat fewer calories but weigh more than those in the early 1900s.*

Diets also were much healthier at the turn of the century. In 1909, carbohydrates accounted for 57% of the total daily caloric intake, 67% of which were complex carbohydrates. Today, carbohydrate intake has decreased to 51%, and complex carbohydrates account for only 24% of the daily carbohydrate intake. The proportion of fat has risen from 32% to 37%. Protein intake has remained unchanged at about 12% of the total caloric intake.

## Nutrient Analysis

The first step in evaluating your diet is to conduct a nutrient analysis. This can be quite an educational experience because most people do not realize how harmful and non-nutritious many common foods are. The analysis covers calories, carbohydrates, fats, cholesterol, and sodium, as well as eight crucial nutrients: protein, calcium, iron, vitamin A, thiamin, riboflavin, niacin, and vitamin C. If the diet has enough of these eight nutrients, the foods consumed in natural form to provide these nutrients typically contain all the other nutrients the human body needs.

To do the nutrient analysis, keep a 3-day record of everything you eat, using the forms in Appendix B, Figure B.1. At the end of each day, look up the nutrient content for those foods in the list of Nutritive Value of Selected Foods, also in Appendix B. Record this information on your listing of foods in Figure B.1. If you do not find a food in the list given in Appendix B, the information often is stated on the food container itself, or you might refer to the references at the end of the list.

When you have recorded the nutritive values for each day, add up each column and write the totals at the bottom of the chart. After the third day use Figure B.2 and compute an average for the 3 days. To rate your diet, compare your figures with those in the recommended dietary allowances (RDA) (Table 7.6). This will give you a good indication of areas of strength and deficiency in your current diet.

**TABLE 7.6**
**Recommended Dietary Allowances (RDA)**

| | Calories | Protein | Fat | Sat. Fat | Choles-terol (mg) | Carbo-hydrates | Calcium (mg) | Iron (mg) | Sodium (mg) | Vit. A (I. U.) | Thiamin (Vit. $B_1$) (mg) | Riboflavin (Vit. $B_2$) (mg) | Niacin (mg) | Vit. C (mg) |
|---|---|---|---|---|---|---|---|---|---|---|---|---|---|---|
| **Men 15–18 years** | See below[a] | See below[b] | < 30%[c] | < 10%[c] | < 300 | 58% >[c] | 1,200 | 12 | 2,400 | 5,000 | 1.5 | 1.8 | 20 | 60 |
| **Men 19–24 years** | | | < 30%[c] | < 10%[c] | < 300 | 58% >[c] | 1,200 | 10 | 2,400 | 5,000 | 1.5 | 1.7 | 19 | 60 |
| **Men 25–50 years** | | | < 30%[c] | < 10%[c] | < 300 | 58% >[c] | 800 | 10 | 2,400 | 5,000 | 1.5 | 1.7 | 19 | 60 |
| **Men 51 +** | | | < 30%[c] | < 10%[c] | < 300 | 58% >[c] | 800 | 10 | 2,400 | 5,000 | 1.2 | 1.4 | 15 | 60 |
| **Women 15–18 years** | | | < 30%[c] | < 10%[c] | < 300 | 58% >[c] | 1,200 | 15 | 2,400 | 4,000 | 1.1 | 1.3 | 15 | 60 |
| **Women 19–24 years** | | | < 30%[c] | < 10%[c] | < 300 | 58% >[c] | 1,200 | 15 | 2,400 | 4,000 | 1.1 | 1.3 | 15 | 60 |
| **Women 25–50 years** | | | < 30%[c] | < 10%[c] | < 300 | 58% >[c] | 800 | 15 | 2,400 | 4,000 | 1.1 | 1.3 | 15 | 60 |
| **Women 51 +** | | | < 30%[c] | < 10%[c] | < 300 | 58% >[c] | 800 | 10 | 2,400 | 4,000 | 1.0 | 1.2 | 13 | 60 |
| **Pregnant** | | | < 30%[c] | < 10%[c] | < 300 | 58% >[c] | 1,200 | 30 | 2,400 | 4,000 | 1.5 | 1.6 | 17 | 70 |
| **Lactating** | | | < 30%[c] | < 10%[c] | < 300 | 58% >[c] | 1,200 | 15 | 2,400 | 6,000 | 1.6 | 1.8 | 20 | 95 |

[a] Use Table 8.1 in Chapter 8 for all categories.
[b] Protein intake should be .8 grams per kilogram of body weight. Pregnant women should consume an additional 15 grams of daily protein; lactating women should have an extra 20 grams.
[c] Percentage of total calories based on recommendations by nutrition experts.
* Adapted from *Recommended Dietary Allowances*, © 1989, by National Academy of Sciences, National Academy Press, Washington DC.

Every 10 years or so, the National Academy of Sciences issues a new RDA based on a review of the most current research on nutrient needs of healthy people. The RDA provides daily nutrient intake recommendations, usually set high enough to encompass 97.5% of the healthy population in the United States. Stated another way, the RDA recommendation for any nutrient is well above almost everyone's actual requirement.

Between the late 1960s and the early 1990s, nutrient information on labels was expressed in terms of the U. S. RDA — a set of standard values for the average consumer — derived from the 1968 edition of the RDA. In 1993 the Food and Drug Administration (FDA) revised food labeling regulations and has replaced the U.S. RDA with Daily Values (see Figure 7.8). These daily values are based on a 2,000-calorie diet and may require adjustments depending on an individual's daily caloric needs.

In setting the Daily Values, the FDA first created two sets of standards: Reference Daily Intakes (RDI) and Daily Reference Values (DRV). For FDA purposes these two sets of standards serve different functions. To avoid consumer confusion in food labeling, however, the FDA combined the RDI and DRV into the Daily Values.

The RDI are reference values for protein, vitamins, and minerals. These are similar in purpose to the old U. S. RDA, but they reflect average allowances based on the 1989 RDA.

The DRV are standards for nutrients and food components that do not have an established RDA. The DRV include carbohydrate, fat, saturated fat, fiber, cholesterol, and sodium. These standards (computed in grams and milligrams based on a 2,000-calorie diet) represent dietary intakes to attain or restrict based on a consensus of critical values associated with health. For example,

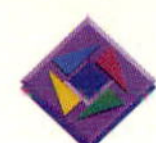

## 1 Better by Design

*How to recognize the new food labels*

The new food labels feature a revamped nutrition panel titled "Nutrition Facts," with nutrient listings that reflect current health concerns. Now you'll be able to find information on fat, fiber and other food components fundamental to lowering your risk of cancer and other chronic diseases. Listings for nutrients like thiamin and riboflavin will no longer be required, because Americans generally eat enough of them these days.

## 2 Size Up the Situation

*All serving sizes are created equal*

Now you can compare similar products and know that their serving sizes are basically identical. So when you realize how much fat is packed into that carton of double-dutch-chocolate-caramel-chew ice cream you're eyeing, you might opt for lowfat frozen yogurt instead. Serving sizes will also be standardized, so manufacturers can't make nutrition claims for unrealistically small portions. That means a chocolate cake, for example, must be divided into 8 servings sized to satisfy the average person — not 16 servings sized to satisfy the average munchkin.

## 3 Look Before You Leap

*Use the Daily Values*

You will find the Daily Values on the bottom half of the "Nutrition Facts" panel. Some represent maximum levels of nutrients that should be consumed each day for a healthful diet (as with fat) while others refer to minimum levels that can be exceeded (as with carbohydrates). They are based on both a 2,000 and 2,500 calorie diet. Your own needs may be more or less, but these figures give you a point from which to compare. For example, the sample label indicates that someone with a 2,000 calorie diet should eat no more than 65 grams of fat per day. This is based on a diet getting 30% of calories as fat. If you normally eat less calories, or want to eat less than 30% of calories as fat, your daily fat consumption will be lower.

## 4 Rate It Right

*Scan the % Daily Values*

The % Daily Values make judging the nutritional quality of a food a snap. For instance, you can look at the % Daily Value column and find that a food has 25% of the Daily Value for fiber. This means the product will give you a substantial portion of the recommended amount of fiber for the day. You can also use this column to compare nutrients in similar products. The % Daily Values are based on a 2,000 calorie diet.

## 5 Trust Adjectives

*Descriptors have legal definitions*

Terms like "low," "high" and "free" have long been used on food labels. What these words actually mean, however, could vary. Thanks to the new labeling laws, such descriptions must now meet legal definitions. For example, you may be shopping for foods high in vitamin A, which has been linked to lower risk of certain cancers. Under the new label laws, a food described as "high" in a particular nutrient must contain 20% or more of the Daily Value for that nutrient. So if the bottle of juice you're thinking of buying says "high in vitamin A,'" you can now feel confident that it really is a good source of the vitamin.

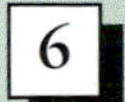

## 6 Read Health Claims with Confidence

*The nutrient link to disease prevention*

You can also expect to see food packages with health claims linking certain nutrients to reduced risk of cancer and other diseases. The federal government has approved three health claims dealing with cancer prevention: a low fat diet may reduce your risk for cancer; high fiber foods may reduce your risk for cancer; and fruits and vegetables may reduce your risk for cancer. A food may not make such a health claim for one nutrient if it contains other nutrients that undermine its health benefits. A high fiber, but high fat, jelly doughnut cannot carry a health claim!

**Nutrition Facts** (1)

Serving Size ½ cup (91g) (2)
Servings Per Container 5

| **Amount Per Serving** | |
|---|---|
| **Calories** 58 | Calories from Fat 0 |
| | **% Daily Value*** (4) |
| **Total Fat** 0g | **0%** |
| Saturated Fat 0g | **0%** |
| **Cholesterol** 0mg | **0%** |
| **Sodium** 45mg | **2%** |
| **Total Carbohydrate** 12g | **4%** |
| Dietary Fiber 3g | **12%** |
| Sugars 3g | |
| **Protein** 3g | |

| Vitamin A | 92% | • | Vitamin C | 16% |
|---|---|---|---|---|
| Calcium | 2% | • | Iron | 5% |

*Percent Daily Values are based on a 2,000 calorie diet. Your daily values may be higher or lower depending on your calorie needs:

| | Calories | 2,000 | 2,500 |
|---|---|---|---|
| Total Fat | Less than | 65g | 80g (3) |
| Sat Fat | Less than | 20g | 25g |
| Cholesterol | Less than | 300mg | 300mg |
| Sodium | Less than | 2,400mg | 2,400mg |
| Total Carbohydrate | | 300g | 375g |
| Fiber | | 25g | 30g |

Calories per gram:
Fat 9 • Carbohydrates 4 • Protein 4

Many factors affect cancer risk. Eating a diet low in fat and high in fiber may lower risk of this disease. (6)

- GOOD SOURCE OF FIBER
- LOWFAT (5)

Reprinted by permission from the American Institute for Cancer Research.

**FIGURE 7.8** ◆ U.S. Recommended Daily Values: A standard for nutrition labeling derived from RDA.

carbohydrate intake should be about 60% of total daily calories (300 grams), and fat intake should be limited to less than 30% (65 grams).

Both the RDA and the Daily Values apply only to healthy people. They are not intended for people who are ill and may require additional nutrients. If you are using the software available with this book to conduct your nutrient analysis, you need only record the foods by code and the number of servings based on the standard amounts given in the list of selected foods in Appendix B (the form provided in Figure B.3). A sample nutrient analysis printout is provided in Figures 7.15 and 7.16 at the end of this chapter.

Some of the most revealing information learned in a nutrient analysis is the source of fat intake in the diet. The average daily fat consumption in the American diet is about 37% of the total caloric intake, which greatly increases the risk for chronic diseases such as cardiovascular disease, cancer, diabetes, and obesity. Less than 30% of total calories should come from fat.

As illustrated in Figure 7.9, each gram of carbohydrates and protein supplies the body with 4 calories, and fat provides 9 calories per gram consumed (alcohol yields 7 calories per gram). In this regard, just looking at the total grams consumed for each type of food can be misleading.

For example, a person who eats 160 grams of carbohydrates, 100 grams of fat, and 70 grams of protein has a total intake of 330 grams of food. This indicates that 33% of the total grams of food is in the form of fat (100 grams of fat ÷ 330 grams of total food × 100). In reality, almost half of that diet is fat calories.

In the sample diet 640 calories are derived from carbohydrates (160 grams × 4 calories per gram), 280 calories from protein (70 grams × 4 calories per gram), and 900 calories from fat (100 grams × 9 calories per gram), for a total of 1,820 calories. If 900 calories are derived from fat, almost half of the total caloric intake is in the form of fat (900 ÷ 1,820 × 100 = 49.5%).

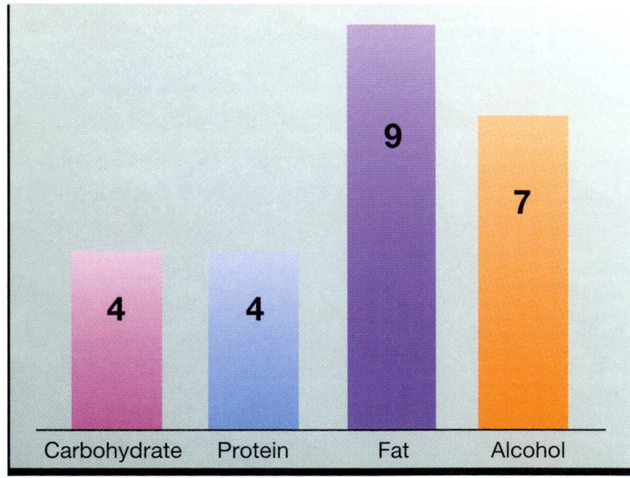


**FIGURE 7.9** ◆ Caloric value of food (fuel nutrients).

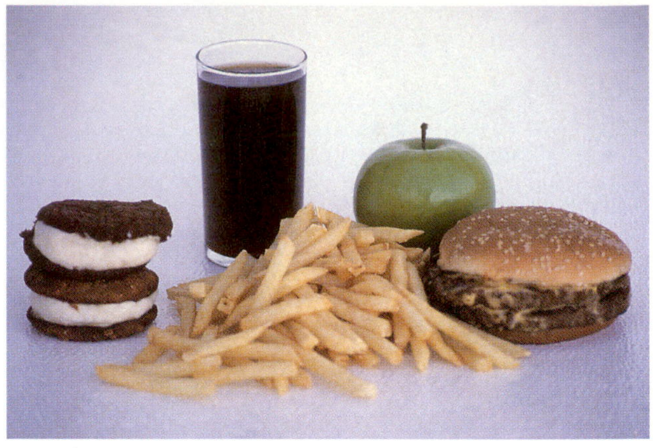

*An apple a day will not keep the doctor away if most meals are high in fat content.*

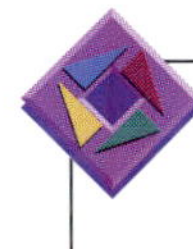

*The RDA provides daily nutrient intake recommendations, usually set high enough to encompass 97.5% of the healthy population in the United States.*

Each gram of fat provides nine calories. A useful guideline when figuring out the fat content of individual foods is shown in Figure 7.10. Multiply the grams of fat by 9 and divide by the total calories in that particular food (per serving). You then multiply that number by 100 to get the percentage. For example, if a food label lists a total of 100 calories and 7 grams of fat, the fat content is 63% of total calories. This simple guideline can help you decrease the fat in your diet. The fat content of selected foods, given in grams and as a percent of total calories, is presented in Figure 7.11. The percentage of fat is further subdivided into saturated, monounsaturated, polyunsaturated, and other fatty acids. Beware of products labeled "97% fat-free." These products use weight and not percent of total calories as a measure of fat. As illustrated in Figure 7.10, many of these foods still are in the range of 30% fat calories.

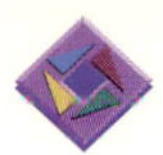

**Nutrition Facts**

Serving Size 1 cup (240 ml)
Servings Per Container 4

| **Amount Per Serving** | |
|---|---|
| **Calories** 120 | Calories from Fat 45 |
| | **% Daily Value*** |
| **Total Fat** 5g | **8%** |
| Saturated Fat 3g | **15%** |
| **Cholesterol** 20mg | **7%** |
| **Sodium** 120mg | **5%** |
| **Total Carbohydrate** 12g | **4%** |
| Dietary Fiber 0g | **0%** |
| Sugars 12g | |
| **Protein** 8g | |

| Vitamin A | 10% | • | Vitamin C | 4% |
|---|---|---|---|---|
| Calcium | 30% | • | Iron | 0% |

*Percent Daily Values are based on a 2,000 calorie diet. Your daily values may be higher or lower depending on your calorie needs:

| | Calories | 2,000 | 2,500 |
|---|---|---|---|
| Total Fat | Less than | 65g | 80g |
| Sat Fat | Less than | 20g | 25g |
| Cholesterol | Less than | 300mg | 300mg |
| Sodium | Less than | 2,400mg | 2,400mg |
| Total Carbohydrate | | 300g | 375g |
| Fiber | | 25g | 30g |

Calories per gram:
Fat 9 • Carbohydrate 4 • Protein 4

**Percent Fat Calories = (gr of fat × 9) ÷ calories per serving × 100**

5 g of fat × 9 calories per g of fat = 45 calories from fat

45 calories from fat ÷ 120 calories per serving × 100 = 38% fat

**FIGURE 7.10** ◆ Computation for fat content in food.

## Achieving a Balanced Diet

Anyone who has completed a nutrient analysis and has given careful attention to Tables 7.4 (vitamins) and 7.5 (minerals) probably will realize that a well-balanced diet entails eating a variety of foods and reducing daily intake of fats and sweets. The Healthy Eating Pyramid contained in Figure 7.12 provides simple and sound instructions for nutrition. The pyramid contains five major food groups, along with fats, oils, and sweets, which are to be used sparingly. The daily recommended number of servings of the five major food groups are:

1. Six to 11 servings of the bread, cereal, rice, and pasta group.
2. Three to five servings of the vegetable group.
3. Two to four servings of the fruit group.
4. Two to three servings of the milk, yogurt, and cheese group.
5. Two to three servings of the meat, poultry, fish, dry beans, eggs, and nuts group.

As illustrated in the Healthy Eating Pyramid, grains, vegetables, and fruits provide the nutritional base for a healthy diet. Daily fruits and vegetables should include as a minimum, one good source of vitamin A (apricots, cantaloupe, broccoli, carrots, pumpkin, dark leafy vegetables) and one good source of vitamin C (citrus fruit, kiwi fruit, cantaloupe, strawberries, broccoli, cabbage, cauliflower, green pepper).

An entirely new field of research with promising results in disease prevention, especially in the fight against cancer, is in the area of *phytochemicals* ("phyto" comes from the Greek word for plant). These compounds, just recently discovered by scientists, are found in large quantities in fruits and vegetables.

The main function of phytochemicals in plants is to protect them from sunlight. In humans, however, they seem to have a powerful ability to block the formation of cancerous tumors. Their actions are so diverse that, at almost every stage of cancer, phytochemicals have the ability to block, disrupt, slow down, or even reverse the process (also see Chapter 10). And these compounds are not found in pills. The message here is to eat a diet with ample fruits and vegetables. The recommendation of five to nine servings of fruits and vegetables daily has absolutely no substitute. People can't expect to eat a poor diet, pop a few pills, and derive the same benefits.

## FAT CONTENT OF SELECTED FOODS

| Food | Calories | Total fat (grams) | % Fat Calories |
|---|---|---|---|
| Avocado/Florida (1) | 340 | 27 | 71.5 |
| Bacon (3 pieces) | 109 | 9 | 74.3 |
| Beef/ground/lean/broiled (4 oz) | 318 | 20 | 56.6 |
| Beef/sirloin (4 oz) | 320 | 21 | 59.1 |
| Beef/T-bone (4 oz) | 338 | 24 | 63.9 |
| Butter (1 tbs) | 102 | 11 | 97.1 |
| Cheese/American (1 oz) | 93 | 7 | 67.7 |
| Cheese/cheddar (1 oz) | 114 | 9 | 71.1 |
| Cheese/cottage 4% (1 cup) | 216 | 9 | 37.5 |
| Cheese/cream (1 oz) | 99 | 10 | 90.9 |
| Cheese/parmesan (1 oz) | 129 | 9 | 62.8 |
| Cheese/Swiss (1 oz) | 106 | 8 | 67.9 |
| Cheeseburger (1) | 305 | 13 | 38.4 |
| Chicken/breast/no skin (4 oz) | 188 | 4 | 19.1 |
| Chicken/thigh/no skin (4 oz) | 232 | 13 | 50.4 |
| Egg/hard-cooked (1) | 77 | 5 | 58.4 |
| Frankfurter/beef & pork (1) | 182 | 17 | 84.1 |
| Halibut/baked (4 oz) | 159 | 3 | 17.0 |
| Hamburger (1) | 255 | 9 | 31.8 |
| Ice cream/vanilla (1 cup) | 267 | 15 | 50.6 |
| Ice milk/vanilla (1 cup) | 182 | 6 | 29.7 |
| Lamb/lean & fat (4 oz) | 293 | 19 | 58.4 |
| Margarine (1 tbs) | 101 | 11 | 98.0 |
| Mayonnaise (1 tbs) | 99 | 11 | 100.0 |
| Milk 2% (1 cup) | 121 | 5 | 37.2 |
| Milk/skim (1 cup) | 85 | .5 | 5.3 |
| Milk/whole (1 cup) | 149 | 8 | 48.3 |
| Nuts/cashew/oil roasted (1 oz) | 163 | 14 | 77.3 |
| Nuts/peanuts/oil roasted (1 oz) | 165 | 14 | 76.4 |
| Oil/canola (1 tbs) | 126 | 14 | 100.0 |
| Oil/olive (1 tbs) | 124 | 14 | 100.0 |
| Salmon/baked (4 oz) | 245 | 12 | 44.1 |
| Sherbet (1 cup) | 266 | 4 | 13.5 |
| Shrimp/boiled (3 oz) | 85 | 1 | 10.6 |
| Tuna/oil/drained (3 oz) | 167 | 7 | 37.7 |
| Tuna/water/drained (3 oz) | 99 | 1 | 9.1 |
| Turkey/dark meat/no skin (4 oz) | 212 | 8 | 34.0 |
| Turkey/light meat/no skin (4 oz) | 117 | 4 | 30.8 |

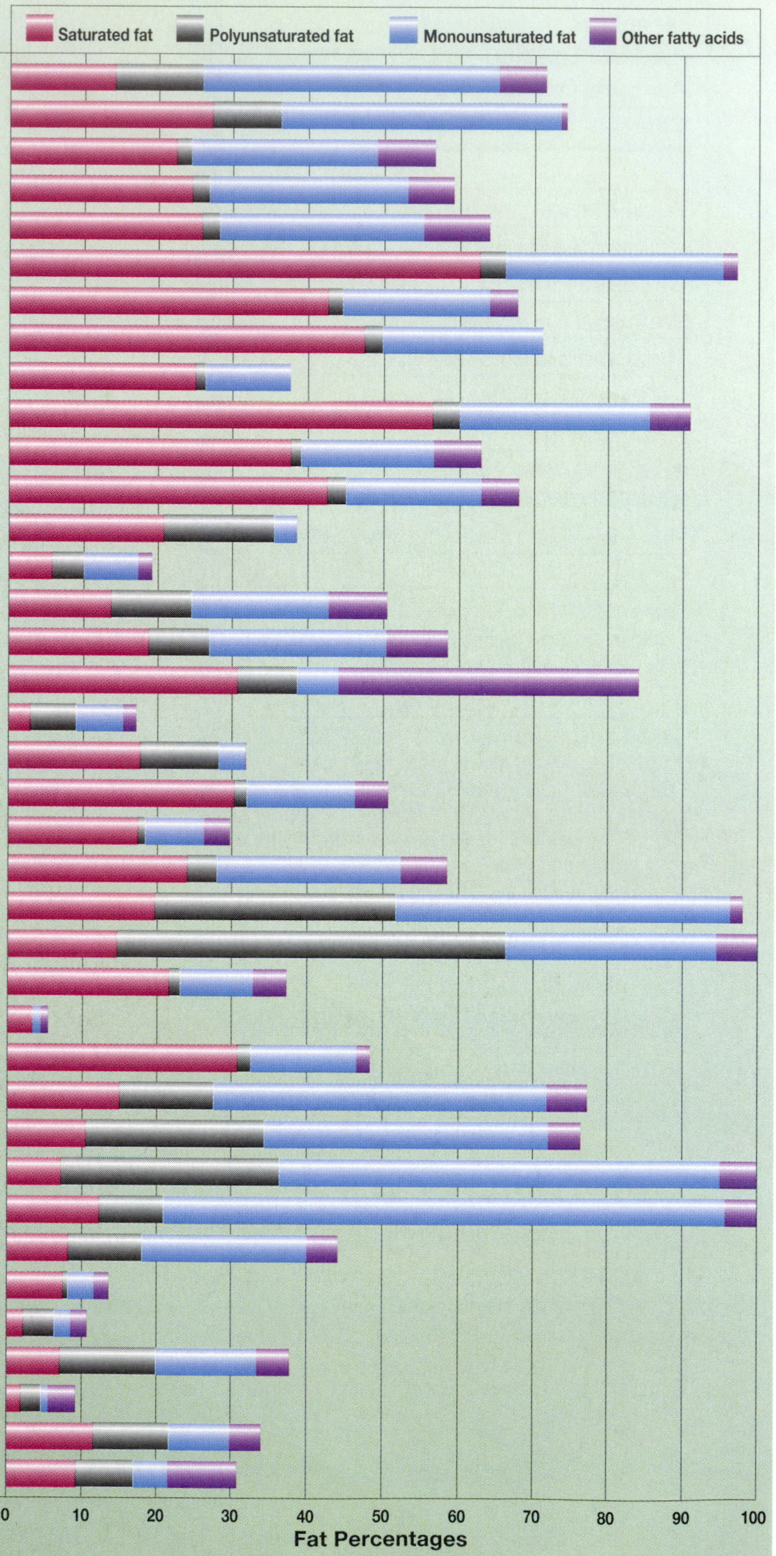

**FIGURE 7.11** ◆ Fat content of selected foods.

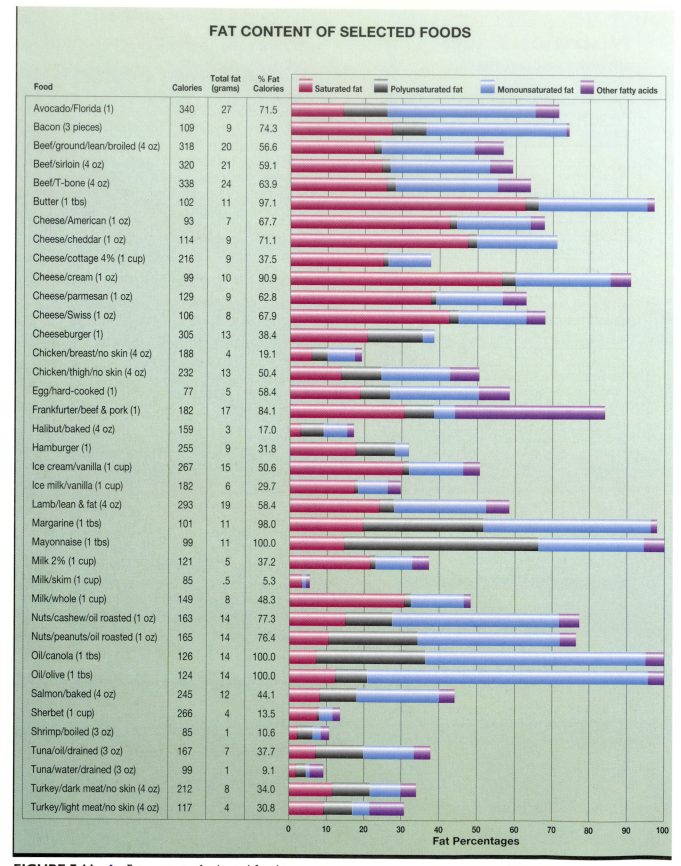

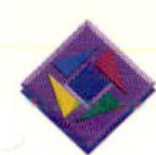

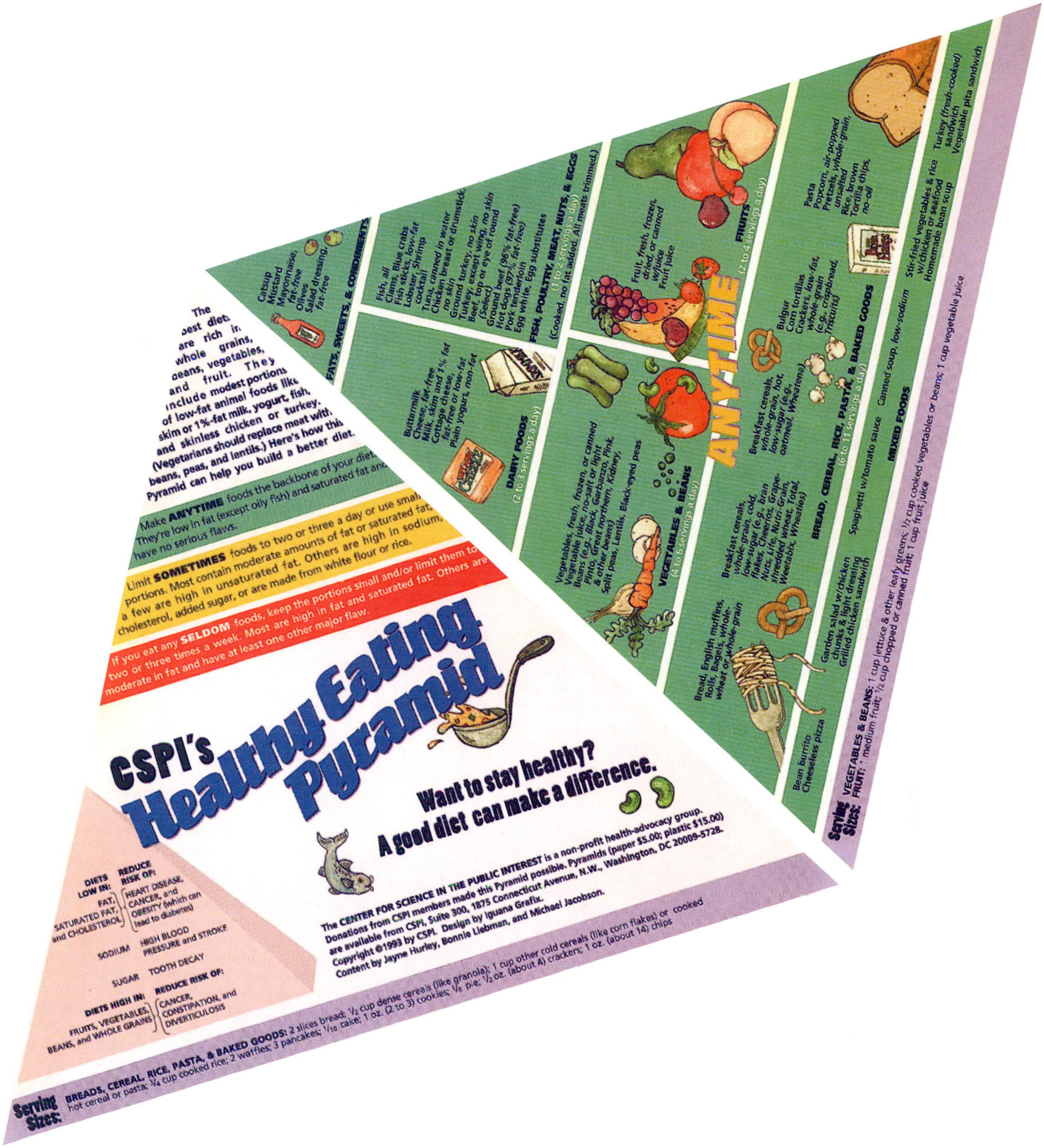

CSPI's Healthy Eating Pyramid

Want to stay healthy? A good diet can make a difference.

The best diets are rich in whole grains, beans, vegetables, and fruit. They include modest portions of low-fat animal foods like skim or 1%-fat milk, yogurt, fish, and skinless chicken or turkey. (Vegetarians should replace meat with beans, peas, and lentils.) Here's how this Pyramid can help you build a better diet.

Make **ANYTIME** foods the backbone of your diet. They're low in fat (except oily fish) and saturated fat and have no serious flaws.

Limit **SOMETIMES** foods to two or three a day or use small portions. Most contain moderate amounts of fat or saturated fat; a few are high in unsaturated fat. Others are high in sodium, cholesterol, added sugar, or are made from white flour or rice.

If you eat any **SELDOM** foods, keep the portions small and/or limit them to two or three times a week. Most are high in fat and saturated fat. Others are moderate in fat and have at least one other major flaw.

**DIETS LOW IN:** FAT, SATURATED FAT, and CHOLESTEROL — **REDUCE RISK OF:** HEART DISEASE, CANCER, and OBESITY (which can lead to diabetes)

SODIUM — HIGH BLOOD PRESSURE and STROKE

SUGAR — TOOTH DECAY

**DIETS HIGH IN:** FRUITS, VEGETABLES, BEANS, and WHOLE GRAINS — **REDUCE RISK OF:** CANCER, CONSTIPATION, and DIVERTICULOSIS

**ANYTIME**

**FATS, SWEETS, & CONDIMENTS:** Catsup, Mustard, Mayonnaise, fat-free, Olives, Salad dressing, fat-free

**FISH, POULTRY, MEAT, NUTS, & EGGS** (1 to 2 servings a day) (Cooked, no fat added. All meats trimmed.): Fish, all; Clams, Blue crabs; Fish sticks, low-fat; Lobster, Shrimp cocktail; Tuna, canned in water; Chicken breast or drumstick, no skin; Ground turkey, no skin; Turkey, except wing, no skin; Beef, top or eye of round (Select); Ground beef (96% fat-free); Hot dogs (97% fat-free); Pork tenderloin; Egg white, Egg substitutes

**DAIRY FOODS** (2 to 3 servings a day): Buttermilk; Cheese, fat-free; Milk, skim and 1% fat; Cottage cheese, fat-free or low-fat; Plain yogurt, non-fat

**FRUITS** (2 to 4 servings a day): Fruit, fresh, frozen, dried, or canned w/juice; Fruit juice

**VEGETABLES & BEANS** (4 to 6 servings a day): Vegetables, fresh, frozen, or canned; Vegetable juice, no-salt or light; Beans (e.g., Black, Garbanzo, Pink, Pinto, Great northern, Kidney, & other beans); Split peas, Lentils, Black-eyed peas

**BREAD, CEREAL, RICE, PASTA, & BAKED GOODS** (6 to 11 servings a day): Bread, English muffins, Rolls, Bagels, whole-wheat or whole-grain; Breakfast cereals, whole-grain, cold, low-sugar (e.g., bran flakes, Cheerios, Grape-Nuts, Life, Nutri-Grain, shredded wheat, Total, Weetabix, Wheaties); Breakfast cereals, whole-grain, hot, low-sugar (e.g., oatmeal, Wheatena); Bulgur; Corn tortillas; Crackers, low-fat, whole-grain (e.g., crispbread, Triscuits); Pasta; Popcorn, air-popped; Pretzels, whole-grain, unsalted; Rice, brown; Tortilla chips, no-oil

**MIXED FOODS:** Bean burrito; Cheeseless pizza; Garden salad w/chicken chunks & light dressing; Grilled chicken sandwich; Spaghetti w/tomato sauce; Canned soup, low-sodium; Stir-fried vegetables & rice w/chicken or seafood; Homemade bean soup; Turkey (fresh-cooked) sandwich; Vegetable pita sandwich

**Serving Sizes: VEGETABLES & BEANS:** 1 cup lettuce & other leafy greens; ½ cup cooked vegetables or beans; 1 cup vegetable juice **FRUIT:** 1 medium fruit; ½ cup chopped or canned fruit; 1 cup fruit juice

**Serving Sizes: BREADS, CEREAL, RICE, PASTA, & BAKED GOODS:** 2 slices bread; ½ cup dense cereals (like granola); 1 cup other cold cereals (like corn flakes) or cooked hot cereal or pasta; ¾ cup cooked rice; 2 waffles; 3 pancakes; 1/10 cake; 1 oz. (2 to 3) cookies; 1/8 pie; ½ oz. (about 4) crackers; 1 oz. (about 14) chips

The CENTER FOR SCIENCE IN THE PUBLIC INTEREST is a non-profit health-advocacy group. Donations from CSPI members made this Pyramid possible. Pyramids (paper $5.00; plastic $15.00) are available from CSPI, Suite 300, 1875 Connecticut Avenue, N.W., Washington, DC 20009-5728. Copyright ©1993 by CSPI. Design by Iguana Grafix. Content by Jayne Hurley, Bonnie Liebman, and Michael Jacobson.

Reprinted with permission from the Center for Science in the Public Interest, 1875 Connecticut Avenue, N.W., Suite 300, Washington, D.C., 20009. The Healthy Eating Pyramid can be obtained for $5.00 from the Center for Science in the Public Interest.

**FIGURE 7.12** ◆ Healthy Eating Pyramid: A guide to daily food choices.

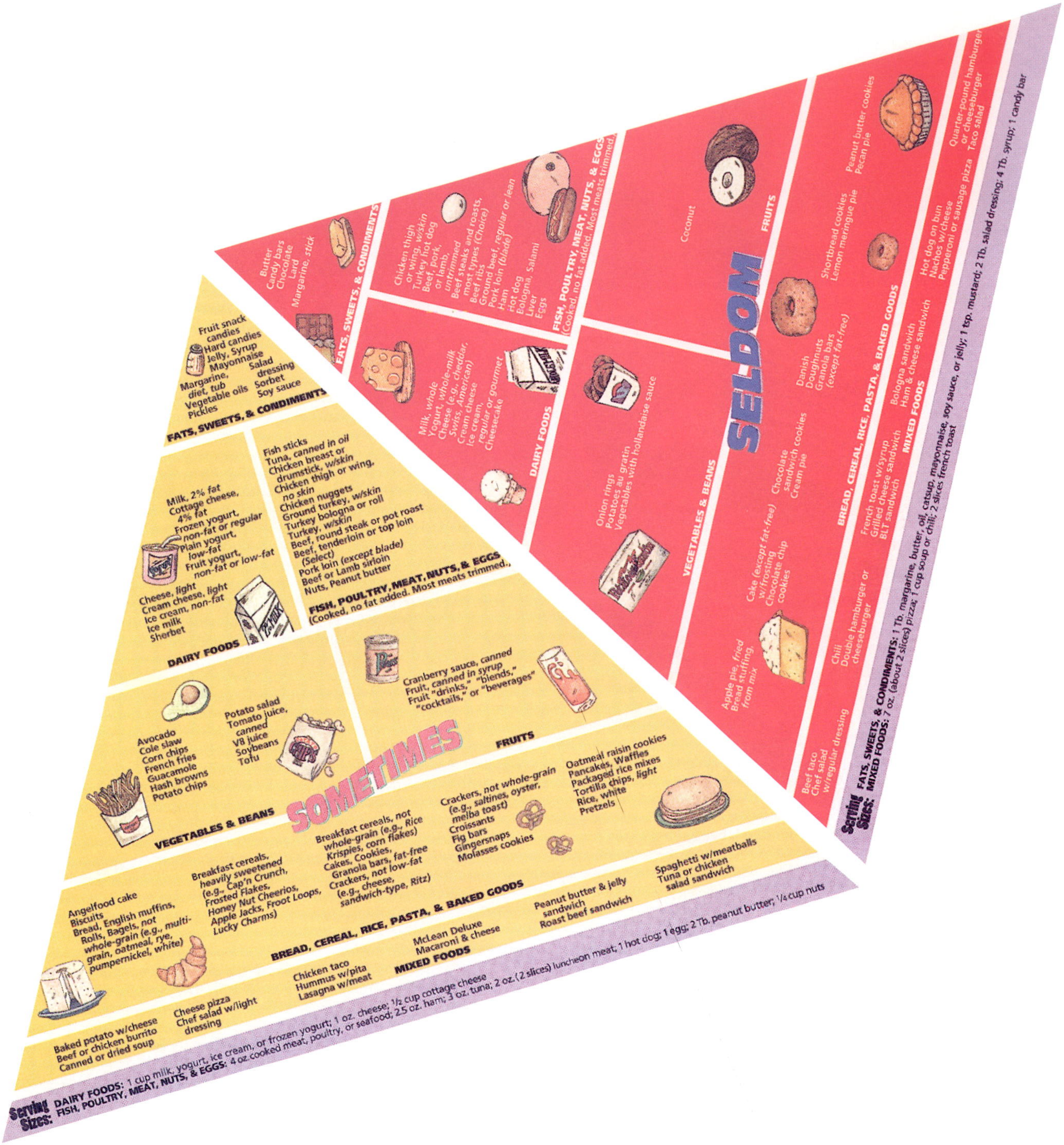

SOMETIMES

FATS, SWEETS, & CONDIMENTS
Fruit snack candies
Hard candies
Jelly, Syrup
Mayonnaise
Salad dressing
Margarine, diet, tub
Sorbet
Vegetable oils
Soy sauce
Pickles

DAIRY FOODS
Milk, 2% fat
Cottage cheese, 4% fat
Frozen yogurt, non-fat or regular
Plain yogurt, low-fat
Fruit yogurt, non-fat or low-fat
Cheese, light
Cream cheese, light
Ice cream, non-fat
Ice milk
Sherbet

FISH, POULTRY, MEAT, NUTS, & EGGS
(Cooked, no fat added. Most meats trimmed.)
Fish sticks
Tuna, canned in oil
Chicken breast or drumstick, w/skin
Chicken thigh or wing, no skin
Chicken nuggets
Ground turkey, w/skin
Turkey bologna or roll
Turkey, w/skin
Beef, round steak or pot roast
Beef, tenderloin or top loin (Select)
Pork loin (except blade)
Beef or Lamb sirloin
Nuts, Peanut butter

VEGETABLES & BEANS
Avocado
Cole slaw
Corn chips
French fries
Guacamole
Hash browns
Potato chips
Potato salad
Tomato juice, canned
V8 juice
Soybeans
Tofu

FRUITS
Cranberry sauce, canned
Fruit, canned in syrup
Fruit "drinks," "blends," "cocktails," or "beverages"

BREAD, CEREAL, RICE, PASTA, & BAKED GOODS
Angelfood cake
Biscuits
Bread, English muffins, Rolls, Bagels, not whole-grain (e.g., multi-grain, oatmeal, rye, pumpernickel, white)
Breakfast cereals, heavily sweetened (e.g., Cap'n Crunch, Frosted Flakes, Honey Nut Cheerios, Apple Jacks, Froot Loops, Lucky Charms)
Breakfast cereals, not whole-grain (e.g., Rice Krispies, corn flakes)
Cakes, Cookies, Granola bars, fat-free
Crackers, not low-fat (e.g., cheese, sandwich-type, Ritz)
Crackers, not whole-grain (e.g., saltines, oyster, melba toast)
Croissants
Fig bars
Gingersnaps
Molasses cookies
Oatmeal raisin cookies
Pancakes, Waffles
Packaged rice mixes
Tortilla chips, light
Rice, white
Pretzels

MIXED FOODS
Baked potato w/cheese
Beef or chicken burrito
Canned or dried soup
Cheese pizza
Chef salad w/light dressing
Chicken taco
Hummus w/pita
Lasagna w/meat
McLean Deluxe
Macaroni & cheese
Peanut butter & jelly sandwich
Roast beef sandwich
Spaghetti w/meatballs
Tuna or chicken salad sandwich

Serving Sizes: DAIRY FOODS: 1 cup milk, yogurt, ice cream, or frozen yogurt; 1 oz. cheese; 1/2 cup cottage cheese
FISH, POULTRY, MEAT, NUTS, & EGGS: 4 oz. cooked meat, poultry, or seafood; 2.5 oz. ham; 3 oz. tuna; 2 oz. (2 slices) luncheon meat; 1 hot dog; 1 egg; 2 Tb. peanut butter; 1/4 cup nuts

SELDOM

FATS, SWEETS, & CONDIMENTS
Butter
Candy bars
Chocolate
Lard
Margarine, stick

FISH, POULTRY, MEAT, NUTS, & EGGS
(Cooked, no fat added. Most meats trimmed.)
Chicken thigh or wing, w/skin
Turkey hot dog
Beef, pork, or lamb, untrimmed
Beef steaks and roasts, most types (Choice)
Beef ribs
Ground beef, regular or lean
Pork loin (blade)
Ham
Hot dog
Bologna, Salami
Liver
Eggs

DAIRY FOODS
Milk, whole
Yogurt, whole-milk
Cheese (e.g., cheddar, Swiss, American)
Cream cheese
Ice cream, regular or gourmet
Cheesecake

FRUITS
Coconut

VEGETABLES & BEANS
Onion rings
Potatoes au gratin
Vegetables with hollandaise sauce

BREAD, CEREAL, RICE, PASTA, & BAKED GOODS
Apple pie, fried
Bread stuffing, from mix
Cake (except fat-free) w/frosting
Chocolate chip cookies
Chocolate sandwich cookies
Cream pie
Danish
Doughnuts
Granola bars (except fat-free)
Shortbread cookies
Lemon meringue pie
Peanut butter cookies
Pecan pie

MIXED FOODS
Beef taco
Chef salad w/regular dressing
Chili
Double hamburger or cheeseburger
French toast w/syrup
Grilled cheese sandwich
BLT sandwich
Bologna sandwich
Ham & cheese sandwich
Hot dog on bun
Nachos w/cheese
Pepperoni or sausage pizza
Quarter-pound hamburger or cheeseburger
Taco salad

Serving Sizes: FATS, SWEETS, & CONDIMENTS: 1 Tb. margarine, butter, oil, catsup, mayonnaise, soy sauce, or jelly; 1 tsp. mustard; 2 Tb. salad dressing; 4 Tb. syrup; 1 candy bar
MIXED FOODS: 7 oz. (about 2 slices) pizza; 1 cup soup or chili; 2 slices french toast

**FIGURE 7.12** ◆ Healthy Eating Pyramid: A guide to daily food choices (continued).

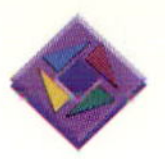

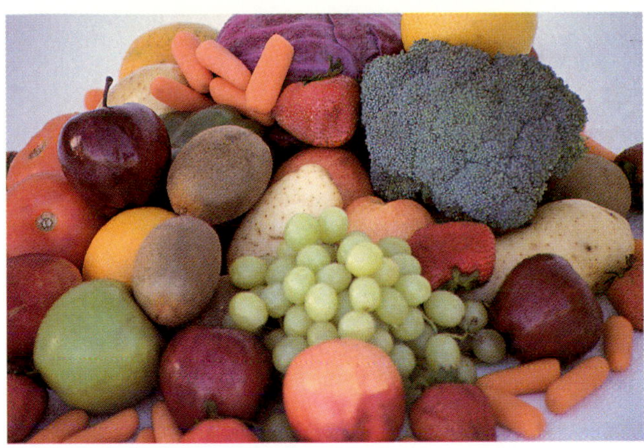

*Fruits and vegetables in general contain large amounts of cancer-prevention phytochemicals.*

Milk, poultry, fish, and meats are to be consumed in moderation. Milk should be skim, and milk products should be low-fat. Three ounces of poultry, fish, or meat and not to exceed 6 ounces daily is the recommendation. All visible fat and skin should be trimmed off meats and poultry before cooking. Egg consumption should be limited to no more than three eggs per week.

As an aid in balancing your diet, the form given in Figure 7.13 enables you to record your daily food intake. This record is much easier to

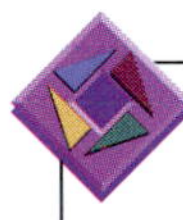

*People cannot expect to eat a poor diet, pop a few pills, and derive the same benefits achieved through a healthy diet.*

keep than the complete nutrient analysis. Make as many copies of this form as the number of days you wish to record. Whenever you have something to eat, record, on Figure 7.13, the food and the amount eaten. Do this immediately after each meal so you will be able to keep track of your actual food intake more easily.

If you eat twice the amount of a standard serving, double the number of servings. Evaluate your diet by checking whether you ate the minimum required servings for each food group. If you meet the minimum required servings at the end of each day, you are doing well in balancing your diet.

Restructure your meals on the plate so rice, pasta, beans, breads, and vegetables are in the center, meats are on the side and are added primarily for flavoring, and desserts consist of fruits. Substitute lowfat or nonfat milk and milk products. This is another strategy to help you enjoy a healthy diet, prevent disease, and improve your overall quality of life.

## NUTRIENT SUPPLEMENTATION

According to the Food and Drug Administration, four of every 10 adults in the United States take nutrient supplements daily, and one in every seven has a nutrient intake almost eight times the RDA. In reality, vitamin and mineral requirements for the body can be met by consuming as few as 1,200 calories per day, as long as the diet contains the recommended servings from the five food groups.

Water-soluble vitamins cannot be stored as long as fat-soluble vitamins. The body readily excretes excessive intakes. Small amounts, however, can be retained for weeks or months in various organs and tissues of the body. Fat-soluble vitamins, on the other hand, are stored in fatty tissue. Therefore, daily intake of these vitamins is not as crucial. Too much vitamin A and vitamin D actually can be detrimental to health.

People should not take megadoses of vitamins. For most vitamins, a megadose is 10 times the RDA or more. For vitamins A and D, it is respectively five and two times the RDA. Mineral doses should not exceed three times the RDA.

Presently, no standard percentage above the RDA is available to guide us in determining the level at which a high dose of a given nutrient may cause health problems. For some nutrients a dose of five times the RDA taken over several months may create problems. For others it may not pose any threat to human health.

Iron deficiency (determined through blood testing) is common in women. Iron supplementation frequently is recommended for these women who have heavy menstrual flow. Some pregnant and lactating women also may require supplements. According to 1990 guidelines by the National Academy of Science, the average pregnant woman who eats an adequate amount of a variety of foods needs only to take a low dose of daily iron supplement. Women who are pregnant with more than one baby may need additional supplements. In the above instances, supplements should be taken under a physician's supervision.

Other people who may benefit from supplementation are alcoholics and street-drug users who do not have a balanced diet, smokers, strict vegetarians, individuals on extremely low-calorie diets, elderly people who don't eat balanced meals regularly, and newborn infants (usually given a single dose of vitamin K to prevent abnormal bleeding). For healthy people with a balanced diet, most supplements do not seem to provide additional benefits. They do not help people run faster, jump higher, relieve stress, improve sexual prowess, cure a common cold, or boost energy levels.

Much research currently is being done to study the effects of antioxidant supplements (vitamins C, E, beta-carotene, and the mineral selenium) in thwarting several chronic diseases (see the discussion on vitamins earlier in this chapter). Antioxidants are believed to offer protection, but the effects and amounts of supplements have not been clearly established yet.

The benefits of antioxidants have been researched mainly through diet alone, by studying people who eat foods high in antioxidants and not through supplements. Researchers do not know if the protective effects are caused by the antioxidants themselves, in combination with other nutrients (such as phytochemicals), or actually by some other nutrients in food that have not yet been investigated. In the case of selenium, excessive amounts may be toxic. A diet with substantial fruits, vegetables, and grains is the best means to obtain ample amounts of antioxidants.

Many people who regularly eat fast foods high in fat content or too many sweets think they need vitamin and mineral supplementation to balance their diet. This is another fallacy about nutrition. The problem in these cases is not a lack of vitamins and minerals but, instead, a diet too high in calories, fat, and sodium. Supplementation will not offset these poor eating habits. Pills are no substitute for common sense.

If you think your diet is not balanced, you first need to conduct a nutrient analysis to determine which nutrients are missing. Use the Healthy Eating Pyramid and the vitamin and mineral charts in this chapter, and eat more of the foods high in antioxidants, phytochemicals, and those with nutrients that are deficient in your diet.

## SPECIFIC NUTRITION CONSIDERATIONS

### Nutrition for Athletes

The two main fuels that supply energy for physical activity are glucose and fat (fatty acids). The body uses amino acids, derived from proteins, as an energy substrate when glucose is low, such as during fasting, prolonged aerobic exercise, or a low carbohydrate diet.

Glucose is derived from foods high in carbohydrates such as breads, cereals, grains, pasta, beans,

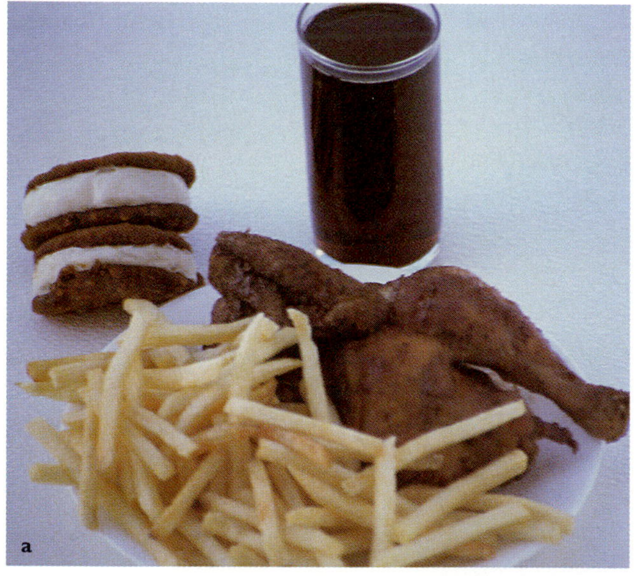


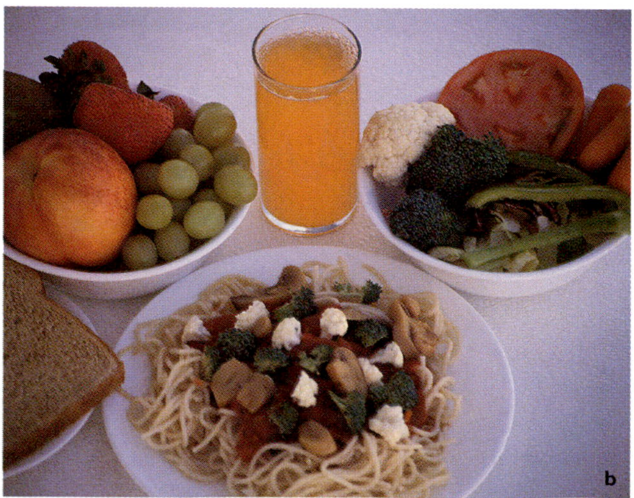


*Traditional (a) and contemporary (b) nutrition concepts. Current concept emphasizes meals high in pasta, rice, beans, breads, and vegetables; meats should be added primarily for flavoring; fruits are used for desserts; and low or nonfat milk products are used.*

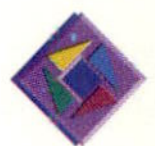

Name: ______________________

| No. | Code* | Food | Amount | Calories | Fat (gm) | Food Groups (servings): Bread, Cereal, Rice & Pasta | Vegetable | Fruit | Milk, Yogurt & Cheese | Meat, Poultry, Fish, Dry Beans, Eggs, & Nuts |
|---|---|---|---|---|---|---|---|---|---|---|
| 1 | | | | | | | | | | |
| 2 | | | | | | | | | | |
| 3 | | | | | | | | | | |
| 4 | | | | | | | | | | |
| 5 | | | | | | | | | | |
| 6 | | | | | | | | | | |
| 7 | | | | | | | | | | |
| 8 | | | | | | | | | | |
| 9 | | | | | | | | | | |
| 10 | | | | | | | | | | |
| 11 | | | | | | | | | | |
| 12 | | | | | | | | | | |
| 13 | | | | | | | | | | |
| 14 | | | | | | | | | | |
| 15 | | | | | | | | | | |
| 16 | | | | | | | | | | |
| 17 | | | | | | | | | | |
| 18 | | | | | | | | | | |
| 19 | | | | | | | | | | |
| 20 | | | | | | | | | | |
| 21 | | | | | | | | | | |
| 22 | | | | | | | | | | |
| 23 | | | | | | | | | | |
| 24 | | | | | | | | | | |
| 25 | | | | | | | | | | |
| 26 | | | | | | | | | | |
| 27 | | | | | | | | | | |
| 28 | | | | | | | | | | |
| 29 | | | | | | | | | | |
| 30 | | | | | | | | | | |
| Totals | | | | | | | | | | |
| Recommended Amount | | | | ** | *** | 6–11 | 3–5 | 2–4 | 2–3 | 2–3 |
| Deficiencies | | | | | | | | | | |

*See list of nutritive value of selected foods in Appendix B.
**Compute using Table 8.1 in Chapter 8.
***Multiply the recommended amount of calories by .30 (30%) and divide by 9 to obtain the recommended amount of grams of fat (if on a diet, multiply by .20 or .10 — see Table 8.3 in Chapter 8).

**FIGURE 7.13** ◆ Daily diet record form.

Name: ______________________

| No. | Code* | Food | Amount | Calories | Fat (gm) | Food Groups (servings) | | | | |
|---|---|---|---|---|---|---|---|---|---|---|
| | | | | | | Bread, Cereal, Rice & Pasta | Vegetable | Fruit | Milk, Yogurt & Cheese | Meat, Poultry, Fish, Dry Beans, Eggs, & Nuts |
| 1 | | | | | | | | | | |
| 2 | | | | | | | | | | |
| 3 | | | | | | | | | | |
| 4 | | | | | | | | | | |
| 5 | | | | | | | | | | |
| 6 | | | | | | | | | | |
| 7 | | | | | | | | | | |
| 8 | | | | | | | | | | |
| 9 | | | | | | | | | | |
| 10 | | | | | | | | | | |
| 11 | | | | | | | | | | |
| 12 | | | | | | | | | | |
| 13 | | | | | | | | | | |
| 14 | | | | | | | | | | |
| 15 | | | | | | | | | | |
| 16 | | | | | | | | | | |
| 17 | | | | | | | | | | |
| 18 | | | | | | | | | | |
| 19 | | | | | | | | | | |
| 20 | | | | | | | | | | |
| 21 | | | | | | | | | | |
| 22 | | | | | | | | | | |
| 23 | | | | | | | | | | |
| 24 | | | | | | | | | | |
| 25 | | | | | | | | | | |
| 26 | | | | | | | | | | |
| 27 | | | | | | | | | | |
| 28 | | | | | | | | | | |
| 29 | | | | | | | | | | |
| 30 | | | | | | | | | | |
| Totals | | | | | | | | | | |
| Recommended Amount | | | | ** | *** | 6–11 | 3–5 | 2–4 | 2–3 | 2–3 |
| Deficiencies | | | | | | | | | | |

*See list of nutritive value of selected foods in Appendix B.
**Compute using Table 8.1 in Chapter 8.
***Multiply the recommended amount of calories by .30 (30%) and divide by 9 to obtain the recommended amount of grams of fat (if on a diet, multiply by .20 or .10 — see Table 8.3 in Chapter 8).

**FIGURE 7.13** ◆ Daily diet record form.

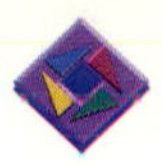

fruits, vegetables, and sweets in general. Glucose is stored in the form of glycogen in muscles and the liver. As noted earlier in the chapter, fatty acids are derived from the breakdown of fats. Unlike glucose, an almost unlimited supply of fatty acids, stored as fat in the body, can be used during exercise.

During resting conditions fat supplies about two-thirds of the energy to sustain the vital processes. During exercise the body uses both glucose and fat in combination to supply the energy demands. The proportion of fat to glucose changes with the intensity of exercise. When exercising below 70% of the individual's maximal work capacity, fat is used as the primary energy substrate. As the intensity of exercise increases, so does the percentage of glucose utilization, up to 100% during maximal work sustained for 2 to 3 minutes.

In general, athletes do not require special supplementation or any other special type of diet. Unless the diet is deficient in basic nutrients, no special, secret, or magic diet will help people perform better or develop faster as a result of what they eat. As long as the diet is balanced, based on a large variety of nutrients from the basic food groups, athletes do not require supplements. Even in strength training and body building, protein in excess of 20% of total daily caloric intake is not necessary.

The main differences between a sedentary person and a highly active individual is in the total number of calories required daily and the amount of carbohydrate intake during bouts of prolonged physical activity. During training, people consume more calories because of the greater energy expenditure required as a result of intense physical training.

### Carbohydrate Loading

While on a regular diet, the body is able to store between 1,500 and 2,000 calories in the form of glycogen. About 75% of this glycogen is stored in muscle tissue. This amount, however, can be increased greatly through carbohydrate loading.

A regular diet should be altered during several days of heavy aerobic training or when a person is going to participate in a long-distance event of more than 90 minutes (for example, marathon, triathlon, road cycling). For events shorter than 90 minutes, carbohydrate loading does not seem to enhance performance.

During prolonged exercise, glycogen is broken down into glucose, which then is readily available to the muscle for energy production. In comparison to fat, glucose frequently is referred to as the "high octane fuel" because it provides about 6% more energy per unit of oxygen consumed.

Heavy training over several consecutive days leads to glycogen depletion faster than it can be replaced through the diet. Glycogen depletion with heavy training is common in athletes. Signs of depletion include chronic fatigue, difficulty in maintaining accustomed exercise intensity, and lower performance.

On consecutive days of exhaustive physical training (several hours daily), a carbohydrate-rich diet, 70% of total daily caloric intake or 8 grams of carbohydrate per 2.2 pounds of body weight, is recommended. This diet often restores glycogen levels in 24 hours. Along with the high-carbohydrate diet, a day of rest often is needed to allow the muscles to recover from glycogen depletion following days of intense training. For people who exercise less than an hour a day, a 60% carbohydrate diet or 6 grams of carbohydrate per 2.2 pounds (1 kilogram) of body weight is enough to restore glycogen stores.

Following an exhaustive workout, eating a combination of carbohydrates and protein (tuna fish sandwich) within 30 minutes of exercise appears to speed up glycogen storage at an even faster rate. Protein intake increases insulin activity, thus enhancing glycogen replenishment. A 70% carbohydrate intake should then be maintained throughout the rest of the day.

By following a special diet/exercise regimen 5 days before a long-distance event, highly trained (aerobically) individuals are capable of storing two to three times the amount of glycogen found in the average person. Athletic performance may be enhanced for long-distance events of more than 90 minutes by eating a regular balanced diet along with intensive physical training the fifth and fourth days before the event, followed by a diet high in carbohydrates (about 70%) and a gradual decrease in training intensity the 3 days before the event.

The amount of glycogen stored as a result of a carbohydrate-rich diet does not seem to be related to the proportion of complex and simple carbohydrates. Intake of simple carbohydrate (sugar) can be raised while on a 70% carbohydrate diet, as long as 48% of the total calories are derived from complex carbohydrates. The latter provide more nutrients and fiber, making them a better choice for a healthier diet.

On the day of the long-distance event, high carbohydrates are still the recommended choice of substrate. But high sugar intake 30 minutes prior to the event might be counterproductive. A "sugar shock" shortly before the event can cause hypoglycemia (low blood glucose). The pancreas responds to high sugar intake with a large production of insulin. Insulin in turn lowers blood glucose. Further, the muscles draw glucose from the blood at the start of exercise, exacerbating the condition.

As a rule of thumb, individuals should consume 1 gram of carbohydrate for each 2.2 pounds of body weight 1 hour prior to exercise. The amount of carbohydrate can be increased to 2, 3, or 4 grams per 2.2 pounds of weight 2, 3, or 4 hours, respectively, before exercise.

During the long-distance event, researchers recommend that 50 to 60 grams of carbohydrate (200 to 240 calories) be consumed every hour. This is best accomplished by drinking 8 ounces of a 6% to 8% carbohydrate sports drink every 15 minutes. This also lessens the chance of dehydration during exercise, which hinders performance and endangers health. The percentage of the carbohydrate drink is determined by dividing the amount of carbohydrate in grams by the amount of fluid, in ml, and multiplying by 100. For example, 18 grams of carbohydrate in 240 ml (8 oz) of fluid yields a drink at 7.5% (18 ÷ 240 × 100).

### Amino Acid Supplements

A myth regarding athletic performance is the unnecessary use of protein (amino acid) supplements to increase muscle mass. The claims and safety of these products have not been proven scientifically. The RDA for protein is .8 grams per kilogram of body weight.

Most athletes, including weight lifters and body builders, increase their caloric intake automatically during intense training. As caloric intake increases, so does the intake of protein, approaching in many instances 2 or more grams per kilogram of body weight. This amount is more than enough to build and repair muscle tissue. Athletes in strength training typically consume between 3 and 4 grams per kilogram of body weight.

People who take costly free-amino acid supplements are led to believe that this contributes to the development of muscle mass. The human body cannot distinguish between amino acids obtained from food or through supplements. Excess protein either is used for energy or is turned into fat. With amino acid supplements, each capsule provides up to 500 milligrams of amino acids and no additional nutrients. Three ounces of meat or fish provide more than 20,000 milligrams of amino acids, along with other essential nutrients such as iron, niacin, and thiamin.

Proponents of free-amino acid supplements further claim that only a small amount of amino acids in food is absorbed and that free-amino acids are absorbed more readily than protein food. Neither claim is correct. The human body absorbs and utilizes between 85% and 99% of all protein from food intake. The body handles whole proteins better than single amino acids predigested in the laboratory setting.

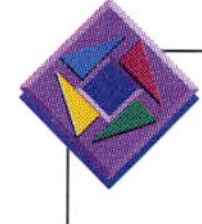

*Expensive protein supplements benefit only those who stand to gain financial benefits from selling them.*

Amino acid supplementation can even be dangerous to the body. Supplementation of a group of chemically similar amino acids often prevents the absorption of other amino acids, potentially causing critical imbalances and toxicities. Long-term risks associated with amino acid supplementation have not been determined.

The rate of absorption provides no additional benefit because building muscle takes hours, not minutes. Muscle overload through heavy training, not supplementation, builds muscle. Expensive protein supplements benefit only those who stand to gain financial benefits from selling them.

## Bone Health and Osteoporosis

*Osteoporosis* has been defined as *the softening, deterioration, or loss of total body bone.* Bones, primarily of the hip, wrist, and spine, become so weak and brittle that they fracture readily. Osteoporosis is preventable. The process begins slowly in the third and fourth decades of life. Women are especially susceptible after menopause because of the accompanying estrogen loss, which increases the rate at which bone mass is broken down.

Approximately 15 to 20 million women in the United States have osteoporosis, and about 1.5 million fractures are attributed to this condition each year. An estimated 30,000 to 60,000 of the 200,000 women with hip fractures die of complications resulting from these fractures. According to Dr. Barbara Drinkwater, a leading researcher in this

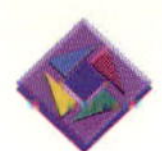

area, "Shocking as these figures are, they cannot adequately convey the pain and deterioration in the quality of life of women who suffer the crippling effects of osteoporotic fractures."[3]

In maximizing bone density in young women and decreasing the rate of bone loss later in life, the importance of normal estrogen levels, adequate calcium intake, and physical activity cannot be overemphasized (see Figure 7.14). All three factors are crucial in preventing osteoporosis. The absence of any one of these three factors leads to bone loss for which the other two factors never completely compensate.

Prevention of osteoporosis begins early in life by having enough calcium in the diet (the RDA is 800 to 1,200 mg per day) and by participating in exercise. The calcium RDA can be met easily through diet alone. Some experts, however, recommend calcium supplements in pre-pubertal children. Along with adequate calcium intake, an additional amount of vitamin D may be needed for optimal calcium absorption. Table 7.7 provides a

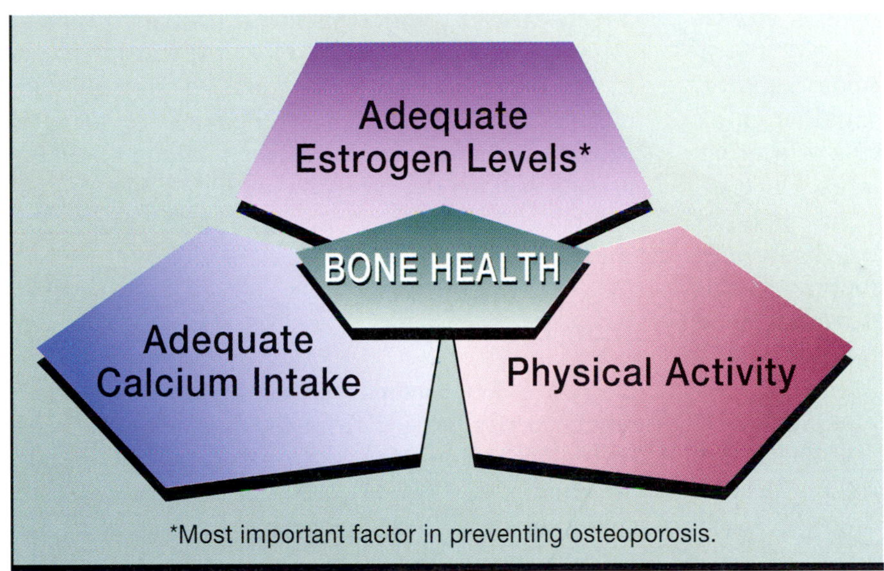


**FIGURE 7.14** ◆ Variables that impact the prevention of osteoporosis.

**TABLE 7.7**
**Low-Fat Calcium-Rich Foods**

| Food | Amount | Calcium (mg) | Calories | Calories From Fat |
|---|---|---|---|---|
| Beans, red kidney, cooked | 1 cup | 70 | 218 | 4% |
| Beet, greens, cooked | 1/2 cup | 72 | 13 | — |
| Broccoli, cooked, drained | 1 sm stalk | 123 | 36 | — |
| Burrito, bean | 1 | 173 | 307 | 28% |
| Cottage cheese, 2% lowfat | 1/2 cup | 78 | 103 | 18% |
| Milk, nonfat, powdered | 1 tbsp | 52 | 27 | 1% |
| Milk, skim | 1 cup | 296 | 88 | 3% |
| Ice milk (vanilla) | 1/2 cup | 102 | 100 | 27% |
| Instant breakfast, whole milk | 1 cup | 301 | 280 | 26% |
| Kale, cooked, drained | 1/2 cup | 103 | 22 | — |
| Okra, cooked, drained | 1/2 cup | 74 | 23 | — |
| Shrimp, boiled | 3 oz. | 99 | 99 | 9% |
| Spinach, raw | 1 cup | 51 | 14 | — |
| Yogurt, fruit | 1 cup | 345 | 231 | 8% |
| Yogurt, lowfat, plain | 1 cup | 271 | 160 | 20% |

list of selected foods and their respective calcium content. A common recommendation is that women after age 45 get 1,500 mg of calcium per day and men, 1,000 mg.

Also, high protein intake may affect calcium absorption by the body. The more protein eaten, the higher the calcium content in the urine. This might be the reason why countries with a high protein intake, including the United States, also have the highest rates of osteoporosis.

The key role of exercise in preventing osteoporosis seems to be related to the decrease in rate of bone density loss following menopause. Active people are able to maintain bone density much more effectively than their inactive counterparts, helping to prevent osteoporosis. A combination of weight-bearing exercises such as walking or jogging and weight training are especially helpful. The benefits of exercise go beyond maintenance of bone density. Exercise strengthens muscles, ligaments, and tendons; all of which provide support to the bones (skeleton). Exercise also improves balance and coordination, which can help prevent falls and injuries.

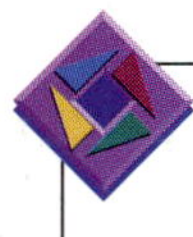

*Sedentary women with normal estrogen levels have better bone mineral density than active amenorrheic athletes.*

Current studies indicate that people who are active have denser bone mineral than inactive people do. Similar to other benefits of participating in exercise, there is no such thing as "bone in the bank." To have good bone health, people need to participate in a regular lifetime exercise program.

Prevailing research also tells us that estrogen is the most important factor in preventing bone loss. In one study lumbar bone density in women who had always had regular menstrual cycles exceeded that of women with a history of oligomenorrhea (irregular cycles) and amenorrhea (cessation of menstruation) interspaced with regular cycles. Furthermore, the lumbar density of these two groups of women was higher than that of women who had never had regular menstrual cycles.

Following menopause, every woman should consider hormone replacement therapy and discuss it with her physician. Women who have estrogen therapy do not lose bone mineral density at the rate of women who do not have estrogen therapy. Neither exercise nor calcium supplementation will offset the damaging effects of lower estrogen levels. Hormone replacement therapy appears to be the only reasonable therapy that post-menopausal women have to prevent osteoporosis in future years.

For instance, amenorrheic athletes (who have lower estrogen levels) have lower bone mineral density than even non-athletes with normal estrogen levels. One study[4] showed that amenorrheic athletes at age 25 have the bones of 52-year-old women. Other research[5] showed four amenorrheic athletes with a bone density equivalent to that of 70- to 80-year-old women. Over the last few years it has become clear that sedentary women with normal estrogen levels have better bone mineral density than active amenorrheic athletes. Many experts believe the best predictor of bone mineral content is the history of menstrual regularity.

## Iron Deficiency

Iron is a key element of hemoglobin in blood, which carries oxygen from the lungs to all tissues of the body. The RDA of iron for adult women is 15 mg per day (10 mg for men). According to a survey by the U.S. Department of Agriculture, 19- to 50-year-old women in the United States consumed only 60% of the RDA for iron. People who do not have enough iron in the body can develop iron deficiency anemia, in which the concentration of hemoglobin in the red blood cells is less than it should be.

Physically active women also may have a greater than average need for iron. Heavy training creates a demand for iron that is higher than the recommended intake because small amounts of iron are lost through sweat, urine, and stools. Mechanical trauma, caused by the pounding of the feet on the pavement during extensive jogging, also may lead to the destruction of iron-containing red blood cells.

A large percentage of female endurance athletes is reported to have iron deficiency. Blood ferritin levels, a measure of stored iron in the human body, should be checked frequently in women who participate in intense physical training.

The rates of iron absorption and iron loss vary from person to person. In most cases, though, people can get enough iron by eating more iron-rich foods such as beans, peas, green leafy vegetables, enriched grain products, egg yolk, fish, and

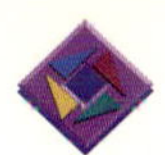

lean meats. Although organ meats, such as liver, are especially good sources, they also are high in cholesterol. A list of foods high in iron content is given in Table 7.8.

## NATIONAL ACADEMY OF SCIENCE'S DIETARY RECOMMENDATIONS

Based on the available scientific research on nutrition and health and the current dietary habits of the American people, the National Academy of Science's Committee on Diet and Health in 1989 issued dietary recommendations for healthy North American adults and children. These guidelines potentially can reduce the risk of developing certain chronic diseases. The committee's recommendations are:[6]

- Reduce fat intake to 30% or less of total calories. Reduce saturated fatty acid intake to less than 10% of total calories and intake of cholesterol to no more than 300 mg daily. Intake of fat and cholesterol can be lowered by substituting fish, poultry without skin, lean meats, and low or nonfat dairy products for fatty meats and whole-milk dairy products; by choosing more vegetables, fruits, cereals, and legumes; and by limiting oils, fats, egg yolks, and fried and other fatty foods.
- Every day eat five or more servings of a combination of vegetables and fruits, especially green and yellow vegetables and citrus fruits. Also, increase intake of starches and other complex carbohydrates by eating six or more servings daily of a combination of breads, cereals, and legumes. An average serving is equal to a half cup for most fresh or cooked vegetables, fruits, dry or cooked cereals and legumes, one medium piece of fresh fruit, one slice of bread, or one roll or muffin. The committee also recommends increasing the intake of carbohydrates to more than 55% of total calories.
- Maintain protein intake at moderate levels (not to exceed 1.6 grams per 2.2 pounds (1 kilogram) of body weight or twice the RDA).
- Balance food intake and physical activity to maintain appropriate body weight (see Chapter 8 for a comprehensive weight control program).
- If you drink alcoholic beverages, limit consumption to the equivalent of less than an ounce of pure alcohol in a single day. This translates into two cans of beer, two small glasses of wine, or two average cocktails. If pregnant, avoid alcoholic beverages altogether.

**TABLE 7.8**
**Iron-Rich Foods**

| Food | Amount | Iron (mg) | Calories | Cholesterol | Calories From Fat |
|---|---|---|---|---|---|
| Beans, red kidney, cooked | 1 cup | 4.4 | 218 | 0 | 4% |
| Beef, ground lean | 3 oz. | 3.0 | 186 | 81 | 48% |
| Beef, sirloin | 3 oz. | 2.5 | 329 | 77 | 74% |
| Beef liver, fried | 3 oz. | 7.5 | 195 | 345 | 42% |
| Beet, greens, cooked | 1/2 cup | 1.4 | 13 | 0 | — |
| Broccoli, cooked, drained | 1 sm stalk | 1.1 | 36 | 0 | — |
| Burrito, bean | 1 | 2.4 | 307 | 14 | 28% |
| Egg, hard, cooked | 1 | 1.0 | 72 | 250 | 63% |
| Farina (Cream of Wheat), cooked | 1/2 cup | 6.0 | 51 | 0 | — |
| Instant breakfast, whole milk | 1 cup | 8.0 | 280 | 33 | 26% |
| Peas, frozen, cooked, drained | 1/2 cup | 1.5 | 55 | 0 | — |
| Shrimp, boiled | 3 oz. | 2.7 | 99 | 128 | 9% |
| Spinach, raw | 1 cup | 1.7 | 14 | 0 | — |
| Vegetables, mixed, cooked | 1 cup | 2.4 | 116 | 0 | — |

- Limit total daily intake of salt to 6 grams or less. Limit the use of salt in cooking, and do not add it to food at the table. Sparingly consume salty, highly processed salty, salt-preserved, and salt-pickled foods.
- Maintain adequate calcium intake.
- Do not take supplements in excess of the RDA in any one day.
- Maintain an optimal intake of fluoride, particularly during the years of primary and secondary tooth formation and growth.

## PROPER NUTRITION: A LIFETIME PRESCRIPTION FOR HEALTHY LIVING

Proper nutrition, a sound exercise program, and quitting smoking (for those who smoke) are the three factors that do the most for health, longevity, and quality of life. Achieving and maintaining a balanced diet is not as difficult as most people would think. If parents were to do a better job of teaching and reinforcing proper nutrition habits in early youth, we would not have the magnitude of nutrition-related health problems that we do. Although the treatment of obesity is important, we should place far greater emphasis in the prevention of obesity in both youth and adults

Children tend to eat the way their parents do. If parents adopt a healthy diet, children most likely will follow. The difficult part for most people is retraining themselves to follow a lifetime healthy nutrition plan — a diet that includes lots of grains, legumes, fruits, vegetables, and low-fat dairy products, with moderate use of animal protein, junk food, sodium, and alcohol.

In spite of the ample scientific evidence linking poor dietary habits to early disease and mortality rates, most people are not willing to change their eating patterns. Even when faced with obesity, elevated blood lipids, hypertension, and other nutrition-related conditions, people do not change. The motivating factor to change one's eating habits seems to be a major health breakdown, such as a heart attack, a stroke, or cancer. By this time the damage already has been done. In many cases it is irreversible and, for some, fatal.

An ounce of prevention is worth a pound of cure. The sooner you implement the dietary guidelines presented in this chapter, the better will be your chances of preventing chronic diseases and reaching a higher state of wellness.

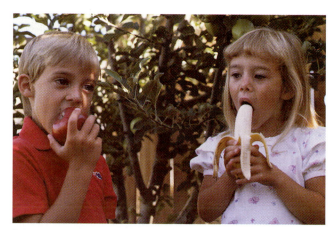

*Positive nutrition habits should be taught and reinforced in early youth.*

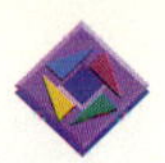

## NOTES

1. D. J. Mela and D. A. Sacchetti, "Sensory Preferences for Fat: Relationships with Diet and Body Composition," *American Journal of Clinical Nutrition,* 53 (1991), 908-915.
2. J. M. Gaziano, and C. H. Hennekens, "A New Look at What Can Unclog Your Arteries," *Executive Health Report* 27:8 (1991), 16.
3. B. L. Drinkwater "Nutrition, Exercise, and Bone Health" (Seattle: Pacific Medical Center, 1990).
4. B. L. Drinkwater "Osteoporosis and the Female Masters Athlete." In J. R. Sutton, and R. M. Brock, editors, *Sports Medicine for the Mature Athlete* (Benchmark Press, (1986), 353-359).
5. K. H. Myburgh, L. K. Bachrach, B. Lewis, K. Kent, and R. Marcus. "Low Bone Mineral Density at Axial and Appendicular Sites in Amenorrheic Athletes." *Medicine and Science in Sports and Exercise, 25:11(1993), 1197-1202.*
6. National Academy of Sciences, "Diet and Health: Implications for Reducing Chronic Disease Risk" (Washington, DC: National Academy Press, 1989).

## SELECT BIBLIOGRAPHY

American Medical Association: Council on Scientific Affairs. "Dietary Fiber and Health." *Journal of the American Medical Association,* 262 (1989), 542-546.

Begley, S. "Beyond Vitamins." *Newsweek*, April 25, 1994, pp. 45–49

Brownell, K., and J. P. Forey. *Handbook of Eating Disorders*. New York: Basic Books, 1986.

Cristian, J. L., and J. L. Greger. *Nutrition for Living*. Menlo Park, CA: Benjamin/Cummings Publishing, 1991.

Coleman, E. *Eating for Endurance*. Palo Alto, CA: Bull Publishing, 1992.

Drinkwater, B. L., B. Bruemner, and C. H. Chestnut III. "Menstrual History as a Determinant of Current Bone Density in Young Athletes." *Journal of the American Medical Association,* 263 (1990), 545-548.

Girdano, D. A., D. Dusek, and G. S. Everly. *Experiencing Health*. Englewood Cliffs, NJ: Prentice Hall, 1985.

"How to Balance Your Diet." *Fit*, April 1983, pp. 46-47.

Hoeger, W. W. K., and S. A. Hoeger. *Lifetime Physical Fitness and Wellness*. Englewood, CO: Morton Publishing, 1992.

Hoeger, W. W. K. *The Complete Guide for the Development & Implementation of Health Promotion Programs*. Englewood, CO: Morton Publishing, 1987.

Kanders, B., D. W. Demster and R. Lindsay. "Interaction of Calcium Nutrition and Physical Activity on Bone Mass in Young Women." *Journal of Bone Mineral Research,* 3 (1988), 145-149.

Kirschmann, J. D. *Nutrition Almanac*. New York: McGraw-Hill Book Company, 1989.

Kleiner, S. M. "Seafood and Your Heart." *Physician and Sportsmedicine,* 18:4 (1990), 19-20.

Morgan, B. L. G. *The Lifelong Nutrition Guide*. Englewood Cliffs, NJ: Prentice Hall, 1983.

National Academy of Sciences: Institute of Medicine. *Eat for Life: The Food and Nutrition Board's Guide to Reducing Your Risk of Chronic Disease*, edited by C. E. Woteki and P. R. Thomas. Washington, DC: National Academy Press, 1992.

"The Fallacies of Taking Supplementation." *Tufts University Diet & Nutrition Letter*, July 1987.

Thornton, J. S. "Feast or Famine: Eating Disorders in Athletes." *Physician and Sportsmedicine,* 18:4 (1990), 116-122.

"Use a Variety of Fibers." *Health Letter*, March 1982.

Whitney, E. N. and S. R. Rolfes. *Understanding Nutrition*. St. Paul: West Publishing, 1993.

NUTRIENT ANALYSIS
FITNESS & WELLNESS SERIES
by Werner W.K. Hoeger & Sharon A. Hoeger
Morton Publishing Company -- Englewood, Colorado

Jane R. Moore
Age: 20
Body Weight: 141 lbs ( 64.0 kg)
Activity Rating: Moderate

Date: 02-12-1992

Food Intake Day One

| Food | Amount | Calories | Protein gm | Fat gm | Sat Fat gm | Cholesterol mg | Carbohydrate gm | Calcium mg | Iron mg | Sodium mg | Vit A I.U. | Thiamin mg | Riboflavin mg | Niacin mg | Vit C mg |
|---|---|---|---|---|---|---|---|---|---|---|---|---|---|---|---|
| Cocoa/hot/with whole milk | 1 cup | 218 | 9.1 | 9 | 6.1 | 33 | 26 | 298 | 0.8 | 123 | 318 | 0.10 | 0.44 | 0.4 | 2 |
| Egg/scrambled w/milk butter | 1 egg(s) | 95 | 6.0 | 7 | 3.0 | 282 | 1 | 54 | 0.9 | 176 | 510 | 0.04 | 0.18 | 0.0 | 0 |
| Bread/white | 2 slice(s) | 136 | 4.4 | 2 | 0.4 | 0 | 26 | 42 | 1.2 | 254 | 0 | 0.12 | 0.10 | 1.2 | 0 |
| Butter | 2 tsp | 72 | 0.0 | 8 | 0.8 | 24 | 0 | 2 | 0.0 | 92 | 320 | 0.00 | 0.00 | 0.0 | 0 |
| Milk/whole | 1 c | 159 | 9.0 | 9 | 5.1 | 34 | 12 | 288 | 0.1 | 120 | 350 | 0.07 | 0.40 | 0.2 | 2 |
| Bread/whole wheat | 2 slice(s) | 122 | 5.2 | 2 | 1.2 | 0 | 24 | 50 | 1.6 | 264 | 0 | 0.12 | 0.06 | 1.4 | 0 |
| Tuna/canned/oil/drained | 1.5 oz. | 84 | 12.5 | 4 | 0.9 | 30 | 0 | 4 | 0.8 | 69 | 35 | 0.02 | 0.05 | 5.1 | 0 |
| Mayonnaise | 2 tsp. | 72 | 0.0 | 8 | 1.4 | 6 | 0 | 2 | 0.0 | 56 | 26 | 0.00 | 0.00 | 0.0 | 0 |
| Pickles/dill | 1 large | 15 | 0.9 | 0 | 0.0 | 0 | 3 | 35 | 1.4 | 1,928 | 140 | 0.00 | 0.03 | 0.0 | 8 |
| Potato/French fried | 20 strips | 428 | 6.8 | 20 | 3.4 | 0 | 56 | 24 | 2.0 | 10 | 0 | 0.20 | 0.12 | 4.8 | 32 |
| Tomato sauce (catsup) | 1 tbsp. | 16 | 0.3 | 0 | 0.0 | 0 | 4 | 3 | 0.1 | 156 | 105 | 0.01 | 0.01 | 0.2 | 2 |
| Apple/raw | 1 med | 80 | 0.3 | 1 | 0.0 | 0 | 20 | 10 | 0.4 | 1 | 120 | 0.04 | 0.03 | 0.1 | 6 |
| Soda pop/root beer | 12 oz. | 140 | 0.0 | 0 | 0.0 | 0 | 36 | 17 | 0.2 | 45 | 0 | 0.00 | 0.00 | 0.0 | 0 |
| Coleslaw | 1 c | 173 | 1.6 | 17 | 1.0 | 5 | 6 | 53 | 0.5 | 144 | 190 | 0.06 | 0.06 | 0.4 | 35 |
| Spaghetti/meat balls/sauce | 1 c | 332 | 18.6 | 12 | 3.0 | 75 | 39 | 124 | 3.7 | 1,009 | 1,590 | 0.25 | 0.30 | 4.0 | 22 |
| Pie/apple | 1 pc. (3.5 in.) | 302 | 2.6 | 13 | 3.5 | 120 | 45 | 9 | 0.4 | 355 | 40 | 0.02 | 0.02 | 0.5 | 1 |
| Totals Day One | | 2,444 | 77.3 | 111 | 29.8 | 609 | 298 | 1,015 | 14.1 | 4,802 | 3,744 | 1.0 | 1.8 | 18.3 | 110 |

**FIGURE 7.15** ◆ Computerized nutrient analysis — sample food list.

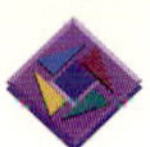

NUTRITIONAL ANALYSIS: DAILY ANALYSIS, AVERAGE, AND RECOMMENDED DIETARY ALLOWANCE (RDA) COMPARISON

| | Calo-ries | Pro-tein gm | Fat % | Sat Fat % | Cho-les-terol mg | Car-bohy-drate % | Cal-cium mg | Iron mg | Sodium mg | Vit A I.U. | Thi-amin mg | Ribo-fla-vin mg | Nia-cin mg | Vit C mg |
|---|---|---|---|---|---|---|---|---|---|---|---|---|---|---|
| Day One | 2,444 | 77.3 | 40 | 11 | 609 | 48 | 1,015 | 14.1 | 4,802 | 3,744 | 1.0 | 1.8 | 18.3 | 110 |
| Day Two | 2,234 | 105.1 | 44 | 12 | 536 | 37 | 639 | 20.6 | 5,719 | 1,902 | 1.1 | 1.7 | 21.6 | 60 |
| Day Three | 2,491 | 92.0 | 43 | 19 | 603 | 43 | 1,787 | 14.7 | 3,919 | 6,351 | 1.6 | 3.5 | 18.2 | 55 |
| Three Day Average | 2,390 | 91.5 | 42 | 14 | 583 | 43 | 1,147 | 16.5 | 4,813 | 3,999 | 1.3 | 2.3 | 19.4 | 75 |
| RDA | 1,904* | 51.2 | <30 | <10 | <300 | 50> | 1,200 | 15.0 | 1,904 | 4,000 | 1.1 | 1.3 | 15.0 | 60 |

*Estimated caloric value based on gender, current body weight, and activity rating (does not include additional calories burned through a physical exercise program).

OBSERVATIONS

Daily caloric intake should be distributed in such a way that 50 to 60 percent of the total calories come from carbohydrates and less than 30 percent of the total calories from fat. Protein intake should be about .8 to 1.5 grams per kilogram of body weight or about 15 to 20 percent of the total calories. Pregnant women need to consume an additional 15 grams of daily protein, while lactating women should have an extra 20 grams of daily protein (these additional grams of protein are already included in the RDA values for pregnant and lactating women). Saturated fats should constitute less than 10 percent of the total daily caloric intake.
Please note that the daily listings of food intake express the amount of carbohydrates, fat, saturated fat, and protein in grams. However, on the daily analysis and the RDA, only the amount of protein is given in grams. The amount of carbohydrates, fat, and saturated fat are expressed in percent of total calories. The final percentages are based on the total grams and total calories for all days analyzed, not from the average of the daily percentages.

If your average intake for protein, fat, saturated fat, cholesterol, or sodium is high, refer to the daily listings and decrease the intake of foods that are high in those nutrients. If your diet is deficient in carbohydrates, calcium, iron, vitamin A, thiamin, riboflavin, niacin, or vitamin C, refer to the statements below and increase your intake of the indicated foods or consult the list of selected foods in your textbook.

Caloric intake may be too high.

Total fat intake is too high.

Saturated fat intake is too high, which increases your risk for coronary heart disease.

Dietary cholesterol intake is too high. An average consumption of dietary cholesterol above 300 mg/day increases the risk for coronary heart disease. Do you know your blood cholesterol level?

Carbohydrate intake is low. Good sources of carbohydrates are whole grain breads and cereals, pasta, rice, fruits, and vegetables such as potatoes and peas.

Calcium intake is low. Good sources of calcium are milk, yogurt, cheese, green leafy vegetables, dried beans, sardines, and salmon.

Sodium intake is high.

Vitamin A intake is low. Foods high in vitamin A include skim milk fortified with vit. A, cheese, butter, fortified margarine, eggs (yolk), liver, and dark green/yellow fruits and vegetables.

**FIGURE 7.16** ◆ Computerized nutrient analysis — RDA comparison

# Principles of Weight Control

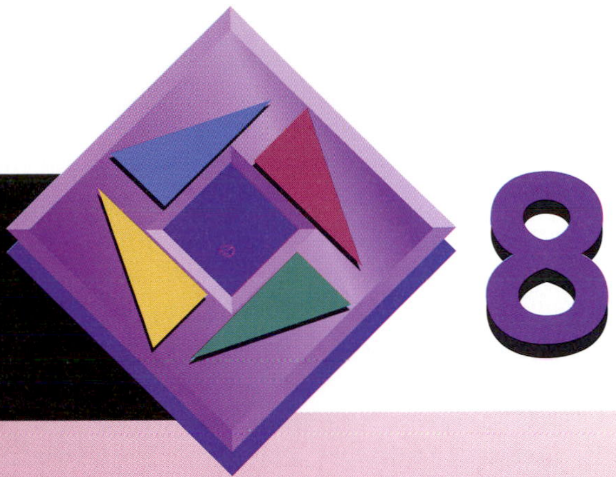


## Key Concepts

Obesity
Overweight
Underweight
Tolerable weight
Anorexia nervosa
Bulimia
Setpoint
Basal metabolic rate

## Objectives

- Understand the health consequences of obesity. Learn about fad diets and other myths and fallacies regarding weight control.
- Become familiar with eating disorders, their associated medical problems and behavior patterns, and understand the need for professional help in treating these conditions.
- Understand the physiology of weight loss, including setpoint theory and the effects of diet on basal metabolic rate.
- Recognize the role of a lifetime exercise program as the key to a successful weight loss and maintenance program.
- Learn how to implement a physiologically sound weight reduction and weight maintenance program.
- Learn behavior modification techniques that help a person adhere to a lifetime weight maintenance program.

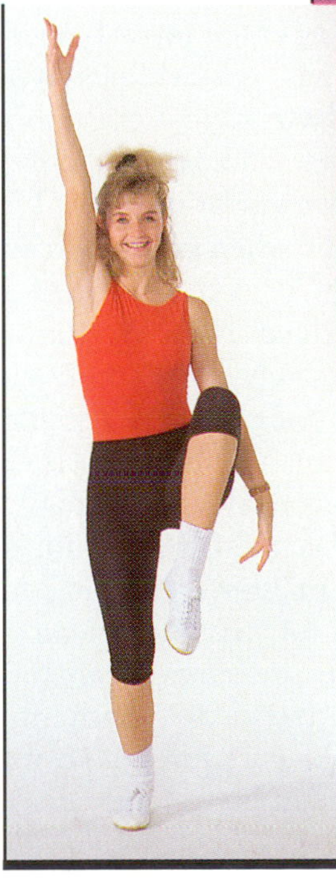

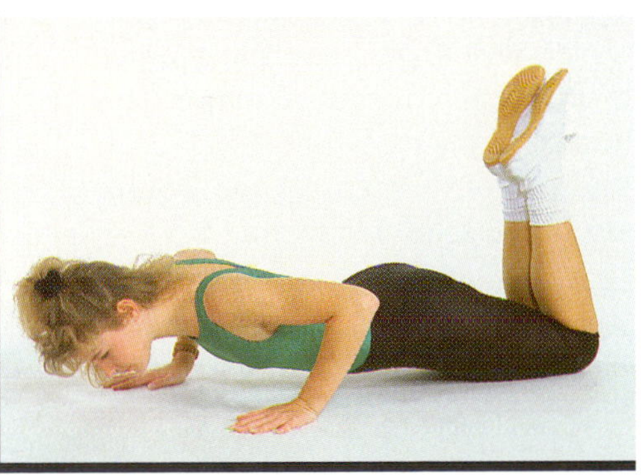

Patty Neavill is a typical example of someone who often tried to change her life around but was unable to do so because she did not know how to implement a sound exercise and weight control program. At age 24 and at 240 pounds, she was discouraged with her weight, level of fitness, self-image, and quality of life in general. She had struggled with her weight most of her life. Like millions of other people, she had made many unsuccessful attempts to lose weight.

Patty put her fears aside and decided to enroll in a fitness course. As part of the course requirement, a battery of fitness tests was administered at the beginning of the semester. Patty's cardiovascular fitness and strength ratings were poor, her flexibility classification was average, and she had 41% body fat.

Following her first fitness assessment, Patty met with her course instructor, who prescribed an exercise and nutrition program like the one in this book. Patty fully committed to carry out the prescription. She walked/jogged five times a week. She enrolled in a weight training course that met twice a week. Her daily caloric intake was set in the range of 1,500 to 1,700 calories.

Determined to become even more active, Patty signed up for recreational volleyball and basketball courses. Besides fun, these classes provided four additional hours of activity per week.

She took care to meet the minimum required servings from the basic food groups each day, which contributed about 1,200 calories to her diet. The remainder of the calories came primarily from complex carbohydrates.

At the end of the 16-week semester, Patty's cardiovascular fitness, strength, and flexibility ratings had all improved to the good category, she lost 50 pounds, and her percent body fat had decreased to 22.5!

Patty was tall. Most people would have thought she was too heavy at 190 pounds. Her percent body fat, however, was lower than the average for college female physical education major students (about 23% body fat).

A thank-you note from Patty to the course instructor at the end of the semester read:

> *Thank you for making me a new person. I truly appreciate the time you spent with me. Without your kindness and motivation, I would have never made it. It is great to be fit and trim. I have never had this feeling before, and I wish everyone could feel like this once in their life.*
>
> *Thank you*
>
> *Your trim Patty!*

Patty never had been taught the principles governing a sound weight loss program. In her case, not only did she need this knowledge, but, like most Americans who never have been involved in the process of becoming physically fit, she needed to be in a structured exercise setting to truly feel the joy of fitness.

Even more significant, Patty maintained her aerobic and strength-training programs. A year after ending her calorie-restricted diet, her weight increased by 10 pounds, but her body fat decreased from 22.5% to 21.2%. As you will see later in this chapter, this weight increase is related mostly to changes in lean tissue, lost during the weight reduction phase.

In spite of only a slight drop in weight during the second year following the calorie-restricted diet, the 2 year follow-up revealed a further decrease in body fat, to 19.5%. Patty understood the new quality of life reaped through a sound fitness program, and, at the same time, she finally learned how to apply the principles that regulate weight maintenance.

Achieving and maintaining recommended body weight is a major objective of a good physical fitness and wellness program. The assessment of recommended body weight was discussed in detail in Chapter 6. Next to poor cardiovascular fitness, obesity is the most frequently encountered problem in fitness and wellness assessments.

Two terms commonly used in reference to people who weigh more than recommended are: overweight and obese. *Overweight* indicates excess weight when compared to a given standard such as height or recommended percent body fat. *Obesity* is defined as a chronic disease characterized by an excessively high amount of body fat in relation to lean body mass. Obesity levels are established at a point at which the excess body fat can lead to serious health problems.

On the other hand, extreme thinness also can lead to life-threatening medical conditions. About 14% of the American people are underweight. Social pressures to attain model-like thinness have contributed to gradually increasing numbers of people who develop eating disorders. Anorexia nervosa and bulimia are discussed later in this chapter.

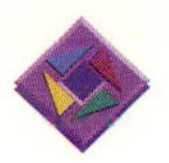

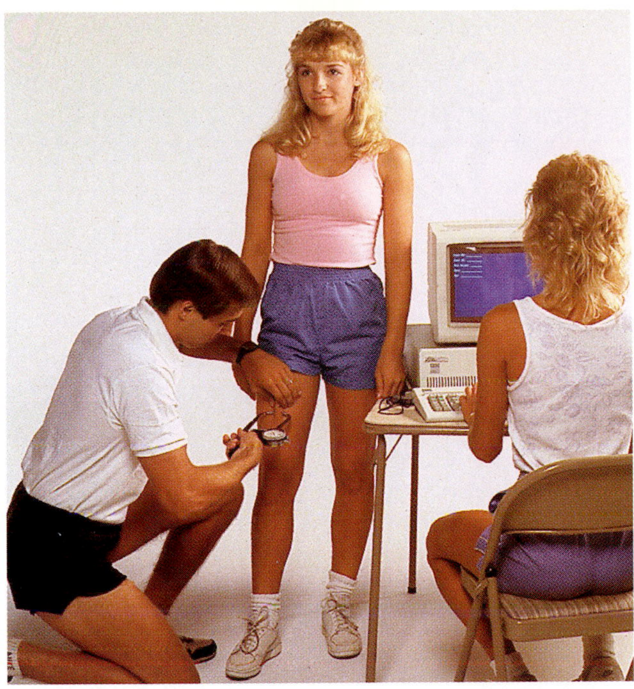

*Recommended body weight is best determined through the assessment of body composition.*

## OBESITY AND OVERWEIGHT

Approximately 65 million Americans are either overweight or consider themselves to be overweight. Of these, 30 million are obese. About 50% of all women and 25% of all men are on diets at any given moment. People spend about $40 billion to $50 billion yearly attempting to lose weight. More than $10 billion goes to memberships in weight reduction centers and another $30 billion to diet food sales.

Overweight and obesity are not the same thing. Most overweight people are not obese. The health consequences of obesity apply primarily to severely overweight individuals.

Granted, genetic differences exist. Some moderately overweight people have health problems, but this is not the case for most. Moderately overweight people with diabetes and other cardiovascular risk factors benefit from weight loss.

### Tolerable Weight

Many people want to lose weight so they will look better. That's a noteworthy goal. The problem, however, is that they have a distorted image of what they really would look like if they were to reduce to what they think is their ideal weight. Hereditary factors play a big role, and only a small fraction of the population has the genes for a "perfect body."

As people set their own target weight, they should be realistic. Attaining the excellent percent body fat figure in Table 6.8, Chapter 6, is extremely difficult for some people. It is even more difficult to maintain, unless they are willing to make a commitment to a vigorous lifetime exercise program and permanent dietary changes. Few people are willing to do that. The moderate percent body fat category may be more realistic for these people.

A question you should ask yourself is: Are you happy with your weight? Part of enjoying a better quality of life is being happy with yourself. If you are not, you either should do something about it or learn to live with it!

If you are above the moderate percent body fat category, you should try to come down and stay in this category, for health reasons. This is the category in which there seems to be no detriment to health.

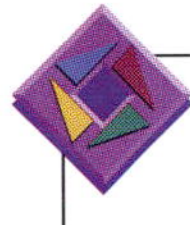

*If you are not willing to change your lifestyle, stop worrying about your weight and deem the moderate percent fat category as tolerable for you.*

If you are in the moderate category but would like to be better, you need to ask yourself a second question: How badly do I want it? Do you want it enough to implement lifetime exercise and dietary changes? If you are not willing to change, you should stop worrying about your weight and deem the moderate category as tolerable for you.

## THE WEIGHT LOSS DILEMMA

Constantly gaining and losing weight — yo-yo dieting — carries as much health risk as being overweight and remaining overweight in the first place. Epidemiological data are beginning to show that frequent fluctuations in weight (up or down) markedly increase the risk of dying from cardiovascular disease.

Based on these findings, quick-fix diets should be replaced by a slow but permanent weight loss program, as described in this chapter. People reap the benefits of recommended body weight when they get to their recommended body weight and stay there throughout life.

Unfortunately, only about 10% of all people who begin a traditional weight loss program, without exercise, are able to lose the desired weight. Worse, only one in 200 is able to keep the weight off. The body is highly resistant to permanent weight changes through caloric restrictions alone.

Traditional diets have failed because few of them incorporate lifetime changes in food selection and exercise as fundamental to successful weight loss. When the diet stops, weight gain begins. The multi-billion dollar diet industry tries to capitalize on the idea that weight can be lost quickly without taking into consideration the consequences of fast weight loss or the importance of lifetime behavioral changes to ensure proper weight loss and maintenance.

In addition, various studies indicate most people, especially obese people, tend to underestimate their energy intake. Those who try to lose weight but apparently fail to do so are referred to as "diet-resistant." A study published in 1992 by Dr. Steven Lichtman and colleagues in the *New England Journal of Medicine* found that, while on a "diet," a group of obese individuals with a self-reported history of diet resistance underreported their average daily caloric intake by almost 50%[1] (1,028 self-reported versus 2,081 actual — see Figure 8.1). These individuals also overestimated their amount of daily physical activity by about 25% (1,022 calories self-reported versus 771 actual calories). These differences represent an additional 1,304 calories of energy unaccounted for by the subjects in the study. These findings suggest that failing to lose weight may be related to misreports of actual food intake and level of physical activity.

Fad diets continue to appeal to people. These diets deceive people and claim that the person indeed will lose weight by following all instructions. Most fad diets are low in calories and deprive the body of certain nutrients, generating a metabolic imbalance. Under these conditions, a lot of the weight lost is in the form of water and protein, and not fat.

On a crash diet close to half the weight loss is in lean (protein) tissue. When the body uses protein instead of a combination of fats and carbohydrates as a source of energy, weight is lost as much as 10 times faster.[2] A gram of protein produces half the amount of energy that fat does. In the case of muscle protein, one-fifth of protein is mixed with four-fifths water. Each pound of muscle yields only one-tenth the amount of energy of a pound of fat. As a result, most of the weight loss is in the form of water, which on the scale, of course, looks good.

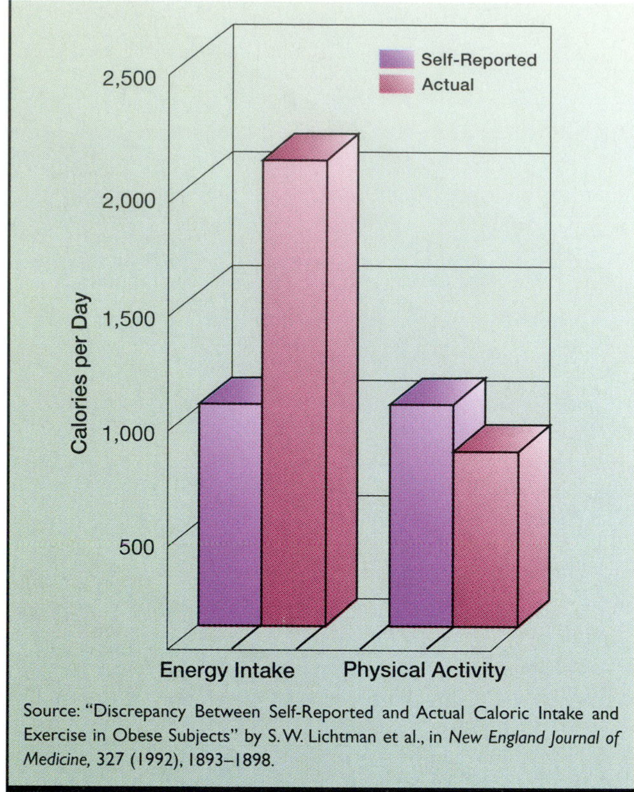


Source: "Discrepancy Between Self-Reported and Actual Caloric Intake and Exercise in Obese Subjects" by S.W. Lichtman et al., in *New England Journal of Medicine*, 327 (1992), 1893–1898.

**FIGURE 8.1** ◆ Differences between self-reported and actual daily caloric intake and exercise.

Some diets allow only certain specialized foods. If people would realize that no magic foods provide all of the necessary nutrients, and that a person has to eat a variety of foods to be well-nourished, the diet industry would not be as successful. Most of these diets create a nutritional deficiency, which at times can be fatal.

The reason some of these diets succeed is that people eventually get tired of eating the same thing day in and day out and start eating less. If they happen to achieve the lower weight but do not make permanent dietary changes, however, they quickly regain the weight once they go back to their old eating habits.

A few diets do recommend exercise along with caloric restrictions. A lot of the weight lost of course is because of the exercise, so the "diet" has achieved its purpose. Unfortunately, if the people do not change their food selection and activity level permanently, they gain back the weight quickly once they discontinue dieting and exercise.

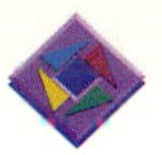

## DISORDERED EATING

Anorexia nervosa and bulimia are physical and emotional problems, thought to develop from individual, family, or social pressures, characterized by an intense fear of becoming fat, which does not disappear even when losing extreme amounts of weight. These medical disorders are increasing steadily in most industrialized nations where society encourages low-calorie diets and thinness.

### Anorexia Nervosa

Anorexia nervosa is *a condition of self-imposed starvation to lose and then maintain very low body weight.* Approximately 19 of every 20 anorexics are young women. An estimated 1% of the female population in the United States is anorexic. Anorexic individuals seem to fear weight gain more than death from starvation. Furthermore, they have a distorted image of their body and think of themselves as being fat even when they are emaciated.

Although a genetic predisposition may contribute, the anorexic person often comes from a mother-dominated home, with possible drug addictions in the family. The syndrome may emerge following a stressful life event and uncertainty about one's ability to cope efficiently.

Because the female role in society is changing more rapidly, women seem to be especially susceptible. Life experiences such as gaining weight, starting menstrual periods, beginning college, losing a boyfriend, having poor self-esteem, being socially rejected, starting a professional career, or becoming a wife or a mother may trigger the syndrome.

These individuals typically begin a diet and at first feel in control and happy about the weight loss, even if they are not overweight. To speed up the weight loss, they frequently combine extreme dieting with exhaustive exercise and overuse of laxatives and diuretics.

Anorexics commonly develop obsessive and compulsive behaviors and emphatically deny their condition. They are preoccupied with food, meal planning, grocery shopping, and unusual eating habits. As they lose weight and their health begins to deteriorate, anorexics feel weak and tired and may realize they have a problem but will not stop the starvation and refuse to consider the behavior as abnormal.

Once they have lost a lot of weight and malnutrition sets in, physical changes become more visible. Some typical changes are amenorrhea (stopping menstruation), digestive problems, extreme sensitivity to cold, hair and skin problems, fluid and electrolyte abnormalities (which may lead to an irregular heartbeat and sudden stopping of the heart), injuries to nerves and tendons, abnormalities of immune function, anemia, growth of fine body hair, mental confusion, inability to concentrate, lethargy, depression, skin dryness, lower skin and body temperature, and osteoporosis.

Many of the changes induced by anorexia nervosa can be reversed. Treatment almost always requires professional help, and the sooner it is started, the better are the chances for reversibility and cure. Therapy consists of a combination of medical and psychological techniques to restore proper nutrition, prevent medical complications, and modify the environment or events that triggered the syndrome.

Seldom are anorexics able to overcome the problem by themselves. Unfortunately, they strongly deny their condition. They are able to hide it and deceive friends and relatives quite effectively. Based on their behavior, many of them meet all of the

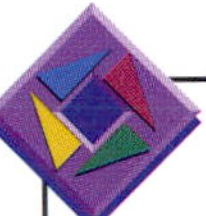

### DIAGNOSTIC CRITERIA FOR ANOREXIA NERVOSA

- Refusal to maintain body weight over a minimal normal weight for age and height (e.g., weight loss leading to maintenance of body weight 15% below that expected; or failure to make expected weight gain during period of growth, leading to body weight 15% below that expected).
- Intense fear of gaining weight or becoming fat, even though underweight.
- Disturbance in the way in which one's body weight, size, or shape is experienced (e.g., the person claims to "feel fat" even when emaciated or believes that one area of the body is "too fat" even when obviously underweight).
- In females, absence of at least three consecutive menstrual cycles when otherwise expected to occur (primary or secondary amenorrhea). (A woman is considered to have amenorrhea if her periods occur only following hormone, e.g., estrogen, administration.)

Source: American Psychiatric Association. *Diagnostic and Statistical Manual of Mental Disorders* (Washington, DC, APA, 1987, p. 67).

characteristics of anorexia nervosa, but it goes undetected because both thinness and dieting are socially acceptable. Only a well-trained clinician is able to make a positive diagnosis.

## Bulimia

A *pattern of binge eating and purging*, bulimia is more prevalent than anorexia nervosa. For many years it was thought to be a variant of anorexia nervosa, but now it is identified as a separate condition. It afflicts mainly young people, and as many as one in every five women on college campuses may be bulimic, according to some estimates. Bulimia also is more prevalent than anorexia nervosa in males.

Bulimics usually are healthy-looking people, well-educated, near recommended body weight, who enjoy food and often socialize around it. In actuality, they are emotionally insecure, rely on others, and lack self-confidence and self-esteem. Recommended weight and food are important to them.

The binge-purge cycle usually occurs in stages. As a result of stressful life events or the simple compulsion to eat, bulimics periodically engage in binge eating that may last an hour or longer.

With some apprehension, bulimics anticipate and plan the cycle. Next they feel an urgency to begin, followed by a large and uncontrollable food consumption during which they may eat several thousand calories (up to 10,000 calories in extreme cases). After a short period of relief and satisfaction, feelings of deep guilt, shame, and intense fear of gaining weight ensue. Purging seems to be an easy answer, as the binging cycle can continue without fear of gaining weight.

The most common form of purging is self-induced vomiting. Bulimics, too, frequently ingest strong laxatives and emetics. Near-fasting diets and strenuous bouts of exercise are common. Medical problems associated with bulimia include cardiac arrhythmias, amenorrhea, kidney and bladder damage, ulcers, colitis, tearing of the esophagus or stomach, tooth erosion, gum damage, and general muscular weakness.

Unlike anorexics, bulimics realize their behavior is abnormal and feel great shame about it. Fearing social rejection, they pursue the binge-purge cycle in secrecy and at unusual hours of the day.

Bulimia can be treated successfully when the person realizes this destructive behavior is not the solution to life's problems. A change in attitude can prevent permanent damage or death.

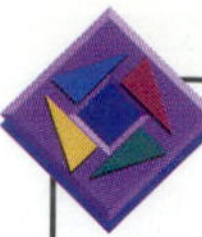

### DIAGNOSTIC CRITERIA FOR BULIMIA

- Recurrent episodes of binge eating (rapid consumption of a large amount of food in a discrete period of time).
- A feeling of lack of control over eating behavior during the eating binges.
- Regular practice of self-induced vomiting or use of laxatives or diuretics, or strict dieting or fasting, or vigorous exercise to prevent weight gain.
- A minimum average of two binge eating episodes a week for at least 3 months.
- Persistent over concern with body shape and weight.

Source: American Psychiatric Association. *Diagnostic and Statistical Manual of Mental Disorders.* (Washington, DC, APA, 1987, pp. 68-69).

Treatment for anorexia nervosa and bulimia are available on most school campuses through the school's counseling center or the health center. Local hospitals also offer treatment for these conditions. Many communities have support groups, frequently led by professional personnel and usually free of charge.

## PHYSIOLOGY OF WEIGHT LOSS

Only a few years ago the principles governing a weight loss and maintenance program seemed to be fairly clear, but we now know the final answers are not in yet. Traditional concepts related to weight control have centered on three assumptions: (a) that balancing food intake against output allows a person to achieve recommended weight, (b) that all fat people just eat too much, and (c) that the human body doesn't care how much (or little) fat it stores. Although these statements have some truth, they are still open to much debate and research.

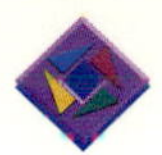

## The Energy-Balancing Equation

The energy-balancing equation basically states that as long as caloric input equals caloric output, the person will not gain or lose weight. If caloric intake exceeds output, the individual gains weight. When output exceeds input, the person loses weight.

This principle is simple. If daily energy requirements could be determined accurately, it seems reasonable that caloric intake could be balanced against output. This is not always the case, though, because genetic and lifestyle-related individual differences determine the number of calories required to maintain or lose body weight.

Table 8.1 (see page 202) offers some general guidelines for estimating daily caloric intake according to lifestyle patterns. This is only an estimated figure and, as discussed later in the chapter, it serves only as a starting point from which individual adjustments have to be made.

One pound of fat equals 3,500 calories. Assuming that a person's basic daily caloric expenditure is 2,500 calories, if this person were to decrease the daily intake by 500 calories per day, it should result in a loss of one pound of fat in 7 days ($500 \times 7 = 3{,}500$). But research has shown, and many dieters probably have experienced, that even when they carefully balance caloric input against caloric output, they do not always lose weight as predicted. Furthermore, two people with similar measured caloric intake and output seldom lose weight at the same rate.

The most common explanation regarding individual differences in weight loss and weight gain has been the variation in human metabolism from one person to another. We are all familiar with people who can eat "all day long" and not gain an ounce of weight, while others cannot even "dream" about food without gaining weight. Because experts did not believe that human metabolism alone could account for such extreme differences, they developed several theories that may better explain these individual variations.

## Setpoint Theory

Results of several research studies point toward a weight-regulating mechanism (WRM) in the hypothalamus of the brain that regulates how much the body should weigh. This mechanism has a setpoint that controls both appetite and the amount of fat stored.

Setpoint is hypothesized to work like a thermostat for body fat, maintaining fairly constant body weight because it knows at all times the exact amount of adipose tissue stored in the fat cells. Some people have high settings; others have low settings.

If body weight decreases (as in dieting), the setpoint senses this change and triggers the WRM to increase the person's appetite or make the body conserve energy to maintain the "set" weight. The opposite also may be true. Some people have a hard time gaining weight. In this case the WRM decreases appetite or causes the body to waste energy to maintain the lower weight.

### Dieting Makes People Fat!

Every person has his or her own certain body fat percentage (as established by the setpoint) that the body attempts to maintain. The genetic instinct to survive tells the body that fat storage is vital, and therefore it sets an acceptable fat level. This level remains somewhat constant or may climb gradually because of poor lifestyle habits.

For instance, under strict calorie reduction the body may make extreme metabolic adjustments in an effort to maintain its setpoint for fat. The basal metabolic rate (amount of energy the body needs to maintain life at complete rest) may drop dramatically against a consistent negative caloric balance, and a person may be on a plateau for days or even weeks without losing much weight. A low metabolic rate compounds a person's problems in maintaining recommended body weight.

Dietary restriction alone will not lower the setpoint, even though the person may lose weight and fat. When the dieter goes back to the normal or even below-normal caloric intake, at which the weight may have been stable for a long time, he or she quickly regains the fat loss as the body strives to regain a comfortable fat store.

Let's use a practical illustration. A person would like to lose some body fat and assumes that a stable body weight has been reached at an average daily caloric intake of 1,800 calories (no weight gain or loss occurs at this daily intake). In an attempt to lose weight rapidly, this person now goes on a strict low-calorie diet, or even worse, a near-fasting diet. Immediately the body activates its survival mechanism and readjusts its metabolism to a lower caloric balance. After a few weeks of dieting at fewer than 400 to 600 calories per day, the body now can maintain its normal functions at 1,000 calories per day.

Having lost the desired weight, the person terminates the diet but realizes the original intake of 1,800 calories per day will have to be lower to maintain the new, lower weight. To adjust to the new, lower body weight, the intake is restricted to about 1,500 calories per day. The individual is surprised to find that, even at this lower daily intake (300 fewer calories), weight comes back at a rate of one pound every 1 to 2 weeks. After ending the diet, this new lowered metabolic rate may take several months to kick back up to its normal level.

From this explanation, individuals clearly should not go on very low-calorie diets. Not only will this slow down resting metabolic rate, but it also will deprive the body of basic daily nutrients required for normal function.

Daily caloric intakes of 1,200 to 1,500 calories provide the necessary nutrients if they are distributed properly over the five basic food groups (meeting the daily required servings from each group). Of course, the individual will have to learn which foods meet the requirements and yet are low in fat and sugar.

Under no circumstances should a person go on a diet that calls for below 1,200 and 1,500 calories for women and men, respectively. Weight (fat) is gained over months and years, not overnight. Likewise, weight loss should be gradual, not abrupt.

### Setpoint and Nutrition

A second way in which the setpoint may work is by keeping track of the nutrients and calories consumed daily. It is thought that the body, like a cash register, records the daily food intake and the brain will not feel satisfied until the calories and nutrients have been "registered."

This setpoint for calories and nutrients seems to work for some people, even when they participate in moderately intense exercise. Some studies have shown that people do not become hungrier with moderate physical activity. Therefore, people can choose to lose weight either by going hungry or by stepping up their daily physical activity. The greater number of calories burned through exercise will help lower body fat.

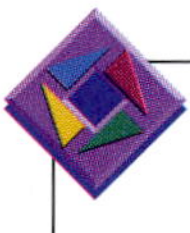

*People can choose to lose weight either by going hungry or by stepping up their daily physical activity.*

The most common question regarding the setpoint is how it can be lowered so the body will feel comfortable at a lesser fat percentage. Several factors seem to affect the setpoint directly by lowering the fat thermostat:

1. Aerobic exercise.
2. A diet high in complex carbohydrates.
3. Nicotine.
4. Amphetamines.

The last two are more destructive than the overfatness, so they are not reasonable alternatives (as far as the extra strain on the heart is concerned, smoking one pack of cigarettes per day is said to be the equivalent of carrying 50 to 75 pounds of excess body fat).

On the other hand, a diet high in fats and refined carbohydrates, near-fasting diets, and perhaps even artificial sweeteners seem to raise the setpoint. Therefore, the only practical and sensible way to lower the setpoint and lose fat weight seems to be a combination of aerobic exercise and a diet high in complex carbohydrates and low in fat.

Because of the effects of proper food management on the body's setpoint, many nutritionists believe the total number of calories should not be the main concern in a weight-control program. Rather, it should be the source of those calories. In this regard, most of the effort is spent in retraining eating habits, increasing the intake of complex carbohydrates and high-fiber foods, and decreasing the consumption of refined carbohydrates (sugars) and fats. In most cases, this change in eating habits will bring about a decrease in total daily caloric intake.

A "diet" is no longer viewed as a temporary tool to aid in weight loss but, instead, as a permanent change in eating behaviors to ensure weight management and better health. The role of increased physical activity also must be considered, because successful weight loss, maintenance, and recommended body composition seldom are attained without a moderate reduction in caloric intake combined with a regular exercise program.

## Diet and Metabolism

Fat can be lost by selecting the proper foods, by exercising or by restricting calories. When a person tries to lose weight by dietary restrictions alone, lean body mass (muscle protein, along with vital

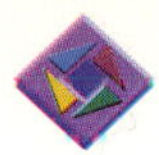

organ protein) always decreases. The amount of lean body mass lost depends entirely on caloric limitation.

When obese people go on a near-fasting diet, up to half of the weight loss is lean body mass and the other half is actual fat loss (see Figure 8.2). When the diet is combined with exercise, close to 100% of the weight loss is in the form of fat, and lean tissue actually may increase. Loss of lean body mass is never good, because it weakens the organs and muscles and slows down metabolism. Large losses in lean tissue can cause disturbances in heart function and damage to other organs. Equally important is not to overindulge (binge) following very-low-calorie diets. This may cause changes in metabolic rate and electrolyte balance, which could trigger fatal cardiac arrhythmias.

Contrary to some beliefs, aging is not the main reason for the lower metabolic rate. It is not so much that metabolism slows down as that people slow down. As people age, we tend to rely more on the amenities of life (remote controls, cellular telephones, intercoms, single-level homes, riding lawn mowers) that lull us into sedentary living.

Basal metabolism is related directly to lean body weight. The more the lean tissue, the higher is the metabolic rate. As a consequence of sedentary living and less physical activity, the lean component decreases and fat tissue increases. The human body, though, requires a certain amount of oxygen per pound of lean body mass. As fat is considered metabolically inert from the point of view of caloric use, the lean tissue uses most of the oxygen, even at rest. As muscle and organ mass (lean body mass) decreases, so do the energy requirements at rest.

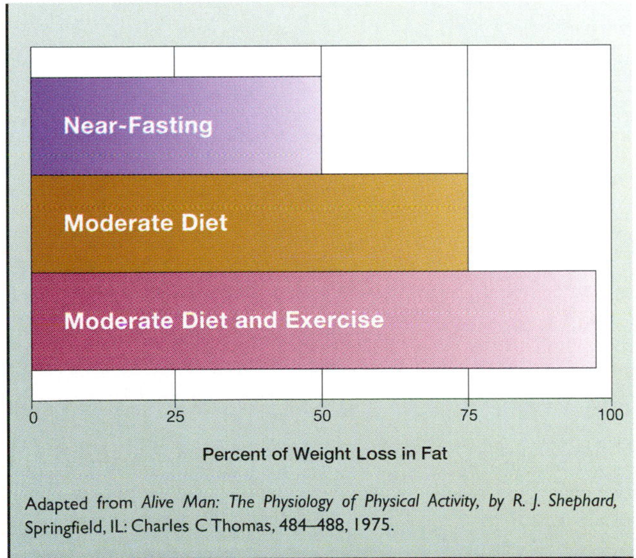


**FIGURE 8.2** ◆ Effects of three forms of diet on fat loss.

Reductions in lean body mass are common in aging people (because of physical inactivity) and those on severely restricted diets. The loss of lean body mass also may account for a lower metabolic rate (described earlier) and the longer time it takes to kick back up.

Diets with caloric intakes below 1,200 to 1,500 calories cannot guarantee the retention of lean body mass. Even at this intake level, some loss is inevitable unless the diet is combined with exercise. Despite the claims of many diets that they do not alter the lean component, the simple truth is that, regardless of what nutrients may be added to the diet, severe caloric restrictions always prompt a loss of lean tissue. Too many people constantly go on low-calorie diets. Every time they do, the metabolic rate slows down as more lean tissue is lost.

You may run across people in their 40s or older who weigh the same as they did when they were 20 and think they are at recommended body weight. During this span of 20 years or more, these people may have dieted many times without participating in an exercise program, thus losing lean body mass. They regain the weight shortly after they terminate each diet, but most of that gain is in fat. Maybe at age 20 they weighed 150 pounds and had only 15% fat. Now at age 40, even though they still weigh 150 pounds, they might be 30% fat. At recommended body weight, they wonder why they are eating very little and still having trouble staying at that weight.

## EXERCISE: THE KEY TO WEIGHT LOSS AND WEIGHT MAINTENANCE

Based on the preceding discussion, exercise is vital to losing weight and maintaining that weight loss. Not only will exercise maintain lean tissue, but advocates of the setpoint theory say that exercise resets the fat thermostat to a new, lower level. This change may be rapid, or it may take time. A few overweight individuals have exercised faithfully almost daily, 60 minutes at a time, for a whole year before weight change is significant. People with a "sticky" setpoint have to be patient and persistent.

If a person is trying to lose weight, a combination of aerobic and strength-training exercises

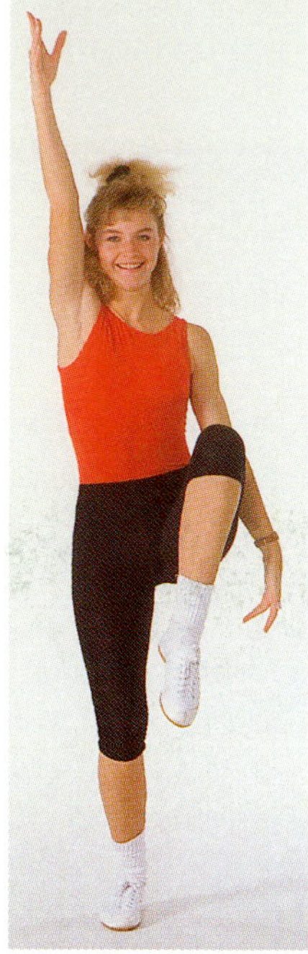

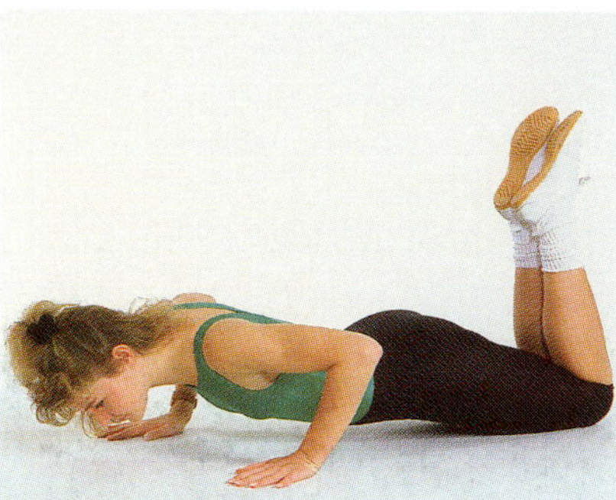

*Regular participation in a combined lifetime aerobic and strength-training-exercise program is the key to successful weight management.*

works best. Aerobic exercise is the best to offset the setpoint, and the continuity and duration of these types of activities cause many calories to be burned in the process. The role of aerobic exercise in successful lifetime weight management cannot be overestimated.

As illustrated in Figure 8.3, more weight loss is achieved by combining a diet with an aerobic exercise program. Of even greater significance, only the individuals who participated in an 18-month post-diet aerobic exercise program were able to keep the weight off. Those who discontinued exercise gained weight. Furthermore, all those who initiated or resumed exercise during the 18-month follow-up were able to lose weight again. Individuals who only dieted and never exercised regained 60% and 92% of their weight loss at the 6- and 18-month follow-up, respectively.

Weight loss comes more rapidly when aerobic exercise is combined with a strength training program. Two exercise groups — a 30-minute aerobic group and a 15-minute aerobic plus 15-minute strength-training (30 minutes total) group — participated in an 8-week, 3-days-per-week study. Both groups followed a dietary plan that consisted of approximately 60% carbohydrates, 20% fats, and 20% proteins.

The aerobic group lost an average of 3½ pounds, 3 of which were fat and the remaining half pound lean tissue. The combined aerobic and strength training group lost an average of 8 pounds. Changes in body composition, however, indicated that the latter group actually lost 10 pounds of fat and gained 2 pounds of lean tissue (see Figure 8.4). These findings indicate that a sensible strength training program helps in losing weight and maintaining or increasing muscle mass and metabolic rate.

Based on estimates, each additional pound of muscle tissue can raise the basal metabolic rate between 30 and 50 calories per day. Using the

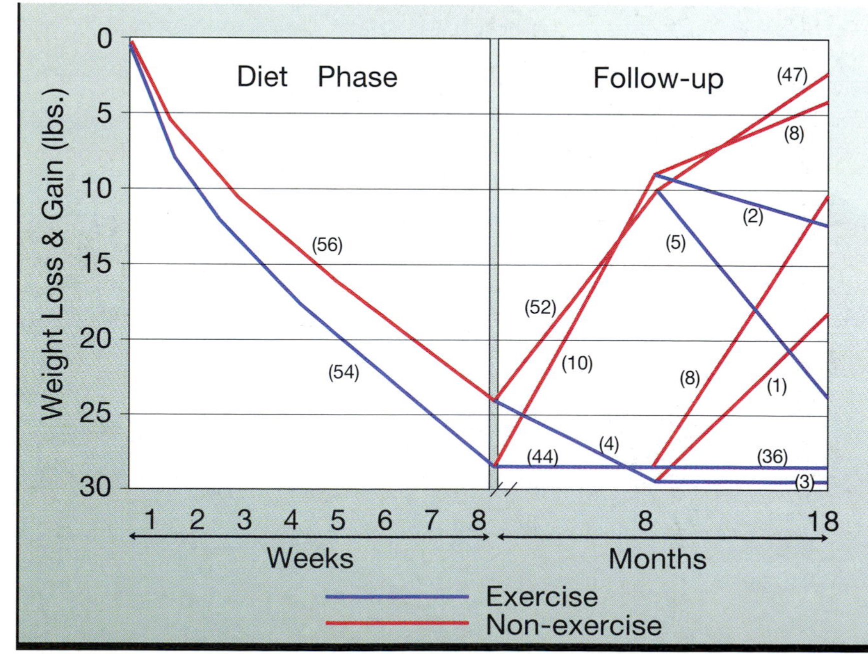


NOTE: Numbers in parentheses indicate number of participants.

Adapted from "Exercise as an Adjunct to Weight Loss and Maintenance in Moderately Obese Subjects, by K. N. Pavlou, S. Krey, and W. P. Steffee," *American Journal of Clinical Nutrition,* 49 (1989), 1115–1123.

**FIGURE 8.3** ◆ Aerobic exercise and weight loss and maintenance in moderately obese individuals.

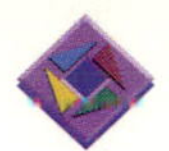

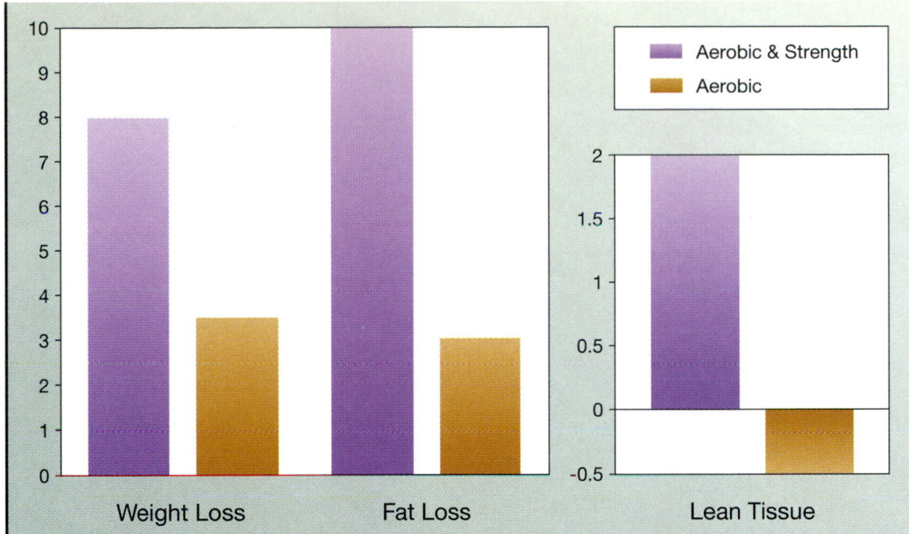


Both groups exercised 30 minutes per session, three times per week, for 12 weeks. The aerobic-plus-strength group performed 15 minutes of aerobic exercise and 15 minutes of strength training.

Source: "You Can Sell Exercise for Weight Loss," by W. L. Wescott, *Fitness Management*, 7:12 (1991), 33–34.

**FIGURE 8.4** ◆ Changes in body composition through an aerobic exercise program and a combined aerobic/strength-training exercise program.

conservative estimate of 30 calories per day, an individual who adds 5 pounds of muscle tissue as a result of strength training increases the basal metabolic rate by 150 calories per day, which equals 54,750 calories per year, or the equivalent of 15.6 pounds of fat.

Strength training is recommended especially for people who think they are at their ideal body weight, yet their body fat percentage is higher than recommended. The number of calories burned during a typical hour-long strength training session is much less than during an hour of aerobic exercise. Because of the high intensity of strength training, the person needs frequent rest intervals to recover from each set of exercise. The average person actually lifts weights only 10 to 12 minutes in each hour of exercise.

Weight can be lost through a regular strength training program, but much more slowly than through aerobics. In the long run, however, the person enjoys the benefits of gains in lean tissue. Guidelines for developing aerobic and strength training programs are given in Chapters 3 and 4.

Because exercise results in more lean body mass, body weight often remains the same or even increases after beginning an exercise program, while inches and percent body fat decrease. More lean tissue means more functional capacity of the human body. With exercise most of the weight loss becomes apparent after a few weeks of training, after the lean component has stabilized.

Although we know now that a negative caloric balance of 3,500 calories does not always result in a loss of exactly 1 pound of fat, the role of exercise in achieving a negative balance by burning additional calories is significant in weight reduction and maintenance programs.

Sadly, some individuals claim that the amount of calories burned during exercise is hardly worth the effort. They think that cutting their daily intake by some 300 calories is easier than participating in some sort of exercise that would burn the same amount of calories. The problem is that the willpower to cut those 300 calories lasts only a few weeks, and then the person goes right back to the old eating patterns.

If a person gets into the habit of exercising regularly, say three times a week, running 3 miles per exercise session (about 300 calories burned), this represents 900 calories in one week, about 3,600 in one month, or 46,800 calories per year. This minimal amount of exercise could mean as many as 13.5 extra pounds of fat in one year, 27 in two, and so on.

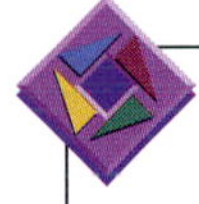

*A combination of both aerobic and strength training exercise are recommended for successful weight loss.*

We tend to forget that our weight creeps up gradually over the years, not just overnight. Hardly worth the effort? And we have not even taken into consideration the increase in lean tissue, the possible resetting of the setpoint, benefits to cardiovascular system and, most important, improved quality of life. The fundamental reasons for overfatness and obesity, few could argue, are lack of physical activity and sedentary living.

In terms of preventing disease, many of the health benefits people try to achieve by losing weight are reaped through exercise alone, even without weight loss. Exercise improves the metabolic profile in spite of no, or only slight, weight loss. Exercise offers protection against premature morbidity and mortality for everyone, including people who already have risk factors for disease (see Chapter 9). The lack of exercise, not the weight problem itself, possibly is the cause of many of the health risks associated with obesity.

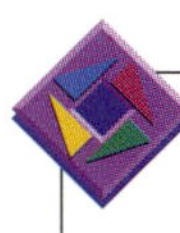

*The lack of exercise, not the weight problem itself, possibly is the cause of many of the health risks associated with obesity.*

## HEALTHY WEIGHT GAIN

"Skinny" people, too, should realize that the only healthy way to gain weight is through exercise (mainly strength training exercises) and a slight increase in caloric intake. Attempting to gain weight just by overeating will raise the fat component and not the lean component — which is not the path to better health. Exercise is the best solution to weight (fat) reduction and weight (lean) gain.

A strength training program such as the one outlined in Chapter 4 is the best approach to add body weight. To produce the most muscle hypertrophy, the training program should include at least two exercises of three to five sets for each major body part (see Principles Involved in Strength Training, Chapter 4). Each set should consist of about 10 repetitions maximum.

Even though the metabolic cost of synthesizing a pound of muscle tissue is still unclear, an estimated addition of 500 calories daily, including 15 grams of protein above the RDA, is recommended to gain an average of 1 pound of muscle tissue per week. Based on the typical American diet, the extra 15 grams of protein are not necessary. Each day, the average American already consumes 30 to 60 grams of protein above the RDA. The extra 500 calories should be in the form of complex carbohydrates, because most diets already are too high in fat. If the higher caloric intake is not accompanied by a strength training program, the gain in body weight will be in the form of fat, not muscle tissue.

## WEIGHT LOSS MYTHS

Spot reducing and losing "cellulite" (as some people refer to the fat deposits that bulge out on certain body parts) are mythical concepts. These deposits are nothing but enlarged fat cells, from accumulated body fat. Doing several sets of daily sit-ups will not get rid of fat in the midsection of the body.

When fat comes off, it does so throughout the entire body, not just the exercised area. The greatest proportion of fat may come off the biggest fat deposits, but the caloric output of a few sets of sit-ups has practically no effect on reducing total body fat. A person has to exercise much longer to really see results.

Other touted means toward quick weight loss — rubberized sweatsuits, steam baths, mechanical vibrators — are misleading. When a person wears a sweatsuit or steps into a sauna, the weight lost is not fat is but merely a significant amount of water. Sure, it looks nice when you step on the scale immediately afterward, but this represents a false loss of weight. As soon as you replace body fluids, you gain back the weight quickly.

Wearing rubberized sweatsuits not only hastens the rate of body fluid loss — fluid that is vital during prolonged exercise — but at the same time raises core temperature. This combination puts a person in danger of dehydration, which impairs cellular function and in extreme cases even can cause death.

Similarly, mechanical vibrators are worthless in a weight control program. Vibrating belts and turning rollers may feel good, but they require no effort whatsoever. Fat cannot be shaken off; it is lost primarily by burning it in muscle tissue.

## LOSING WEIGHT THE SOUND AND SENSIBLE WAY

Dieting never has been fun and never will be. People who are overweight and are serious about losing weight, however, have to include regular

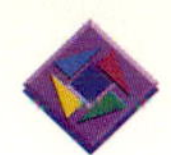

exercise in their life along with proper food management and a sensible reduction in caloric intake.

Some precautions are in order, as excessive body fat is a risk factor for cardiovascular disease. Depending on the extent of the weight problem, a medical examination and possibly a stress ECG (see Chapter 9) may be a good idea before undertaking the exercise program. A physician should be consulted in this regard.

Significantly overweight individuals also may have to choose activities in which they will not have to support their own body weight but that still will be effective in burning calories. Joint and muscle injuries are common in overweight individuals who participate in weight-bearing exercises such as walking, jogging, and aerobics.

Swimming may not be a good exercise either. More body fat makes a person more buoyant, and most people are not at the skill level to swim fast enough to get the best training effect. They tend to just float along, limiting the amount of calories burned, as well as the benefits to the cardiovascular system.

Some better alternatives are riding a bicycle (either road or stationary), walking in a shallow pool, or running in place in deep water (treading water). These forms of water exercise are gaining popularity and have proven to be effective in weight reduction without the "pain" and fear of injuries. Through the caloric expenditure of selected physical activities given in Table 8.2, you will be able to determine your own daily caloric requirement using Figure 8.5.

How long should each exercise session last? To develop and maintain cardiovascular fitness, 20 to 30 minutes of exercise at the ideal target rate, three to five times per week, is suggested (see Chapter 3). For weight loss, many experts recommend exercise at least 45 minutes at a time, five to six times a week .

A person should not try to do too much too fast. Unconditioned beginners should start with about 15 minutes of aerobic exercise three times a week, gradually increasing the duration by approximately 5 minutes each week and the frequency by one day per week during the next 3 to 4 weeks.

One final benefit of exercise for weight control is that it allows fat to be burned more efficiently. As both carbohydrates and fats are sources of energy, when the glucose levels begin to drop during prolonged exercise, more fat is used as energy substrate.

Equally important is that fat-burning enzymes increase with aerobic training. Essentially, fat is lost by burning it in muscle. Therefore, as the concentration of the enzymes increases, so does the ability to burn fat.[3]

In addition to exercise and adequate food management, sensible adjustments in caloric intake are recommended. Most research finds that a negative caloric balance is required to lose weight. Perhaps the only exception is in people who are eating too few calories. A nutrient analysis (see Chapter 7) often reveals that faithful dieters are not consuming enough calories. These people actually need to increase their daily caloric intake (combined with an exercise program) to get metabolism to kick back up to a normal level.

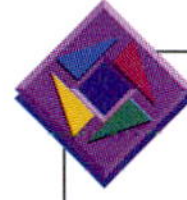

*Successful weight loss requires moderate caloric restriction and regular physical activity.*

The reasons for prescribing a lower caloric figure to lose weight are:

1. Most people underestimate their caloric intake and are eating more than they should be eating.
2. Developing new behaviors takes time, and some people have trouble changing and adjusting to new eating habits.
3. Many individuals are in such poor physical condition that they take a long time to increase their activity level enough to offset the setpoint and burn enough calories to aid in body fat loss.
4. Some dieters have difficulty succeeding unless they can count calories.
5. A few people simply will not alter their food selection. For those who will not change their food selection (which still will increase the risk for chronic diseases), a large increase in physical activity, a negative caloric balance, or a combination of the two is the only solution to lose weight successfully.

The daily caloric requirement can be estimated by consulting Tables 8.1 and 8.2 and Figure 8.5. As this is only an estimated value, individual adjustments related to many of the factors discussed in this chapter may be necessary to establish a more precise value. Nevertheless, the estimated value does offer a beginning guideline for weight control or reduction.

The average daily caloric requirement without exercise is based on typical lifestyle patterns, total body weight, and gender. Individuals who hold jobs that require heavy manual labor burn more calories during the day than those who have sedentary jobs such as working behind a desk.

To find your activity level:

1. Refer to Table 8.1 and rate yourself accordingly. The number given in Table 8.1 is per pound of body weight, so you should multiply your current weight by that number. For example, the typical caloric requirement to maintain body weight for a moderately active male who weighs 160 pounds is 2,400 calories (160 lbs × 15 calories per pound.

**TABLE 8.1**
**Average Caloric Requirement Per Pound of Body Weight Based on Lifestyle Patterns and Sex**

| | Calories Per Pound | |
|---|---|---|
| | Men | Women* |
| Sedentary — Limited physical activity | 13.0 | 12.0 |
| Moderate physical activity | 15.0 | 13.5 |
| Hard Labor — Strenuous physical effort | 17.0 | 15.0 |

*Pregnant or lactating women add three calories to these values.

**TABLE 8.2**
**Caloric Expenditure of Selected Physical Activities**

| Activity* | Cal/lb/min** | Activity* | Cal/lb/min** | Activity* | Cal/lb/min** |
|---|---|---|---|---|---|
| Aerobelt Exercise | | Dance | | StairMaster | |
| Aero-belt Jogging/6 mph | 0.098 | Moderate | 0.030 | Moderate | 0.070 |
| Aero-belt Step-Aerobics/8" | 0.105 | Vigorous | 0.055 | Vigorous | 0.090 |
| Aero-belt Walking/4 mph | 0.073 | Golf | 0.030 | Stationary Cycling | |
| Aerobics | | Gymnastics | | Moderate | 0.055 |
| Moderate | 0.065 | Light | 0.030 | Vigorous | 0.070 |
| Vigorous | 0.095 | Heavy | 0.056 | Strength Training | 0.050 |
| Step-Aerobics | 0.070 | Handball | 0.064 | Swimming (crawl) | |
| Archery | 0.030 | Hiking | 0.040 | 20 yds/min | 0.031 |
| Badminton | | Judo/Karate | 0.086 | 25 yds/min | 0.040 |
| Recreation | 0.038 | Racquetball | 0.065 | 45 yds/min | 0.057 |
| Competition | 0.065 | Rope Jumping | 0.060 | 50 yds/min | 0.070 |
| Baseball | 0.031 | Rowing (vigorous) | 0.090 | Table Tennis | 0.030 |
| Basketball | | Running | | Tennis | |
| Moderate | 0.046 | 11.0 min/mile | 0.070 | Moderate | 0.045 |
| Competition | 0.063 | 8.5 min/mile | 0.090 | Competition | 0.064 |
| Bowling | 0.030 | 7.0 min/mile | 0.102 | Volleyball | 0.030 |
| Calisthenics | 0.033 | 6.0 min/mile | 0.114 | Walking | |
| Cycling (level) | | Deep water*** | 0.100 | 4.5 mph | 0.045 |
| 5.5 mph | 0.033 | Skating (moderate) | 0.038 | Shallow pool | 0.090 |
| 10.0 mph | 0.050 | Skiing | | Water Aerobics | |
| 13.0 mph | 0.071 | Downhill | 0.060 | Moderate | 0.050 |
| | | Level (5 mph) | 0.078 | Vigorous | 0.070 |
| | | Soccer | 0.059 | Wrestling | 0.085 |

*Values are only for actual time engaged in the activity.
**Cal/lb/min = calories per pound of body weight per minute of activity
***Treading water

Adapted from *Fitness for Life: An Individualized Approach*, by P. E. Allsen, J. M. Harrison, and B. Vance (Dubuque, IA: Wm. C. Brown, 1989); *Fitness for College and Life*, by C. A. Bucher, and W. E. Prentice (St. Louis: Times Mirror/Mosby College Publishing, 1989); *Physiological Measurements of Metabolic Functions in Man*, by C. F. Consolazio, R. E. Johnson, and L. J. Pecora (New York: McGraw-Hill, 1963); *Physical Fitness: The Pathway to Healthful Living*, by R. V. Hockey (St. Louis: Times Mirror/Mosby College Publishing, 1989); and research conducted at Boise State University by W. W. K. Hoeger et al, 1986–1993.

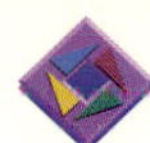

| | | |
|---|---|---|
| A. | Current body weight | ________ |
| B. | Caloric requirement per pound of body weight (use Table 8.1) | ________ |
| C. | Typical daily caloric requirement without exercise to maintain body weight (A × B) | ________ |
| D. | Selected physical activity (e.g., jogging)* | ________ |
| E. | Number of exercise sessions per week | ________ |
| F. | Duration of exercise session (in minutes) | ________ |
| G. | Total weekly exercise time in minutes (E × F) | ________ |
| H. | Average daily exercise time in minutes (G ÷ 7) | ________ |
| I. | Caloric expenditure per pound per minute (cal/lb/min) of physical activity (use Table 8.2) | ________ |
| J. | Total calories burned per minute of physical activity (A × I) | ________ |
| K. | Average daily calories burned as a result of the exercise program (H × J) | ________ |
| L. | Total daily caloric requirement with exercise to maintain body weight (C + K) | ________ |
| M. | Number of calories to subtract from daily requirement to achieve a negative caloric balance** | ________ |
| N. | Target caloric intake to lose weight (L − M) | ________ |

* If more than one physical activity is selected, you will need to estimate the average daily calories burned as a result of each additional activity (steps D through K) and add all of these figures to L above.

** Subtract 500 calories if the total daily requirement with exercise (L) is below 3,000 calories. As many as 1,000 calories may be subtracted for daily requirements above 3,000 calories.

**FIGURE 8.5** ◆ Computation form for daily caloric requirement.

2. Determine the average number of calories burned daily as a result of exercise. To get this number, figure out the total number of minutes you exercise weekly, and then figure the daily average exercise time. For instance, a person cycling at 13 miles per hour, five times a week, 30 minutes each time, exercises 150 minutes per week (5 × 30). The average daily exercise time is 21 minutes (150 ÷ 7). Round off to the lowest unit.
3. Referring to Table 8.2, find the energy requirement for the activity (or activities) chosen for the exercise program. In the case of cycling (13 miles per hour), the requirement is .071 calories per pound of body weight per minute of activity (cal/lb/min). With a body weight of 160 pounds, this man burns 11.4 calories each minute (body weight × .071, or 160 × .071). In 21 minutes he burns approximately 240 calories (21 × 1.4).
4. Obtain the estimated total caloric requirement, with exercise, needed to maintain body weight. To do this, add the typical daily requirement (without exercise) and the average calories burned through exercise. In our example it is 2,640 calories (2,400 + 240). If a negative caloric balance is recommended to lose weight, this person has to consume fewer than 2,640 calories daily to achieve the objective. Because of the many factors that play a role in weight control, the previous value is only an estimated daily requirement.

Furthermore, to lose weight, a person can't predict that exactly one pound of fat will be lost in one week by reducing daily intake by 500 calories (500 × 7 = 3,500 calories, or the equivalent of one pound of fat). The estimated daily caloric figure provides only a target guideline for weight control. Periodic readjustments are necessary because individuals differ, and the estimated daily cost changes as you lose weight and modify your exercise habits.

The recommended number of calories to be subtracted from the daily intake to obtain a negative caloric balance depends on the typical daily requirement. At this point, the best recommendation is to decrease the daily intake moderately, never below 1,200 calories for women and 1,500 for men.

A good rule to follow is to restrict the intake by no more than 500 calories if the daily requirement is below 3,000 calories. For caloric requirements in excess of 3,000, as many as 1,000 calories per day may be subtracted from the total intake. The daily distribution should be approximately 60% carbohydrates (mostly complex carbohydrates), less than 30% fat, and about 12% protein.

Many experts believe that a person may take off weight more efficiently by reducing the amount of daily fat intake to 10% to 20% of the total daily caloric intake. Because 1 gram of fat supplies more than twice the amount of calories that carbohydrates and protein do, the general tendency is not to overeat.

Further, it takes only 3% to 5% of ingested calories to store fat as fat, whereas it takes approximately 25% of ingested calories to convert carbohydrates to fat. Other research points to the fact that if people eat the same amount of calories as carbohydrate or fat, those on the fat diet will store more fat. Successful weight-loss programs allow only small amounts of fat in the diet.

Many people have trouble adhering to a 10% to 20% fat-calorie diet. During weight-loss periods, however, you are encouraged strongly to do so. Start with a 20% fat-calorie diet. Refer to Table 8.3 to aid you in determining the grams of fat at 10%, 20%, and 30% of the total calories for selected energy intakes. Also use the form provided in Figure 7.13, Chapter 7, to monitor your daily fat intake.

**TABLE 8.3**
**Grams of Fat at 10%, 20%, and 30% of Total Calories for Selected Energy Intakes**

| Caloric Intake | Grams of Fat 10% | 20% | 30% |
|---|---|---|---|
| 1,300 | 14 | 29 | 43 |
| 1,400 | 16 | 31 | 47 |
| 1,500 | 17 | 33 | 50 |
| 1,600 | 18 | 36 | 53 |
| 1,700 | 19 | 38 | 57 |
| 1,800 | 20 | 40 | 60 |
| 1,900 | 21 | 42 | 63 |
| 2,000 | 22 | 44 | 67 |
| 2,100 | 23 | 47 | 70 |
| 2,200 | 24 | 49 | 73 |
| 2,300 | 26 | 51 | 77 |
| 2,400 | 27 | 53 | 80 |
| 2,500 | 28 | 56 | 83 |
| 2,600 | 29 | 58 | 87 |
| 2,700 | 30 | 60 | 90 |
| 2,800 | 31 | 62 | 93 |
| 2,900 | 32 | 64 | 97 |
| 3,000 | 33 | 67 | 100 |

The time of day when food is consumed also may play a part in weight reduction. A study conducted at the Aerobics Research Center in Dallas, Texas, indicated that, when a person is on a diet, weight is lost most effectively if most of the calories are consumed before 1:00 p.m. and not during the evening meal. This center recommends that, when a person is attempting to lose weight, intake should consist of a minimum of 25% of the total daily calories for breakfast, 50% for lunch, and 25% or less at dinner.

Other experts have reported that, if most of the daily calories are consumed during one meal, the body may perceive that something is wrong and will slow down the metabolism so it can store more calories in the form of fat. Eating most of the calories in one meal also causes a person to go hungry the rest of the day, making the diet more difficult to follow.

The principle of consuming most of the calories earlier in the day not only seems helpful in losing weight but also in managing atherosclerosis. The time of day when most of the fats and cholesterol are consumed can influence blood lipids and coronary heart disease. Peak digestion time following a heavy meal is about 7 hours after that meal. If most lipids are consumed during the evening meal, digestion peaks while the person is sound asleep, when the metabolism is at it slowest rate. Consequently, the body may not metabolize fats and cholesterol as well, leading to a higher blood lipid count and increasing the risk for atherosclerosis and coronary heart disease.

To monitor daily progress, you may use a form such as given in Figure 7.13. Meeting the basic requirements from each food group should get top priority. The caloric content for each food is given in the Nutritive Value of Selected Foods list in Appendix B. For a more precise record, the

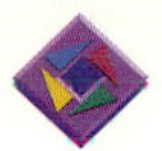

information should be recorded immediately after each meal. According to the person's progress, adjustments can be made in the typical daily requirement or the exercise program, or both.

## TIPS FOR BEHAVIOR MODIFICATION AND ADHERENCE TO A WEIGHT MANAGEMENT PROGRAM

Achieving and maintaining recommended body composition is by no means impossible, but it does require desire and commitment. If weight management is to become a priority in life, people must realize they have to retrain behavior to some extent.

Modifying old habits and developing new, positive behaviors take time. Individuals have applied the following management techniques to change detrimental behavior successfully and adhere to a positive lifetime weight-control program. In developing a retraining program, people are not expected to incorporate all of the strategies listed but should note the ones that apply to them. The form provided in Figure 8.6 allows you to evaluate and monitor your own weight management behaviors.

1. **Make a commitment to change.** The first ingredient to modify behavior is the desire to do so. The reasons for change must be more compelling than those for continuing present lifestyle patterns. People must accept the fact that they have a problem and decide by themselves whether they really want to change. If a sincere commitment is there, the chances for success are enhanced already.

2. **Set realistic goals.** Most people with a weight problem would like to lose weight in a relatively short time but fail to realize that the weight problem developed over a span of several years. A sound weight reduction and maintenance program can be accomplished only by establishing new lifetime eating and exercise habits, both of which take time to develop. In setting a realistic long-term goal, short-term objectives also should be planned. The long-term goal may be to decrease body fat to 20% of total body weight. The short-term objective may be to decrease body fat 1% each month. Objectives like these allow for regular evaluation and help maintain motivation and renewed commitment to attain the long-term goal.

3. **Incorporate exercise into the program.** Choosing enjoyable activities, places, times, equipment, and people to exercise with helps a person adhere to an exercise program. Details on developing a complete exercise program are found in Chapters 3 (cardiovascular), 4 (strength), and 5 (flexibility).

4. **Develop healthy eating patterns.** Plan to eat three regular meals per day consistent with the body's nutritional requirements. Learn to differentiate hunger from appetite. Hunger is the actual physical need for food. Appetite is a desire for food, usually triggered by factors such as stress, habit, boredom, depression, food availability, or just the thought of food itself. Eat only when you have a physical need. In this regard, developing and sticking to a regular meal pattern helps control hunger.

5. **Avoid automatic eating.** Many people associate certain daily activities with eating. For example, people eat while cooking, watching television, reading, talking on the telephone, or visiting with neighbors. Most of the time, the foods consumed in these situations lack nutritional value or are high in sugar and fat.

6. **Stay busy.** People tend to eat more when they sit around and do nothing. Occupying the mind and body with activities not associated with eating helps take away the desire to eat. Try walking, cycling, playing sports, gardening, sewing, or visiting a library, a museum, a park. Develop other skills and interests, or try something new and exciting to break the routine of life.

7. **Plan your meals ahead of time.** Sensible shopping is required to accomplish this objective (by the way, shop on a full stomach, because hungry shoppers tend to buy unhealthy foods impulsively and then snack on the way home). Include whole-grain breads and cereals, fruits and vegetables, low-fat milk and dairy products, lean meats, fish, and poultry.

8. **Cook wisely.** Use less fat and refined foods when preparing food. Trim all visible fat off meats, and remove skin from poultry before cooking. Skim the fat off gravies and soups. Bake, broil, and boil instead of frying. Use

Name: ______________________________

| **Strategy** **Date:** | | | | | | | | | | | | | | | |
|---|---|---|---|---|---|---|---|---|---|---|---|---|---|---|---|
| 1. I made a commitment to change | | | | | | | | | | | | | | | |
| 2. I set realistic goals | | | | | | | | | | | | | | | |
| 3. I exercise regularly | | | | | | | | | | | | | | | |
| 4. I have healthy eating patterns | | | | | | | | | | | | | | | |
| 5. I avoid automatic eating | | | | | | | | | | | | | | | |
| 6. I stay busy | | | | | | | | | | | | | | | |
| 7. I plan meals ahead of time | | | | | | | | | | | | | | | |
| 8. I cook wisely | | | | | | | | | | | | | | | |
| 9. I do not serve more food than I should eat | | | | | | | | | | | | | | | |
| 10. I eat slowly and at the table only | | | | | | | | | | | | | | | |
| 11. I avoid social binges | | | | | | | | | | | | | | | |
| 12. I avoid refrigerator and cookie-jar raids | | | | | | | | | | | | | | | |
| 13. I avoid eating out. If I do, I eat low fat meals | | | | | | | | | | | | | | | |
| 14. I practice stress management | | | | | | | | | | | | | | | |
| 15. I monitor behavior changes | | | | | | | | | | | | | | | |
| 16. I reward my accomplishments | | | | | | | | | | | | | | | |
| 17. I think positive | | | | | | | | | | | | | | | |

**FIGURE 8.6** ◆ Behavioral modification progress form for weight management.

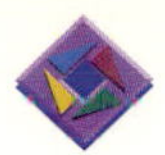

butter, cream, mayonnaise, and salad dressings sparingly. Avoid coconut oil, palm oil, and cocoa butter. Prepare plenty of bulky foods. Include whole-grain breads and cereals, vegetables, and legumes in most meals. Try fruits for dessert. Beware of soda pop, fruit juices, and fruit-flavored drinks. Cut down on sugar and other refined carbohydrates such as corn syrup, malt sugar, dextrose, and fructose. Drink plenty of water — at least eight glasses a day.

9. **Do not serve more food than you should eat.** Measure the food portions and keep serving dishes away from the table. This means you will eat less, have a harder time getting seconds, and have less appetite because food is not visible. People should not be forced to eat when they are satisfied (including children after they have already had a healthy, nutritious serving).

10. **Eat slowly and at the table only.** Eating is one of the pleasures of life, and we need to take time to enjoy it. Eating on the run is not good because the body doesn't have enough time to "register" nutritive and caloric consumption, and people overeat before the body perceives the signal of fullness. Always eating at the table also forces people to take time out to eat, and it deters snacking between meals, primarily because of the extra time and effort required to sit down and eat. When done eating, do not sit around the table. Clean up and put away the food to keep from unnecessary snacking.

11. **Avoid social binges.** Social gatherings commonly entice self-defeating behavior. Plan ahead and visualize yourself in that gathering. Do not feel pressured to eat or drink, and don't rationalize in these situations. Choose low-calorie foods, and entertain yourself with other activities such as dancing and talking.

12. **Beware of raids on the refrigerator and the cookie jar.** When you find yourself in these tempting situations, take control. Stop and think what is happening. If you have the propensity for raids, try environmental management. Do not bring high-calorie, high-sugar, or high-fat foods into the house. If they are in the house already, store them where they are hard to get to or see. If they are out of sight or not readily available, the temptation is less. Keeping food in places such as the garage and the basement tends to discourage people from taking the time and effort to get them. By no means should you have to completely eliminate treats, but all things should be done in moderation.

13. **Avoid eating out.** Most meals served at restaurants (especially fast food restaurants) are high in calories and fat. People who eat out regularly tend to have a difficult time managing weight. When eating out, plan your choices ahead of time by selecting low-fat and low-calorie meals.

14. **Practice stress management techniques.** Many people snack and increase their food consumption in stressful situations. Eating is not a stress-releasing activity and actually can aggravate the problem if weight control is an issue. Several stress management techniques are set forth in Chapter 11.

15. **Monitor changes and reward accomplishments.** Feedback on fat loss, lean tissue gain, and weight loss is a reward in itself. Awareness of changes in body composition also helps reinforce new behaviors. Being able to exercise without interruption for 15, 20, 30, 60 minutes, cycling a certain distance, running a mile — all these accomplishments deserve recognition. Meeting objectives calls for rewards, but not related to eating. Buy new clothing, a tennis racquet, a bicycle, exercise shoes, or something else that is special and you would not have acquired otherwise.

16. **Think positive.** Avoid negative thoughts on how difficult changing your past behaviors might be. Instead, think of the benefits you will reap, such as feeling, looking, and functioning better, plus enjoying better health and improving your quality of life. Attempt to stay away from negative environments and people who will not be supportive. Avoid those who do not have the same desires and who encourage self-defeating behaviors.

## IN CONCLUSION

There is no simple and quick way to take off excessive body fat and keep it off for good. Weight management is accomplished by making a lifetime commitment to physical activity and selecting foods properly. When taking part in a weight (fat) reduction program, people also have to moderately decrease their caloric intake and implement strategies to modify unhealthy eating behaviors.

During the process of behavior modification, relapses into past negative behaviors are almost inevitable. The three most common reasons for relapse are:

1. Stress-related factors (major life changes, depression, job changes, illness).
2. Social reasons (entertaining, eating out, business travel).
3. Self-enticing behaviors (placing yourself in a situation to see how much you can get away with: "One small taste won't hurt," leading to, "I'll eat just one slice," and finally, "I haven't done so well, so I might as well eat some more").

Making mistakes is human and does not necessarily mean failure. Failure comes to those who give up and do not use previous experiences to build upon and, in turn, develop skills that will prevent self-defeating behaviors in the future. Where there's a will, there's a way, and those who persist will reap the rewards.

## NOTES

1. S. W. Lichtman, et al., "Discrepancy Between Self-Reported and Actual Caloric Intake and Exercise in Obese Subjects." *The New England Journal of Medicine*, 327:27 (1992), 1893-1898.
2. D. Remington, A. G. Fisher, and E. A. Parent., *How to Lower Your Fat Thermostat* (Provo, UT: Vitality House International, 1983).
3. Remington, Fisher, and Parent.

## SELECT BIBLIOGRAPHY

Anderson, A. J., et al. "Body Fat Distribution, Plasma Lipids and Lipoproteins." *Arteriosclerosis* 8 (1988), 88-94.

Bennett, W., and J. Gurin. "Do Diets Really Work?" *Science*, March 1982, pp. 42-50.

"Brown Fat is Good Fat." *Health Letter*, December 11, 1981.

Committee on Diet and Health, Food and Nutrition Board. *Diet and Health: Implications for Reducing Chronic Disease Risk*. Washington, DC: National Academy Press, 1989.

Hafen, B. Q., A. L. Thygerson, and K. J. Frandsen. *Behavioral Guidelines for Health & Wellness*. Englewood, CO: Morton Publishing, 1988.

Health Implications of Obesity: National Institutes of Health Consensus Development Conference. *Annals of Internal Medicine*, 103 (1985), 977-1077.

Jenkins, D. J. A., et al. "Nibbling Versus Gorging: Metabolic Advantages of Increased Meal Frequency." *New England Journal of Medicine* 321:14 (1989), 929-934.

Morgan, B. L. G. *The Lifelong Nutrition Guide*. Englewood Cliffs, NJ: Prentice Hall, 1983.

National Academy of Sciences. *Diet and Health: Implications for Reducing Chronic Disease Risk*. Washington, DC: National Academy Press, 1989.

Perkins, K. A., L. H. Epstein, B. L. Marks, R. L. Stiller, and R. G. Jacob. "The Effect of Nicotine on Energy Expenditure During Light Physical Activity." *New England Journal of Medicine* 320:14 (1989), 898-903

Sims, E. A. H. "Obesity is Hazardous to Your Health: Affirmative." *Debates in Medicine* 2 (1989), 103-137.

Steen, S. N., R. A. Oppliger, and K. D. Brownell. "Metabolic Effects of Repeated Weight Loss and Regain in Adolescent Wrestlers." *Journal of the American Medical Association*, 260 (1988), 47-50.

Stunkard, A. J., T. I. A. Sorensen, C. Hanis, T. W. Teasdale, R. Chakraborty, W. J. Schull, and F. Schulsinger. "An Adoption Study of Human Obesity." *New England Journal of Medicine* 314:4 (1986), 193-198.

Wadden, T. A., T. B. Van Itallie, and G. L. Blackburn. "Responsible and Irresponsible Use of Very-Low-Calorie Diets in the Treatment of Obesity." *Journal of the American Medical Association*, 263 (1990), 83-85.

Westcott, W. "Why Every Adult Should Strength Train." *Nautilus*, Summer 1994, pp. 18-20.

Whitney, E. N., and E. V. N. Hamilton. *Understanding Nutrition*. St. Paul: West Publishing, 1994.

Wolf, M. D. "The Battle Against Body Fat." *Fitness Management*, 3:3 (1987), 48-49.

# Cardiovascular Disease Prevention

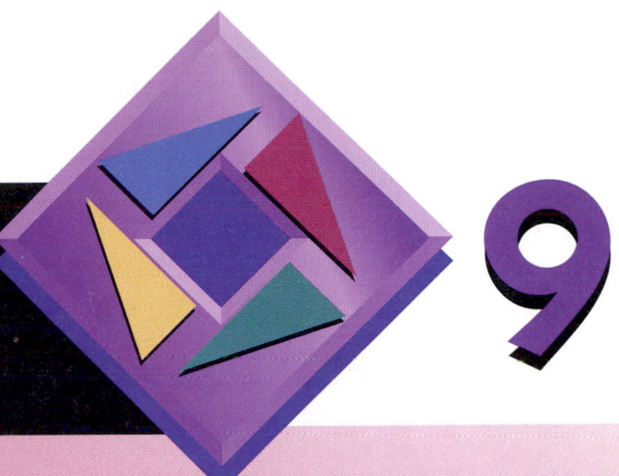


## Key Concepts

Cardiovascular disease
Coronary heart disease
Risk factor
Electrocardiogram
Stress ECG
Cholesterol
HDL-cholesterol
LDL-cholesterol
Atherosclerosis
Triglycerides
Diabetes
Hypertension
Stress

## Objectives

- Define cardiovascular disease and coronary heart disease
- Understand the importance of a healthy lifestyle in preventing cardiovascular disease.
- Assess your own risk for developing coronary heart disease.
- Discuss the major risk factors that lead to coronary heart disease, including physical inactivity, hypertension, smoking, and abnormal cholesterol profile.
- Be introduced to a comprehensive program for reducing the risk for coronary heart disease managing the overall risk for cardiovascular disease

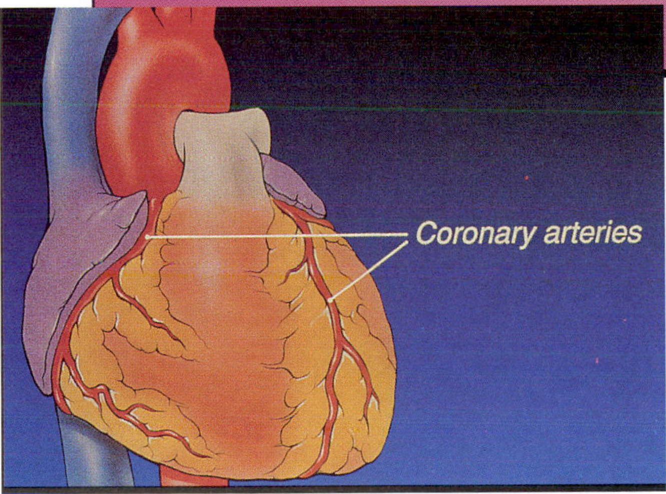


From *Heart of a Healthy Life*. Courtesy of the American Heart Association, © 1992.

Cardiovascular disease is the leading cause of death in the United States, accounting for nearly half of the total mortality rate in 1990. The disease encompasses any pathological condition that affects the heart and the circulatory system (blood vessels). Some examples of cardiovascular disease are coronary heart disease, peripheral vascular disease, congenital heart disease, rheumatic heart disease, stroke, high blood pressure, congestive heart failure, and atherosclerosis (fatty/cholesterol deposits in the walls of the arteries leading to formation of plaque). Cardiovascular disease alone now costs the nation well over $135 billion annually.

Although heart and blood vessel disease is still the number-one health problem in the United States, the incidence has declined by 36% in the last two decades (see Figure 9.1), mainly because of health education. More people now are aware of the risk factors for cardiovascular disease and are changing their lifestyle to lower their own potential risk for this disease.

The major form of cardiovascular disease is coronary heart disease (CHD), a condition in which the arteries that supply the heart muscle with oxygen and nutrients are narrowed by fatty deposits such as cholesterol and triglycerides. Narrowing of the coronary arteries diminishes the blood supply to the heart muscle, which can precipitate a heart attack (see Figure 9.2).

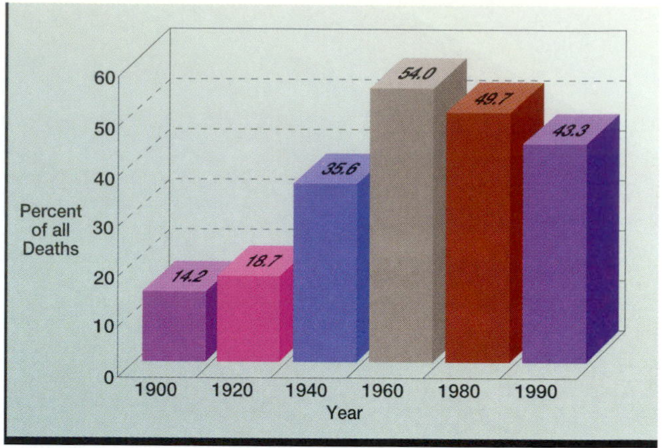


**FIGURE 9.1** ◆ Incidence of cardiovascular disease in the United States for selected years: 1900–1990.

CHD is the single leading cause of death in the United States, accounting for approximately a third of all deaths and more than half of all cardiovascular deaths. Oddly enough, almost all of the risk factors for CHD are preventable and reversible, and the individual can reduce that risk.

Each year more than 330,000 coronary bypass operations and 190,000 coronary angioplasty procedures are performed in the United States. Angioplasty involves inserting a balloon-tipped catheter to widen the inner lumen of the arteries. Health-care costs for coronary bypass range between $30,000 and $40,000, and, for an angioplasty

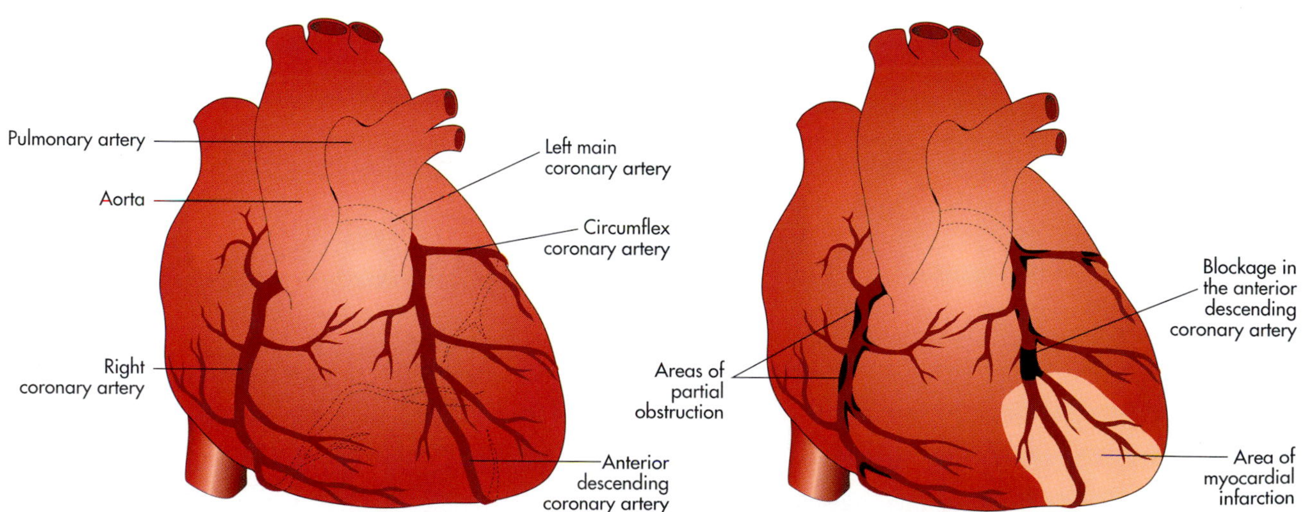


**FIGURE 9.2** ◆

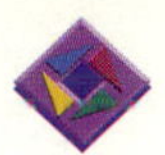

procedure, $7,500 — or about $11 billion per year for coronary heart disease surgery.

## CORONARY HEART DISEASE RISK PROFILE

Although genetic inheritance plays a role in CHD, the most important determinant is personal lifestyle. A CHD risk factor analysis is administered to evaluate the impact of a person's lifestyle and genetic endowment as potential factors contributing to the development of coronary disease. The specific objectives of a CHD risk factor analysis are:

- To screen individuals who may be at high risk for the disease.
- To educate regarding the leading risk factors for developing CHD.
- To implement programs aimed at reducing the risk.
- To use the analysis as a starting point from which to compare changes induced by the intervention program.

The leading risk factors contributing to CHD are listed in Table 9.1. A self-assessment CHD risk factor analysis is given in Figure 9.3. This CHD risk factor analysis can be done by people with little or no medical information about their cardiovascular health, as well as by those who have had a thorough medical examination. The guidelines for zero risk are outlined for each factor, making this self-assessment analysis a valuable tool in managing CHD risk factors.

For example, a person who fills out the form knows that the ideal blood pressure is around 120/80 or lower, that risk is reduced by smoking less or quitting altogether, that HDL-cholesterol should be 45 mg/dl (milligrams per deciliter) or higher for men and 55 mg/dl or higher for women, and that LDL-cholesterol should be less than 170 mg/dl (if unknown, basic nutritional guidelines also are given). The role of HDL- and LDL-cholesterol in protection against heart disease is discussed later in this chapter.

To provide a meaningful CHD risk score, a weighting system* was developed to show the impact of each risk factor on developing the disease. This weighting system is based on research and on the work done at leading preventive medicine facilities in the United States. The most significant risk factors are given the heaviest numeric weight.

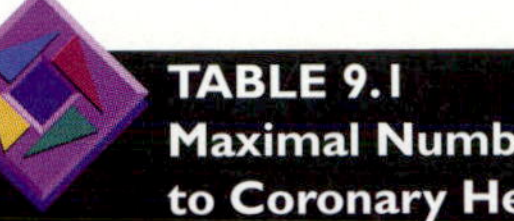

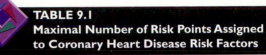

**TABLE 9.1**
**Maximal Number of Risk Points Assigned to Coronary Heart Disease Risk Factors**

| Risk Factors | Maximal Risk Points |
|---|---|
| Abnormal cholesterol profile | 12 |
| Low HDL-cholesterol | 6 |
| High LDL-cholesterol | 6 |
| Abnormal stress electrocardiogram | 8 |
| Smoking | 8 |
| Personal history of heart disease | 8 |
| Hypertension | 8 |
| Systolic blood pressure | 4 |
| Diastolic blood pressure | 4 |
| Physical inactivity | 8 |
| Diabetes | 6 |
| High blood glucose | 3 |
| Known diabetic | 3 |
| Family history of heart disease | 6 |
| Age | 4 |
| Excessive body fat | 3 |
| Tension and stress | 3 |
| Abnormal resting electrocardiogram | 3 |
| Elevated triglycerides | 2 |

For example, a poor cholesterol profile seems to be the best predictor for developing CHD. Up to 12 risk points are assigned to individuals with "very high" LDL-cholesterol levels and "very low" HDL-cholesterol levels. On the other hand, the least heavily weighted risk factor is triglycerides. A maximum of only 2 risk points is assigned to this factor. Each risk factor also is assigned a zero risk level, the level at which it does not appear to increase the risk for disease at all.

Based on actual test results, a person receives a score anywhere from zero to the maximum number of points for each factor. When the risk points from all of the risk factors are totaled, the final number is used to rate an individual in one of five overall risk categories for potential development of CHD.

*The weighting system for the CHD risk factor analysis has been adapted with permission from *The Complete Guide for the Development and Implementation of Health Promotion Programs*, by W. W. K Hoeger (Englewood, CO: Morton Publishing, 1987).

A "very low" CHD risk category designates the group at lowest risk for developing heart disease based on age and sex. "Low" CHD suggests that, even though people in this category are taking good care of their cardiovascular health, they still can improve it (unless all of the risk points come from age and family history). "Moderate" CHD risk means people can definitely improve their lifestyle to lower the risk for disease, or medical treatment may be required. A score in the "high" or "very high" CHD risk category points to a strong probability of developing heart disease within the next few years and calls for immediate implementation of a personal risk reduction program, including medical, nutritional, and exercise intervention by professional staff.

## LEADING RISK FACTORS

With the exception of age, family history of heart disease, and certain electrocardiogram (ECG) abnormalities, the risk factors are preventable and reversible. The leading risk factors for CHD are discussed next, along with the general recommendations for reducing that risk.

### Physical Inactivity

Physical inactivity is responsible for low levels of cardiovascular endurance, previously defined as the ability of the heart, lungs, and blood vessels to deliver enough oxygen to the cells to meet the demands of prolonged physical activity. The level of cardiovascular endurance (or fitness) is given most commonly by the maximal amount of oxygen (in milliliters) that every kilogram (2.2 pounds) of body weight is able to utilize per minute of physical activity (ml/kg/min). As maximal oxygen uptake increases, so does the efficiency of the cardiovascular system.

Even though physical inactivity has not been assigned the most risk points (8 points for a poor level of fitness, as compared to 12 for a poor cholesterol profile, see Table 9.1), improving cardiovascular endurance through aerobic exercise has a great impact in reducing the overall risk for heart disease.

Although specific recommendations can be followed to improve each risk factor, a regular aerobic exercise program helps to control most of the major risk factors that lead to heart disease. Aerobic exercise will:

- Increase cardiovascular endurance.
- Decrease and control blood pressure.
- Reduce body fat.
- Lower blood lipids (cholesterol and triglycerides).
- Improve HDL-cholesterol.
- Help control diabetes.
- Increase and maintain good heart function, sometimes improving certain ECG abnormalities.
- Motivate toward smoking cessation.
- Alleviate tension and stress.
- Counteract a personal history of heart disease.

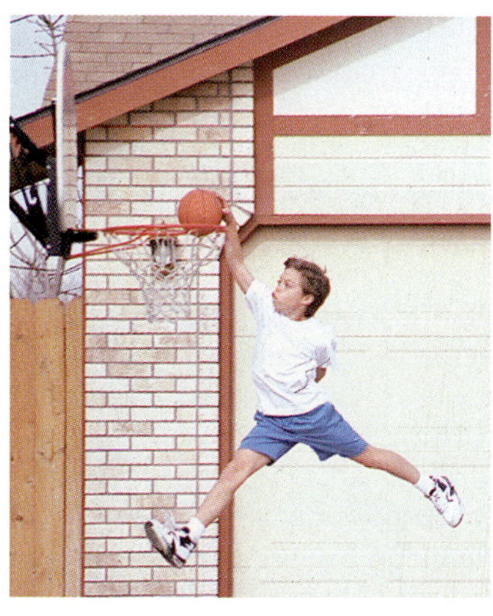

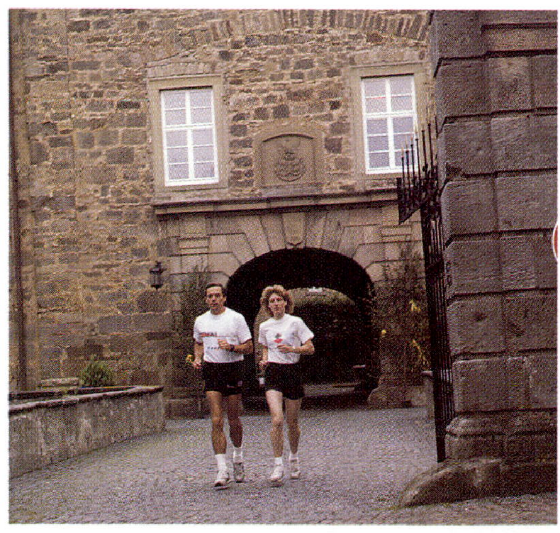

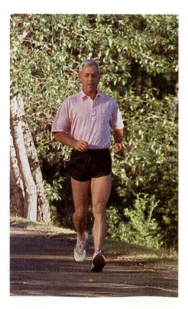

*Lifetime participation in aerobic activities is one of the most important factors in preventing cardiovascular disease.*

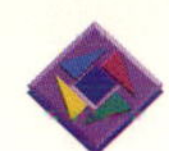

## SELF-ASSESSMENT CORONARY HEART DISEASE RISK FACTOR ANALYSIS

| Risk Factor | | | | | Score |
|---|---|---|---|---|---|
| 1. Physical Activity | Do you participate in a regular aerobic exercise program (brisk walking, jogging, swimming, bicycling, aerobics, etc.) for more than 20 minutes: | | | | |
| | Once a week or less | | | 8 | |
| | Two times per week | | | 3 | |
| | Three or more times per week | | | 0 | 0 |
| 2. Resting and Stress Electrocardiograms (ECG) | Add scores for both ECGs | | | | |
| | ECG | Resting | Stress | | |
| | Normal | (0) | (0) | 0 | |
| | Equivocal | (1) | (4) | 1-5 | |
| | Abnormal | (3) | (8) | 3-11 | 0 |
| 3. HDL-Cholesterol (If unknown, answer question 6) | | Men | Women | | |
| | | ≥ 45 | ≥ 55 | 0 | |
| | | 36–44 | 46–54 | 3 | |
| | | ≤ 35 | ≤ 45 | 6 | 0 |
| 4. LDL-Cholesterol (If unknown, answer question 6) | ≤ 129 | | | 0 | |
| | 130-159 | | | 3 | |
| | ≥ 160 | | | 6 | 3 |
| 5. Triglycerides (If unknown, answer question 6) | ≤ 125 | | | 0 | |
| | 126-499 | | | 1 | |
| | ≥ 500 | | | 2 | 1 |
| 6. Diet (Do not answer if questions 3, 4 and 5 have been answered) | Does your regular diet include (high score if all apply): | | | | |
| | One or more daily servings of red meat; 7 or more eggs/week; daily butter, cheese, whole milk, sweets and alcohol | | | 10-14 | |
| | Four to six servings of red meat/week, 4-6 eggs per week, margarine, 1% or 2% milk, some cheese, sweets, and alcohol | | | 4-10 | |
| | Fish, poultry, red meat less than three times/week, less than 3 eggs/week, skim milk and skim milk products, moderate sweets and alcohol | | | 0-3 | |
| 7. Diabetes/Glucose | ≤120 | | | 0 | |
| | 121-128 | | | 1 | |
| | 129-136 | | | 1.5 | |
| | 137-144 | | | 2 | |
| | 145-149 | | | 2.5 | |
| | >150 | | | 3 | |
| | Diabetics add another 3 points | | | 3 | 2 |
| 8. Blood Pressure | Score applies to each reading (e.g. 144/88 score = 4) | | | | |
| | | Systolic | Diastolic | | |
| | | ≤120 (0) | ≤80 (0) | 0 | |
| | | 121-130 (1) | 81-90 (1) | 1-2 | |
| | | 131-140 (2) | 91-98 (2) | 2-4 | |
| | | 141-150 (3) | 99-106 (3) | 3-6 | |
| | | ≥151 (4) | ≥107 (4) | 4-8 | 1 |
| | | | | Subtotal Risk Score: | 7 |

**FIGURE 9.3** ◆

| | | Men | Women | Points | Score |
|---|---|---|---|---|---|
| 9. | Percent Body Fat | 12-17% | 18-22% | 0 | |
| | | 18-22% | 23-27% | 1 | |
| | | 23-27% | 28-32% | 2 | |
| | | ≥28% | ≥33% | 3 | 2 |

| | | | Points | Score |
|---|---|---|---|---|
| 10. | Smoking | Lifetime nonsmoker | 0 | |
| | | Ex-smoker over one year | 0 | |
| | | Ex-smoker less than one year | 1 | |
| | | Smoke less than 1 cigarette/day | 1 | |
| | | Nonsmoker, but live or work in smoking environment | 2 | |
| | | Pipe, cigar smoker, or chew tobacco | 2 | |
| | | Smoke 1-9 cigarettes/day | 3 | |
| | | Smoke 10-19 cigarettes/day | 4 | |
| | | Smoke 20-29 cigarettes/day | 5 | |
| | | Smoke 30-39 cigarettes/day | 6 | |
| | | Smoke 40 or more cigarettes/day | 8 | 0 |
| 11. | Tension and Stress | Are you: | | |
| | | Sometimes tense | 0 | |
| | | Often tense | 1 | |
| | | Nearly always tense | 2 | |
| | | Always tense | 3 | 0 |
| 12. | Personal History | Have you ever had a heart attack, stroke, coronary disease, or any known heart problem: | | |
| | | During the last year | 8 | |
| | | 1-2 years ago | 5 | |
| | | 2-5 years ago | 3 | |
| | | More than 5 years ago | 2 | |
| | | Never suffered from heart disease | 0 | 0 |
| 13. | Family History | Have any of your blood relatives (parents, uncles, brothers, sisters, grandparents) suffered from cardiovascular disease (heart attack, strokes, bypass surgery): | | |
| | | One or more before age 51 | 6 | |
| | | One or more between 51 and 60 | 3 | |
| | | One or more after age 60 | 1 | |
| | | None have suffered from cardiovascular disease | 0 | 1 |
| 14. | Age | 29 or younger | 0 | |
| | | 30-39 | 1 | |
| | | 40-49 | 2 | |
| | | 50-59 | 3 | |
| | | ≥60 | 4 | 4 |

Total Risk Score: 14

**Risk Categories**

| | |
|---|---|
| Very Low | 5 or less points |
| Low | Between 6 and 15 points |
| Moderate | Between 16 and 25 points |
| High | Between 26 and 35 points |
| Very High | 36 or more points |

**FIGURE 9.3** ◆ *Continued.*

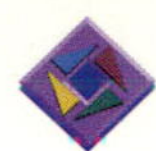

The significance of physical inactivity in contributing to cardiovascular risk was clearly shown in 1992 when the American Heart Association added physical inactivity as one of the four major risk factors for cardiovascular disease. The other three are smoking, a poor cholesterol profile, and high blood pressure. Based on the overwhelming amount of scientific data in this area, the evidence of the benefits of aerobic exercise in reducing heart disease is far too impressive to be ignored.

Research at the Institute for Aerobics Research in Dallas, Texas,[1] clearly shows the tie between cardiovascular fitness and mortality, regardless of age and other risk factors (see Figure 1.7 in Chapter 1 and Figures 9.9 and 9.10 in this chapter). A higher level of physical fitness benefits even those who have other risk factors such as high blood pressure, abnormal cholesterol, cigarette smoking, and a family history of heart disease. In most cases unfit people in the study (group 1) without these risk factors had higher death rates than fit people (groups 4 and 5) with these same risk factors.

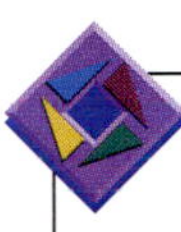

*Physical inactivity, smoking, a poor cholesterol profile, and high blood pressure are the four most significant risk factors for coronary heart disease.*

Although the findings show that the higher the level of cardiovascular fitness, the longer the life, the largest drop in premature death is seen between the unfit and the moderately fit groups. Even small improvements in cardiovascular endurance decrease the risk for cardiovascular mortality. Most adults who participate in a moderate exercise program can attain these fitness levels easily. The researchers recommended minimum exercise for adults to achieve moderate fitness. This minimum dose is presented in Figure 9.4.

Subsequent research published in 1993 in the *New England Journal of Medicine* substantiated the importance of exercise in preventing CHD.[2] Dr. Ralph Paffenbarger and his colleagues indicated that the benefits of starting a moderate to vigorous physical activity program (by previously inactive adults) were as important as quitting smoking, managing blood pressure, or controlling cholesterol. The increase in physical activity led to the same decrease as giving up cigarette smoking in relative risk for death from CHD.

Even though aerobically fit individuals have a lower incidence of cardiovascular disease, a regular aerobic exercise program by itself does not guarantee a lifetime free of cardiovascular problems. Poor lifestyle habits, such as smoking, eating too many fatty/salty/sweet foods, being overweight, and having high stress levels, increase cardiovascular risk and will not be eliminated completely through aerobic exercise.

Overall management of risk factors is the key to lowering the risk for cardiovascular disease. Still, aerobic exercise is one of the most important activities in preventing and reducing cardiovascular problems. The basic principles for cardiovascular exercise are given in Chapter 3.

## Abnormal Electrocardiogram

The electrocardiogram is a valuable measure of the heart's function. The ECG provides a record of the electrical impulses that stimulate the heart to contract (see Figure 9.5). In reading an ECG, five general areas are interpreted: heart rate, heart rhythm,

| | Activity | Distance (miles) | Time (min.) | Frequency (days/week) |
|---|---|---|---|---|
| **Women** | | | | |
| Program I: | Walking | 3 or more | 30 or less | 3 or more |
| Program II: | Walking | 2 | 30–40 | 5–6 |
| **Men** | | | | |
| Program I: | Walking | 2 | 27 or less | 3 or more |
| Program II: | Walking | 2 | 30–40 | 6–7 |

From *Fitness and Mortality* by S. N. Blair (Dallas: Aerobics Research Center, 1991).

**FIGURE 9.4** ◆ Minimum aerobic exercise dose for moderate fitness.

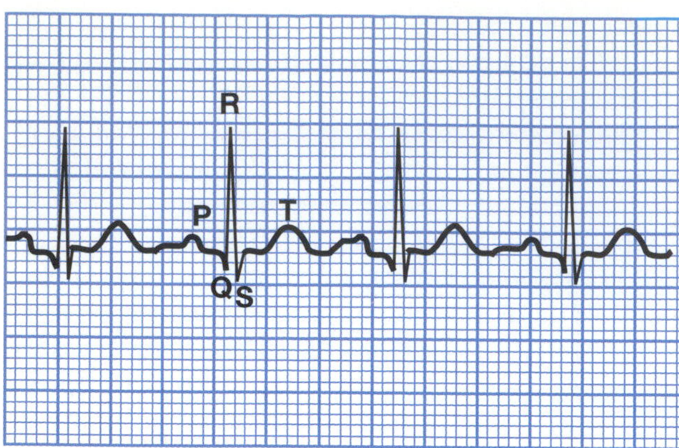


**FIGURE 9.5** ◆ Normal electrocardiogram.

axis of the heart, enlargement or hypertrophy of the heart, and myocardial infarction or heart attack.

On a standard 12-lead ECG, 10 electrodes are placed on the person's chest. From these 10 electrodes, 12 leads or "pictures" of the electrical impulses as they travel through the heart muscle (myocardium) are studied from 12 different positions. By looking at ECG tracings, abnormalities in heart functioning can be identified. Based on the findings, the ECG may be interpreted as normal, equivocal, or abnormal. An ECG will not always identify problems, so a normal tracing is not an absolute guarantee. On the other hand, an abnormal tracing does not necessarily signal a serious condition. The abnormality in Figure 9.6 is seen commonly during exercise in patients with CHD.

ECGs are taken at rest, during the stress of exercise, and during recovery. An exercise ECG also is known as a graded exercise stress test or a maximal exercise tolerance test. Similar to a high-speed test on a car, a *stress ECG* reveals the tolerance of the heart to increased physical activity. It is a much better test than a *resting ECG* to discover CHD.

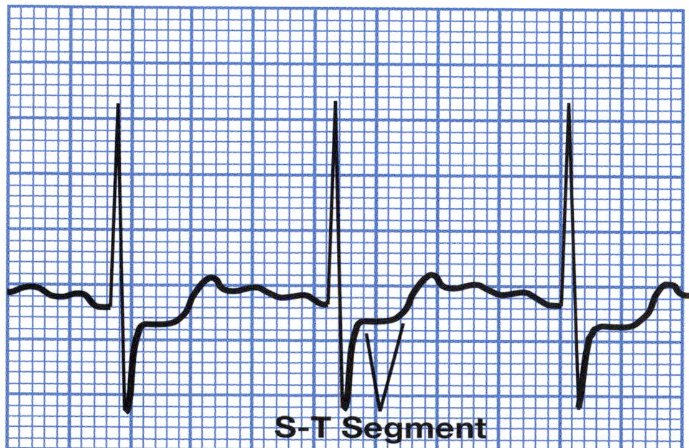


**FIGURE 9.6** ◆ Abnormal electrocardiogram showing depressed S-T segment.

Stress ECGs also are used to assess cardiovascular fitness levels, to screen persons for preventive and cardiac rehabilitation programs, to detect abnormal blood pressure response during exercise, and to establish actual or functional maximal heart rate for exercise prescription. The *recovery ECG* is another important diagnostic tool in monitoring the return of the heart's activity to normal conditions.

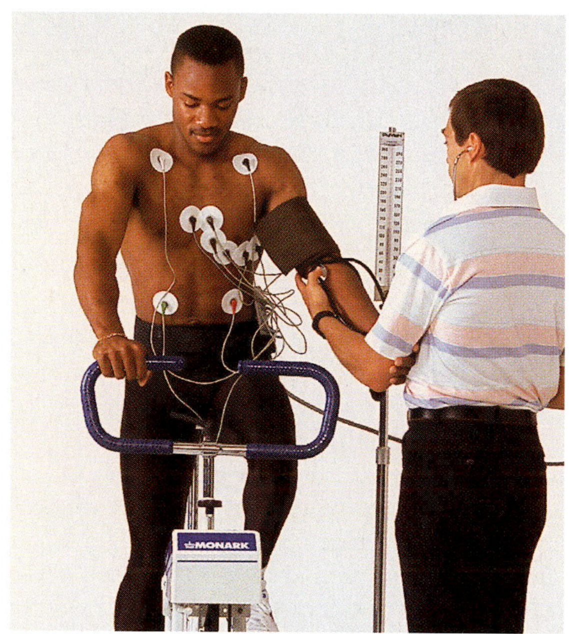


*Exercise tolerance test with 12-lead electrocardiographic monitoring (exercise stress-ECG).*

Not every adult who wishes to start or continue in an exercise program needs a stress ECG. It should be administered under the following guidelines:

1. Men over age 40 and women over age 50.
2. A total cholesterol level above 200 mg/dl or an HDL-cholesterol below 35 mg/dl.
3. Hypertensive and diabetic patients.
4. Cigarette smokers.
5. Individuals with a family history of CHD, syncope, or sudden death before age 60.
6. People with an abnormal resting ECG.

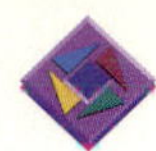

7. All individuals with symptoms of chest discomfort, dysrhythmias, syncope, or chronotropic incompetence (heart rate that increases slowly during exercise and never reaches maximum).

At times the stress ECG has been questioned as a reliable predictor of CHD, but it remains the most practical, inexpensive, noninvasive procedure available to diagnose latent (undiagnosed/ unknown) CHD. The test is accurate in diagnosing CHD about 65% of the time.

Part of the problem with reliability is that many times those who administer stress ECGs do it without clearly understanding the test's indications and limitations. Nevertheless, sensitivity of the test increases along with severity of the disease. The test also produces more accurate results in people who are at high risk for cardiovascular disease, in particular men over age 40 and women over 50 with a poor cholesterol profile, high blood pressure, or a family history of heart disease.

Test protocols, number of leads, electrocardiographic criteria, and the skill of technicians administering the test also affect its sensitivity. Despite its limitations, it is still a useful tool in identifying people who have high risk for exercise-related sudden death.

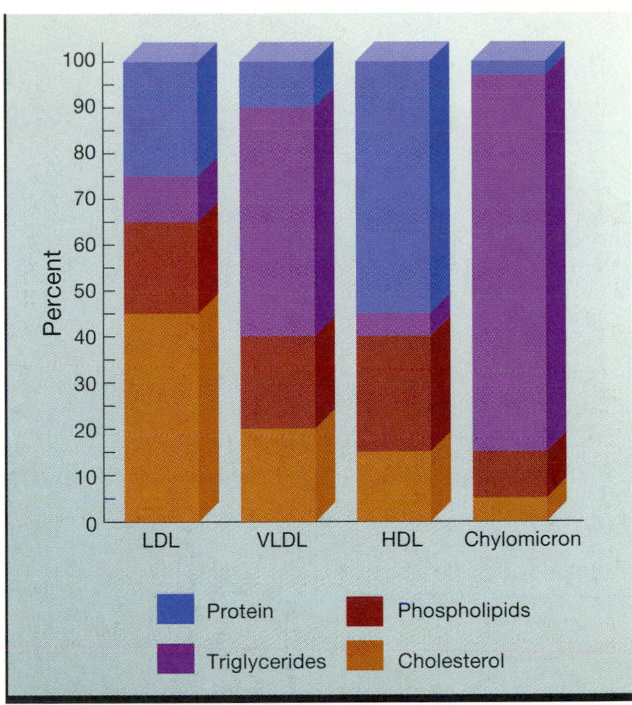


**FIGURE 9.7** ◆ Approximate content of the four major types of lipoproteins.

## Abnormal Cholesterol Profile

The term *blood lipids* (fats) is used mainly in reference to cholesterol and triglycerides. These lipids are carried in the bloodstream by molecules of protein known as high-density lipoproteins (HDLs), low-density lipoproteins (LDLs), very low-density lipoproteins (VLDLs), and chylomicrons (see Figure 9.7). Although subcategories of these lipoproteins have been identified recently, the discussion here focuses primarily on the four major categories.

Cholesterol has received much attention because direct relationships have been established between high total cholesterol, high LDL-cholesterol, low HDL-cholesterol, and the rate of CHD in men and women. Total blood cholesterol levels are considered too high in more than 65 million Americans.

Cholesterol is a waxy substance, technically a steroid alcohol, found only in animal fats and oil. This fatty substance is used in making cell membranes, as a building block for some hormones, in the fatty sheath around nerve fibers, and in other necessary substances.

An abnormal cholesterol profile contributes to atherosclerotic plaque, the buildup of fatty tissue in the walls of the arteries (see Figure 9.8). As the plaque builds up, it blocks the blood vessels that supply the heart muscle (myocardium) with oxygen and nutrients, and these obstructions can trigger a mycardial infarction or heart attack.

Unfortunately, the heart disguises its problems quite well, and typical symptoms of heart disease, such as angina pectoris or chest pain, do not start until the arteries are about 75% blocked. In many cases the first symptom is sudden death. Based on the research conducted at the Institute for Aerobics Research in Dallas, Texas, the relative risk for all causes of mortality by physical fitness and total cholesterol levels is given in Figure 9.9.

The general recommendation by the National Cholesterol Education Program (NCEP) is to keep total cholesterol levels below 200 mg/dl. Other health professionals recommend that total cholesterol in individuals age 30 and younger should not be higher than 180 mg/dl, and for children the level should be below 170mg/dl. Cholesterol levels between 200 and 239 mg/dl are borderline high, and levels of 240 mg/dl and above indicate high risk for disease (see Table 9.2).

Many practitioners of preventive medicine recommend a range between 160 and 180 mg/dl as

## THE ATHEROSCLEROTIC PROCESS

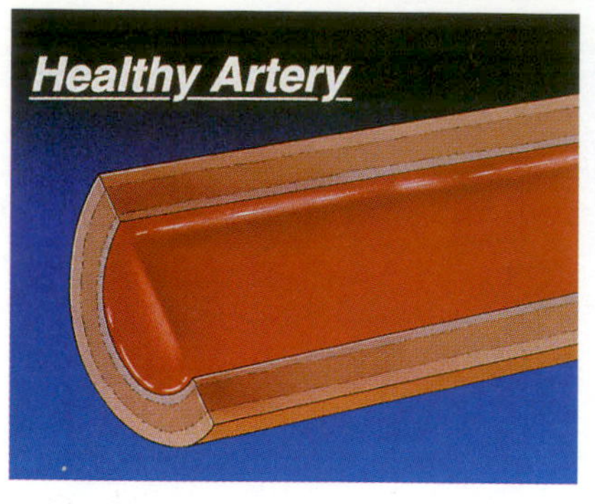


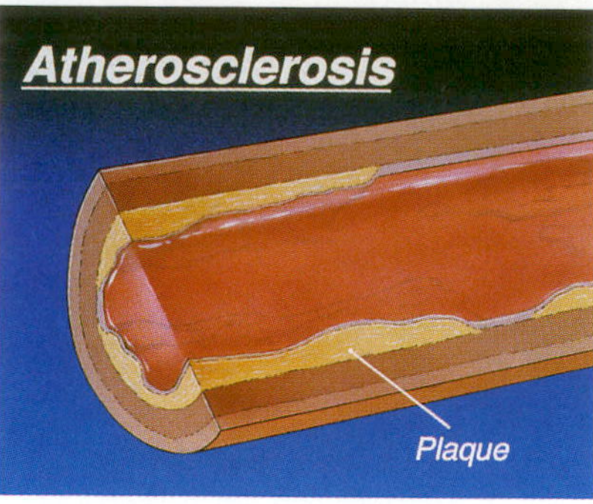


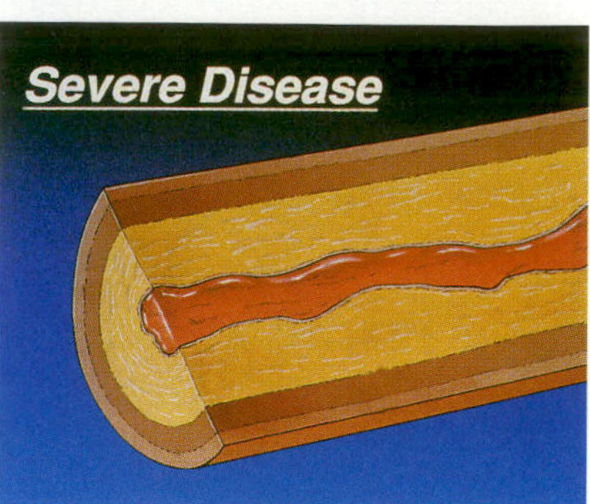


From *Heart of a Healthy Life*. Courtesy of the American Heart Association, © 1992.

**FIGURE 9.8** ◆

the ideal level of total cholesterol. In the Framingham Heart Study, a 40-year ongoing project in the community of Framingham, Massachusetts, not a single individual with a total cholesterol level of 125 mg/dl or lower has had a heart attack. Dr. William Castelli, director of the Framingham Study, recommends a total cholesterol level of less than 150 mg/dl for possible plaque regression in people with atherosclerosis.

As important as it is, total cholesterol no longer is the best predictor for cardiovascular risk. Many heart attacks occur in people with only slightly elevated total cholesterol. More significant is the way in which cholesterol is carried in the

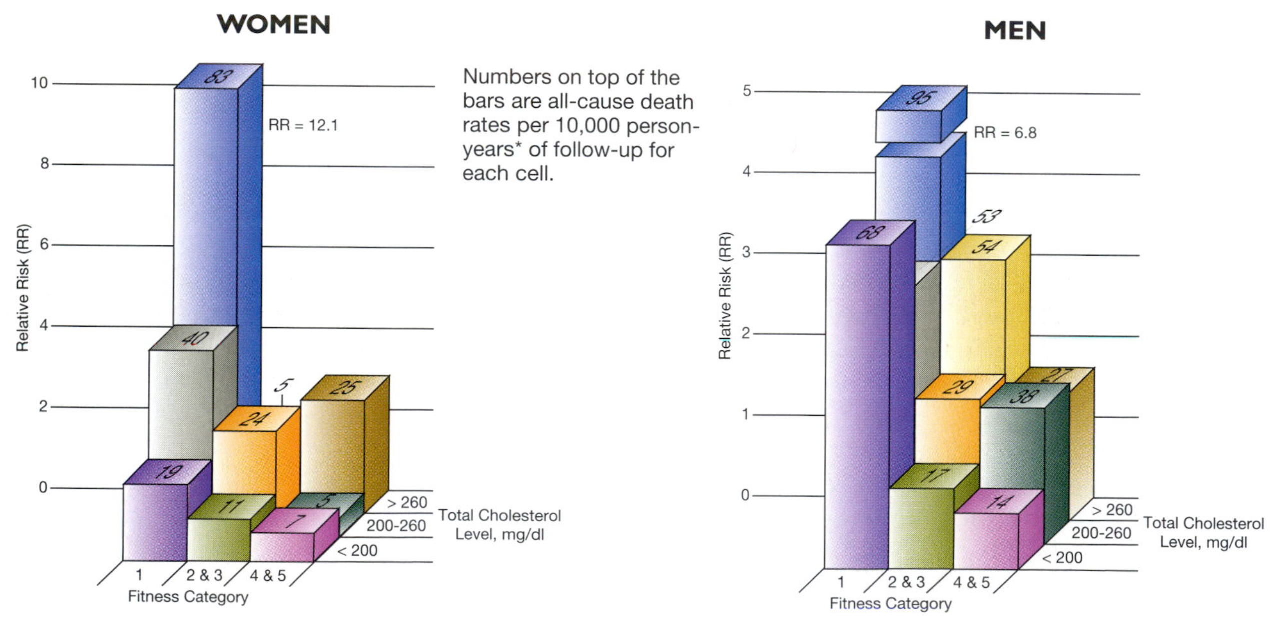


*One person-year indicates one person who was followed up one year later.

Source: *Physical Fitness and All-Cause Mortality: A Prospective Study of Healthy Men and Women*, by S. N. Blair, H. W. Kohl III, R. S. Paffenbarger, Jr., D. G. Clark, K. H. Cooper, and L. W. Gibbons, in *Journal of the American Medical Association,* 262 (1989), 2395–2401. © American Medical Association. Reproduced by permission.

**FIGURE 9.9** ◆ Relative risks of all-cause mortality by physical fitness and serum cholesterol level.

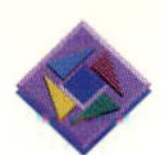

bloodstream. Cholesterol is transported primarily in the form of high-density lipoprotein cholesterol (HDL-cholesterol) and low-density lipoprotein cholesterol (LDL-cholesterol).

In a process known as *reverse cholesterol transport*, HDL molecules tend to attract cholesterol, which is carried to the liver, changed to bile, and eventually excreted in the stool. HDLs act as "scavengers," removing cholesterol from the body and preventing plaque from forming in the arteries. The strength of HDL is in the protein molecules found in their coatings. When HDL comes in contact with cholesterol-filled cells, these protein molecules attach to the cells and take their cholesterol.

LDL-cholesterol, on the other hand, tends to release cholesterol, which then may penetrate the lining of the arteries and speed up the process of atherosclerosis. The NCEP guidelines state that an LDL-cholesterol value below 130 mg/dl is desirable, between 130 and 159 mg/dl is borderline-high, and 160 mg/dl and above is high risk for cardiovascular disease. For people with atherosclerosis, Dr. William Castelli, director of the Framingham Study, recommends an LDL-cholesterol level of 90 mg/dl or lower. A recently discovered subcategory of LDL-cholesterol, a smaller and denser LDL particle, is noteworthy because this type of particle is a bigger culprit in atherosclerosis than the regular LDL particle.

The more HDL-cholesterol (particularly the subcategory $HDL_2$), the better. HDL-cholesterol, the "good cholesterol," offers some protection against heart disease. In fact, low levels of HDL-cholesterol could be the best predictor of CHD and may be more significant than the total value. A low level of HDL-cholesterol has the strongest relationship to CHD at all levels of total cholesterol, including levels below 200 mg/dl.[3]

Researchers at the 1988 annual American Heart Association meeting indicated that people with low total cholesterol (less than 200 mg/dl) and also low HDL-cholesterol (under 40 mg/dl) may have three times greater heart disease risk than those with high cholesterol but with good HDL-cholesterol levels. Other research based on 797 patients whose total cholesterol was less than 200mg/dl showed that 60% of the patients had heart disease, and almost 75% of this group had HDL-cholesterol levels below 40 mg/dl. The recommended HDL-cholesterol values to minimize the risk for CHD is 45 mg/dl or higher in men and 55 mg/dl or higher in women. HDL-cholesterol levels above 60 md/dl actually may reduce the risk for CHD. Guidelines for the various types of cholesterol are given in Table 9.2.

For the most part, HDL-cholesterol is determined genetically. Generally, women have higher levels than men. The female sex hormone estrogen tends to raise HDL, so premenopausal women have a much lower incidence of heart disease. Black children and adult Black men have higher values than Caucasians. HDL-cholesterol also decreases with age.

Increasing HDL-cholesterol improves the cholesterol profile and lessens the risk for CHD. Habitual aerobic exercise, weight loss, and quitting smoking raise HDL-cholesterol.[4] Beta-carotene[5] and drug therapy also promote higher HDL-cholesterol levels. Rapid weight loss, however, causes a drop

**TABLE 9.2**
**Cholesterol Guidelines**

| | Amount | | Rating |
|---|---|---|---|
| **Total Cholesterol** | <200 mg/dl | | Desirable |
| | 200–239 mg/dl | | Borderline high |
| | ≥240 mg/dl | | High risk |
| **LDL-Cholesterol** | <130 mg/dl | | Desirable |
| | 130-159 mg/dl | | Borderline high |
| | ≥160 mg/dl | | High risk |
| | **Men** | **Women** | |
| **HDL-Cholesterol** | ≥45 mg/dl | ≥55 mg/dl | Desirable |
| | 36–44 mg/dl | 46–54 mg/dl | Moderate risk |
| | ≤35 mg/dl | ≤45 mg/dl | High risk |

in HDL-cholesterol. Once weight loss stabilizes, HDL-cholesterol increases again, but it does not reach the pre-weight loss level.

HDL-cholesterol and a regular aerobic exercise program clearly are related. The intensity of exercise is not crucial, but rather the total amount of exercise is the key to change blood lipids. Exercising 30 minutes five times a week appears to be sufficient to alter the lipid profile (decrease LDL and increase HDL). Individual responses to aerobic exercise differ, but, generally, the more the exercise, the higher the HDL-cholesterol level.

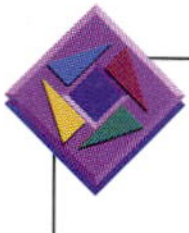

*Just thinking and planning an exercise program does not help raise HDL-cholesterol!*

Even when more LDL-cholesterol is present than the cells can use, cholesterol seems not to cause a problem until it is oxidized by free radicals. When oxidized, white blood cells invade the arterial wall, take up the cholesterol, and form the lesions that clog the arteries.

As discussed in Chapter 7, the antioxidant effect of vitamins C and E and beta-carotene can reduce the risk for CHD.[6] New information suggests that a single unstable free radical (oxygen compound produced in normal metabolism) can damage LDL particles. Vitamin C seems to inactivate free radicals, and vitamin E protects LDL from oxidation. Beta-carotene not only absorbs free radicals, keeping them from causing damage, but it also seems to increase HDL levels.

Certain cholesterol-lowering drugs also may help raise HDL levels. These agents include colestipol, niacin, cholestyramine, and gemfibrozil.[7] Cholesterol-lowering drugs decrease absorption in the intestines or block cholesterol formation by the cells. Some experts believe HDL levels below 40 mg/dl in combination with triglycerides above 150 mg/dl should be treated with medication.

Some authorities also believe the ratio of LDL-cholesterol to HDL-cholesterol is a strong indicator of potential risk for cardiovascular disease. An LDL-cholesterol to HDL-cholesterol ratio of 3.5 or lower is excellent for men, and 3.0 or lower is best for women. For instance, 50 mg/dl of HDL-cholesterol, as compared to 150 mg/dl of LDL-cholesterol, translates to a ratio of 3.0 ($150 \div 50 = 3.0$).

Although the average American consumes between 400 and 500 mg of cholesterol daily, the body actually manufactures more than that. Saturated fats raise cholesterol levels more than anything else in the diet. Saturated fats produce approximately 1000 mg of cholesterol per day.[8] Because of individual differences, some people can have a higher than normal intake of saturated fats and still maintain normal levels. Others who have a lower intake can have abnormally high levels.

Saturated fats are found mostly in meats and dairy products but seldom in foods of plant origin (see Table 9.3 and Figure 7.11 in Chapter 7). Poultry and fish contain less saturated fat than beef but should be eaten in moderation (about 3 to 6 ounces per day — see Chapter 7). Unsaturated fats are mainly of plant origin and cannot be converted to cholesterol.

If LDL-cholesterol is higher than ideal, it can be lowered by losing body fat, manipulating the diet, and taking medication. A diet low in fat, saturated fat, and cholesterol and high in fiber is recommended to decrease LDL-cholesterol. The NCEP recommends replacing saturated fat with monounsaturated fat (for example, olive, canola, peanut, and sesame oils), because the latter does not cause a reduction in HDL-cholesterol (also see the discussion on saturated fatty acids in Chapter 7).

Many experts believe that, to have a real effect in lowering LDL-cholesterol, total fat consumption must be much lower than the current 30% of total daily caloric intake guideline. Saturated fat consumption has to be under 10% of the total daily caloric intake, and the average cholesterol consumption should be much lower than 300 mg per day.

Research studies on the effects of a 30% fat diet have shown that it has little or no effect in lowering cholesterol, and that CHD actually continues to progress in people who have the disease.

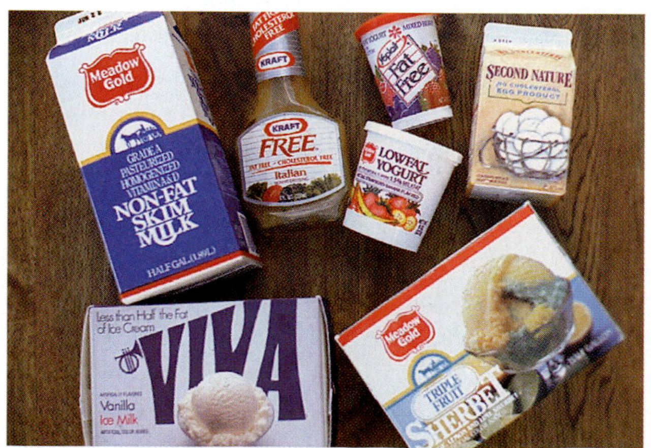


*Substituting low-fat for high-fat products in the diet decreases the risk for disease.*

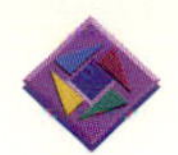

**TABLE 9.3**
**Cholesterol and Saturated Fat Content of Selected Foods**

| Food | Serving Size | Choles-terol (mg.) | Sat. Fat (gr.) |
|---|---|---|---|
| Avocado | 1/8 med. | — | 3.2 |
| Bacon | 2 slc. | 30 | 2.7 |
| Beans (all types) | any | — | — |
| Beef — Lean, fat trimmed off | 3 oz. | 75 | 6.0 |
| Beef — Heart (cooked) | 3 oz. | 150 | 1.6 |
| Beef — Liver (cooked) | 3 oz. | 255 | 1.3 |
| Butter | 1 tsp. | 12 | 0.4 |
| Caviar | 1 oz. | 85 | — |
| Cheese — American | 2 oz. | 54 | 11.2 |
| Cheese — Cheddar | 2 oz. | 60 | 12.0 |
| Cheese — Cottage (1% fat) | 1 cup | 10 | 0.4 |
| Cheese — Cottage (4% fat) | 1 cup | 31 | 6.0 |
| Cheese — Cream | 2 oz. | 62 | 6.0 |
| Cheese — Muenster | 2 oz. | 54 | 10.8 |
| Cheese — Parmesan | 2 oz. | 38 | 9.3 |
| Cheese — Swiss | 2 oz. | 52 | 10.0 |
| Chicken (no skin) | 3 oz. | 45 | 0.4 |
| Chicken — Liver | 3 oz. | 472 | 1.1 |
| Chicken — Thigh, Wing | 3 oz. | 69 | 3.3 |
| Egg (yolk) | 1 | 250 | 1.8 |
| Frankfurter | 2 | 90 | 11.2 |
| Fruits | any | — | — |
| Grains (all types) | any | — | — |
| Halibut, Flounder | 3 oz. | 43 | 0.7 |
| Ice Cream | 1/2 cup | 27 | 4.4 |
| Lamb | 3 oz. | 60 | 7.2 |
| Lard | 1 tsp. | 5 | 1.9 |
| Lobster | 3 oz. | 170 | 0.5 |
| Margarine (all vegetable) | 1 tsp. | — | 0.7 |
| Mayonnaise | 1 tbsp. | 10 | 2.1 |
| Milk — Skim | 1 cup | 5 | 0.3 |
| Milk — Low Fat (2%) | 1 cup | 18 | 2.9 |
| Milk — Whole | 1 cup | 34 | 5.1 |
| Nuts | 1 oz. | — | 1.0 |
| Oysters | 3 oz. | 42 | — |
| Salmon | 3 oz. | 30 | 0.8 |
| Scallops | 3 oz. | 29 | — |
| Sherbet | 1/2 cup | 7 | 1.2 |
| Shrimp | 3 oz. | 128 | 0.1 |
| Trout | 3 oz. | 45 | 2.1 |
| Tuna (canned — drained) | 3 oz. | 55 | — |
| Turkey — Dark Meat | 3 oz. | 60 | 0.6 |
| Turkey — Light Meat | 3 oz. | 50 | 0.4 |
| Vegetables (except avocado) | any | — | — |

The good news comes from a 1991 study published in the *Archives of Internal Medicine.*[9] Men and women in the study lowered their cholesterol by an average of 23% in only 3 weeks following a 10% or less fat-calorie diet combined with a regular aerobic exercise program, primarily walking. In this diet cholesterol intake was lower than 25 mg/day. The author of the study concluded that the exact percent-fat guideline (10% or 15%) is unknown (it also varies from individual to individual), but that 30% total fat calories is definitely too high when attempting to lower cholesterol.

A daily 10%-total-fat diet requires the person to limit fat intake to an absolute minimum. Some health-care professionals contend that a diet like this is difficult to follow in definitely. People with high cholesterol levels, however, may not need to follow that diet indefinitely but should adopt the 10%-fat diet while attempting to lower cholesterol. Thereafter, eating a 30%-fat-diet may be adequate to maintain recommended cholesterol levels (1991 national data indicate that current fat consumption in the United States averages 37% of total calories; see Figure 7.7, Chapter 7).

A drawback of very low fat diets (less than 25% fat) is that they tend to lower HDL-cholesterol and increase triglycerides. If HDL-cholesterol is already low, monounsaturated fat should be added to the diet. Olive oil and nuts are sample food items that are high in monounsaturated fat. A specialized nutrition book should be consulted to determine food items that are high in monounsaturated fat.

To lower LDL-cholesterol levels, the following general dietary guidelines are recommended:

1. Consume fewer than three eggs per week.
2. Eat red meats (3 ounces per serving) fewer than three times per week, and no organ meats (such as liver and kidneys).
3. Do not eat commercially baked foods.
4. Drink lowfat milk (1% or less fat, preferably) and lowfat dairy products.
5. Do not use coconut oil, palm oil, or cocoa butter.
6. Eat fish instead of red meat.
7. Bake, broil, grill, poach, or steam food instead of frying.
8. Refrigerate cooked meat before adding to other dishes. Remove fat hardened in the refrigerator before mixing the meat with other foods.

9. Avoid fatty sauces made with butter, cream, or cheese.
10. Maintain recommended body weight.

A combination of a healthy diet, a sound aerobic exercise program, and weight control is the best prescription for controlling blood lipids. If this does not work, a physician can administer a blood test to break down the lipoproteins into their various subcategories. Most U. S. laboratories do not conduct these tests. The American Heart Association, however, has established six Lipid Disorder Training Centers that administer comprehensive blood tests. Your local American Heart Association can provide further information.

The NCEP guidelines recommend that people consider drug therapy if, after 6 months on a low-cholesterol, low-fat diet, cholesterol remains unacceptably high. An unacceptable level is above 190 mg/dl for people with fewer than two risk factors and no signs of heart disease. For people with more than two risk factors and with a history of heart disease, LDL-cholesterol above 160 mg/dl is unacceptable.

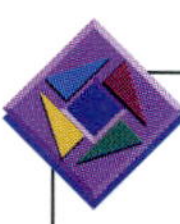

*A healthy diet, a sound aerobic exercise program, and weight control is the best prescription for controlling blood lipids.*

## Elevated Triglycerides

Triglycerides are also known as *free fatty acids*. In combination with cholesterol, triglycerides speed up formation of plaque in the arteries. They appear to be a more significant CHD risk factor in women than in men. Triglycerides are carried in the bloodstream primarily by very low-density lipoproteins (VLDLs) and chylomicrons.

Although they are found in poultry skin, lunch meats, and shellfish, these fatty acids are manufactured mainly in the liver, from refined sugars, starches, and alcohol. High intake of alcohol and sugars (honey included) significantly raises triglyceride levels. Triglycerides can be lowered by cutting down on these foods along with reducing weight (if overweight) and doing aerobic exercise. An optimal blood triglyceride level is less than 125mg/dl (see Table 9.4).

**TABLE 9.4**
**Triglycerides Guidelines**

| Amount | Rating |
|---|---|
| ≤125 mg/dl | Desirable |
| 126–499 mg/dl | Borderline high |
| ≥500 mg/dl | High risk |

Some people consistently have slightly elevated triglyceride levels (above 140 mg/dl) and HDL-cholesterol levels below 35 mg/dl. About 80% of these people have a genetic condition called LDL phenotype B (approximately 40% of the U. S. population falls in this category). Although the blood lipids may not be notably high, these people are at higher risk for atherosclerosis and CHD.[10]

People who have never had a blood chemistry test should do so, to establish a baseline for future reference. The blood test should include the HDL-cholesterol component.

No definitive guidelines have been set forth, but if the person follows an initial normal baseline test and adheres to the recommended dietary and exercise guidelines, a blood analysis every 3 years prior to age of 40 should suffice. Thereafter, a blood lipid test is recommended every year, in conjunction with a regular preventive medicine physical examination.

A single baseline test is not necessarily a valid measure. Cholesterol levels vary from month to month and sometimes even from day to day. If the first test reveals cholesterol abnormalities, the test should be repeated within a few weeks to confirm the results.

## Diabetes

Diabetes mellitus is a condition in which the blood glucose is unable to enter the cells because the pancreas either totally stops producing insulin or does not produce enough to meet the body's needs. As a result, glucose absorption by the cells and the liver is low, leading to high glucose levels in the blood.

The incidence of cardiovascular disease and death in the diabetic population is quite high. People with chronically high blood glucose levels also may have problems metabolizing fats, making them more susceptible to atherosclerosis, increasing the risk for coronary disease and contributing to other conditions such as vision loss and kidney damage.

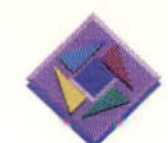

Fasting blood glucose levels above 120 mg/dl may be an early sign of diabetes and should be brought to a physician's attention. Many health care practitioners consider blood glucose levels around 150 to 160 mg/dl as borderline diabetes (see Table 9.5).

**TABLE 9.5**
**Blood Glucose Guidelines**

| Amount | Rating |
|---|---|
| ≤120 | Desirable |
| 121-159 | Borderline high |
| ≥160 | High |

Diabetes is of two types:

1. Type I, or insulin-dependent diabetes
2. Type II, or non-insulin-dependent diabetes.

Type I also is called *juvenile diabetes* because it is found mainly in young people. In insulin-dependent diabetes, the pancreas produces little or no insulin. In Type II, often referred to as *adult-onset diabetes*, the insulin-producing cells function adequately but the body is unable to use insulin correctly.

Although some people have a genetic predisposition to diabetes, adult-onset diabetes is related closely to overeating, obesity, and lack of physical activity. Approximately 70% of Type II diabetics are overweight or have a history of obesity. In most cases this condition can be corrected through a special diet, a weight-loss program, and a regular exercise program. A diet high in water-soluble fibers (found in fruits, vegetables, oats, and beans) is helpful in treating diabetes. A simple aerobic exercise program (walking, cycling, or swimming four to five times a week) often is prescribed because it makes the body more sensitive to insulin. Individuals who have high blood glucose levels should consult a physician to decide on the best treatment.

According to research published in 1991 in the *New England Journal of Medicine*,[11] aerobic exercise helps prevent diabetes in middle-aged men. The protective effect is even greater in those with risk factors such as obesity, high blood pressure, and family propensity.

The preventive effect is attributed to less body fat and better sugar and fat metabolism resulting from the regular exercise program. At 3,500 calories per week, the risk was cut in half, as compared to sedentary men. This preventive effect, according to one of the authors of the study, should hold for women, too.

## Hypertension

Some 60,000 miles of blood vessels run through the human body. As the heart forces the blood through these vessels, the fluid is under pressure. Blood pressure is a measure of the force exerted against the walls of the vessels by the blood flowing through them.

Blood pressure is assessed using a sphygmomanometer and a stethoscope. The sphygmomanometer consists of an inflatable bladder contained within a cuff and a mercury gravity manometer or an aneroid manometer from which the pressure is read. The pressure is measured in milliliters of mercury (mmHg), usually expressed in two numbers. The higher number reflects the pressure exerted during the forceful contraction of the heart or systole (therefore, the term systolic pressure), and the lower pressure is taken during the heart's relaxation, or diastolic phase, when no blood is being ejected. Ideal blood pressure is 120/80 or below (see Table 9.6).

**TABLE 9.6**
**Blood Pressure Guidelines**

| Rating | Systolic | Diastolic |
|---|---|---|
| Ideal | ≤120 | ≤80 mmHg |
| Borderline high | 121–139 | 81–89 mmHg |
| Hypertension | ≥140 | ≥90 mmHg |

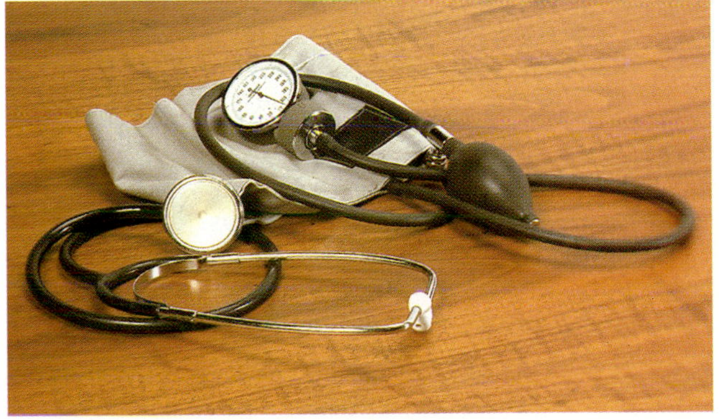

*Aneroid blood pressure gauge and stethoscope.*

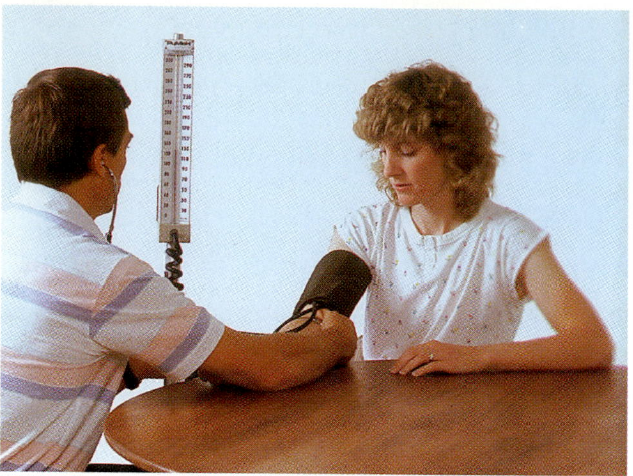

*Blood pressure assessment using a mercury gravity manometer.*

The procedure for blood pressure assessment is outlined in Appendix D. If blood pressure equipment is available, you should take the opportunity to assess your blood pressure in the near future. A form to record your blood pressure readings is also provided in Appendix D (see Figure D.1).

### Standards

A few years ago a systolic pressure of 100 plus your age was the acceptable standard. Hypertension was viewed as the point at which the pressure doubled the mortality risk, about 160/96. Readings between 140/90 and 160/96 (either number being in that range) were classified as mild hypertension.

This is no longer the case. Statistical evidence now indicates that blood pressure readings above 140/90 increase the risk for disease and premature death. Consequently, all blood pressures above 140/90 are viewed as hypertension.

Even though the threshold for hypertension has been set at 140/90, many experts believe that the lower the blood pressure, the better. Even if the pressure is around 90/50, as long as that person does not have any symptoms of low blood pressure, or *hypotension*, he or she need not be concerned. Typical hypotension symptoms are dizziness, light-headedness, and fainting.

Blood pressure also may fluctuate during a regular day. Many factors affect blood pressure, and one single reading may not be a true indicator of your real pressure. For example, physical activity and stress raise blood pressure, and rest and relaxation lower it. Consequently, several measurements should be taken before diagnosing high pressure.

Based on 1994 estimates by the American Heart Association, nearly 50 million Americans aged 6 and older are hypertensive. As a disease, hypertension has been referred to as "the silent killer." It does not hurt, it does not make you feel sick, and, unless you check it, years may go by before you even realize you have a problem. High blood pressure is a risk factor not only for CHD but also for congestive heart failure, stroke, and kidney failure. The relative risk for all-cause mortality by systolic blood pressure and various fitness levels is shown in Figure 9.10.

### What Makes Hypertension a Killer

All inner walls of arteries are lined by a layer of smooth endothelial cells. Blood lipids cannot penetrate the lining and build up unless damage is done to the cells. High blood pressure is thought to be a leading contributor to destruction of this lining. As blood pressure rises, so does the risk for atherosclerosis. The higher the pressure, the greater is the damage to the arterial wall, making the vessels susceptible to fat deposits, especially if serum cholesterol also is high. Blockage of the coronary vessels decreases blood supply to the heart muscle and can lead to a heart attack. When brain arteries are involved, a stroke may follow.

A clear example of the connection between high blood pressure and atherosclerosis can be seen by comparing blood vessels in the human body. Even when atherosclerosis is present throughout major arteries, fatty plaques rarely are seen in the pulmonary artery, which goes from the right part of the heart to the lungs. The pressure in this artery normally is below 40 mmHg, and at such low pressure significant deposits do not occur. This is one of the reasons people with low blood pressure have a lower incidence of cardiovascular disease.

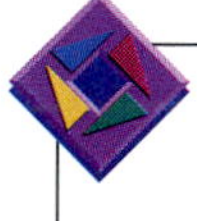

*High blood pressure is a risk factor for coronary heart disease, congestive heart failure, stroke, and kidney failure.*

Constant high blood pressure also causes the heart to work much harder. At first the heart does well, but in time this continual strain produces an enlarged heart, followed by congestive heart failure. Furthermore, high blood pressure damages blood vessels to the kidneys and eyes, which may result in kidney failure and loss of vision.

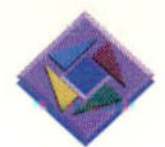

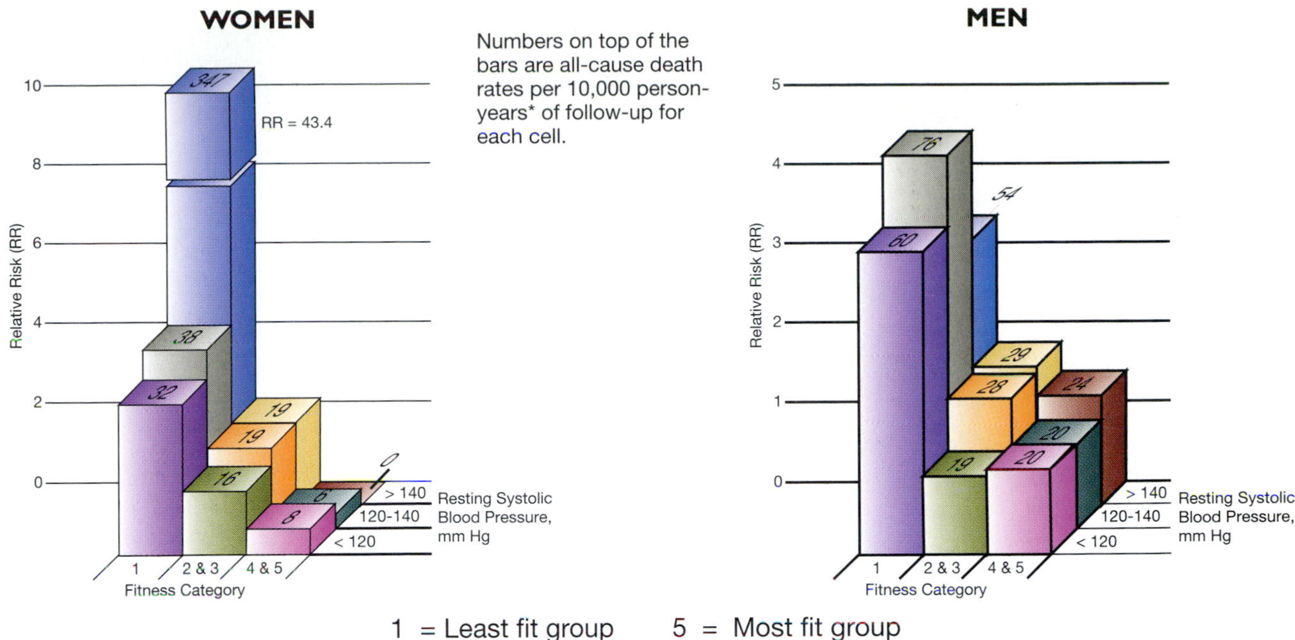


Source: *Physical Fitness and All-Cause Mortality: A Prospective Study of Healthy Men and Women*, by S. N. Blair, H. W. Kohl III, R. S. Paffenbarger, Jr., D. G. Clark, K. H. Cooper, and L. W. Gibbons, in *Journal of the American Medical Association*, 262 (1989), 239–240. © American Medical Association. Reproduced by permission.

**FIGURE 9.10** ◆ Relative risks of all-cause mortality by physical fitness and systolic blood pressure.

### Treatment

Of all hypertension, 90% has no definite cause. Referred to as *essential hypertension*, this type is treatable. Effective treatments include aerobic exercise, weight reduction, a low-sodium/ high-potassium diet, reduction in stress, no smoking, a diet designed to lower blood lipids, lower caffeine and alcohol intake, and antihypertensive medication. The remaining 10% of hypertensive cases is caused by pathological conditions such as narrowing of the kidney arteries, glomerulonephritis (a kidney disease), tumors of the adrenal glands, and narrowing of the aortic artery. With this type of hypertension, the pathological cause has to be treated before the blood pressure problem can be corrected.

Antihypertensive medicines often are the first choice of treatment, but they produce many side effects, including lethargy, sleepiness, sexual difficulties, higher blood cholesterol and glucose levels, lower potassium levels, and elevated uric acid levels. A physician may end up treating these side effects as much as the hypertension itself. Because of the multiple side effects, about half of the patients stop taking the medication within the first year of treatment.

Another factor contributing to high blood pressure is too much sodium in the diet (salt, or sodium chloride, contains approximately 40% sodium). With high sodium intake the body retains more water, which increases the blood volume and, in turn, drives up the pressure. On the other hand, high intake of potassium seems to regulate water retention and lower the pressure slightly.

Although sodium is essential for normal body functions, the body can function with as little as 200 mg, or a tenth of a teaspoon daily. Even under strenuous conditions of job and sports participation that incite heavy perspiration, the amount of sodium required seldom is more than 3,000 mg per day. Yet, sodium intake in the typical American diet ranges between 6,000 and 20,000 mg per day!

In underdeveloped countries and American Indian tribes where no salt is used in cooking or added at the table, and the only sodium comes from food in its natural form, daily intake rarely is more than 2,000 mg. Blood pressure in these people does not increase with age, and hypertension is practically unknown. These findings suggest that the human body may be able to handle 2,000 mg per day, but intakes higher than that over the years may cause a gradual rise in blood pressure.

Where does all the sodium come from? The answer is found in Table 9.7. Most people do not realize the amount of sodium in various foods (the list in Table 9.7 does not include salt added at the table).

When treating high blood pressure (unless it is extremely high), before recommending medication many sports medicine physicians recommend a combination of aerobic exercise, weight loss, and less sodium in the diet. In most instances this treatment brings blood pressure under control.

The link between hypertension and obesity has been well-established. Not only does blood volume increase with excess body fat, but every additional pound of fat requires an estimated extra mile of blood vessels to feed this tissue. Furthermore, blood capillaries are constricted by the adipose tissues as these vessels run through them. As a result, the heart muscle must work harder to pump the blood through a longer, constricted network of blood vessels.

The role of aerobic exercise in managing blood pressure is becoming more important each day. On the average, cardiovascularly fit individuals have lower blood pressures than unfit people do. An 18-year follow-up study[12] on exercising and nonexercising subjects showed much lower blood pressures in the active group. The exercise group had an average resting blood pressure of 120/78 as compared to 150/90 for the nonexercise group (see Table 9.8).

Aerobic exercise often is prescribed for hypertensive

**TABLE 9.7**
**Sodium and Potassium Levels of Selected Foods**

| Food | Serving Size | Sodium (mg) | Potassium (mg) |
|---|---|---|---|
| Apple | 1 med. | 1 | 182 |
| Asparagus | 1 cup | 2 | 330 |
| Avocado | 1/2 | 4 | 680 |
| Banana | 1 med. | 1 | 440 |
| Bologna | 3 oz. | 1,107 | 133 |
| Bouillon Cube | 1 | 960 | 4 |
| Cantaloupe | 1/4 | 17 | 341 |
| Carrot (raw) | 1 | 34 | 225 |
| Cheese | | | |
| American | 2 oz. | 614 | 93 |
| Cheddar | 2 oz. | 342 | 56 |
| Muenster | 2 oz. | 356 | 77 |
| Parmesan | 2 oz. | 1,056 | 53 |
| Swiss | 2 oz. | 148 | 64 |
| Chicken (light meat) | 6 oz. | 108 | 700 |
| Corn (canned) | 1/2 cup | 195 | 80 |
| Corn (natural) | 1/2 cup | 3 | 136 |
| Frankfurter | 1 | 627 | 136 |
| Haddock | 6 oz. | 300 | 594 |
| Hamburger (reg) | 1 | 500 | 321 |
| Lamb (leg) | 6 oz. | 108 | 700 |
| Milk (whole) | 1 cup | 120 | 351 |
| Milk (skim) | 1 cup | 126 | 406 |
| Orange | 1 med. | 1 | 263 |
| Orange Juice | 1 cup | 1 | 200 |
| Peach | 1 med. | 2 | 308 |
| Pear | 1 med. | 2 | 130 |
| Peas (canned) | 1/2 cup | 200 | 82 |
| Peas (boiled-natural) | 1/2 cup | 2 | 178 |
| Pizza (cheese - 14" diam.) | 1/8 | 456 | 85 |
| Potato | 1 med. | 6 | 763 |
| Potato Chips | 10 | 150 | 226 |
| Potato (french fries) | 10 | 5 | 427 |
| Pork | 6 oz. | 96 | 438 |
| Roast Beef | 6 oz. | 98 | 448 |
| Salami | 3 oz. | 1,047 | 170 |
| Salmon (canned) | 6 oz. | 198 | 756 |
| Salt | 1 tsp. | 2,132 | 0 |
| Soups | | | |
| Chicken Noodle | 1 cup | 979 | 55 |
| Clam Chowder (New England) | 1 cup | 914 | 146 |
| Cream of Mushroom | 1 cup | 955 | 98 |
| Vegetable Beef | 1 cup | 1,046 | 162 |
| Soy Sauce | 1 tsp. | 1,123 | 22 |
| Spaghetti (tomato sauce and cheese) | 6 oz. | 648 | 276 |
| Strawberries | 1 cup | 1 | 244 |
| Tomato (raw) | 1 med. | 3 | 444 |
| Tuna (drained) | 3 oz. | 38 | 255 |

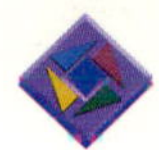

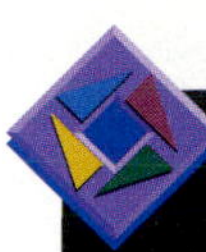

**TABLE 9.8**
**Effects of a Regular Aerobic Exercise Program* on Resting Blood Pressure**

| | Initial | Final |
|---|---|---|
| **Exercise Group** | | |
| Age | 44.6 | 68.0 |
| Blood Pressure | 120/79 | 120/78 |
| **Nonexercise Group** | | |
| Age | 51.6 | 69.7 |
| Blood Pressure | 135/85 | 150/90 |

* The aerobic exercise program consisted of an average four training sessions per week, each 66 minutes long, at about 76 percent of heart rate reserve.

Based on data from "The Effect of Physical Activity on Aerobic Power in Older Men (A Longitudinal Study)," by F. W. Kash, J. L. Boyer, S. P. Van Camp, L. S. Verity, and J. P. Wallace. *Physician and Sports Medicine,* 18:4 (1990), 73–83 (an 18-year follow-up study).

patients. Several well-documented studies have shown that nearly 90% of hypertensive patients who begin a moderate aerobic exercise program can expect a notable decrease in blood pressure after only a few weeks of training. The research data also show that exercise, not weight loss, is the main contributor to the lowered blood pressure of exercisers. If aerobic exercise is discontinued, these changes are not maintained.

Research presented by Dr. Larry Gibbons (Institute for Aerobics Research, Dallas, Texas) at the 1990 American College of Sports Medicine meeting also indicates that exercise programs for hypertensive patients should be of moderate intensity. Training at about 50% of heart rate reserve seems to have the same effect in lowering blood pressure as training at a 70% heart rate reserve. High-intensity training in hypertensive patients actually may cause the blood pressure to rise slightly. Even so, a person may be better off to be highly fit and have high blood pressure than to be unfit and have low blood pressure. As illustrated in Figure 9.10, the death rates for unfit individuals with low systolic blood pressure are much higher than highly fit people with high systolic blood pressure.

Most important is a preventive approach. Keeping blood pressure under control is easier than trying to bring it down once it is high. Regardless of your past blood pressure history, high or low, you should check it routinely. Regular physical exercise, weight control, a low-salt diet, no smoking, and stress management are the keys to controlling blood pressure.

Those who are taking medication for hypertension should not stop unless the prescribing physician gives the go-ahead. If it is not treated properly, high blood pressure can kill. By combining medication with the other treatments, drug therapy eventually maybe reduced or completely eliminated.

## Excessive Body Fat

Body composition refers to the ratio of lean body weight to fat weight. If the body contains too much fat, the person is considered obese (see guidelines in Chapter 6, Table 6.8).

Obesity has long been recognized as a risk factor for CHD. Until a few years ago experts believed that CHD actually was brought on by some of the other risk factors that usually accompany obesity (higher cholesterol and triglycerides, hypertension, diabetes, lower level of cardiovascular fitness). More recent evidence, however, suggests that too much body fat is a coronary risk factor in and of itself. Even when all of the other risk factors are in good range, people with high body fat have a higher incidence of cardiovascular disease.

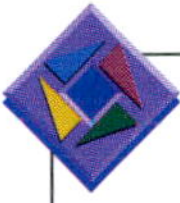

*The only sure way to lose body fat and keep it off is through a healthy diet accompanied by a lifetime aerobic and strength-training program.*

Attaining recommended body composition is important not only in lowering the risk for cardiovascular disease but also in reaching a better state of health and wellness. The only positive thing that can be said about too much body fat is that it can be lost through a combination of diet and exercise. Dieting by itself seldom works.

If you have a weight problem and want to get down to you recommended weight, you must:

1. Increase your physical activity and participate in aerobic and strength-training programs.
2. Follow a diet low in fat and refined sugars and high in complex carbohydrates and fiber.
3. Reduce your total caloric intake moderately while still getting the necessary nutrients to sustain normal body functions.

Additional recommendations for weight reduction and weight control are discussed in Chapter 8.

## Smoking

More than 48 million adults and 3.5 million adolescents in the United States smoke. Cigarette smoking is the single largest preventable cause of illness and premature death in the United States. Smoking has been linked to cardiovascular disease, cancer, bronchitis, emphysema, and peptic ulcers. In relation to coronary disease, not only does smoking speed up the process of atherosclerosis, but it also carries a threefold increase in the risk of sudden death following a myocardial infarction.

Smoking prompts the release of nicotine and some other 1,200 toxic compounds into the bloodstream. Similar to hypertension, many of these substances are destructive to the inner membrane that protects the walls of the arteries. As mentioned, once the lining is damaged, cholesterol and triglycerides can be deposited readily in the arterial wall (see Figure 9.11). As the plaque builds up, it obstructs blood flow through the arteries.

Furthermore, smoking encourages the formation of blood clots, which can completely block an artery already narrowed by atherosclerosis. In addition, carbon monoxide, a by product of cigarette smoke, decreases the blood's oxygen-carrying capacity. A combination of obstructed arteries, less oxygen, and nicotine in the heart muscle heightens the risk for a serious heart problem.

Smoking also increases heart rate, raises blood pressure, and irritates the heart, which can trigger fatal cardiac arrhythmias (irregular heart rhythms). Another harmful effect is a decrease in HDL-cholesterol, the "good" type that helps control blood lipids. Smoking actually presents a much greater risk of death from heart disease than from lung disease.

Pipe and cigar smoking and chewing tobacco also increase the risk for heart disease. Even if the smoker inhales no smoke, he or she absorbs toxic substances through the membranes of the mouth, and these end up in the bloodstream. Individuals who use tobacco in any of these three forms also have a much greater risk for cancer of the oral cavity.

The risk for both cardiovascular disease and cancer starts to decrease the moment you quit smoking. The risk approaches that of a lifetime nonsmoker 10 and 15 years, respectively, after quitting. A more thorough discussion of the harmful effects of cigarette smoking, the benefits of quitting, and a complete program for quitting are detailed in Chapter 12.

## Tension and Stress

Tension and stress have become a part of life. Everyone has to deal daily with goals, deadlines, responsibilities, pressures. Almost everything in life (whether positive or negative) is a source of stress. The stressor itself is not what creates the health hazard but, rather, the individual's response to it.

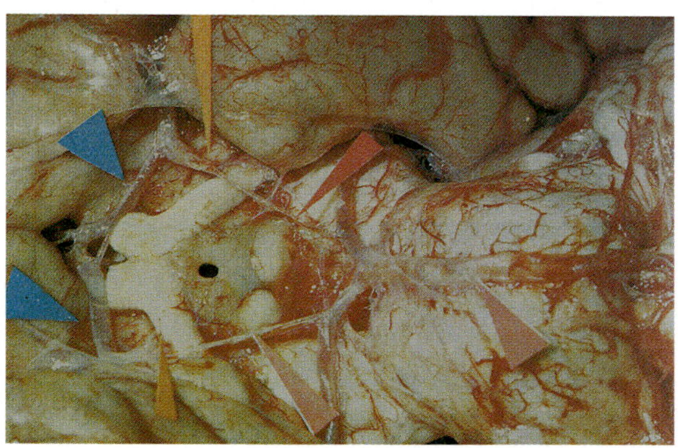

Healthy artery

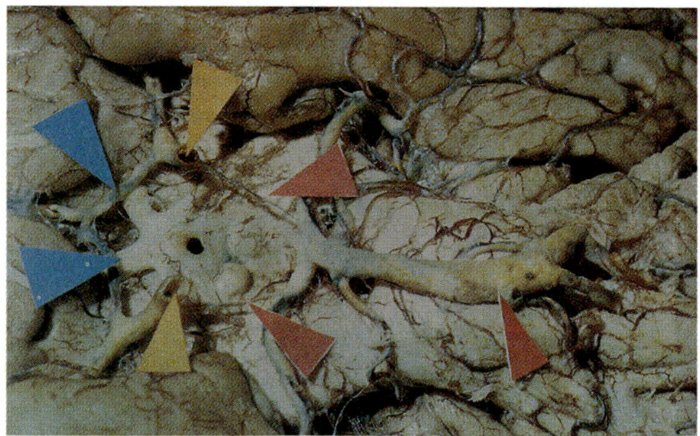

Obstruction of the same artery by fatty substances in a chronic smoker

Reproduced by permission from "If You Smoke" slide show by Gordon Hewlett.

**FIGURE 9.11** ◆ Comparison of normal and atherosclerotic arteries at the base of the brain.

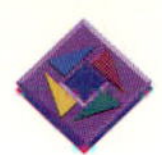

The human body responds to stress by producing more catecholamines (hormones) to prepare the body for "fight or flight." These hormones increase heart rate, blood pressure, and blood glucose levels, enabling the person to take action. If the person fights or flees, higher levels of catecholamines are metabolized and the body is able to return to a normal state. If, however, a person is under constant stress and unable to take action (as in the death of a close relative or friend, loss of a job, trouble at work, financial insecurity), the catecholamines remain high in the bloodstream.

People who are not able to relax place a constant low-level strain on the cardiovascular system that could manifest itself in heart disease. In addition, when a person is in a stressful situation, the coronary arteries that feed the heart muscle constrict, reducing the oxygen supply to the heart. If the blood vessels are largely blocked by atherosclerosis, abnormal heart rhythms or even a heart attack may follow.

Individuals who are under a lot of stress and do not cope well with it need to take measures to counteract the effects of stress in their lives. One way is to identify the sources of stress and learn how to cope with them. People need to take control of themselves, examine and act upon the things that are most important in their lives, and ignore less meaningful details.

Physical activity is one of the best ways to relieve stress.When a person takes part in physical activity, the body metabolizes excess catecholamines and is able to return to a normal state. Exercise also steps up muscular activity, which contributes to muscular relaxation after completing the physical activity.

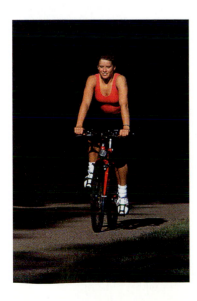

*Physical activity, one of the best ways to relieve stress.*

Many executives in large cities are choosing the evening hours for their physical activity program, stopping after work at the health or fitness club. In doing this, they are able to "burn up" the excess tension accumulated during the day and enjoy the evening hours. This has proven to be one of the best stress management techniques. More information on stress control is presented in Chapter 11.

## Personal and Family History

Individuals who have had cardiovascular problems are at higher risk than those who have never had a problem. People with this history should control the other risk factors as much as they can. Most risk factors are reversible, so this will greatly decrease the risk for future problems. The more time that has passed since the cardiovascular problem occurred, the lower is the risk for recurrence.

Genetic predisposition toward heart disease has been demonstrated clearly and seems to be gaining in importance. All other factors being equal, a person with blood relatives who now have or did have heart disease before age 60 runs a greater risk than someone with no such history. The younger the age at which the cardiovascular incident happened to the relative, the greater is the risk for the disease.

In many cases there is no way of knowing whether a person's true genetic predisposition or simply poor lifestyle habits led to a heart problem. A person may have been physically inactive, overweight, have smoked, and had bad dietary habits, leading to a heart attack. Regardless, blood relatives fall in the family history category. Because we have no reliable way to differentiate all the factors contributing to cardiovascular disease, a person with a family history should watch all other factors closely and maintain as low a risk level as possible. In addition, the person should have a blood chemistry analysis each year to make sure the body is handling blood lipids properly.

## Age

Age is a risk factor because of the higher incidence of heart disease in older people. This tendency may be induced partly by other factors stemming from changes in lifestyle as we get older — less physical activity, poor nutrition, obesity, and so on.

Young people should not think they are exempt from heart disease, though. The process begins early in life. Autopsies conducted on soldiers killed at age 22 and younger revealed that approximately 70% had early stages of atherosclerosis. Other studies found elevated blood cholesterol levels in children as young as 10 years old.

Although the aging process cannot be stopped, it certainly can be slowed down. Physiological versus chronological age is important in preventing disease. Some individuals in their 60s or older have the body of a 20-year-old. And 20-year-olds often are in such poor condition and health that they almost seem to have the body of a 60-year-old. Risk factor management and positive lifestyle habits are the best ways to slow down the natural aging process.

## A FINAL WORD ON CORONARY RISK REDUCTION

Most of the risk factors for CHD are reversible and preventable. The fact that a person has a family history of heart disease and possibly some of the other risk factors because of neglect in lifestyle does not mean this person is doomed. A healthier lifestyle — free of cardiovascular problems — is something over which you have much control. You are encouraged to be persistent. Will power and commitment are required to develop patterns that eventually will turn into healthy habits contributing to total well-being.

## NOTES

1. S. N. Blair, H. W. Kohl III, R. S. Paffenbarger, Jr, D. G. Clark, K. H. Cooper, and L. W. Gibbons, "Physical Fitness and All-Cause Mortality: A Prospective Study of Healthy Men and Women." *Journal of the American Medical Association* 262 (1989), 2395-2401.
2. R. S. Paffenbarger, Jr, R. T. Hyde, A. L. Wing, I. Lee, D. L. Jung, and J. B. Kampert, "The Association of Changes in Physical-Activity Level and Other Lifestyle Characteristics with Mortality Among Men." *New England Journal of Medicine*, 328 (1993), 538-545.
3. P. A. Romm, M. K. Hong, and C. E. Rackley. "High-Density-Lipoprotein Cholesterol and Risk of Coronary Heart Disease," *Practical Cardiology* 16 (1990), 28-40.
4. C. J. Gluek, "Nonpharmacologic and Pharmacologic Alteration of High Density Lipoprotein Cholesterol: Therapeutic Approaches to Prevention of Atherosclerosis," *American Heart Journal* 110 (1985), 1107-1115.
5. J. M. Gaziano and C. H. Hennekens. "A New Look at What Can Unclog Your Arteries," *Executive Health Report* 27:8 (1991), 16.
6. Gaziano and Hennekens.
7. Romm et al.
8. American Heart Association, *Heart and Stroke Facts*. (Dallas: AHA, 1993).
9. R. J. Barnard, "Effects of Lifestyle Modification on Serum Lipids," *Archives of Internal Medicine* 151 (1991), 1389-1394.
10. R. Superko, "Platelets and Lipid Interaction with a Vessel Wall," symposium presented at American College of Sports Medicine Annual Meeting, 1991.
11. S. P. Superko, D. R. Ragland, R. W. Leung, and R. S. Paffenbarger. "Physical Activity and Reduced Occurrences of Non-Insulin-Dependent Diabetes Mellitus," *New England Journal of Medicine* 325 (1991), 147-152.
12. F. W. Kash, J. L. Boyer, S. P. Van Camp, L. S. Verity, and J. P. Wallace, "The Effect of Physical Activity on Aerobic Power in Older Men (A Longitudinal Study)," *Physician and Sports Medicine* 18:4 (1990), 73-83.

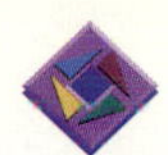

# SELECT BIBLIOGRAPHY


American Heart Association. *Heart and Stroke Facts*: 1994 (Statistical Supplement). Dallas: AHA, 1993.

Blair, S. N., K. H. Cooper, L. W. Gibbons, L. R. Gettman, S. Lewis, and N. N. Goodyear. "Changes in Coronary Heart Disease Risk Factors Associated with Increased Treadmill Time in 753 Men." *American Journal of Epidemiology* 3 (1983), 352-359.

Blair, S. N., N. N. Goodyear, L. W. Gibbons, and K. H. Cooper. "Physical Fitness and Incidence of Hypertension in Healthy Normotensive Men and Women." *Journal of the American Medical Association* 252 (1984), 487-490.

Blankenhorn, D. H., et al. "Beneficial Effects of Combined Colestipol-Niacin Therapy on Coronary Atherosclerosis and Coronary Venous Bypass Grafts. *Journal of the American Medical Association* 257 (1987), 3233-3240.

Blankenhorn, D. H., and H. N. Hodis. "Status Report on Coronary Atherosclerosis Regression: Clinical Implications." *Practical Cardiology* 16:11 (1990), 41-56.

Cristian, J. L., and J. L. Greger. *Nutrition for Living*. Menlo Park, CA: Benjamin/Cummings Publishing, 1991.

Cooper, K. H. *The Aerobics Program for Total Well-Being*. New York: Mount Evans and Co., 1982.

Cooper, K. H. *Running Without Fear*. New York: Mount Evans and Co., 1985.

Dietrich, E. B. *The Arizona Heart Institute's Heart Test*. New York: International Heart Foundation, 1981.

Frick, M. H., et al. "Helsinki Heart Study: Primary-Prevention Trial with Gemfibrozil in Middle-Aged Men with Dyslipidemia." *New England Journal of Medicine* 317 (1987), 1237-1245.

Gibbons, L. W., S. Blair, K. H. Cooper, and M. Smith. "Association Between Coronary Heart Disease Risk Factors and Physical Fitness in Healthy Adult Women." *Circulation* 5 (1993), 977-983.

Gordon, D. J., et al. "High-Density Lipoprotein Cholesterol and Coronary Heart Disease in Hypercholesterolemic Men: The Lipid Research Clinics Coronary Primary Prevention Trial." *Circulation* 74 (1986), 1217-1225.

Guss, S. B. "Heart Attack Risk Score." *Cardiac Alert*, 1983.

Hoeger, W. W. K. *Ejercicio, Salud y Vida* [Exercise, Health and Life]. Caracas, Venezuela: Editorial Arte, 1980.

Hoeger, W. W. K. *The Complete Guide for the Development & Implementation of Health Promotion Programs*. Englewood, CO: Morton Publishing, 1987.

Hoeger, W. W. K. "Self-Assessment of Cardiovascular Risk." *Corporate Fitness & Recreation* 5:6 (1986), 1316.

"How Good is 'Good' Cholesterol?" *Health Letter*, April 9, 1982.

Hubert, H. B., M. Feinleib, P. M. MacNamara, and W. P. Castelli. "Obesity as an Independent Risk Factor for Cardiovascular Disease: A 26-year Follow-up of Participants in the Framingham Heart Study." *Circulation* 5 (1983), 968-977.

Johnson, L. C. *Interpreting Your Test Results*. Chattanooga, TN: Blue Cross/Blue Shield of Tennessee, 1990.

Kannel, W. B., D. McGee, and T. Gordon. "A General Cardiovascular Risk Profile: The Framingham Study." *American Journal of Cardiology* 7 (1976), 46-51.

Kostas, G. "Three Nutrients May Help Control Blood Pressure." *Aerobics News* 1:7 (1986), 6.

Leon, A., J. Connett, D. R. Jacobs, and R. Rauramaa. "Leisure-time Physical Activity Levels and Risk of Coronary Heart Disease and Death: The Multiple Risk Factor Intervention Trial." *Journal of the American Medical Association* 258 (1987), 2388-2395.

Manninen, V., et al. "Lipid Alterations and Decline in the Incidence of Coronary Heart Disease in the Helsinki Heart Study." *Journal of the American Medical Association* 260 (1988), 641-651.

Multiple Risk Factor Intervention Trial Research Group." Risk Factor Changes and Mortality Results." *Journal of the American Medical Association* 248 (1982), 1465-1477.

Neufeld, H. N., and U. Gouldbourt. "Coronary Heart Disease: Genetic Aspects." *Circulation*, 5 (1983), 943-954.

Ornish, D. S., E. Brown, L. W. Scherwitz, et al., "Can Lifestyle Changes Reverse Coronary Heart Disease? Lifestyle Heart Trial." *Lancet*. 336 129-133.

Page, L. B. "On Making Sense of Salt and Your Blood Pressure." *Executive Health*, August 1982.

Peters, R. K., L. D. Cady, Jr., D. P. Bischoff, L. Bernstein, and M.C. Pike. "Physical Fitness and Subsequent Mycardial Infarction in Healthy Workers." *Journal of the American Medical Association* 249 (1983), 3052-3056.

Powell, K. E., P. D. Thompson, C. J. Caspersen, and J. S. Kendrick. "Physical Activity and the Evidence of Coronary Heart Disease." *Public Health Reviews* 8 (1987), 253-287.

Romm, P. A., M. K. Hong, and C. E. Rackley. "High-Density-Lipoprotein Cholesterol and Risk of Coronary Heart Disease." *Practical Cardiology* 16 (1990), 28-40.

Sandvik, L., J. Erikssen, E. Thaulow, G. Erikssen, R. Mundal, and K. Rodahl. "Physical Fitness as a Predictor of Mortality Among Healthy, Middle-Aged Norwegian Men." *New England Journal of Medicine*, 328 (1993), 533-537.

Sobolski, J., et al. "Protection Against Ischemic Heart Disease in the Belgian Physical Fitness Study: Physical Fitness Rather than Physical Activity." *American Journal of Epidemiology* 125 (1987), 601-610.

Van Camp, S. P. "The Fixx Tragedy: A Cardiologist's Perspective." *Physician and Sportsmedicine* 12 (1984), 153-155.

Wiley, J. A., and T. C. Camacho. "Lifestyle and Future Health: Evidence from the Alameda County Study." *Preventive Medicine* 9 (1980), 121.

# Cancer Risk Management

## Key Concepts

Cancer
Malignant tumor
Benign tumor
DNA
Phytochemicals
Telomeres
Telomerase
Angiogenesis
Carcinoma in situ
Metastasis
Nonmelanoma
Cruciferous vegetables
Nitrosamines
Antioxidants
UVB
Warning signals

## Objectives

- Be able to define cancer and how it starts and spreads
- Recognize the importance of health education in a cancer prevention program.
- Become acquainted with the American Cancer Society's guidelines for cancer prevention.
- Learn to recognize early warning signs of possible serious illness.
- Become familiar with major risk factors that lead to specific types of cancer.
- Assess the risk for developing certain types of cancer.

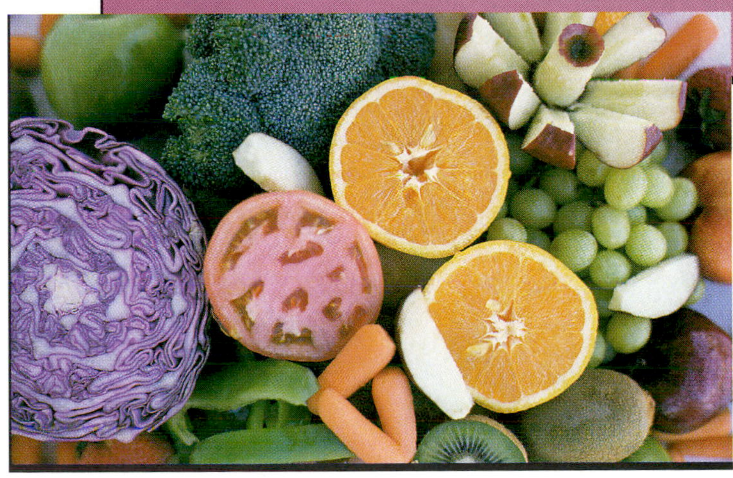

The human body has approximately 100 trillion cells. Under normal conditions these cells reproduce themselves in an orderly way. Cell growth takes place so old, worn-out tissue can be replaced and injuries can be repaired.

Cell growth is controlled by deoxyribonucleic acid (DNA) and ribonucleic acid (RNA), found in the nucleus of each cell. When nuclei lose their ability to regulate and control cell growth, cell division is disrupted, and mutant cells may develop (see Figure 10.1). Some of these cells may grow uncontrollably and abnormally, forming a mass of tissue called a tumor, which can be either benign or malignant. Benign tumors do not invade other tissues. They can interfere with normal bodily functions, but they rarely cause death. A malignant tumor is a cancer. More than 100 types of cancer can develop in any tissue or organ of the human body.

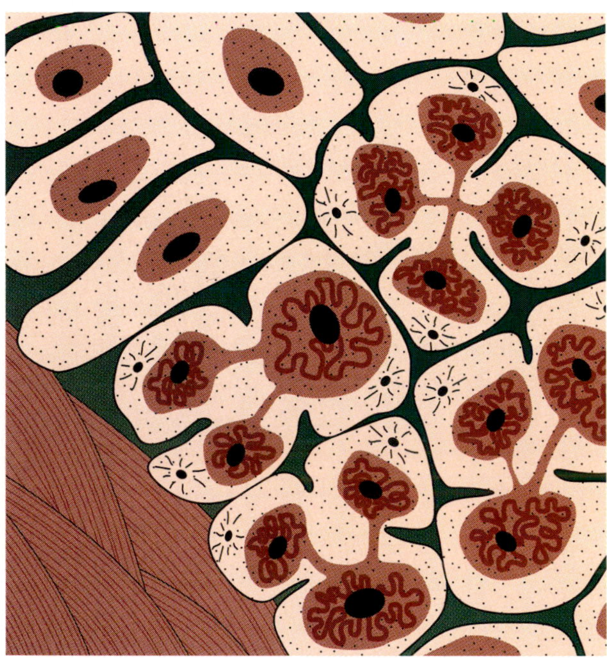

Illustration courtesy of American Cancer Society (contained in *Youth Looks at Cancer.* New York: American Cancer Society, p. 4, 1982).

**FIGURE 10.1** ◆ Cancer cells divide erratically and crowd out normal cells.

The process of cancer actually begins with an alteration in *DNA, the molecule that bears the cell's genetic code.* Found within DNA are oncogenes (cancer genes) and tumor suppressor genes, which normally work together to repair and replace cells. *Oncogenes initiate the process of cell division. Suppressor genes deactivate the process.* Defects in these genes, caused by external factors such as radiation, chemicals, and viruses, as well as internal factors such as immune conditions, hormones, and genetic mutations, ultimately allow the cell to grow into a tumor.

A cell may duplicate as many as 100 times. Normally, the DNA molecule is duplicated perfectly during cell division. In a few cases the DNA molecule is not replicated exactly, but repairs are made quickly by specialized enzymes. Occasionally cells with defective DNA keep dividing and ultimately form a small tumor. As more mutations occur, the altered cells continue to divide and can become malignant. A decade or more can pass between carcinogenic exposure or mutations and the time cancer is diagnosed.

The process of abnormal cell division is related indirectly to a strand of molecules referred to as *telomeres*, found at both ends of a chromosome (see Figure 10.2). Each time a cell divides, chromosomes lose some telomeres. After many cell divisions, chromosomes eventually run out of telomeres and the cell invariably dies.

In 1994 scientists discovered that human tumors make an enzyme known as *telomerase*, which allows cancer cells to reproduce indefinitely. In these cells telomerase keeps the chromosome

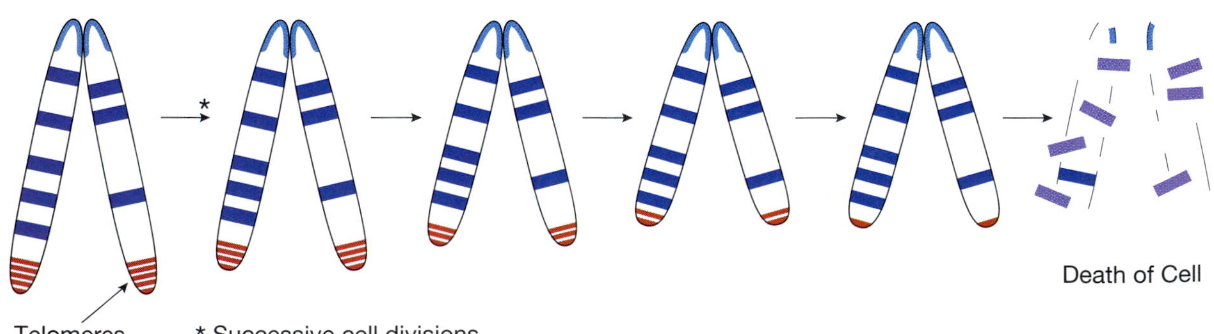


**FIGURE 10.2** ◆ Erosion of chromosome telomeres in normal cells until none is left. At this point cells die and are replaced.

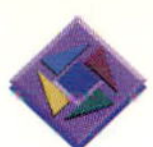

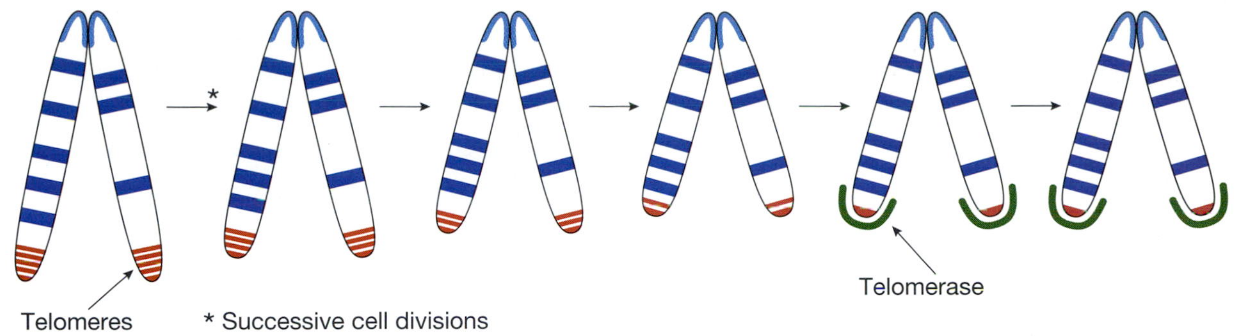


**FIGURE 10.3** ◆ The enzyme telomerase, found in cancerous cells prevents the complete erosion of telomeres. These cells reproduce indefinitely, eventually developing into tumors.

from running out of telomeres entirely. The shortened strand of telomeres (see Figure 10.3) now allows cells to reproduce indefinitely.[1]

After many cell divisions, by nature cancer cells grow old, but telomerase keeps them from dying. If scientists can confirm that telomerase plays such a crucial role in the formation of tumors, research efforts will be directed to finding a way to block the action of telomerase, thereby making cancerous cells die.

Cancer starts with the abnormal growth of one cell, which then can multiply into billions of cancerous cells (see Figure 10.4). A critical turning point in the development of cancer is when a tumor reaches about one million cells. At this stage, it is referred to as *carcinoma in situ* (an encapsulated malignant tumor that is found at an early stage and has not spread).

If undetected, the tumor may go for months and years without any significant growth. While

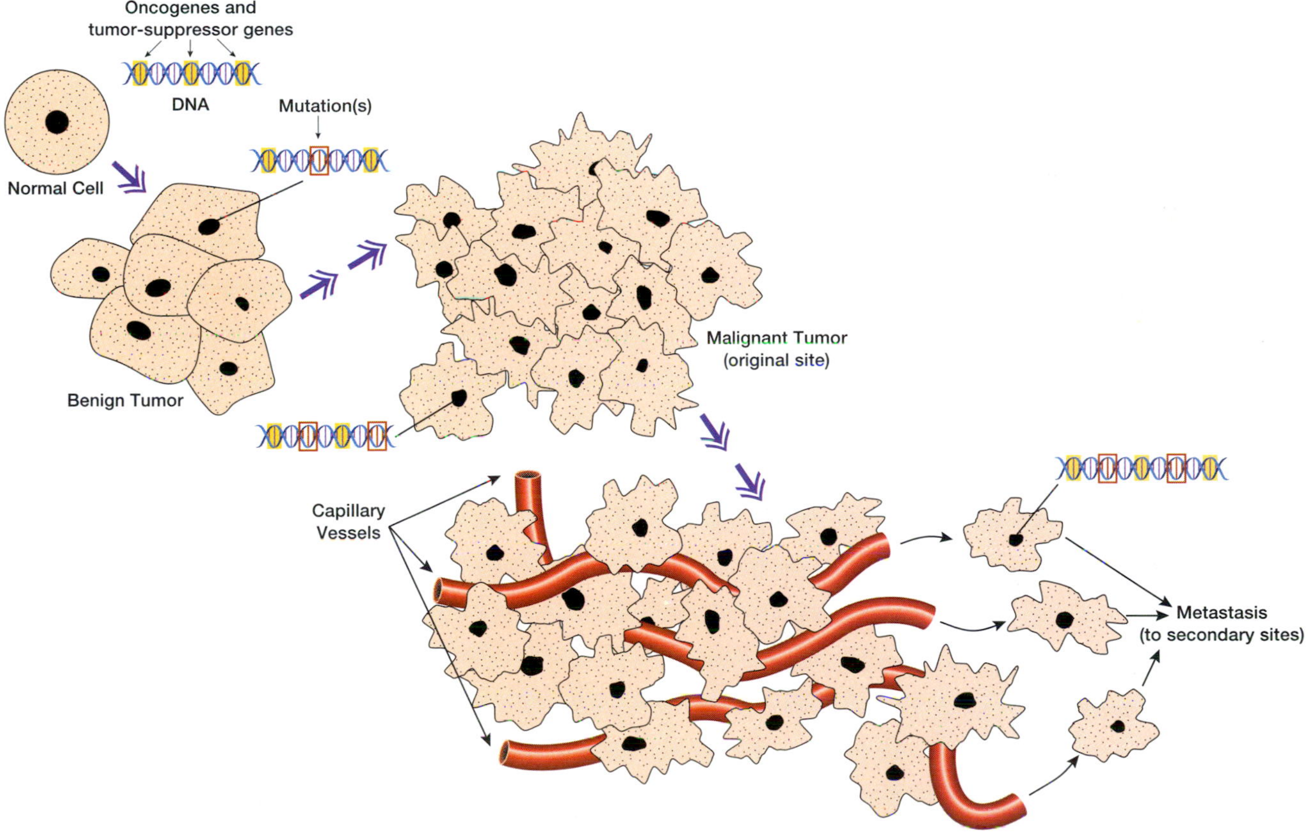


**FIGURE 10.4** ◆ How cancer starts and spreads.

encapsulated it does not pose a serious threat to human health. To grow, the tumor requires more oxygen and nutrients. In time a few of the cancer cells start producing chemicals that enhance *angiogenesis* or capillary (blood vessel) formation into the tumor. Angiogenesis is the precursor of *metastasis*, the movement of bacteria or body cells from one part of the body to another. Through these new vessels, cells now can break away from a malignant tumor and migrate to other parts of the body, where they can cause new cancer (Figure 10.4).

Most adults have precancerous or cancerous cells in their bodies. By middle age our bodies contain millions of precancerous cells. Although the immune system and the blood turbulence destroy most cancer cells, only one abnormal cell lodging elsewhere can start a new cancer. These cells also will grow and multiply uncontrollably, destroying normal tissue. The rate at which cancer cells grow varies from one type to another. Some types grow fast; others take years. In contrast, benign tumors do not invade other tissue. They can interfere with normal bodily functions, but they rarely cause death.

Once cancer cells metastasize, treatment becomes more difficult. Therapy can kill most cancer cells, but a few cells may become resistant to treatment. These cells then can grow into a new tumor that will not respond to the same treatment.

## INCIDENCE OF CANCER

According to a 1990 report by the National Center for Health Statistics, cancer was the cause of 23.5% of all deaths in the United States. It is the second leading cause of death in the country and the leading cause in children between ages 1 and 14.

Estimates indicate that the number of people with cancer will double in this decade as the population ages. This means that 85 million Americans, based on the total 1993 population, will develop cancer in their lifetime, striking approximately three of every four families. By the year 2000, cancer is expected to replace heart disease as the number-one killer in the United States. About 538,000 people died from the disease in 1994, and approximately 1,208,000 new cases were diagnosed that same year.[2]

The 1994 statistical estimates of cancer incidence and deaths by sex and site are given in Figure 10.5.

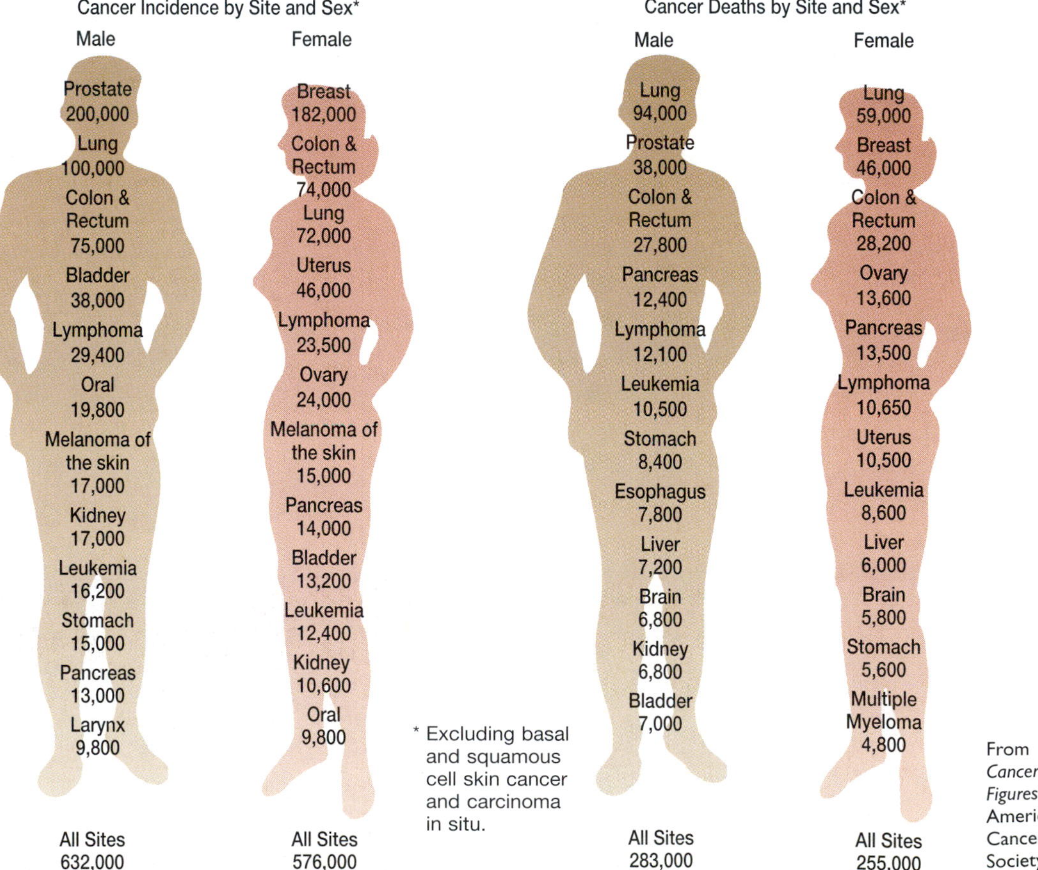


**FIGURE 10.5** ◆ Cancer incidence and deaths by site and gender: 1994.

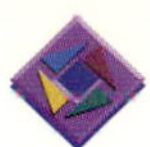

These estimates exclude *nonmelanoma skin cancer* (cancer that spreads or grows directly from the original site but does not metastasize to other regions of the body) and carcinoma in situ.

As with coronary heart disease, cancer is largely preventable. As much as 80% of all human cancer is related to lifestyle or environmental factors (including diet, tobacco use, excessive use of alcohol, sexual and reproductive history, and exposure to occupational hazards — see Figure 10.6). Most of these cancers could be prevented through positive lifestyle habits.

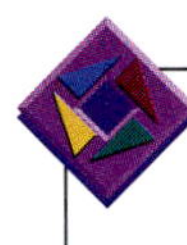

*The number of people with cancer may double this decade. Yet, many cancers are preventable through healthy lifestyle choices.*

Research sponsored by the American Cancer Society and the National Cancer Institute showed that individuals who have a healthy lifestyle have some of the lowest cancer mortality rates ever reported in scientific studies[3] (also see the discussion on wellness, fitness, and longevity in Chapter 1). A group of about 10,000 members of the Church of Jesus Christ of Latter Day Saints (commonly referred to as the Mormon church) in California was reported to have only about one-third (men) to one-half (women) the rate of cancer mortality as the general White population (Figure 10.7). In this study the investigators looked at three general health habits in the participants: lifetime abstinence from smoking, regular physical activity, and sleep. In addition, healthy lifestyle guidelines instituted by the church since 1833 include abstaining from all forms of tobacco, alcohol, caffeine, and drugs, and adhering to a well-balanced diet based on grains, fruits, and vegetables, and moderate amounts of poultry and red meat.

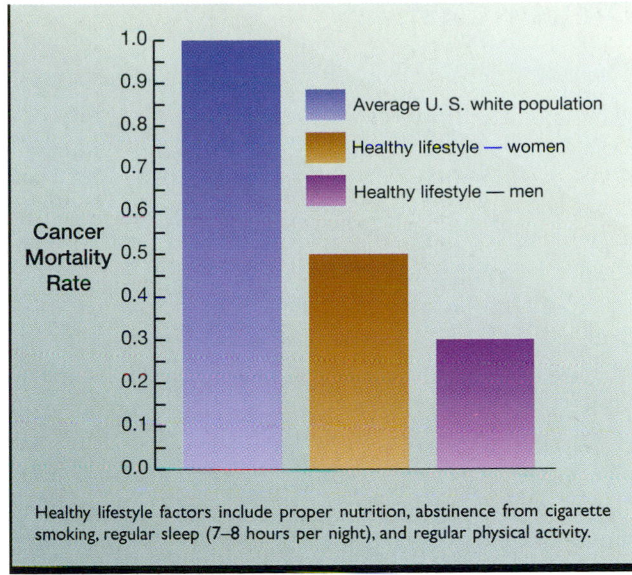


Healthy lifestyle factors include proper nutrition, abstinence from cigarette smoking, regular sleep (7–8 hours per night), and regular physical activity.

**FIGURE 10.7** ◆ Effects of a healthy lifestyle on cancer mortality rate.[3]

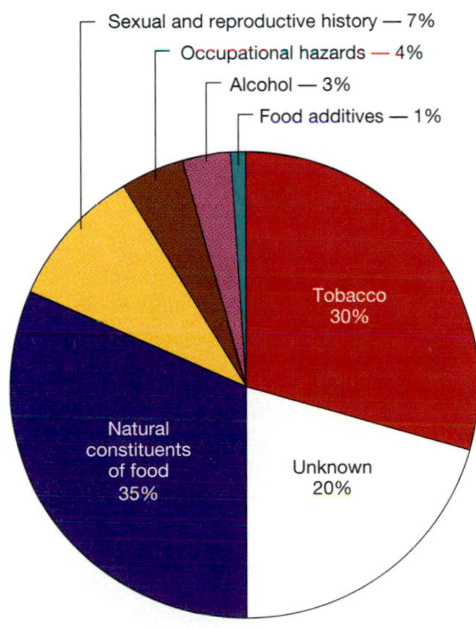


**FIGURE 10.6** ◆ Estimate of the relative role of the major factors that cause cancer.

Equally important is that more than 8 million Americans with a history of cancer were alive in 1994, nearly 5 million of whom were considered cured. For most patients, "cured" means 5 years without symptoms after treatments stop. Life expectancy for these individuals is the same as for those who never have had cancer.[4]

## GUIDELINES FOR CANCER PREVENTION

The biggest factor in fighting cancer today is health education. People need to be informed about the risk factors for cancer and the guidelines for early detection. The most effective way to protect against cancer is to change negative lifestyle habits and behaviors. Following are guidelines for preventing cancer.

## Dietary Changes

The diet should be low in fat and high in fiber, and contain vitamins A and C from natural sources. Protein intake should be within the RDA guidelines. *Cruciferous vegetables* (plants that produce cross-shaped leaves) are encouraged. Alcohol should be consumed in moderation, and obesity should be avoided.

High fat intake has been linked primarily to breast, colon, and prostate cancers. Low intake of fiber seems to increase the risk for colon cancer. Foods high in vitamins A and C may deter larynx, esophagus, and lung cancers. Salt-cured, smoked, and nitrite-cured foods have been associated with cancer of the esophagus and stomach. Vitamin C seems to discourage the formation of *nitrosamines* (cancer-causing substances formed from eating cured meats).

Carrots, squash, sweet potatoes, and cruciferous vegetables (cauliflower, broccoli, cabbage, Brussels sprouts, and kohlrabi) seem to protect against cancer. These vegetables contain a lot of beta-carotene (a precursor to vitamin A) and vitamin C. Researchers believe the antioxidant effect of these vitamins protects the body from oxygen free radicals.

As discussed in Chapter 7, during normal metabolism most of the oxygen in the human body is converted into stable forms of carbon dioxide and water. A small amount, however, ends up in an unstable form known as oxygen free radicals, which are thought to attack and damage the cell membrane and DNA, leading to the formation of cancers. Antioxidants absorb free radicals before they can cause damage, and they also interrupt the sequence of reactions once damage has begun.[5]

A promising new horizon in cancer prevention is the recent discovery of phytochemicals (also see Chapter 7). These chemical compounds, found in abundance in fruits and vegetables, appear to exert a powerful effect in cancer prevention by blocking the formation of cancerous tumors and disrupting the process at almost every step of the way. Phytochemicals exert their protective action in several ways:[6]

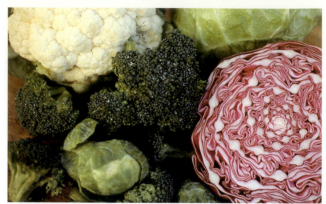

*Cruciferous vegetables are recommended in a cancer-prevention diet.*

- Removing carcinogens from cells before they cause damage.
- Activating enzymes that detoxify cancer-causing agents.
- Keeping carcinogens from locking onto cells.
- Preventing carcinogens from binding to DNA.
- Breaking up cancer-causing precursors to benign forms.
- Disrupting the chemical combination of cell molecules that can produce carcinogens.
- Keeping small tumors from accessing capillaries to get oxygen and nutrients.

As examples of phytochemicals: Sulforaphane (found in broccoli) removes carcinogens from cells; PEITC (broccoli) and Capsaicin (hot chili peppers)

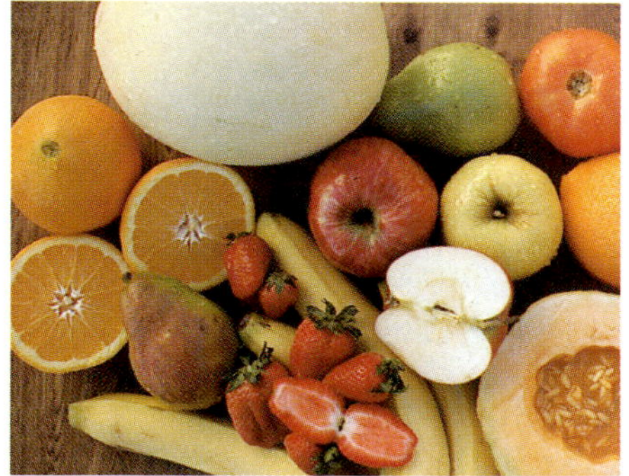

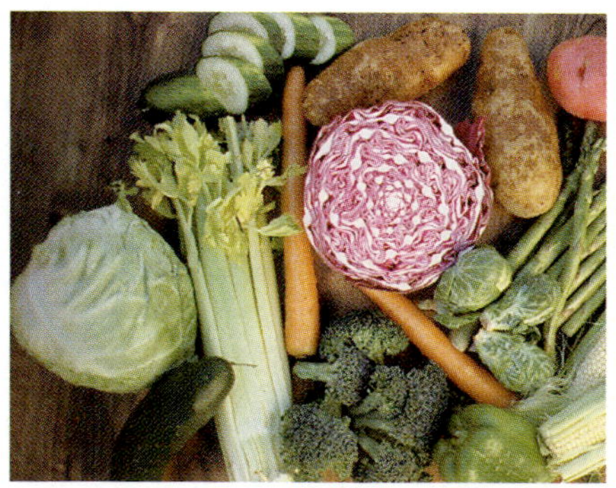

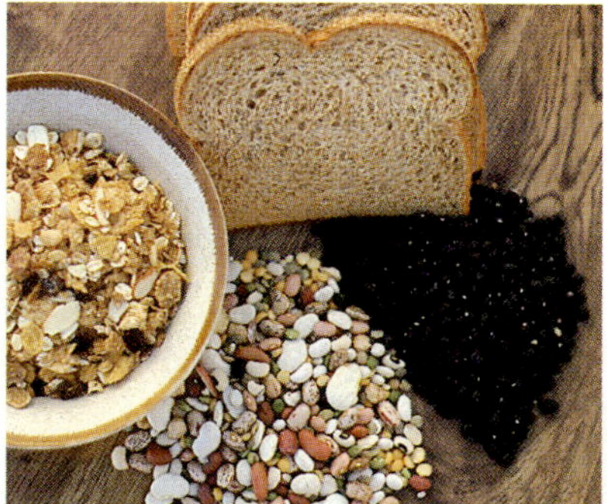

*Nutrition guidelines for a cancer prevention program include a diet low in fat and high in fiber, with ample amounts of vitamins A and C from natural sources.*

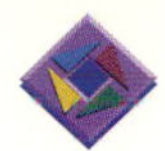

keep carcinogens from binding to DNA; Genistein (soybeans) prevents small tumors from accessing capillaries to get oxygen and nutrients, Flavenoids (most fruits and vegetables) help keep cancer-causing hormones from locking on to cells; and p-coumaric and chlorogenic acids (strawberries, green peppers, tomatoes, and pineapples) seem to disrupt the chemical combination of cell molecules that can produce carcinogens.

Nutritional guidelines also recommend avoiding excessive protein intake. Daily protein intake for some Americans is almost twice the amount the human body needs. Too much animal protein seems to decrease blood enzymes that prevent precancerous cells from developing into tumors.

Some research suggests that grilling protein (fat or lean) at high temperatures for a long time increases the formation of carcinogenic substances on the skin or surface of the meat. Microwaving the meat for a couple of minutes before barbecuing decreases the risk, as long as the fluid released by the meat is discarded. Most potential carcinogens collect in this solution. Removing the skin before serving and cooking at lower heat to a medium stage rather than well done also seems to lower the risk.

Alcohol should be consumed in moderation, as too much alcohol raises the risk for developing certain cancers, especially when it is combined with tobacco smoking or smokeless tobacco. In combination, these substances significantly increase the risk for mouth, larynx, throat, esophagus, and liver cancers. Approximately 17,000 cancer deaths yearly are attributed to excessive use of alcohol, often in combination with smoking. The combined action of heavy use of alcohol and tobacco can increase cancer of the oral cavity fifteenfold.

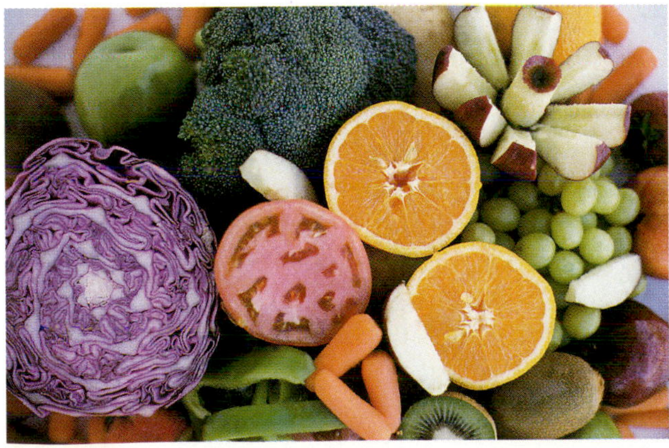

*Phytochemicals found in abundance in fruits and vegetables seem to have a powerful effect in decreasing cancer risk.*

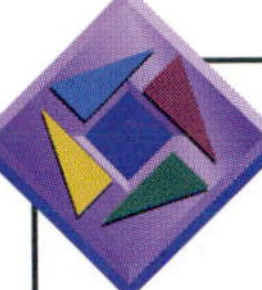

## IDEAS FOR A HEALTHY, CANCER-FIGHTING DIET

**Increase intake of phytochemicals, fiber, cruciferous vegetables, and more antioxidants by:**

- Eating more fruits and vegetables in general
- Including broccoli, cauliflower, kale, turnips, cabbage, kohlrabi, Brussels sprouts, hot chili peppers, red and green peppers, carrots, sweet potatoes, winter squash, spinach, garlic, onions, strawberries, tomatoes, pineapples, and citrus fruits in your regular diet.
- Eating vegetables raw or quickly cooked by steaming or stir-frying.
- Substituting fruit and vegetable juices for coffee, tea, and soda
- Eating whole grain flour breads
- Using whole wheat flour instead of refined white flour in baking
- Using brown-unpolished rice instead of white-polished rice

**Decrease daily fat intake to less than 30% of total caloric intake by:**

- Trimming all visible fat from meat and removing skin from poultry prior to cooking
- Decreasing the amount of fat and oils used in cooking
- Substituting low fat for high fat dairy products
- Using salad dressing sparingly
- Using only half to three-quarters the amount of fat required in baking recipes
- Cutting down on nuts and seeds consumption
- Limiting consumption of beef, poultry, or fish to no more than 3 to 6 ounces per day (about the size of a deck of cards)

Maintaining recommended body weight also is encouraged. Obesity has been associated with cancers of the colon, rectum, breast, prostate, gallbladder, ovary, and uterus.

## Abstaining From Tobacco

Smoking is the culprit in 83% of lung cancers and 30% of all cancers. Smokeless tobacco also increases the risk for mouth, larynx, throat, and esophagus cancers. About 138,600 cancer deaths each year stem from tobacco use.

Cigarette smoking by itself is a major health hazard. When considering all related deaths, cigarette smoking is responsible for about 450,000 unnecessary deaths each year. The average life expectancy for a chronic smoker is up to 18 years less than for a nonsmoker.

## Avoiding Excessive Sun Exposure

Too much exposure to sunlight (or any ultraviolet source, including tanning booths) is a major contributor to skin cancer. The most common sites of skin cancer are those exposed to the sun most often (face, neck, and back of the hands).

The three types of skin cancer are:

1. Basal cell carcinoma
2. Squamous cell carcinoma
3. Malignant melanoma.

The latter is the most deadly, causing approximately 6,900 deaths in 1993.

Nearly 90% of the 700,000 cases of skin cancer reported yearly in the United States could have been prevented by protecting the skin from the sun's rays. One in every six Americans eventually will develop some type of skin cancer.

Nothing is healthy about a "healthy tan." Tanning of the skin is the body's natural reaction to permanent and irreversible damage from too much exposure to the sun. Even small doses of sunlight add up to a greater risk for skin cancer and premature aging. The tan fades at the end of the summer season, but the underlying skin damage does not disappear. In particular, people with sensitive skin should avoid sun exposure between 10:00 a.m. and 3:00 p.m.

The stinging sunburn comes from ultraviolet B rays (UVB), which also are thought to be the main cause of premature wrinkling and skin aging, roughened/leathery/sagging skin, and skin cancer. Unfortunately, the damage may not become evident until up to 20 years later. In comparison, skin that has not been overexposed to the sun remains smooth and unblemished, and, over time, shows less evidence of aging.

Sunscreen lotion should be applied about 30 minutes before lengthy exposure to the sun because the skin takes that long to absorb the protective ingredients. A sun protection factor (SPF) of at least 15 is recommended. SPF 15 means the skin takes 15 times longer to burn than with no lotion. If you ordinarily get a mild sunburn after 20 minutes of noonday sun, an SPF 15 allows you to remain in the sun about 300 minutes before burning. The higher the number, the more the protection. When swimming or sweating, waterproof sunscreens should be reapplied more often because all sunscreens lose strength when they are diluted.

## Estrogen, Radiation Exposure, and Potential Occupational Hazards

Estrogen intake has been linked to endometrial cancer but can be taken safely under careful supervision by a physician. Although radiation exposure increases the risk for cancer, the benefits of x-rays may outweigh the risk involved, and most medical facilities use the lowest dose possible to keep the risk to a minimum. Occupational hazards, such as asbestos fibers, nickel and uranium dusts, chromium compounds, vinyl chloride, and bischlormethyl ether, increase the risk for cancer. Cigarette smoking magnifies the risk from occupational hazards.

## Physical Activity

A more active lifestyle also seem to offer a protective effect against cancer. Although the mechanism is not clear, physical fitness and cancer mortality in men and women may have a graded and consistent inverse relationship[7] (see Figure 10.8). A moderately intense lifetime exercise program has been shown to lower the risk for cancers of the breast, colon, and reproductive system. In addition, growing evidence suggests that the body's autoimmune system may play a role in preventing cancer. Studies have indicated that exercise improves the autoimmune system.

## Other Factors

The contribution of many of the other much-publicized factors is not as significant as those just

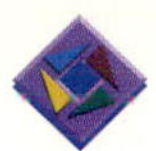

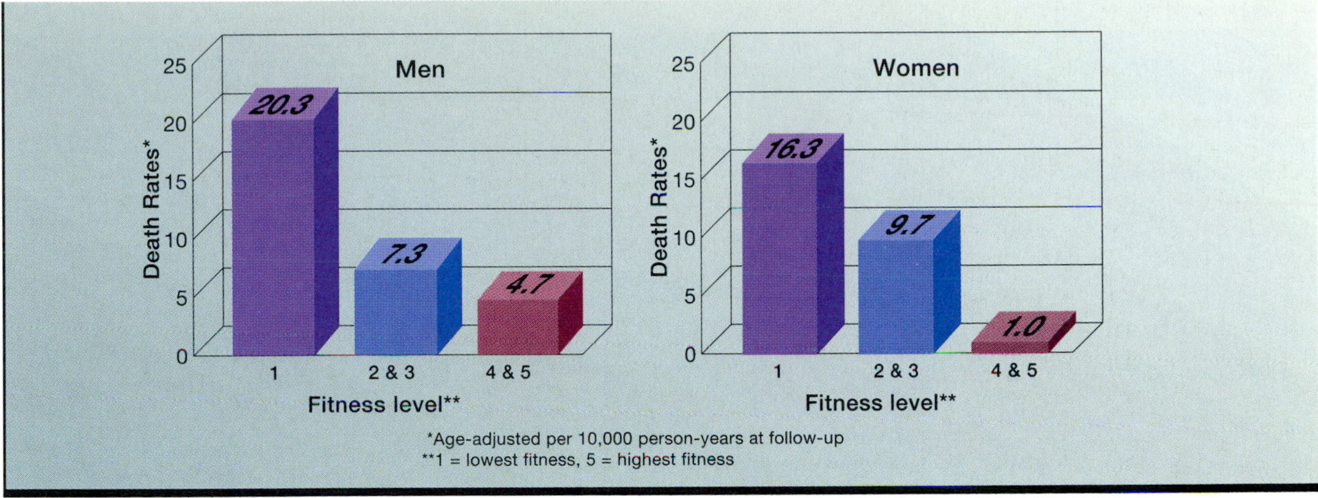


**FIGURE 10.8** ◆ Association between physical activity and cancer.[7]

pointed out. Intentional food additives, saccharin, processing agents, pesticides, and packaging materials currently used in the United States and other developed countries seem to have minimal consequences. High levels of tension and stress and poor coping may affect the autoimmune system negatively and render the body less effective in dealing with the various cancers.

Genetics plays a role in susceptibility in about 10% of all cancers. Most of the effect is seen in the early childhood years. Some cancers are a combination of genetic and environmental liability. Genetics may add to the environmental risk of certain types of cancers. The biggest carcinogenic exposure in the workplace is cigarette smoke. Environment, however, means more than pollution and smoke. It incorporates diet, lifestyle-related events, viruses, and physical agents such as x-rays and exposure to the sun.

## Early Detection

Fortunately, through early detection many cancers can be controlled or cured. The real problem comes when cancerous cells spread, because they are difficult to wipe out then. Therefore, effective prevention, or at least early detection, is crucial. Herein lies the importance of periodic screening.

Everyone should become familiar with the following seven warning signals for cancer and bring them to a physician's attention if any are present:

1. Change in bowel or bladder habits.
2. Sore that does not heal.
3. Unusual bleeding or discharge.
4. Thickening or lump in breast or elsewhere.
5. Indigestion or difficulty in swallowing.
6. Obvious change in wart or mole.
7. Nagging cough or hoarseness.

Furthermore, the American Medical Association has developed a questionnaire to alert people to symptoms that may indicate a serious health problem. The questionnaire is given at the end of this chapter, in Figure 10.11. Although in most cases nothing serious will be found, any of the symptoms calls for a physician's attention as soon as possible. Finally, the Guidelines for Screening Recommendations by the American Cancer Society, outlined in Table 10.1, should be included in regular physical examinations as part of a cancer prevention program.

Scientific evidence and testing procedures for prevention and early detection of cancer do change. Studies continue to provide new information about cancer prevention and detection. The intent of cancer prevention programs is to educate and guide individuals toward a lifestyle that will help prevent cancer and enable early detection of malignancy. Treatment of cancer always should be left to specialized physicians and cancer clinics. Current treatment modalities include surgery, radiation, radioactive substances, chemotherapy, hormones, and immunotherapy.

**TABLE 10.1**
**Guidelines for Cancer Screening**

| Test | Age | Frequency |
|---|---|---|
| Breast physical examination | 20-40 | Every 3 yrs |
| | Over 40 | Annually |
| Breast self-examination | Over 20 | Monthly |
| Chest x-ray | No specific recommendation | No specific recommendation |
| Digital rectal examination | Over 40 | Annually |
| Endometrial tissue examination | At menopause[a] | At menopause |
| Mammography | 35-40 | One baseline |
| | 40-49 | Every 1-2 yrs |
| | Over 50 | Annually |
| Pap smear | 20-65 and sexually active teenagers | 2 consecutive yrs, then every 3 yrs |
| Pelvic examination | 20-40 | Every 3 yrs |
| | Over 40 | Annually |
| | At menopause | |
| Sigmoidoscopy | Over 50 | 2 consecutive yrs, then every 3-5 yrs |
| Sputum cytology | No specific recommendation | No specific recommendation |
| Stool guaiac | Over 50 | Annually |
| Health counseling and cancer check-up[b] | Over 20 | Every 3 yrs |
| | Over 40 | Every yr |

From *Guidelines for the Cancer-Related Checkup: Recommendations and Rationale* (New York: American Cancer Society, July/August 1980). Reproduced by permission.

[a] Recommended for obese women with a history of involuntary infertility, failure of ovulation, abnormal uterine bleeding, or estrogen therapy.

[b] To include examinations for cancers of the thyroid, testicles, prostate, ovaries, lymph nodes, oral region, and skin.

## CANCER QUESTIONNAIRE: ASSESSING YOUR RISKS*

The Texas Division of the American Cancer Society designed a simple self-testing questionnaire to help people assess their risk for cancer. Some people have a greater than average risk for developing certain cancers. These people are identified by risk factors for certain common types of cancer. These are the major risk factors and by no means represent the only ones that might be involved. The instructions given to people who take this questionnaire are:

> Read each question concerning each site and its specific risk factors. Be honest in your responses. Place the number in parentheses (risk points) in the correct space provided to the left of each question. For example, Question #2 on lung cancer: If you are 53 years old (age 50 to 59), then enter 5 (risk points) as your score on the left. At the end of each site, total your number of points for that site. Record the final number of points in your cancer profile (Figure 10.10) and in the fitness and wellness profile in Appendix A. Figure A.1

Men should complete the questions for lung, colon-rectum, and skin cancer. In addition, three major cancer sites for women are included with space to enter the score totals.

Check your own risks against the answers contained on this questionnaire. Individual numbers for specific questions are not to be interpreted as a precise measure of relative risk, but the totals for a given site should give you a general indication of your risk. An explanation of the risk factors for each type of cancer follows the questionnaire. If

* Cancer Questionnaire: Assessing Your Risks obtained from the Texas Division of the American Cancer Society and reproduced with permission. (NOTE: This questionnaire is not available nationwide; distribution is limited to Texas residents only.)

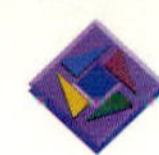

you are at higher risk, you are advised to discuss the results with your physician.

## Lung Cancer

_____ 1. Sex
- a. Male (2)
- b. Female (1)

_____ 2. Age
- a. 39 or less (1)
- b. 40-49 (2)
- c. 50-59 (5)
- d. 60+ (7)

_____ 3. Smoking status
- a. Smoker (8)
- b. Nonsmoker (1)

_____ 4. Type of smoking
- a. Current cigarettes or little cigars (10)
- b. Pipe and/or cigar, but not cigarettes (3)
- c. Ex-cigarette smoker (2)

_____ 5. Amount of cigarettes smoked per day
- a. 0 cigarettes (1)
- b. Less than 1 pack per day (5)
- c. 1 pack (9)
- d. 1-2 packs (15)
- e. 2+ packs (20)

_____ 6. Type of cigarette
- a. High tar/nicotine (10)*
- b. Medium T/N (9)
- c. Low T/N (7)
- d. Nonsmoker (1)

_____ 7. Duration of smoking
- a. Never smoked (1)
- b. Ex-smoker (3)
- c. Up to 15 years (5)
- d. 15-25 years (10)
- e. 25+ years (20)

_____ 8. Type of industrial work
- a. Mining (3)
- b. Asbestos (7)
- c. Uranium and radioactive products

_____ Total

## Colon-Rectum Cancer

_____ 1. Age
- a. 39 or less (10)
- b. 40-59 (20)
- c. 60+ (50)

_____ 2. Has anyone in your immediate family ever had:
- a. Colon cancer (20)
- b. One or more polyps of the colon (10)
- c. Neither (1)

_____ 3. Have you ever had:
- a. Colon cancer (100)
- b. One or more polyps of the colon (40)
- c. Ulcerative colitis (20)
- d. Cancer of the breast or uterus (10)
- e. None (1)

_____ 4. Bleeding from the rectum (other than obvious hemorrhoids or piles)
- a. Yes (75)
- b. No (1)

_____ Total

## Skin Cancer

_____ 1. Frequent work or play in the sun:
- a. Yes (10)
- b. No (1)

_____ 2. Work in mines, around coal tars, or around radioactivity:
- a. Yes (10)
- b. No (1)

_____ 3. Complexion — fair and/or light skin:
- a. Yes (10)
- b. No (1)

_____ Total

## Breast Cancer

_____ 1. Age group
   a. 20-34 (10)
   b. 35-49 (40)
   c. 50+ (90)

_____ 2. Race group
   a. Oriental (5)
   b. Black (20)
   c. White (25)
   d. Mexican American (10)

_____ 3. Family history
   a. Mother, sister, aunt, or grandmother with breast cancer (30)
   b. None (10)

_____ 4. Your History
   a. Previous lumps or cysts (25)
   b. No breast disease (10)
   c. Previous breast cancer (100)

_____ 5. Maternity
   a. 1st pregnancy before 25 (10)
   b. 1st pregnancy after 25 (15)
   c. No pregnancies (20)

_____ Total

## Cervical Cancer

(Lower portion of uterus. These questions would not apply to a woman who has had a total hysterectomy.)

_____ 1. Age group
   a. Less than 25 (10)
   b. 25-39 (20)
   c. 40-54 (30)
   d. 55+ (30)

_____ 2. Race
   a. Oriental (10)
   b. Puerto Rican (20)
   c. Black (20)
   d. White (10)
   e. Mexican American (20)

_____ 3. Number of pregnancies
   a. 0 (10)
   b. 1-3 (20)
   c. 4 and over (30)

_____ 4. Viral infections
   a. Herpes and other viral infections or ulcer formations on the vagina (10)
   b. Never (1)

_____ 5. Age at first intercourse
   a. Before 15 (40)
   b. 15-19 (30)
   c. 20-24 (20)
   d. 25 and over (10)
   e. Never (5)

_____ 6. Bleeding between periods or after intercourse
   a. Yes (40)
   b. No (1)

_____ Total

## Endometrial Cancer

(Body of uterus. These questions do not apply to a woman who has had a total hysterectomy.)

_____ 1. Age group
   a. 39 or less (5)
   b. 40-49 (20)
   c. 50+ (60)

_____ 2. Race
   a. Oriental (10)
   b. Black (10)
   c. White (20)
   d. Mexican American (10)

_____ 3. Births
   a. None (15)
   b. 1 to 4 (7)
   c. 5 or more (5)

_____ 4. Weight
   a. 50 or more pounds overweight (50)
   b. 20-49 pounds overweight (15)
   c. Underweight for height (10)
   d. Normal (10)

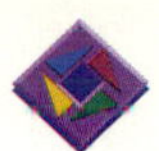

_____ 5. Diabetes (elevated blood sugar)
   a. Yes (3)
   b. No (1)

_____ 6. Estrogen hormone intake
   a. Yes, regularly (15)
   b. Yes, occasionally (12)
   c. None (10)

_____ 7. Abnormal uterine bleeding
   a. Yes (40)
   b. No (1)

_____ 8. Hypertension (high blood pressure)
   a. Yes (3)
   b. No (1)

_____ Total

## CANCER QUESTIONNAIRE INTERPRETATION

The following interpretation of the cancer questionnaire is to summarize, explain new evidence, and provide valuable information on the individual risk that a person may have for each type of cancer. Potential cancer risk is based on individual lifestyle and medical history.

### Lung Cancer

1. **Sex.** Men have a higher risk of lung cancer than women, equating them for type, amount and duration of smoking. Since more women are smoking cigarettes for a longer duration than previously, their incidence of lung and upper respiratory tract (mouth, tongue, and larynx) cancer is increasing.
2. **Age.** The occurrence of lung and upper respiratory tract cancer increases with age.
3. **Smoking status.** Cigarette smokers have up to twenty times or even greater risk than non-smokers. However, the rates of ex-smokers who have not smoked for ten years approach those of non-smokers.
4. **Type of smoking.** Pipe and cigar smokers are at a higher risk for lung cancer than nonsmokers. Cigarette smokers are at a much higher risk than nonsmokers or pipe and cigar smokers. All forms of tobacco, including chewing, markedly increase the user's risk of developing cancer of the mouth.
5. **Amount of cigarettes smoked per day.** Male smokers of less than one-half pack per day have five times higher lung cancer rates than nonsmokers. Male smokers of one to two packs per day have fifteen times higher lung cancer rates than nonsmokers. Smokers of more than two packs per day are twenty times more likely to develop lung cancer than nonsmokers.
6. **Type of cigarette.** Smokers of low-tar/nicotine cigarettes have slightly lower lung cancer rates.
7. **Duration of smoking.** The frequency of lung and upper respiratory tract cancer increases with the duration of smoking.
8. **Type of industrial work.** Exposures to materials used in the industries mentioned in the questionnaire have been demonstrated to be associated with lung cancer. Smokers who work in these industries may have greatly increased risks. Exposures to materials in other industries may also carry a higher risk.

**Total Risk:**

24 or less .... You have a low risk for lung cancer (low risk category).

25-49 ....... You may be a light smoker and would have a good chance of kicking the habit (light risk).

50-74 ....... As a moderate smoker, your risks of lung and upper respiratory tract cancer are increased. If you stop smoking now, these risks will decrease (moderate risk).

75 or over .... As a heavy cigarette smoker, your chances of getting lung and upper respiratory tract cancer are greatly increased. Your best bet is to stop smoking now — for the health of it. See your doctor if you have a nagging cough, hoarseness, persistent pain, or a sore in the mouth or throat (high risk).

### Colon-Rectum Cancer

1. **Age.** Colon cancer occurs more frequently after the age of 50.

2. **Family predisposition.** Colon cancer is more common in families with a previous history of this disease.
3. **Personal history.** Polyps and bowel diseases are associated with colon cancer.
4. **Rectal bleeding.** Rectal bleeding may be a sign of colorectal cancer.

### Total Risk:

29 or less . . . . You are at a low risk for colon-rectal cancer.

30-69 . . . . . . . This is a moderate risk category. Testing by your physician may be indicated.

70 or over . . . . This is a high-risk category. You should see your physician for the following tests: digital rectal exam, guaiac slide test, and protoscopic exam.

In addition to the risk factors mentioned in the questionnaire, a diet high in fat and low in fiber as well as a history of breast or endometrial cancer also increase the risk for colon-rectum cancer.

## Skin Cancer

1. **Sun exposure.** Excessive ultraviolet light causes cancer of the skin. Protect yourself with a sun screen medication.
2. **Work environment.** Working in mines, around coal tar, or around radioactive materials can cause cancer of the skin.
3. **Complexion.** Persons with light complexions need more protection than others.

### Total Risk:

Numerical risks for skin cancer are difficult to state. For instance, a person with a dark complexion can work longer in the sun and be less likely to develop cancer than a light-complected person. Furthermore, a person wearing a long sleeved shirt and wide-brimmed hat may work in the sun and be less at risk than a person who wears a bathing suit for only a short period. The risk greatly increases with age.

If you answer "yes" to any question, you need to protect your skin from the sun or any other toxic material. Changes in moles, warts, or skin sores are very important and should be seen by your doctor.

## Breast Cancer

1. **Age.** The risk for breast cancer significantly increases after age fifty.
2. **Race.** Breast cancer occurs more frequently in white women than any other group.
3. **Family history.** The risk for breast cancer is higher in women with a family history of this type of cancer. The risk is even higher if more than one family member has developed breast cancer, and is also enhanced by the closeness in terms of immediacy, e.g., mother, sister, aunt, or grandmother.
4. **Personal history.** A previous history of breast or ovarian cancer would indicate a greater risk.
5. **Maternity.** The risk is greater in women who have never had children and in women who bear children after age thirty.

### Total Risk:

Under 100 . . . . Low-risk women should practice monthly breast self-examination (BSE — see Figure 10.9) and have their breasts examined by a doctor as a part of a cancer-related checkup.

100-199 . . . . . Moderate-risk women should practice monthly BSE and have their breasts examined by a doctor as part of a cancer-related checkup. Periodic breast x-rays should be included as your doctor may advise.

200 or over . . . High-risk women should practice monthly BSE and have the above examinations more often. See your doctor for the recommended (frequency of breast physical examinations and x-ray) examinations related to you.

Other possible risk factors for breast cancer not listed in the questionnaire are a diet high in fat, onset of menstruation prior to age 13, chronic cystic disease, and ionizing radiation.

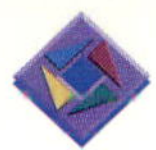

## HOW TO EXAMINE YOUR BREASTS

**1**

In the shower: Check for any lump or thickening.

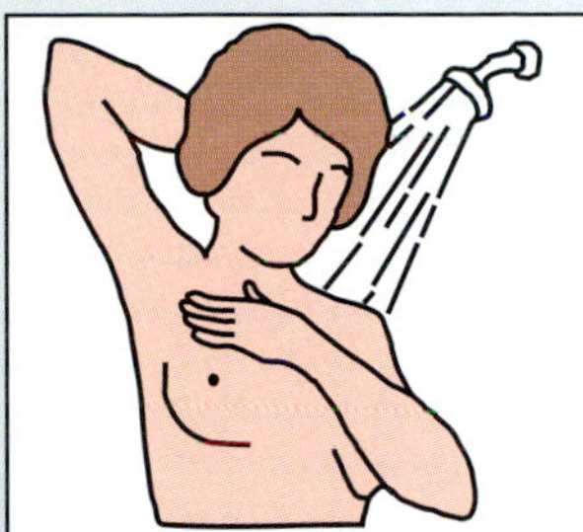

**2**

Before a mirror: Look for any changes in contour of your breasts, a swelling or dimple in the skin.

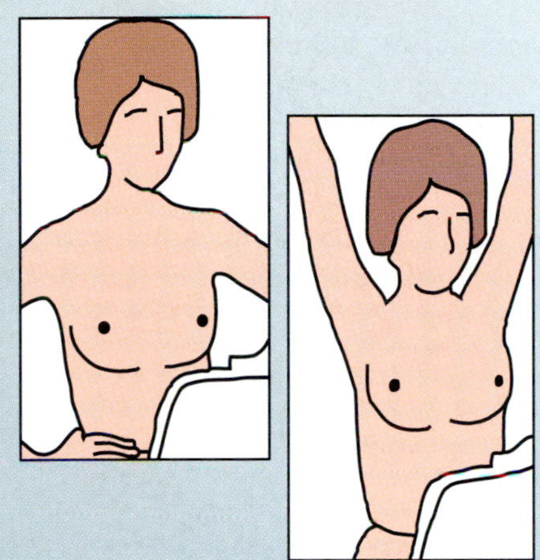

**3**

Lying down: Put pillow under right shoulder. With fingers flat, examine right breast, press gently in small circular motions; then squeeze nipple to check for discharge. Now do left breast.

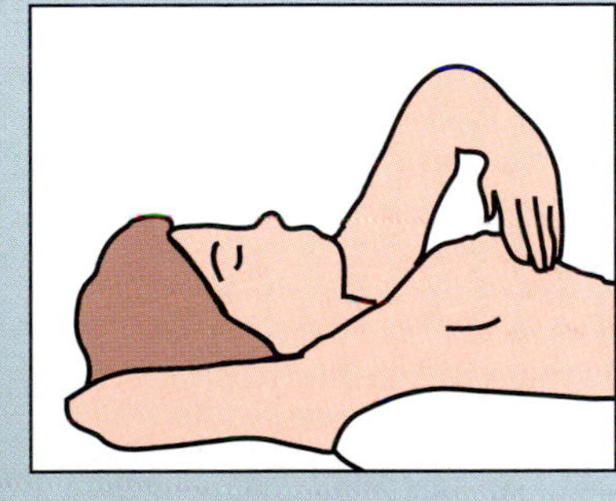

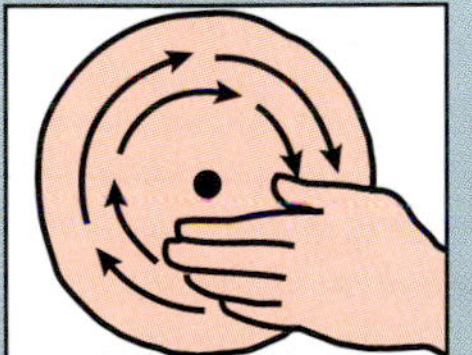

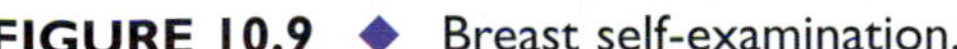

Reproduced by permission from American Cancer Society, Atlanta, GA.

**FIGURE 10.9** ◆ Breast self-examination.

## Cervical Cancer

1. **Age.** The highest occurrence is in the 40 and over age group. The numbers represent the relative rates of cancer for different age groups. A 45-year-old woman has a risk three times higher than a 20-year-old.
2. **Race.** Puerto Ricans, Blacks, and Mexican Americans have higher rates of cervical cancer.
3. **Number of pregnancies.** Women who have delivered more children have a higher occurrence.
4. **Viral infections.** Viral infections of the cervix and vagina are associated with cervical cancer.
5. **Age at first intercourse.** Women with earlier intercourse and with more sexual partners are at a higher risk.
6. **Bleeding.** Irregular bleeding may be a sign of uterine cancer.

### Total Risk:

40-69 ....... This is a low-risk group. Ask your doctor for a pap test. You will be advised how often you should be tested after your first test.

70-99 ....... In this moderate-risk group, more frequent pap tests may be required.

100 or over ... You are in a high-risk group and should have a pap test (and pelvic exam) as advised by your doctor.

## Endometrial Cancer

1. **Age.** Endometrial cancer is seen in older age groups. The numbers by the age groups represent relative rates of endometrial cancer at different ages. A 50-year-old woman has a risk twelve times higher than a 35-year-old woman.
2. **Race.** Caucasians have a higher occurrence.
3. **Births.** The fewer children one has delivered, the greater the risk of endometrial cancer.
4. **Weight.** Women who are overweight are at greater risk.
5. **Diabetes.** Cancer of the endometrium is associated with diabetes.
6. **Estrogen use.** Cancer of the endometrium may be associated with prolonged continuous estrogen hormone intake. This occurs in only a small

number of women. You should consult your physician before starting or stopping any estrogen medication.

7. **Abnormal bleeding.** Women who do not have cyclic regular menstrual periods are at greater risk.
8. **Hypertension.** Cancer of the endometrium is associated with high blood pressure.

### Total Risk:

49-59 ....... You are at low risk for developing endometrial cancer.

60-99 ....... Your risks are slightly higher (moderate risk). Report any abnormal bleeding immediately to your doctor. Tissue sampling at menopause is recommended.

100 or over ... Your risks are much greater (high risk). See your doctor for tests as appropriate.

Additional risk factors that may be associated with endometrial cancer, not included in the questionnaire, are infertility, a prolonged history of failure to ovulate, and menopause after age 55.

## OTHER CANCER SITES

Risk factors and prevention techniques for other types of cancer not contained in the cancer questionnaire have been outlined in *The American Cancer Society Cancer Book* and in a series of pamphlets on "Facts on Cancer" (one each for selected cancer sites). These types of cancer are listed next, along with the risk factors associated with each type and preventive techniques to decrease risk. Unlike the previous questionnaire, no numeric weights for the different risk factors have been assigned. However, as you read the information, rate yourself on a scale from 1 to 3 (1 = low risk, 2 = moderate risk, 3 = high risk) for each cancer site, and record your results in Figure 10.10.

## Prostate Cancer

The prostate gland is actually a cluster of smaller glands that encircles the top section of the urethra (urinary channel) at the point where it leaves the bladder. The function of the prostate is not quite clear, but the muscles of these small glands help squeeze prostatic secretions into the urethra.

### Risk Factors

1. **Advancing age.** The highest incidence of prostate cancer is found in men over 55. The incidence is also higher among Blacks than Whites, and more married than single men develop this type of cancer.
2. **A history of venereal disease.** Herpes Simplex Virus Type 2 and Cytomegalovirus (herpes virus) have been linked to prostate cancer.
3. **A history of prostate infections** (more than two).
4. **A diet high in fat.**

### Prevention and Warning Signals

Prostate cancer is difficult to control because the causes are not known. Death rates can be lowered through early detection and awareness of the warning signals. Detection is made by a rectal exam of the gland and should be conducted once a year after the age of 40. Possible warning signals include: difficulties in urination (especially at night), painful urination, blood in the urine, and constant pain in the lower back or hip area.

## Testicular Cancer

Testicular cancer accounts for only one percent of all male cancers. However, it is the most common type of cancer seen in men between ages 25 and 35. The incidence is slightly higher in Whites than Blacks, and it is rarely seen in middle-aged and older men. The malignancy rate of testicular tumors is 96%, but this type of cancer is highly curable if it is diagnosed early.

### Risk Factors

1. Undescended testicle not corrected before age 6.
2. Atrophy of the testicle following mumps or virus infection.
3. Family history of testicular cancer.
4. Recurrent injury to the testicle.
5. Abnormalities of the endocrine system (e.g., high hormone levels of pituitary gonadotropin or androgens).
6. Incomplete testicular development.

### Prevention and Warning Signals

The incidence of testicular cancer is quite high in males born with an undescended testicle. Therefore, this condition should be corrected early in

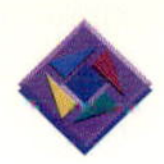

life. Parents of infant males need to make sure that the child is checked by a physician to ensure that the testes have descended into the scrotum. Testicular self-examination (TSE) once a month following a warm bath or shower (when the scrotal skin is relaxed) is recommended. Each testicle is gently examined by rolling it between the thumb and fingers. The individual should feel for a firm lump about the size of a pea. Although most lumps are noncancerous, if detected, a physician should be promptly consulted.

Some of the warning signs associated with testicular cancer are: a small lump found on the testicle, slight enlargement (usually painless) and change in consistency of the testis, sudden build-up of blood or fluid in the scrotum, groin and lower abdominal pain or discomfort accompanied by a sensation of dragging and heaviness, breast enlargement or tenderness, and enlarged lymph glands.

Early diagnosis of testicular cancer is essential, as this type of cancer spreads rapidly to other parts of the body. Because in most cases no early symptoms or pain are associated with testicular cancer, most people do not see a physician for months following the discovery of a lump or a slightly enlarged testis. Unfortunately, this delay allows almost 90% of testicular cancer to metastasize (spread) before a diagnosis is made.

## Pancreatic Cancer

The pancreas is a thin gland that lies behind the stomach. This gland releases insulin and pancreatic juice. Insulin regulates blood sugar, and pancreatic juice contains enzymes that aid in food digestion.

### Possible Risk Factors

1. Increased incidence between ages 35 and 70, but significantly higher around age 55.
2. Cigarette smoking.
3. High cholesterol diet.
4. Exposure to unspecified environmental agents.

### Prevention and Warning Signals

Detection of pancreatic cancer is difficult because (a) no symptoms are evoked in the early disease process, and (b) advanced disease symptoms are similar to those of other diseases. Warning signals that may be related to pancreatic cancer include pain in the abdomen or lower back, jaundice, loss of weight and appetite, nausea, weakness, agitated depression, loss of energy and feeling weary, dizziness, chills, muscles spasms, double vision, and coma.

## Kidney and Bladder Cancer

The kidneys are the organs that filter the urine, and the bladder stores and empties the urine. Most of these two types of cancer are caused by environmental factors. Bladder cancer occurs most frequently between the ages of 50 and 70. Eighty percent of bladder cancers are seen in men, and the incidence is twice as high in White males as compared to Black males.

### Risk Factors

1. Congenital (inborn) abnormalities of either organ (these conditions are detected by a physician).
2. Exposure to certain chemical compounds such as aniline dyes, naphthalenes, or benzidines.
3. Heavy cigarette smoking.
4. History of schistosomiasis (a parasitic bladder infection).
5. Frequent urinary tract infections, particularly after age 50.

### Prevention and Warning Signals

Avoiding cigarette smoking and occupational exposure to cancer-causing chemicals is important to decrease risk. Bloody urine, especially repeated occurrences, is always a warning sign and requires immediate evaluation.

## Oral Cancer

Oral cancer includes the mouth, lips, tongue, salivary glands, pharynx, larynx, and floor of the mouth. Most of these cancers seem to be related to cigarette smoking and excessive alcohol consumption.

### Risk Factors

1. Heavy smoking and/or drinking.
2. Broken or ill-fitting dentures.
3. Broken tooth that irritates the inside of the mouth.

4. Chewing and dipping tobacco.
5. Excessive sun exposure (lip cancer).

### Prevention and Warning Signals

Regular examinations and good dental hygiene help in the prevention and early detection of oral cancer. Warning signals may include: a nonhealing sore or white patch in the mouth, a lump, problems with chewing and swallowing, a constant feeling of having "something" in the throat. A person with any of those conditions should be evaluated by a physician or dentist. A tissue biopsy is normally conducted to diagnose the presence of cancer.

## Esophageal and Stomach Cancer

The incidence of gastric cancer in the United States has dropped about 40% in the last 30 years. Cancer experts attribute this drastic decrease to changes in dietary habits and more refrigeration. This type of cancer is more common in men, and the incidence is also higher in Black males than in White males.

### Risk Factors

1. A diet high in starch and low in fresh fruits and vegetables.
2. High consumption of salt-cured, smoked, and nitrate-cured foods.
3. Stomach acid imbalance.
4. History of pernicious anemia.
5. Chronic gastritis or gastric polyps.
6. Family history of these types of cancer.

### Prevention and Warning Signals

Prevention is accomplished primarily by increasing dietary intake of complex carbohydrates and fiber and decreasing the intake of salt-cured, smoked, and nitrate-cured foods. In addition, regular guaiac testing for occult blood (hemoccult test) is recommended. Warning signals for this type of cancer include: indigestion for two weeks or longer, blood in the stools, vomiting, rapid weight loss.

## Ovarian Cancer

The ovaries are part of the female reproductive system that produces and releases the egg and the hormone estrogen. Ovarian cancer develops more frequently after menopause, and the highest incidence is seen between ages 55 and 64.

### Risk Factors

1. Women over 50 years old.
2. History of ovarian problems.
3. Extensive history of menstrual irregularities.
4. Family history of ovarian cancer.
5. Personal history of breast, bowel, or endometrial cancer.
6. Nulliparity (not having given birth to a child).

### Prevention and Warning Signals

In most cases, there are no signs or symptoms related to ovarian cancer. Therefore, regular pelvic examinations to detect signs of enlargement or other abnormalities are highly recommended. Some warning signals may be: an enlarged abdomen, abnormal vaginal bleeding, unexplained digestive disturbances in women over 40, normal-sized ovaries (premenopause size) after menopause.

## Thyroid Cancer

The thyroid gland, located in the lower portion of the front of the neck, helps regulate growth and metabolism. Thyroid cancer occurs almost twice as often in women as in men, and the incidence is also higher in Whites than Blacks.

### Risk Factors

1. Increased age.
2. Radiation therapy of the head and neck region received in childhood or adolescence.
3. Family history of thyroid cancer.

### Prevention and Warning Signals

Regular inspection for thyroid tumors is done by palpation of the gland and surrounding areas during a physical examination. Thyroid cancer is slow-growing; therefore, it is highly treatable. However, any unusual lumps in front of the neck should be promptly reported to a physician. Although thyroid cancer does not have many warning signals (besides a lump), these may include: difficulty in swallowing, choking, labored breathing, persistent hoarseness.

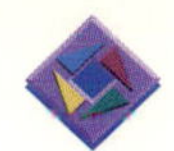

## Liver Cancer

The incidence of liver cancer in the United States is very low. Men are more prone to liver cancer, and the disease is more common after age 60.

### Risk Factors

1. History of cirrhosis of the liver.
2. History of hepatitis B virus.
3. Exposure to vinyl chloride (industrial gas used in plastics manufacturing) and aflatoxin (natural food contaminant).

### Prevention and Warning Signals

Prevention consists primarily of avoiding the risk factors and being aware of warning signals. Possible signs and symptoms are a lump or pain in the upper right abdomen (which may radiate into the back and the shoulder), fever, nausea, rapidly deteriorating health, jaundice, and liver tenderness.

## Leukemia

Leukemia is a type of cancer that interferes with blood-forming tissues (bone marrow, lymph nodes, and spleen), by producing too many immature white blood cells. People who have leukemia cannot fight infection very well. The causes of leukemia are mostly unknown, although suspected risk factors have been identified.

### Risk Factors

1. Inherited susceptibility, but not directly transmitted from parent to child.
2. Greater incidence in children with Down syndrome (mongolism) and a few other genetic abnormalities.
3. Excessive exposure to ionizing radiation.
4. Environmental exposure to chemicals such as benzene.

### Prevention and Warning Signals

Detection is not easy because early symptoms may be associated with serious ailments. Early warning signals include: fatigue, pallor, weight loss, easy bruising, nose bleeds, paleness, loss of appetite, repeated infections, hemorrhages, night sweats, bone and joint pain, fever. At a more advanced stage, fatigue increases, hemorrhages become more severe, pain and high fever continue, the gums swell, and various skin disorders occur.

## Lymphomas

Lymphomas are cancer of the lymphatic system. The lymphatic system consists of lymph nodes found throughout the body and a network of vessels that link these nodes. The lymphatic system participates in the body's immune reaction to foreign cells, substances, and infectious agents.

### Risk Factors

As with leukemia, the causes of lymphomas are unknown at this time. Some researchers suspect that a form of herpes virus, referred to as Epstein-Barr, is active in the initial stages of lymphosarcomas. Other researchers suggest that certain external factors may alter the immune system, making it more susceptible to the development and multiplication of cancer cells.

### Prevention and Warning Signals

Prevention of lymphomas is limited because little is known about its causes. Enlargement of a lymph node or cluster of lymph nodes is the first sign of lymphoma. Other signs and symptoms may be: enlarged spleen or liver, weakness, fever, back or abdominal pain, nausea/vomiting, unexplained weight loss, unexplained itching and sweating, fever at night that lasts for a long time.

## WHAT CAN YOU DO?

If you are at high risk for any of the cancer sites, you are advised to discuss this with your physician. An ounce of prevention is worth a pound of cure. Although cardiovascular disease is the number-one killer in the country, cancer is the number-one fear. Of all cancers, 60% to 80% are preventable, and about 50% are curable. Most cancers are lifestyle-related, so being aware of the risk factors and following the screening guidelines (Table 10.1) and basic recommendations for cancer prevention will greatly decrease the risk for developing cancer.

## NOTES

1. G. Cowley, "The Secrets of a Cancer Cell's Success," *Newsweek,* April 25, 1994, pp. 48-49.
2. American Cancer Society, *Cancer Facts & Figures – 1994* (New York: ACS, 1994).
3. J. E. Enstrom, "Health Practices and Cancer Mortality Among Active California Mormons," *Journal of the National Cancer Institute,* 81 (1989), 1807-1814.
4. American Cancer Society.
5. J. M. Gaziano and C. H. Hennekens, "A New Look at What Can Unclog Your Arteries," *Executive Health Report,* 27:8 (1991), 16.
6. S. Begley, "Beyond Vitamins" *Newsweek,* April 25, 1994, pp. 45-49.
7. S. N. Blair, H. W. Kohl III, R. S. Paffenbarger, Jr., D. G. Clark, K. H. Cooper, and L. W. Gibbons, "Physical Fitness and All-Cause Mortality: A Prospective Study of Healthy Men and Women," *Journal of the American Medical Association,* 262 (1989), 2395-2401.

## SELECT BIBLIOGRAPHY

American Cancer Society, Texas Division. *Cancer: Assessing Your Risk.* Dallas: ACS, 1982.

American Cancer Society. *Cancer Book.* New York: ACS, 1986.

American Cancer Society, *Guidelines for the Cancer-Related Checkup: Recommendations and Rationale.* New York: ACS, 1980.

American Cancer Society. Pamphlets, Facts on "selected" cancer sites. New York: ACS, 1978 and 1983.

Greenwald, P. "Assessment of Risk Factors for Cancer." *Preventive Medicine,* 9 (1980), 260-263.

Hammond, E. C., and H. Seidman. "Smoking and Cancer in the United States." *Preventive Medicine,* 9 (1980), 169-173.

Higginson, J. "Proportion of Cancers Due to Occupation." *Preventive Medicine,* 9 (1980), 180-188.

Paffenbarger, R. S., R. T. Hyde, A. L. Wing, and C. H. Steinmetz. "A Natural History of Athleticism and Cardiovascular Health." *Journal of the American Medical Association,* 252 (1984), 491-495.

Rothman, K. J. "The Proportion of Cancer Attributable to Alcohol Consumption." *Preventive Medicine,* 9 (1980), 174-179.

Weisburger, J. H., D. M. Hegsted, G. B. Gori, and B. Lewis. "Extending the Prudent Diet to Cancer Prevention." *Preventive Medicine,* 9 (1980), 297-304.

Williams, C. L. "Primary Prevention of Cancer Beginning in Childhood." *Preventive Medicine,* 9 (1980), 275-280.

Williams, P. A. "A Productive History and Physical Examination in the Prevention and Early Detection of Cancer." *Cancer,* 47 (1981), 1146-1150.

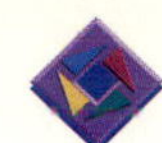

Name:______________________ Date: ______________________

| **Cancer Site** | **Total Points** Men | Women | **Risk Category** |
|---|---|---|---|
| Lung | ______ | ______ | ______ |
| Colon-Rectum | ______ | ______ | ______ |
| Skin | ______ | ______ | ______ |
| Breast | | ______ | ______ |
| Cervical | | ______ | ______ |
| Endometrial | | ______ | ______ |
| Prostate | ______ | | ______ |
| Testicular | ______ | | ______ |
| Pancreatic | ______ | ______ | ______ |
| Kidney and Bladder | ______ | ______ | ______ |
| Oral | ______ | ______ | ______ |
| Esophageal and Stomach | ______ | ______ | ______ |
| Ovarian | ______ | ______ | ______ |
| Thyroid | ______ | ______ | ______ |
| Liver | ______ | ______ | ______ |
| Leukemia | ______ | ______ | ______ |
| Lymphomas | ______ | ______ | ______ |

**FIGURE 10.10** ◆ Cancer profile.

## EARLY WARNING SIGNS OF POSSIBLE SERIOUS ILLNESS

Many serious illnesses begin with apparently minor or localized symptoms that, if they are recognized early, can alert you to act in time for the disease to be cured or controlled. In most cases, of course, nothing is seriously wrong. **If you experience any of the following symptoms, discuss the problem with your physician without delay.** Only check conditions that apply.

- ☐ 1. Rapid loss of weight—more than about 4 kg (10 lbs) in ten weeks—without apparent cause.
- ☐ 2. A sore, scab, or ulcer, in the mouth, or on the body, that fails to heal within weeks.
- ☐ 3. A skin blemish or mole that begins to bleed or itch, or that changes color, size, or shape.
- ☐ 4. Severe headaches that develop for no obvious reason.
- ☐ 5. Sudden attacks of vomiting, without preceding nausea.
- ☐ 6. Fainting spells for no apparent reason.
- ☐ 7. Visual problems such as seeing "haloes" around lights, or intermittently blurred vision, especially in dim light.
- ☐ 8. Increasing difficulty with swallowing.
- ☐ 9. Hoarseness without apparent cause that lasts for a week or more.
- ☐ 10. A "smoker's" cough or any other nagging cough that has been getting worse.
- ☐ 11. Blood in coughed-up phlegm, or sputum.
- ☐ 12. Constantly swollen ankles.
- ☐ 13. A bluish tinge to the lips, the insides of the eyelids, or the nailbeds.
- ☐ 14. Extreme shortness of breath for no apparent reason.
- ☐ 15. Vomiting of blood or a substance that resembles coffee grounds.
- ☐ 16. Persistent indigestion or abdominal pain.
- ☐ 17. A marked change in normal bowel habits, such as alternating attacks of diarrhea and constipation.
- ☐ 18. Bowel movements that look black and tarry.
- ☐ 19. Rectal bleeding.
- ☐ 20. Unusually cloudy, pink, red, or smoky-looking urine.
- ☐ 21. In men, discomfort or difficulty when urinating.
- ☐ 22. In men, discharge from the tip of the penis.
- ☐ 23. In women, a lump or unusual thickening of a breast or any alteration in breast shape such as flattening, bulging, or puckering of skin.
- ☐ 24. In women, bleeding or unusual discharge from the nipple.
- ☐ 25. In women, vaginal bleeding or "spotting" that occurs between usual menstrual periods or after menopause.



**FIGURE 10.11** ◆

# Stress Assessment and Management Techniques

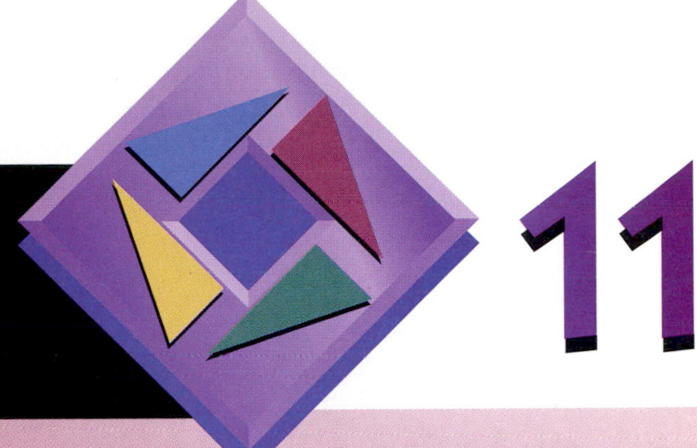

11

## Key Concepts

Stress
Stressor
Eustress
Distress
Life Experiences Survey
Type A
Type B
Type C
Structured Interview
Stress vulnerability
Social support
Time management
Fight or flight
Biofeedback
Progressive muscle relaxation
Breathing exercise
Autogenic training
Meditation

## Objectives

- Define stress, eustress, and distress.
- Explain the role of stress in maintaining health and optimal performance.
- Identify the major sources of stress in life.
- Define the two types of behavior patterns.
- Learn to lower your vulnerability to stress.
- Develop time-management skills.
- Define the role of physical exercise in reducing stress.
- Learn to use various stress management techniques.

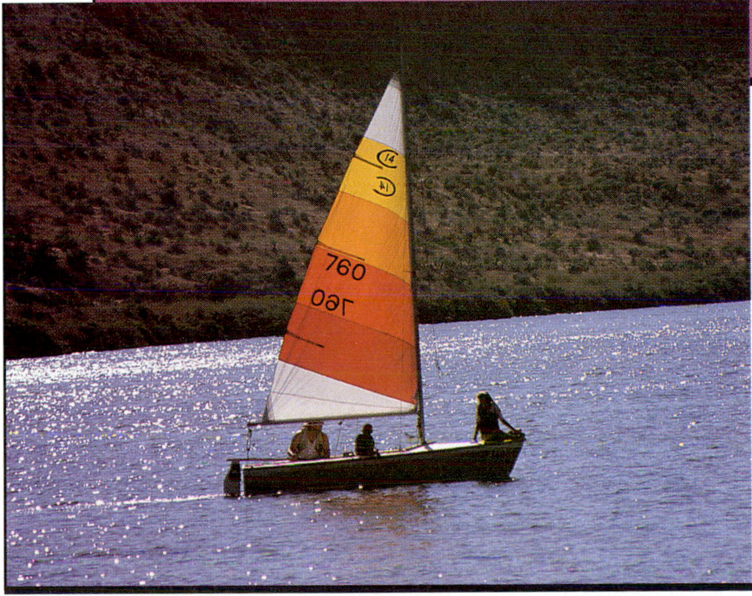

Learning to live and get ahead today is nearly impossible without stress. To succeed in an unpredictable world that changes with every new day, working under pressure is the rule rather than the exception for most people. As a result, stress is one of the most common problems we face these days. According to current estimates the annual cost of stress and stress-related diseases in the United States exceeds $100 billion, a direct result of health care costs, lost productivity, and absenteeism.

The good news is that stress can be self-controlled. Most people have accepted stress as a normal part of daily life. Even though everyone has to deal with it, few seem to understand it and know how to cope effectively. People should not avoid stress entirely, as a certain amount of stress is necessary for optimum health, performance, and well-being. To succeed and have fun in life without "hits, runs, and errors" is difficult.

Just what is stress? Dr. Hans Selye, one of the foremost authorities on stress, defined stress as *the nonspecific response of the human organism to any demand placed upon it.*[1] "Nonspecific" indicates that the body reacts the same regardless of the nature of the event that leads to the stress response. In simpler terms, stress is the body's mental, emotional, and physiological response to any situation that is new, threatening, frightening, or exciting.

The body's response to stress has been the same ever since humans were first put on the earth. Stress prepares the organism to react to the stress-causing event, also called the *stressor*. The problem, though, is the way in which we react to stress. Many people thrive under stress; others under similar circumstances are unable to handle it. An individual's reaction to a stress-causing agent determines whether stress is positive or negative.

Dr. Selye defined the ways in which we react to stress as either eustress or distress. In both cases, the nonspecific response is almost the same. In the case of *eustress, health and performance continue to improve even as stress increases.* On the other hand, *distress* refers to *the unpleasant or harmful stress under which health and performance begin to deteriorate.* The relationship between stress and performance is illustrated in Figure 11.1.

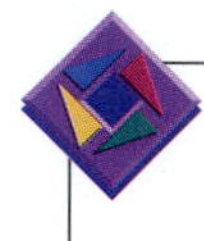

*Stress is the nonspecific response of the human organism to any demand placed upon it.*

Stress is a fact of modern life, and every person does need an optimal level of stress that is most conducive to adequate health and performance. When stress levels reach mental, emotional, and physiological limits, however, stress becomes distress and the person no longer functions effectively.

Chronic distress raises the risk for many health disorders, including coronary heart disease, hypertension, eating disorders, ulcers, diabetes, asthma, depression, migraine headaches, sleep disorders, and chronic fatigue and may even play a role in the development of certain types of cancers. Recognizing this turning point and overcoming the problem quickly and efficiently are crucial in maintaining emotional and physiological stability.

## SOURCES OF STRESS

During recent years several instruments have been developed to assess sources of stress in life. One of the instruments used most often is the Life

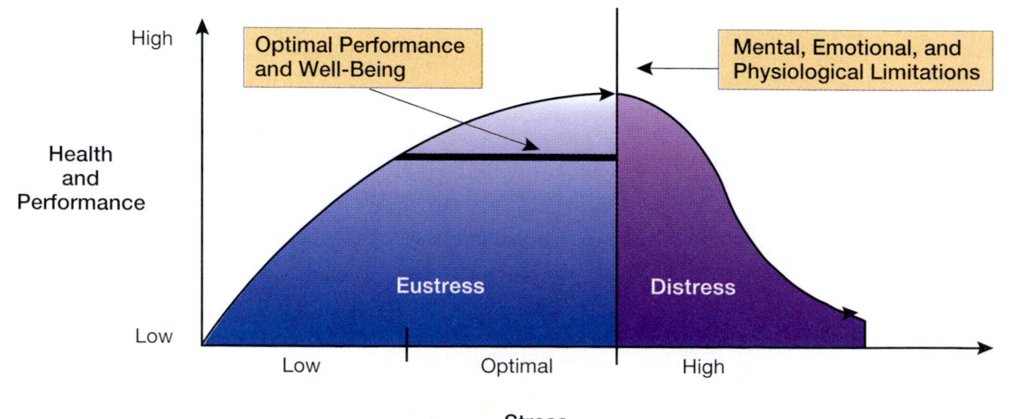


**FIGURE 11.1** Relationship between stress and health and performance.

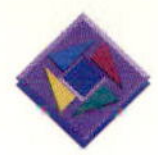

Experiences Survey, presented in Figure 11.2. This survey identifies a person's life changes within the last 12 months that may have an impact on that person's physical and psychological well-being.

The Life Experiences Survey is divided into two sections. Section 1, to be completed by all respondents, contains a list of 47 life events plus three blank spaces for other events experienced but not listed in the survey. Section 2 contains an additional 10 questions designed for students only (students should fill out both sections).

The survey requires the person to rate the extent to which the life events he or she experienced had a positive or negative impact on his or her life at the time these events occurred. The ratings are on a 7-point scale. A rating of –3 indicates an extremely undesirable impact. A rating of zero (0) suggests neither a positive nor a negative impact. A rating of +3 indicates an extremely desirable impact.

After determining the life events that have taken place, the negative and the positive points are added together separately. Both scores are expressed as positive numbers (for example — positive ratings: 2, 1, 3, 3 = 9 points positive score; negative ratings: –3, –2, –2, –1, –2 = 10 points negative score). A final "total life change" score can be obtained by adding the positive score and the negative score together as positive numbers (total life change score: 9 + 10 = 19 points).

Because negative and positive changes alike can produce nonspecific responses, the total life change score is a good indicator of total life stress. Most research in this area, however, suggests that the negative change score is a better predictor of potential physical and psychological illness than the total change score.

More research is necessary to establish the role of total change and the role of the ratio of positive to negative stress. Therefore, only the negative score is used as part of the stress profile. To obtain a stress rating, the end of Figure 11.2 presents the various stress categories based on the survey's results.

## BEHAVIOR PATTERNS

Common life events are not the only source of stress in life. All too often individuals bring on stress as a result of their behavior patterns. The two main types of behavior patterns are Type A and Type B. Each type is based on several characteristics that are used to classify people into one of these behavioral patterns.

Several attempts have been made to develop an objective scale to identify Type A individuals properly, but these questionnaires are not as valid and reliable as researchers would like them to be. Consequently, the main assessment tool to determine behavioral type is still the *Structured Interview*. During the Structured Interview a person is asked to reply to several questions that describe Type A and Type B behavior patterns. The interviewer notes not only the responses to the questions but also mental, emotional, and physical behaviors the individual exhibits as he or she replies to each question.

Based on the answers and the associated behaviors, the interviewer rates the person along a continuum, ranging from Type A to Type B. Along this continuum behavioral patterns are classified into five categories: A-1, A-2, X (a mix of Type A and Type B), B-3, and B-4. The Type A-1 exhibits all of the Type A characteristics, and the B-4 shows a relative absence of Type A behaviors. The Type A-2 does not exhibit a complete Type A pattern, and the Type B-3 exhibits only a few Type A characteristics.

*Type A behavior characterizes a primarily hard-driving, overambitious, aggressive, at times hostile and overly competitive person.* Type A individuals often set their own goals, are self-motivated, try to accomplish many tasks at the same time, are excessively achievement-oriented, and have a high degree of time urgency.

In contrast, *Type B behavior is characteristic of calm, casual, relaxed, easy-going individuals.* Type B people take one thing at a time, do not feel pressured or hurried, and seldom set their own deadlines.

Over the years, experts have indicated that individuals classified as Type A are under too much stress and have a significantly higher incidence of coronary heart disease. Based on these findings, Type A individuals have been counseled to lower their stress level by modifying many of their Type A behaviors.

Many of the Type A characteristics are learned behaviors. Consequently, if people can learn to identify the sources of stress and make changes in their behavioral responses, they can move along the continuum and respond more like Type B's. The debate, however, has centered on which Type A behaviors should be changed, because not all of them are undesirable.

## THE LIFE EXPERIENCES SURVEY

**Section I**

| | | | | | | | |
|---|---|---|---|---|---|---|---|
| 1. Marriage | –3 | –2 | –1 | 0 | +1 | +2 | +3 |
| 2. Detention in jail or comparable institution | –3 | –2 | –1 | 0 | +1 | +2 | +3 |
| 3. Death of spouse | –3 | –2 | –1 | 0 | +1 | +2 | +3 |
| 4. Major change in sleeping habits (much more or much less sleep) | –3 | –2 | –1 | 0 | +1 | +2 | +3 |
| 5. Death of close family member: | | | | | | | |
| a. mother | –3 | –2 | –1 | 0 | +1 | +2 | +3 |
| b. father | –3 | –2 | –1 | 0 | +1 | +2 | +3 |
| c. brother | –3 | –2 | –1 | 0 | +1 | +2 | +3 |
| d. sister | –3 | –2 | –1 | 0 | +1 | +2 | +3 |
| e. grandmother | –3 | –2 | –1 | 0 | +1 | +2 | +3 |
| f. grandfather | –3 | –2 | –1 | 0 | +1 | +2 | +3 |
| g. other (specify) | –3 | –2 | –1 | 0 | +1 | +2 | +3 |
| 6. Major change in eating habits (much more or much less food intake) | –3 | –2 | –1 | 0 | +1 | +2 | +3 |
| 7. Foreclosure on mortgage or loan | –3 | –2 | –1 | 0 | +1 | +2 | +3 |
| 8. Death of close friend | –3 | –2 | –1 | 0 | +1 | +2 | +3 |
| 9. Outstanding personal achievement | –3 | –2 | –1 | 0 | +1 | +2 | +3 |
| 10. Minor law violations (traffic tickets, disturbing the peace, etc.) | –3 | –2 | –1 | 0 | +1 | +2 | +3 |
| 11. Male: Wife/girlfriend's pregnancy | –3 | –2 | –1 | 0 | +1 | +2 | +3 |
| 12. Female: Pregnancy | –3 | –2 | –1 | 0 | +1 | +2 | +3 |
| 13. Changed work situation (different work responsibility, major change in working conditions, working hours, etc.) | –3 | –2 | –1 | 0 | +1 | +2 | +3 |
| 14. New job | –3 | –2 | –1 | 0 | +1 | +2 | +3 |
| 15. Serious illness or injury of close family member: | | | | | | | |
| a. father | –3 | –2 | –1 | 0 | +1 | +2 | +3 |
| b. mother | –3 | –2 | –1 | 0 | +1 | +2 | +3 |
| c. sister | –3 | –2 | –1 | 0 | +1 | +2 | +3 |
| d. brother | –3 | –2 | –1 | 0 | +1 | +2 | +3 |
| e. grandfather | –3 | –2 | –1 | 0 | +1 | +2 | +3 |
| f. grandmother | –3 | –2 | –1 | 0 | +1 | +2 | +3 |
| g. spouse | –3 | –2 | –1 | 0 | +1 | +2 | +3 |
| h. other (specify) | –3 | –2 | –1 | 0 | +1 | +2 | +3 |
| 16. Sexual difficulties | –3 | –2 | –1 | 0 | +1 | +2 | +3 |
| 17. Trouble with employer (in danger of losing job, being suspended, demoted, etc.) | –3 | –2 | –1 | 0 | +1 | +2 | +3 |
| 18. Trouble with in-laws | –3 | –2 | –1 | 0 | +1 | +2 | +3 |
| 19. Major change in financial status (a lot better off or a lot worse off) | –3 | –2 | –1 | 0 | +1 | +2 | +3 |
| 20. Major change in closeness of family members (increased or decreased closeness) | –3 | –2 | –1 | 0 | +1 | +2 | +3 |
| 21. Gaining a new family member (through birth, adoption, family member moving in, etc.) | –3 | –2 | –1 | 0 | +1 | +2 | +3 |
| 22. Change of residence | –3 | –2 | –1 | 0 | +1 | +2 | +3 |
| 23. Marital separation from mate (due to conflict) | –3 | –2 | –1 | 0 | +1 | +2 | +3 |
| 24. Major change in church activities (increased or decreased attendance) | –3 | –2 | –1 | 0 | +1 | +2 | +3 |
| 25. Marital reconciliation with mate | –3 | –2 | –1 | 0 | +1 | +2 | +3 |
| 26. Major change in number of arguments with spouse (a lot more or a lot less arguments) | –3 | –2 | –1 | 0 | +1 | +2 | +3 |
| 27. Married Male: Change in wife's work outside the home (beginning work, ceasing work, changing to a new job, etc.) | –3 | –2 | –1 | 0 | +1 | +2 | +3 |

*(Continued)*

From "Assessing the Impact of Life Changes: Development of the Life Experiences Survey," by I. G. Sarason, *Journal of Consulting and Clinical Psychology* 46 (1978), 932–946. 

**FIGURE 11.2** ◆

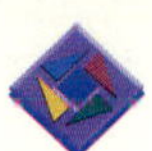

## THE LIFE EXPERIENCES SURVEY

| | | | | | | | | |
|---|---|---|---|---|---|---|---|---|
| 28. | Married Female: Change in husband's work (loss of job, beginning new job, retirement, etc.) | −3 | −2 | −1 | 0 | +1 | +2 | +3 |
| 29. | Major change in usual type and/or amount of recreation | −3 | −2 | −1 | 0 | +1 | +2 | +3 |
| 30. | Borrowing more than $10,000 (buying home, business etc.) | −3 | −2 | −1 | 0 | +1 | +2 | +3 |
| 31. | Borrowing less than $ 10,000 (buying car, TV, getting school loan, etc.) | −3 | −2 | −1 | 0 | +1 | +2 | +3 |
| 32. | Being fired from job | −3 | −2 | −1 | 0 | +1 | +2 | +3 |
| 33. | Male: Wife/girlfriend having abortion | −3 | −2 | −1 | 0 | +1 | +2 | +3 |
| 34. | Female: Having abortion | −3 | −2 | −1 | 0 | +1 | +2 | +3 |
| 35. | Major personal illness or injury | −3 | −2 | −1 | 0 | +1 | +2 | +3 |
| 36. | Major change in social activities, e.g., parties, movies, visiting (increased or decreased participation) | −3 | −2 | −1 | 0 | +1 | +2 | +3 |
| 37. | Major change in living conditions of family (building new home, remodeling, deterioration of home, neighborhood, etc.) | −3 | −2 | −1 | 0 | +1 | +2 | +3 |
| 38. | Divorce | −3 | −2 | −1 | 0 | +1 | +2 | +3 |
| 39. | Serious injury or illness of close friend | −3 | −2 | −1 | 0 | +1 | +2 | +3 |
| 40. | Retirement from work | −3 | −2 | −1 | 0 | +1 | +2 | +3 |
| 41. | Son or daughter leaving home (due to marriage, college, etc.) | −3 | −2 | −1 | 0 | +1 | +2 | +3 |
| 42. | Ending of formal schooling | −3 | −2 | −1 | 0 | +1 | +2 | +3 |
| 43. | Separation from spouse (due to work, travel, etc.) | −3 | −2 | −1 | 0 | +1 | +2 | +3 |
| 44. | Engagement | −3 | −2 | −1 | 0 | +1 | +2 | +3 |
| 45. | Breaking up with boyfriend/girlfriend | −3 | −2 | −1 | 0 | +1 | +2 | +3 |
| 46. | Leaving home for the first time | −3 | −2 | −1 | 0 | +1 | +2 | +3 |
| 47. | Reconciliation with boyfriend/girlfriend | −3 | −2 | −1 | 0 | +1 | +2 | +3 |
| 48. | Others ______________________ | −3 | −2 | −1 | 0 | +1 | +2 | +3 |
| 49 | ______________________ | −3 | −2 | −1 | 0 | +1 | +2 | +3 |
| 50. | ______________________ | −3 | −2 | −1 | 0 | +1 | +2 | +3 |

**Section 2**

| | | | | | | | | |
|---|---|---|---|---|---|---|---|---|
| 51. | Beginning a new school experience at a higher academic level (college, graduate school, professional school, etc.) | −3 | −2 | −1 | 0 | +1 | +2 | +3 |
| 52. | Changing to a new school at the same academic level undergraduate, graduate, etc.) | −3 | −2 | −1 | 0 | +1 | +2 | +3 |
| 53. | Academic probation | −3 | −2 | −1 | 0 | +1 | +2 | +3 |
| 54. | Being dismissed from dormitory or other residence | −3 | −2 | −1 | 0 | +1 | +2 | +3 |
| 55. | Failing an important exam | −3 | −2 | −1 | 0 | +1 | +2 | +3 |
| 56. | Changing a major | −3 | −2 | −1 | 0 | +1 | +2 | +3 |
| 57. | Failing a course | −3 | −2 | −1 | 0 | +1 | +2 | +3 |
| 58. | Dropping a course | −3 | −2 | −1 | 0 | +1 | +2 | +3 |
| 59. | Joining a fraternity/sorority | −3 | −2 | −1 | 0 | +1 | +2 | +3 |
| 60. | Financial problems concerning school (in danger of not having sufficient money to continue) | −3 | −2 | −1 | 0 | +1 | +2 | +3 |

Total Negative Points: ☐

Total Positive Points: ☐

| Category | Negative Score | | Total Score | |
|---|---|---|---|---|
| | Men | Women | Men | Women |
| Poor | ≥13 | ≥15 | ≥27 | ≥27 |
| Fair | 7–12 | 8–14 | 17–26 | 18–26 |
| Average | 6 | 7 | 16 | 17 |
| Good | 1–5 | 1–6 | 5–15 | 6–16 |
| Excellent | 0 | 0 | 1–4 | 1–5 |

**FIGURE 11.2** ◆ *(continued)*

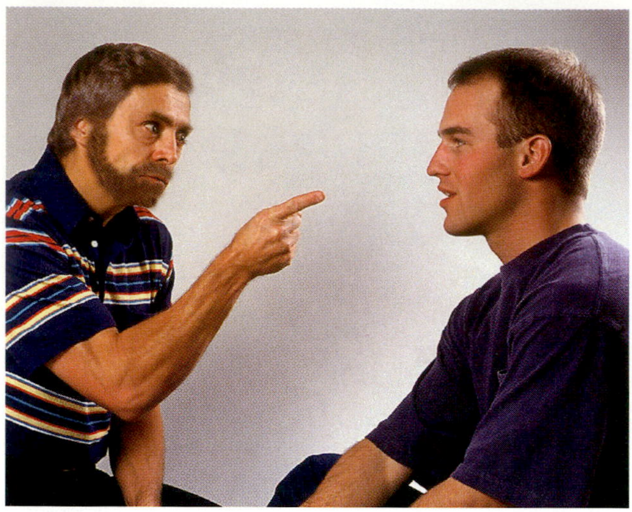

*Angry and hostile behaviors increase the risk for disease.*

New scientific evidence further indicates that not all typical Type A people are at higher risk for disease. Type A individuals who commonly express anger and hostility are the ones at higher risk. Therefore, many behavioral modification counselors now work on changing the latter behaviors to prevent disease.

We also know that many individuals perform well under pressure. They typically are classified as Type A but do not demonstrate any of the detrimental effects of stress. Drs. Robert and Marilyn Kriegel came up with the term Type C to characterize people with these behaviors.[2]

*Type C* individuals are just as highly stressed as Type A's but do not seem to be at higher risk for disease than Type B's. *The keys to successful Type C performance seem to be commitment, confidence, and control.* Type C people are highly committed to what they are doing, have a great deal of confidence in their ability to do their work, and are in constant control of their actions. In addition, they enjoy their work and maintain themselves in top physical condition to be able to meet the mental and physical demands of their work.

Because of the results of recent studies, Type A behavior by itself is no longer viewed as a major risk factor for coronary heart disease. Many experts now believe that emotional stress is far more likely to trigger a heart attack than physical stress. People who are impatient and readily annoyed when they have to wait for someone or something — an employee, a traffic light, in a restaurant line — are especially vulnerable.

Research also is focusing on individuals who have anxiety, depression, and feelings of helplessness when they encounter setbacks and failures in life. People who lose control of their lives, those who give up on their dreams in life, knowing that they could and should be doing better, probably are more likely to have heart attacks than hard-driving people who enjoy their work.

## VULNERABILITY TO STRESS

Researchers have identified a number of factors that can affect the way in which people handle stress. How people deal with these factors actually can increase or decrease vulnerability to stress. The questionnaire provided in Figure 11.3 lists these factors so you can determine your vulnerability rating. Many of the items on this questionnaire are related to health, social support, self-worth, and nurturance (sense of being needed). All of the factors are crucial for a person's physical, social, mental, and emotional well-being. The questionnaire will help you identify specific areas in which you can make improvements to help you cope more efficiently.

The benefits of physical fitness are discussed extensively in this book. Further, social support, self-worth, and nurturance are essential to cope effectively with stressful life events. These factors render a supportive and protective role in people's lives. The more integrated people are in society, the less vulnerable they are to stress and illness.

Positive correlations have been found between social support and health outcomes. People can draw upon social support to weather crises. Knowing that someone else cares, that people are there to lean on, that support is out there, is valuable for survival (or growth) in times of need.

As you take the test, you will notice that many of the items describe situations and behaviors that are within your own control. To make yourself less vulnerable to stress, you will want to improve the behaviors that make you more vulnerable to stress. You should start by modifying the behaviors that are easiest to change before undertaking some of the most difficult ones. After completing the questionnaire, record the results in Figure 11.4 and in your fitness and wellness profile in Appendix A.

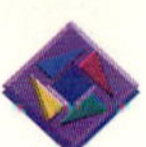

## STRESS VULNERABILITY QUESTIONNAIRE

| Item | Strongly Agree | Mildly Agree | Mildly Disagree | Strongly Disagree |
|---|---|---|---|---|
| 1. I try to incorporate as much physical activity* as possible in my daily schedule. | 1 | 2 | 3 | 4 |
| 2. I exercise aerobically 20 minutes or more at least three times per week. | 1 | 2 | 3 | 4 |
| 3. I regularly sleep 7 to 8 hours per night. | 1 | 2 | 3 | 4 |
| 4. I take my time eating at least one hot, balanced meal a day. | 1 | 2 | 3 | 4 |
| 5. I drink fewer than two cups of coffee (or equivalent) per day. | 1 | 2 | 3 | 4 |
| 6. I am at recommended body weight. | 1 | 2 | 3 | 4 |
| 7. I enjoy good health. | 1 | 2 | 3 | 4 |
| 8 I do not use tobacco in any form. | 1 | 2 | 3 | 4 |
| 9. I limit my alcohol intake to no more than one drink per day. | 1 | 2 | 3 | 4 |
| 10. I do not use hard drugs (chemical dependency). | 1 | 2 | 3 | 4 |
| 11. I have someone I love, trust, and can rely on for help if I have a problem or need to make an essential decision. | 1 | 2 | 3 | 4 |
| 12. There is love in my family. | 1 | 2 | 3 | 4 |
| 13. I routinely give and receive affection. | 1 | 2 | 3 | 4 |
| 14. I have close personal relationships with other people who provide me with a sense of emotional security. | 1 | 2 | 3 | 4 |
| 15. There are people close by whom I can turn to for guidance in time of stress. | 1 | 2 | 3 | 4 |
| 16. I can speak openly about feelings, emotions, and problems with people I trust. | 1 | 2 | 3 | 4 |
| 17. Other people rely on me for help. | 1 | 2 | 3 | 4 |
| 18. I am able to keep my feelings of anger and hostility under control. | 1 | 2 | 3 | 4 |
| 19. I have a network of friends who enjoy the same social activities I do. | 1 | 2 | 3 | 4 |
| 20. I take time to do something fun at least once a week. | 1 | 2 | 3 | 4 |
| 21. My religious beliefs provide guidance and strength to my life. | 1 | 2 | 3 | 4 |
| 22. I often provide service to others. | 1 | 2 | 3 | 4 |
| 23. I enjoy my job (major or school). | 1 | 2 | 3 | 4 |
| 24. I am a competent worker. | 1 | 2 | 3 | 4 |
| 25. I get along well with co-workers (or students). | 1 | 2 | 3 | 4 |
| 26. My income is sufficient for my needs. | 1 | 2 | 3 | 4 |
| 27. I manage time adequately. | 1 | 2 | 3 | 4 |
| 28. I have learned to say "no" to additional commitments when I am already pressed for time. | 1 | 2 | 3 | 4 |
| 29. I take daily quiet time for myself. | 1 | 2 | 3 | 4 |
| 30. I practice stress management as needed. | 1 | 2 | 3 | 4 |

Total Points: ______

**Scoring:**

0–30 points . . . . . . . . .Excellent (great resistance to stress)
31–40 points . . . . . . . . .Good (little vulnerability to stress)
41–50 points . . . . . . . . .Average (somewhat vulnerable to stress)
51–60 points . . . . . . . . .Fair (vulnerable to stress)
≥61 points . . . . . . . . .Poor (highly vulnerable to stress)

*Walk instead of driving, avoid escalators and elevators, or walk to neighboring offices, homes, and stores.

**FIGURE 11.3** ◆

Name:______________________________

| | Date | ______ | ______ | ______ |
|---|---|---|---|---|
| Life Experiences Survey | | | | |
| Score (negative) | | ______ | ______ | ______ |
| Stress Rating | | ______ | ______ | ______ |
| Stress Vulnerability Questionnaire | | | | |
| Score | | ______ | ______ | ______ |
| Rating | | ______ | ______ | ______ |
| Stress Management Technique(s) to be used | | ______ | ______ | ______ |

**FIGURE 11.4** ◆ Stress profile.

## TIME MANAGEMENT

According to Benjamin Franklin, "Time is the stuff life is made of." The present "hurry-up" style of life of the American people is not conducive to wellness. The hassles involved in getting through a routine day often lead to stress-related illnesses. People who do not manage their time properly will quickly experience chronic stress, fatigue, despair, discouragement, and illness.

Based on a 1990 Gallup Poll, almost 80% of Americans reported that time moves too fast for them, 54% felt they had to get everything done. The younger the respondents, the more they struggled with lack of time. Almost half wished they had more time for exercise and recreation, hobbies, and family.

Healthy and successful people are good time managers, able to maintain a pace of life within their comfort zone. In a survey of 1954 Harvard graduates from the school of business, only 27% had reached the goals they established in college. Every one had rated himself as a superior time manager, and only 8% of the remaining graduates perceived themselves as superior time managers. The successful graduates attributed their success to "smart work," not necessarily "hard work."

### Five Steps to Time Management

Trying to achieve one or more goals in a limited time can create a tremendous amount of stress. Many people just don't seem to have enough hours in the day to accomplish their tasks. The greatest demands on our time, nonetheless, frequently are self-imposed: trying to do too much, too fast, too soon. You can follow five basic steps to make better use of your time:

1. **Find the time killers.** Common time killers are listed below. Granted, some of these activities (such as eating, sleeping, and recreation) are

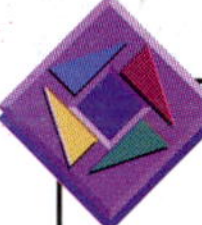

**COMMON TIME KILLERS**

- watching television
- listening to radio/music
- sleeping
- eating
- daydreaming
- shopping
- socializing/parties
- recreation
- talking on the telephone
- worrying
- procrastination
- drop-in visitors
- confusion (unclear goals)
- indecision (what to do next)
- interruptions
- perfectionism (every detail must be done)

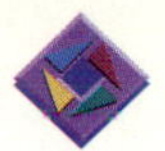

Keep a 4- to 7-day log, and record at half-hour intervals the activities you do (make additional copies of this form as needed). Record the activities as you go through your typical day, so you will remember them all. At the end of each day, decide when you wasted time. Using a highlighter, identify the time killers on this form and plan necessary changes for the next day.

Name: ______________________________ Date: ____________________

| | |
|---|---|
| 6:00 | |
| 6:30 | |
| 7:00 | |
| 7:30 | |
| 8:00 | |
| 8:30 | |
| 9:00 | |
| 9:30 | |
| 10:00 | |
| 10:30 | |
| 11:00 | |
| 11:30 | |
| 12:00 | |
| 12:30 | |
| 1:00 | |
| 1:30 | |
| 2:00 | |
| 2:30 | |
| 3:00 | |
| 3:30 | |
| 4:00 | |
| 4:30 | |
| 5:00 | |
| 5:30 | |
| 6:00 | |
| 6:30 | |
| 7:00 | |
| 7:30 | |
| 8:00 | |
| 8:30 | |
| 9:00 | |
| 9:30 | |
| 10:00 | |
| 10:30 | |
| 11:00 | |
| 11:30 | |
| 12:00 | |

**FIGURE 11.5** ◆ Finding your time killers.

necessary for health and wellness, but in excess they'll lead to stress in life.

Many people do not know how they spend each part of the day. Try to keep a 4- to 7-day log, and record your activities at half-hour intervals. A form is provided in Figure 11.5 to do this (make as many copies as the number of days you wish to evaluate). As you go through your typical day, record the activities so you will remember all of them. At the end of each day, decide when you wasted time. You may be shocked by the amount of time you spent on the phone, sleeping (more than 8 hours per night), or watching television.

2. **Set long-range and short-range goals.** Setting goals requires some in-depth thinking and helps put your life and daily tasks in perspective. What do I want out of life? Where do I want to be 10 years from now? Next year? Next week? Tomorrow? You can use the form provided in Figure 11.6 to list these goals.

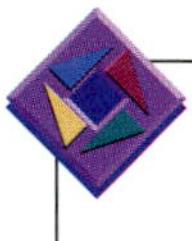

*Learn to say no to activities that keep you from getting your top priorities done.*

3. **Identify your immediate goals,** and prioritize them for today and this week (use Figure 11.7 — make as many copies as necessary). Each day sit down and determine what you need to accomplish that day and that week. Rank your "today" and "this week" tasks in four categories: (a) top-priority, (b) medium-priority, (c) low-priority, and (d) "trash."

   Top-priority tasks are the most important ones. If you were to reap most of your productivity from 30% of your activities, which would they be? Medium-priority activities are those that must be done but can wait a day or two. Low-priority activities are those to be done only upon completing all top- and middle-priority activities. Trash are activities that are not worth your time (for example, cruising the hallways).

4. **Use a daily planner to help you organize and simplify your day.** In this way you can access your priority list, appointments, notes, references, names, places, phone numbers, and addresses conveniently from your coat pocket or purse. Many individuals think that planning daily and weekly activities is a waste of time. A few minutes to schedule your time each day, however, may pay off in hours saved.

   As you plan your day, be realistic and find your comfort zone. Determine what is the best way to organize your day. Which is the most productive time for work, study, errands? Are you a morning person, or are you getting most of your work done when people are quitting for the day? Pick your best hours for top-priority activities. Be sure to schedule enough time for exercise and relaxation. Recreation is not necessarily wasted time. You need to take care of your physical and emotional well-being. Otherwise your life will be seriously imbalanced.

5. **Nightly audits.** Take 10 minutes each night to figure out how well you accomplished your goals that day. Successful time managers evaluate themselves daily. This simple task will help you see the entire picture. Cross off the goals you accomplished, and carry over to the next day those you did not get done. You also may realize that some goals can be moved down to low-priority or be trashed.

## Time-Management Skills

In addition to the five major steps, the following can help you make better use of your time:

- **Delegate.** If possible, delegate activities that someone else can do for you. Having another person type your paper while you prepare for an exam might be well worth the expense and your time.
- **Say "no."** Learn to say *no* to activities that keep you from getting your top priorities done. You can do only so much in a single day. Nobody has enough time to do everything he or she would like to get done. Don't overload either. Many people are afraid to say no because they feel guilty if they do. Think ahead, and think of the consequences. Are you doing it to please others? What will it do to your well-being? Can you handle one more task? At some point you have to balance your activities and look at life and time realistically.
- **Protect against boredom.** Doing nothing can be a source of stress. People need to feel that they are contributing and that they are productive members of society. It also is good for self-esteem and self-worth. Set realistic goals, and work toward them each day.

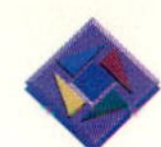

In the spaces provided below, list your goals as indicated. You may want to keep this form and review it in years to come.

I. List three goals you wish to accomplish in this life:

1. ______________________________
2. ______________________________
3. ______________________________

II. List three goals you wish to see accomplished 10 years from now:

1. ______________________________
2. ______________________________
3. ______________________________

III. List three goals you wish to accomplish this year:

1. ______________________________
2. ______________________________
3. ______________________________

IV. List three goals you wish to accomplish this month:

1. ______________________________
2. ______________________________
3. ______________________________

V. List three goals you wish to accomplish this week:

1. ______________________________
2. ______________________________
3. ______________________________

Signature: ______________________ Date: ______________

**FIGURE 11.6** ◆ Planning your long- and short-range goals.

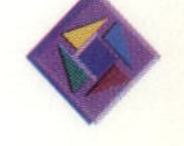



Take 10 minutes each morning and write down the goals or tasks you wish to accomplish that day. Rank them as top, medium, low, or "trash" priorities (Make as many copies of this form as needed). At the end of the day, evaluate how well you accomplished your tasks for the day. Cross off the goals you accomplished, and carry over to the next day those you did not get done.

Date: ____________ Day of the Week: ____________

Top-Priority Goals

1. ____________
2. ____________
3. ____________
4. ____________

Medium-Priority Goals

1. ____________
2. ____________
3. ____________
4. ____________

Low-Priority Goals

1. ____________
2. ____________
3. ____________
4. ____________

Trash (do only after all other goals have been accomplished)

1. ____________
2. ____________
3. ____________
4. ____________

Take a few minutes each Sunday night and write down the goals or tasks you wish to accomplish during the upcoming week. As with your daily goals, rank them as top, medium, low, or "trash" priorities (Make as many copies of this form as needed). At the end of the week, evaluate how well you accomplished your goals. Cross off the goals you accomplished, and carry over to the next week those you did not get done.

Week: ____/____/199__ to ____/____/199__

Top -Priority Goals

1. ____________
2. ____________
3. ____________
4. ____________

Medium-Priority Goals

1. ____________
2. ____________
3. ____________
4. ____________

Low Priority-Goals

1. ____________
2. ____________
3. ____________
4. ____________

Trash (do only after all other goals have been accomplished)

1. ____________
2. ____________
3. ____________
4. ____________

**FIGURE 11.7** ◆ Listing of daily and weekly goals and priorities.

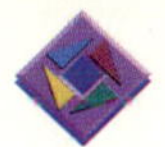

- **Plan ahead for disruptions.** Even a careful plan of action can be disrupted. An unexpected phone call or visitor can ruin your schedule. Planning your response ahead will help you deal with these saboteurs.
- **Get it done.** Select only one task at a time, concentrate on it, and see it through. Many people do a little here, do a little there, then do something else. In the end, nothing gets done. An exception to working on just one task at a time is when you are doing a difficult task. Rather than "killing yourself," interchange with another activity that is not as hard.
- **Eliminate distractions.** If you have trouble adhering to a set plan, remove distractions and trash activities from your eyesight. Television, radio, magazines, open doors, or studying in a park might distract you and become time killers.
- **Set aside "overtimes."** Regularly schedule time you did not think you would need as overtime to complete unfinished projects. Most people underschedule rather than overschedule time. The result is usually late-night burnout! If you schedule overtimes and get your tasks done, enjoy some leisure time, get ahead on another project, or work on some of your trash priorities.
- **Plan time for you.** Set aside special time for yourself daily. Life is not meant to be all work. Use your time to walk, read, or listen to your favorite music.
- **Reward yourself.** As with any other healthy behavior, positive change or a job well done deserves a reward. We often overlook the value of rewards, even if they are self-given. People practice behaviors that are rewarded and discontinue those that are not.

One more activity that you should perform weekly is to go through the list of strategies in Figure 11.8 to determine if you are becoming a good time manager. Provide a yes or no answer to each statement. If you are able to answer yes to most questions, congratulations. You are becoming a good time manager.

## COPING WITH STRESS

The way in which people perceive and cope with stress seems to be more important in the development of disease than the amount and type of stress itself. If individuals perceive stress as a definite problem in their lives, when it interferes with optimal level of health and performance, several excellent stress management techniques can help them cope more effectively.

First, of course, the person must recognize that a problem exists. Many people either do not want to believe they are under too much stress or they fail to recognize some of the typical symptoms of distress. Noting some of the stress-related symptoms (see below) will help a person respond more objectively and initiate an adequate coping response.

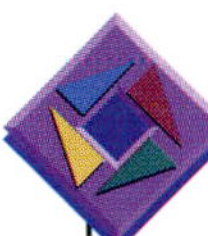

### COMMON SYMPTOMS OF STRESS

- headaches
- muscular aches (mainly in neck, shoulders, and back)
- grinding teeth
- nervous tick, finger tapping, toe tapping
- increased sweating
- increase in or loss of appetite
- insomnia
- nightmares
- fatigue
- dry mouth
- stuttering
- high blood pressure
- tightness or pain in the chest
- impotence
- hives
- dizziness
- depression
- irritation
- anger
- hostility
- fear, panic, anxiety
- stomach pain, flutters
- nausea
- cold, clammy hands
- poor concentration
- pacing
- restlessness
- rapid heart rate
- low-grade infection
- loss of sex drive
- rash or acne

On a weekly basis, go through the list of strategies given below and write a "Yes" or "No" in response to each statement. If you are able to answer "Yes" to most questions, congratulations. You are becoming a good time manager.

| **Strategy** **Date:** | | | | | | | | | | | | | | | |
|---|---|---|---|---|---|---|---|---|---|---|---|---|---|---|---|
| 1. I evaluate my time killers periodically | | | | | | | | | | | | | | | |
| 2. I have written down my long-range goals | | | | | | | | | | | | | | | |
| 3. I have written down my short-range goals | | | | | | | | | | | | | | | |
| 4. I use a daily planner | | | | | | | | | | | | | | | |
| 5. I conduct nightly audits | | | | | | | | | | | | | | | |
| 6. I conduct weekly audits | | | | | | | | | | | | | | | |
| 7. I delegate activities that others can do | | | | | | | | | | | | | | | |
| 8. I have learned to say no to additional tasks when I'm already in "overload" | | | | | | | | | | | | | | | |
| 9. I plan activities to avoid boredom | | | | | | | | | | | | | | | |
| 10. I plan ahead for distractions | | | | | | | | | | | | | | | |
| 11. I work on one task at a time until it's done | | | | | | | | | | | | | | | |
| 12. I have removed distractions from my work | | | | | | | | | | | | | | | |
| 13. I set aside "overtimes" | | | | | | | | | | | | | | | |
| 14. I set aside special time for myself daily | | | | | | | | | | | | | | | |
| 15. I reward myself for a job well done | | | | | | | | | | | | | | | |

**FIGURE 11.8** ◆ Evaluation of time-management skills.

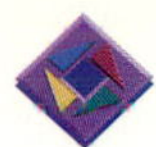

When people have stress-related symptoms, they first should try to identify and remove the stressor or stress-causing agent. This is not as simple as it may seem, because in some situations eliminating the stressor is not possible, or a person may not even know the exact causing agent. If the cause is unknown, keeping a log of the time and days when the symptoms occur, as well as the events preceding and following the onset of symptoms, may be helpful.

For instance, a couple noted that every afternoon around 6 o'clock, the wife became nauseated and had abdominal pain. After seeking professional help, both were instructed to keep a log of daily events. It soon became clear that the symptoms did not occur on weekends but always started just before the husband came home from work during the week. Following some personal interviews with the couple, it was determined that the wife felt a lack of attention from her husband and responded subconsciously by becoming ill to the point at which she required personal care and affection from her husband. Once the stressor was identified, appropriate behavior changes were initiated to correct the situation.

In many instances, however, the stressor cannot be removed. Examples of situations in which little or nothing can be done to eliminate the stress-causing agent are the death of a close family member, first year on the job, an intolerable boss, a change in work responsibility. Nevertheless, stress can be managed through relaxation techniques.

The body responds to stress by activating the *fight-or-flight* mechanism, which prepares a person to take action by stimulating the vital defense systems. This stimulation originates in the hypothalamus and the pituitary gland in the brain. The hypothalamus activates the sympathetic nervous system, and the pituitary activates the release of catecholamines (hormones) from the adrenal glands.

These hormonal changes increase heart rate, blood pressure, blood flow to active muscles and the brain, glucose levels, oxygen consumption, and strength — all necessary for the body to fight or flee. For the body to relax, one of these actions must take place. If the person fights or flees, the body relaxes and stress dissipates but if the person is unable to take action, the muscles tense up and tighten (see Figure 11.9). This increased tension and tightening can be dissipated effectively through some coping techniques.

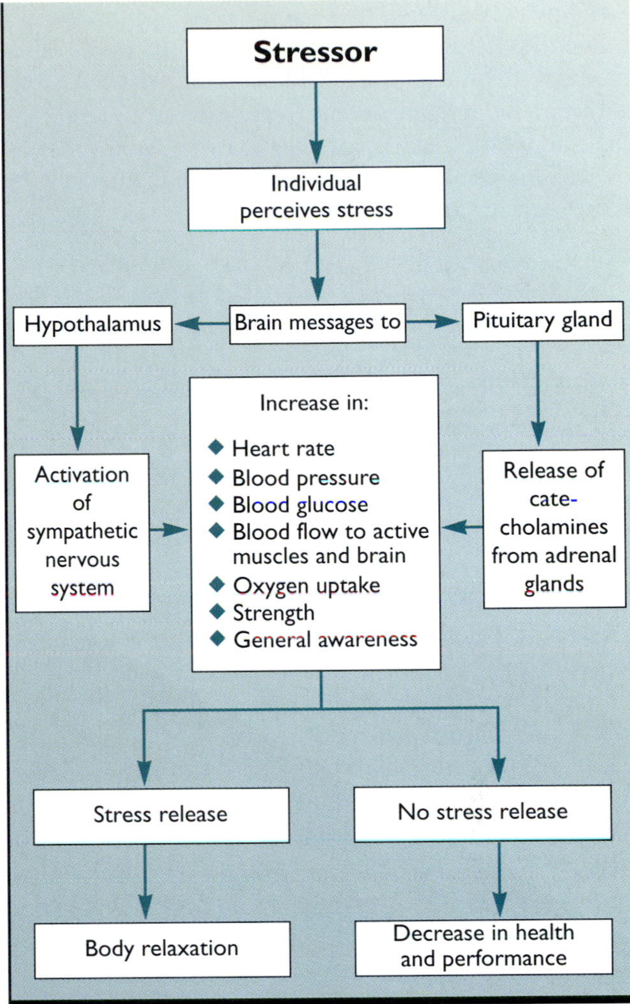


**FIGURE 11.9** ◆ Physiological response to stress: fight or flight mechanism.

## RELAXATION TECHNIQUES

Benefits are reaped immediately after engaging in any of several relaxation techniques. Several months of regular practice, however, may be necessary for total mastery. The relaxation exercises that follow should not be considered cure-alls or panaceas. If these exercises do not prove to be effective, more specialized textbooks and professional help are called for. In some instances a person's symptoms may not be caused by stress but, rather, may be related to a different medical disorder.

### Biofeedback

Clinical application of biofeedback in treating various medical disorders has become popular in the last few years. Besides its successful application in managing stress, it is used commonly in treating medical disorders such as essential hypertension, asthma, heart rhythm and rate disturbances, cardiac neurosis, eczematous dermatitis, fecal incontinence, insomnia, and stuttering. Biofeedback as a treatment modality has been defined as:[3]

> A process in which a person learns to reliably influence physiological responses of two kinds: either responses which are not ordinarily under voluntary control or responses which ordinarily are easily regulated but for which regulation has broken down due to trauma or disease.

In simpler terms biofeedback is the interaction with the interior self. This interaction allows a person to learn the relationship between the mind and the biological response. The person actually can "feel" how thought processes influence biological responses, (such as heart rate, blood pressure, body temperature, and muscle tension, and how biological responses influence the thought process.

As an illustration of this process, consider the association between a strange noise in the middle of a dark, quiet night and the heart rate response. At first the heart rate shoots up because of the stress the unknown noise induces. The individual may even feel the heart palpitating in the chest and, while still uncertain about the noise, attempts not to panic to prevent an even faster heart rate. Upon realizing that all is well, the person can take control and influence the heart rate to come down. The mind now is able to exert almost complete control over the biological response.

Complex electronic instruments are required to conduct biofeedback. The process itself entails a three-stage, closed-loop feedback system:

1. A biological response to a stressor is detected and amplified.
2. The response is processed.
3. Results of the response are fed back to the individual immediately.

The person uses this new input and attempts to change the physiological response voluntarily, which, in turn, is detected, amplified, and processed. The results then are fed back to the person. The process continues with the intent of teaching the person to reliably influence for the better the physiological response (see Figure 11.10). The most common methods used to measure physiological responses are heart rate, finger temperature, blood pressure equipment, electromyograms, and electroencephalograms.

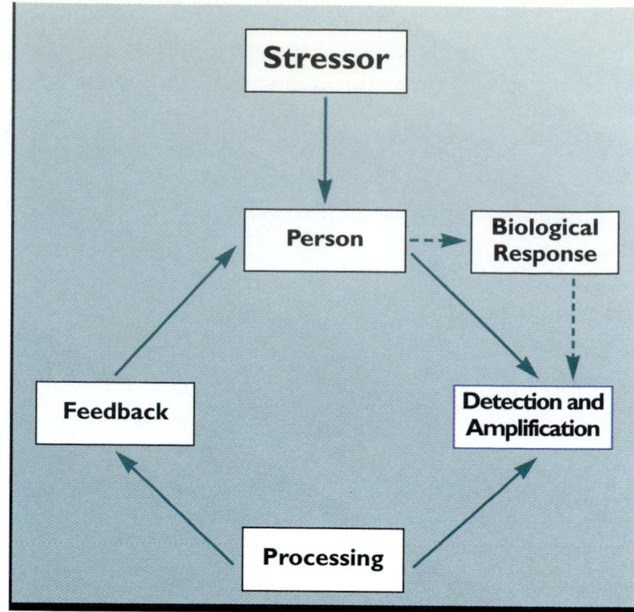


**FIGURE 11.10** ◆ Biofeedback mechanism.

Although biofeedback has significant applications in treating various medical disorders, including stress, it requires adequately trained personnel and, in many cases, costly equipment. Therefore, several alternative methods that yield similar results frequently are substituted for biofeedback. For example, research has shown that physical exercise and progressive muscle relaxation, used successfully in stress management, seem to be just as effective as biofeedback in treating essential hypertension.

## Physical Activity

Physical activity is one of the simplest tools to control stress. The value of exercise in reducing stress is related to several factors, the main one being a decrease in muscular tension. For example, a person can be distressed because he or she has had a miserable 8 hours of work in a smoke-filled room with an intolerable boss. To make matters worse, it is late and on the way home the car in front is going much slower than the speed limit. The fight-or-flight mechanism is activated, catecholamines rise, heart rate and blood pressure shoot up, breathing quickens and deepens, muscles tense up, and all systems say "go." No action can be initiated or stress dissipated, though, because the person just cannot hit the boss or the car in front.

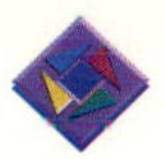

A real remedy would be to take action by "hitting" the swimming pool, the tennis ball, the weights, or the jogging trail. By engaging in physical activity, a person is able to reduce the muscular tension and metabolize the increased catecholamines that brought about the physiological changes triggering the fight-or-flight mechanism. Although exercise does not solve problems at work or take care of slow drivers on the road, it certainly can help a person cope with stress, preventing it from becoming a chronic problem.

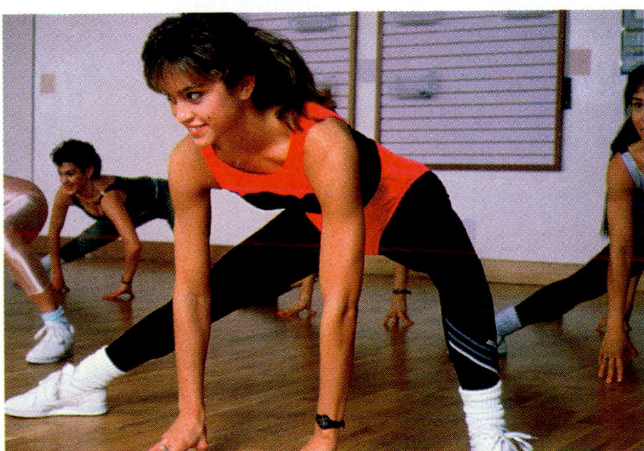

*Physical activity is an excellent tool to control stress.*

The early evening hours are becoming the most popular time to exercise for a lot of highly stressed executives. On the way home from work, they stop at the health club or the fitness center. Exercising at this time helps them to dissipate the stress accumulated during the day.

Most people can relate to exercise as a means of managing stress by remembering how good they felt the last time they concluded a strenuous exercise session after a long, difficult day at the office. A fatigued muscle is a relaxed muscle. For this reason, many people have said that the best part of exercise is the shower afterward.

Not only does evening exercise help to get rid of the stress, but it also provides an opportunity to enjoy the evening more. At home, the family will appreciate Dad or Mom coming home more relaxed, leaving work problems behind, and being able to dedicate all energy to family activities.

Research also has shown that physical exercise requiring continuous and rhythmic muscular activity, such as aerobic exercise, stimulates alpha-wave activity in the brain. These are the same wave patterns seen commonly during meditation and relaxation.

Further, during vigorous aerobic exercise lasting 30 minutes or longer, morphine-like substances referred to as endorphines are thought to be released from the pituitary gland in the brain. These substances not only act as painkillers but also seem to induce the soothing, calming effect often associated with aerobic exercise.

Another way that exercise helps to lower stress is by deliberately diverting stress to various body systems. Dr. Hans Selye explains in his book, *Stress Without Distress*,[4] that when accomplishing one specific task becomes difficult, a change in activity can be as good or better than rest itself. For example, if a person is having trouble with a task and does not seem to be getting anywhere, jogging or swimming for a while is better than sitting around and getting frustrated. In this way the mental strain is diverted to the working muscles, and one system helps the other to relax.

Other psychologists indicate that when muscular tension is removed from the emotional strain, the emotional strain disappears. In many cases the change of activity suddenly clears the mind and helps put the pieces together. Researchers have found that physical exercise gives people a psychological boost because exercise:

- Lessens feelings of anxiety, depression, frustration, aggression, anger, and hostility.
- Alleviates insomnia.
- Provides an opportunity to meet social needs and develop new friendships.
- Allows the person to share common interests and problems.
- Develops discipline.
- Provides the opportunity to do something enjoyable and constructive that will lead to better health and total well-being.

Beyond the short-term benefits of exercise in lessening stress, another benefit of a regular aerobic exercise program is in actually strengthening the cardiovascular system itself. Because the cardiovascular system seems to be affected seriously by stress, a stronger system should be able to cope more effectively. For instance, good cardiovascular endurance has been shown to lower resting heart rate and blood pressure. Because both heart rate and blood pressure rise in stressful situations, initiating the stress response at a lower baseline will counteract the negative effects of stress. Cardiovascularly fit individuals can cope more effectively and are less affected by the stresses of daily living.

## Progressive Muscle Relaxation

Progressive muscle relaxation was developed by Dr. Edmund Jacobsen in the 1930s. This technique enables individuals to relearn the sensation of deep relaxation. The technique involves *progressively contracting and relaxing muscle groups throughout the body*. As chronic stress leads to high levels of muscular tension, acute awareness of how progressively tightening and relaxing the muscles feels releases the tension on the muscles and teaches the body to relax at will.

Feeling the tension during the exercises also helps the person to be more alert to signs of distress because this tension is similar to that experienced in stressful situations. In everyday life these feelings then can cue the person to do relaxation exercises.

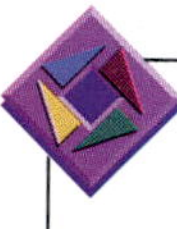

*Progressively tightening and relaxing the muscles releases tension and teaches the body to relax at will.*

Relaxation exercises should be done in a quiet, warm, well-ventilated room. The recommended exercises and the duration of the routine vary from one person to the next. Most important is that the individual pay attention to the sensation he or she feels each time the muscles are tensed and relaxed.

The exercises should encompass all muscle groups of the body. An example of a sequence of progressive muscle relaxation exercises is given next. The instructions for these exercises can be read to the person or memorized or tape-recorded. At least 20 minutes should be set aside to complete the entire sequence. Doing the exercises any faster will defeat their purpose. Ideally, the sequence should be done twice a day.

The individual performing the exercises stretches out comfortably on the floor, face up, with a pillow under the knees, and assumes a passive attitude, allowing the body to relax as much as possible. Each muscle group is to be contracted in sequence, taking care to avoid any strain. Muscles should be tightened to only about 70% of the total possible tension to avoid cramping or some type of injury to the muscle itself.

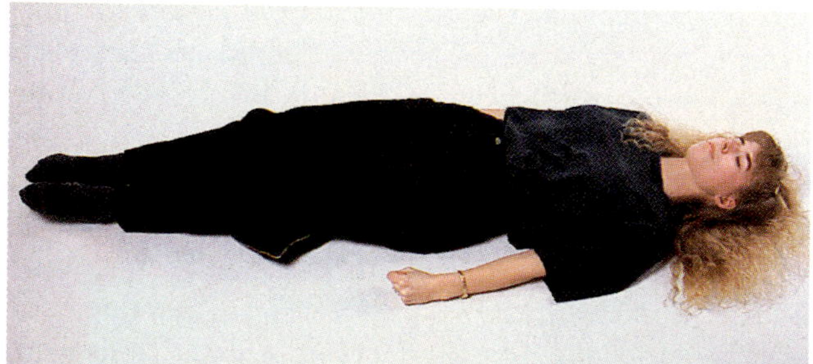

*Practicing regular progressive muscle relaxation helps reduce stress.*

To produce the relaxation effects, the person must pay attention to the sensation of tensing up and relaxing. The person holds each contraction about 5 seconds and then allows the muscles to go totally limp. The person should take enough time to contract and relax each muscle group before going on to the next. An example of a complete progressive muscle relaxation sequence is:

1. Point your feet, curling the toes downward. Study the tension in the arches and the top of the feet. Hold, and continue to note the tension, then relax. Repeat once again.
2. Flex the feet upward toward the face, and note the tension in your feet and calves. Hold, and relax. Repeat once more.
3. Push your heels down against the floor as if burying them in the sand. Hold, and note the tension at the back of the thigh. Relax. Repeat once more.
4. Contract the right thigh by straightening the leg, gently raising the leg off the floor. Hold, and study the tension. Relax. Repeat with the left leg. Hold and relax. Repeat each leg again.
5. Tense the buttocks by raising your hips ever so slightly off the floor. Hold, and note the tension. Relax. Repeat once again.
6. Contract the abdominal muscles. Hold them tight and note the tension. Relax. Repeat one more time.
7. Suck in your stomach. Try to make it reach your spine. Flatten your lower back to the floor. Hold, and feel the tension in the stomach and lower back. Relax. Repeat once more.
8. Take a deep breath and hold it, then exhale. Repeat. Note your breathing becoming slower and more relaxed.
9. Place your arms at the side of your body and clench both fists. Hold, study the tension, and relax. Repeat a second time.
10. Flex the elbow by bringing both hands to the shoulders. Hold tight and study the tension in the biceps. Relax. Repeat one more time.

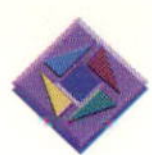

11. Place your arms flat on the floor, palms up, and push the forearms hard against the floor. Note the tension on the triceps. Hold, and relax. Repeat once more.
12. Shrug your shoulders, raising them as high as possible. Hold, and note the tension. Relax. Repeat once again.
13. Gently push your head backward. Note the tension in the back of the neck. Hold, relax. Repeat one more time.
14. Gently bring the head against the chest, push forward, hold, and note the tension in the neck. Relax. Repeat a second time.
15. Press your tongue toward the roof of your mouth. Hold, study the tension, and relax. Repeat once more.

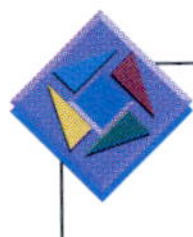

*Each muscle contraction should be performed at 70% of maximal capacity for about five seconds.*

16. Press your teeth together. Hold, and study the tension. Relax. Repeat one more time.
17. Close your eyes tightly. Hold them closed and note the tension. Relax, leaving your eyes closed. Do this one more time.
18. Wrinkle your forehead and note the tension. Hold, and relax. Repeat one more time.

When time is a factor during the daily routine and an individual is not able to go through the entire sequence, he or she may do only the exercises specific to the area that feels most tense. Performing a partial sequence is better than not doing the exercises at all. Completing the entire sequence, of course, yields the best results.

## Breathing Techniques For Relaxation

Breathing exercises also can be an antidote to stress. These exercises have been used for centuries in the Orient and India to improve mental, physical, and emotional stamina. In breathing exercises the person concentrates on "breathing away" the tension and inhaling fresh air to the entire body. Breathing exercises can be learned in only a few minutes and require considerably less time than the progressive muscle relaxation exercises.

As with any other relaxation technique, these exercises should be done in a quiet, pleasant, well-ventilated room. Any of the three examples of breathing exercises presented here will help relieve tension induced by stress.

1. **Deep breathing.** Lie with your back flat against the floor, and place a pillow under your knees, feet slightly separated, with toes pointing outward. (The exercise also may be done while sitting up in a chair or standing straight up). Place one hand on your abdomen and the other hand on your chest.

   Slowly breathe in and out so the hand on your abdomen rises when you inhale and falls as you exhale. The hand on the chest should not move much at all. Repeat the exercise about 10 times. Next, scan your body for tension, and compare your present tension with the tension you felt at the beginning of the exercise. Repeat the entire process once or twice more.
2. **Sighing.** Using the abdominal breathing technique, breathe in through your nose to a specific count (e.g., 4, 5, or 6). Now exhale through pursed lips to double the intake count (e.g., 8, 10, or 12). Repeat the exercise eight to 10 times whenever you feel tense.
3. **Complete natural breathing.** Sit in an upright position or stand straight up. Breathing through your nose, gradually fill your lungs from the bottom up. Hold your breath for several seconds. Now exhale slowly by allowing your chest and abdomen to relax completely. Repeat the exercise eight to 10 times.

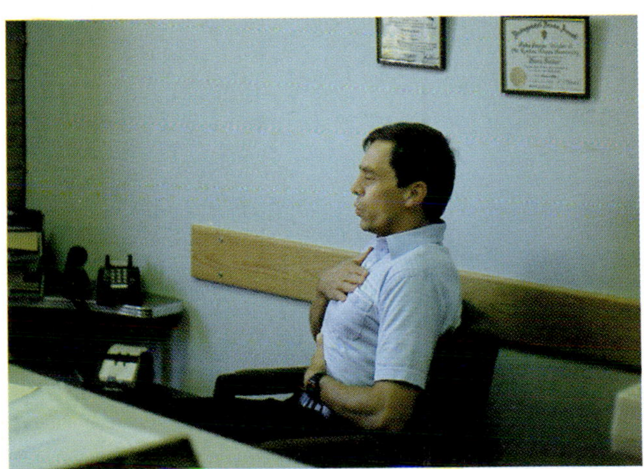

*Breathing exercises help dissipate stress.*

## Autogenic Training

Autogenic training is basically *a form of self-suggestion, in which people are able to place themselves in an autohypnotic state* by repeating and concentrating on feelings of heaviness and warmth in the extremities. This technique was developed by Johannes Schultz, a German psychiatrist, who noted that hypnotized individuals developed sensations of warmth and heaviness in the limbs and torso. The sensation of warmth is caused by dilation of blood vessels, which increases blood flow to the limbs. Muscular relaxation produces the feeling of heaviness.

In this technique the person lies down or sits in a comfortable position, eyes closed, and concentrates progressively on six fundamental stages:

1. **Heaviness**

   My right (left) arm is heavy.
   Both arms are heavy.
   My right (left) leg is heavy.
   Both legs are heavy.
   My arms and legs are heavy.

2. **Warmth**

   My right (left) arm is warm.
   Both arms are warm.
   My right (left) leg is warm.
   Both legs are warm.
   My arms and legs are warm.

3. **Heart**

   My heartbeat is calm and regular (repeat four or five times).

4. **Respiration**

   My body breathes itself (repeat four or five times).

5. **Abdomen**

   My abdomen is warm (repeat four or five times).

6. **Forehead**

   My forehead is cool (repeat four or five times).

The autogenic training technique is more difficult to master than any of those mentioned previously. The person should not move too fast through the entire exercise, as this actually may interfere with learning and relaxation. Each stage must be mastered before proceeding to the next.

## Meditation

Meditation is *a mental exercise that can bring about psychological and physical benefits.* The objective of meditation is to gain control over one's attention, clearing the mind and blocking out the stressor(s) responsible for the higher tension. This technique can be learned rather quickly and can be used frequently during times of increased tension and stress.

Initially the person who is learning to meditate should choose a room that is comfortable, quiet, and free of all disturbances (including telephones). After learning the technique, the person will be able to meditate just about anywhere. A time block of approximately 15 minutes, twice a day, is needed to meditate.

1. Sit in a chair in an upright position with the hands resting either in your lap or on the arms of the chair. Close your eyes and focus on your breathing. Allow your body to relax as much as possible. Do not try to consciously relax, because trying means work. Rather, assume a passive attitude and concentrate on your breathing.
2. Allow the body to breathe regularly, at its own rhythm, and repeat in your mind the word "one" every time you inhale, and the word "two" every time you exhale. Paying attention to these two words keeps distressing thoughts from entering into your mind.
3. Continue to breathe in this way about 15 minutes. Because the objective of meditation is to bring about a hypometabolic state leading to body relaxation, do not use an alarm clock to remind you that the 15 minutes have expired. The alarm will only trigger your stress response again, defeating the purpose of the exercise. Opening your eyes once in a while to keep track of the time is fine, but do not rush or anticipate the end of the 15 minutes. This time has been set aside for meditation, and you need to relax, take your time, and enjoy the exercise.

## Which Technique Is Best?

Each person reacts to stress differently. Therefore, the best coping strategy depends mostly on the individual. Which technique is used does not really matter as long as it works. An individual may want to experiment with all of them to find out which

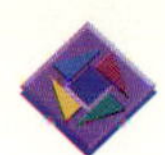

works best. A combination of two or more works best for many people.

All of the coping strategies discussed here help to block out stressors and promote mental and physical relaxation by diverting the attention to a different, nonthreatening action. Some of the techniques are easier to learn and may take less time per session. Regardless of which technique you select, the time spent doing stress management exercises (several times a day, as needed) is well worth the effort when stress becomes a significant problem in life.

People need to learn to relax and take time out for themselves. Stress is not what makes people ill but, rather, the way they react to the stress-causing agent. Individuals who learn to be diligent and start taking control of themselves find that they can enjoy a better, happier, and healthier life.

## NOTES

1. H. Selye, *Stress Without Distress.* New York: Signet, 1974.
2. R. J. Kriegel and M. H. Kriegel, *The C Zone: Peak Performance Under Stress* (Garden City, NY: Anchor Press/Doubleday, 1984).
3. E. B. Blanchard and L. H. Epstein. *A Biofeedback Primer* (Reading, MA: Addison-Wesley, 1978).
4. H. Selye.

## SELECT BIBLIOGRAPHY


Andrasik, F., D. Coleman, and L. H. Epstein. "Biofeedback: Clinical and Research Considerations." In *Behavioral Medicine: Assessment and Treatment Strategies*, edited by D. M. Doleys, R. L. Meredith, and A. R. Ciminero. New York: Plenum Press, 1982.

Blue Cross Association. *Stress.* Chicago: BCA, 1974.

Brown, B. *New Mind, New Body.* New York: Harper & Row, 1974.

Chesney, M. A., J. R. Eagleston, and R. H. Roseman. "Type A Assessment and Intervention." In *Medical Psychology: Contributions to Behavioral Medicine*, edited by C. K. Prokop and L. A. Bradley. New York: Academic Press, 1981.

Gauron, E. F. *Mental Training for Peak Performance.* Lansing, NY: Sport Science Associates, 1984.

Girdano, D., and G. Everly. *Controlling Stress and Tension: A Holistic Approach.* Englewood Cliffs, NJ: Prentice Hall, 1990.

Greenberg, J. S. *Comprehensive Stress Management.* Dubuque, IA: Wm. C. Brown Co., 1987.

Luthe, W. "Autogenic Training: Method, Research and Applications in Medicine." *American Journal of Psychotherapy,* 17 (1963), 174-195.

McKay, M., M. Davis, and P. Fanning. *Thoughts and Feelings: The Act of Cognitive Stress Intervention.* Richmond, CA: New Harbinger Publications, 1981.

Miller, L. H., and A. D. Smith. "Vulnerability Scale." *Stress Audit,* 1983.

Sarason, I. G., J. H. Johnson, and J. M. Siegel. "Assessing the Impact of Life Changes: Development of the Life Experiences Survey." *Journal of Consulting and Clinical Psychology,* 46 (1978), 932-946.

Schafer, W. *Stress Management for Wellness.* Fort Worth, TX: HBJ College Publishers, 1992.

Selye, H. *The Stress of Life.* New York: McGraw-Hill Book Co., 1978.

Smith, J. S. *Creative Stress Management: The 1-2-3 Cope System.* Englewood Cliffs, NJ: Prentice Hall, 1993.

Staff. "How Running Relieves Stress." *Runner* 8:11 (1986), 38-43, 82.

Turk, D. C., and R. D. Kerns. "Assessment in Health Psychology: A Cognitive-Behavioral Perspective." In *Measurement Strategies in Health Psychology*, edited by P. Karoly. New York: John Wiley & Sons, 1985.

# Smoking Cessation

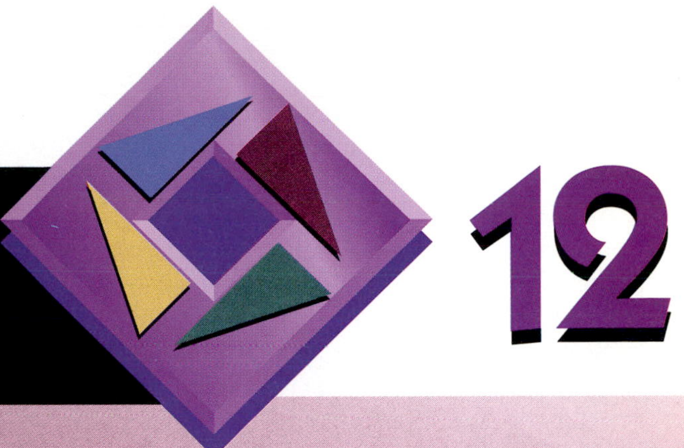


## Key Concepts

Alveoli
Carcinogens
Nicotine
Tar
Secondhand smoke
Stimulation
Handling
Accentuation
Crutch
Dependence
Habit
Aesthetics
Mastery
Cold turkey
Tapering off

## Objectives

- Understand the detrimental health effects of tobacco use in general.
- Recognize cigarette smoking as the largest preventable cause of premature illness and death in the United States.
- Learn the fundamental reasons why people smoke.
- Understand the benefits and the significance of a smoking cessation program.
- Learn how to implement a smoking cessation program, either for yourself (if you smoke) or to help others go through the quitting process.

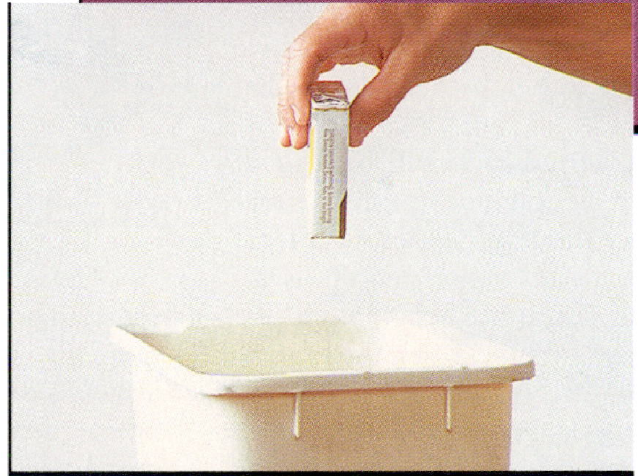

People throughout the world have used tobacco for hundreds of years. Before the 18th century they smoked tobacco primarily in the form of pipes or cigars. Cigarette smoking per se did not become popular until the mid-1800s, and its use started to increase dramatically at the turn of the century.

In 1915, 18 billion cigarettes were consumed in the United States, as compared to 640 billion in 1981. This figure dropped to 538 billion in 1989. Nonetheless, more than 48 million Americans over age 17 still smoke an average of one and one-half packs of cigarettes per day.

The harmful effects of cigarette smoking and tobacco use in general were not exactly known until the early 1960s, when researchers began to show a link between tobacco usage and disease. In 1964, the U.S. Surgeon General issued the first major report presenting scientific evidence that cigarettes are indeed a major health hazard in our society.

Tobacco use in all its forms now is considered a significant threat to life. An estimated 10% of the 5 billion people presently living on the earth will die as a result of smoking-related illnesses, killing approximately 3 million people each year.

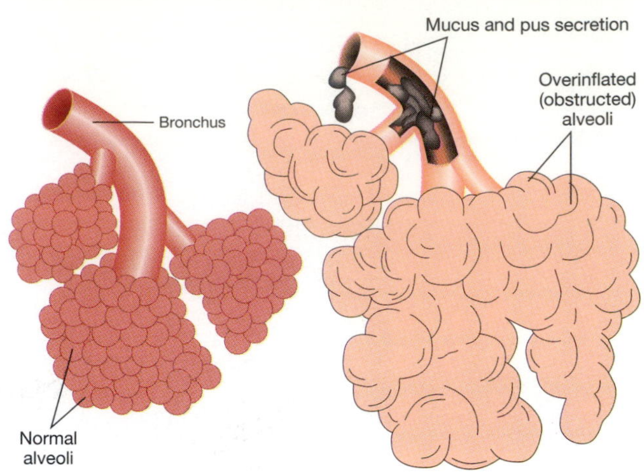


**FIGURE 12.1** ◆ Normal and diseased alveoli in the lungs.

## CIGARETTE SMOKING

Illegal drug overdoses kill about 17,500 people per year in the United States. Drug felonies and drug-related murders kill another 1,600 people each year. This brings drug-related deaths to a grand total of 19,100. Citizens and the government have mounted a tremendous campaign to eradicate illegal drug use in America.

A drug-free society certainly would be a great accomplishment for our people and future generations. At the same time, though, cigarettes, a legal drug, kill about 26 times as many people as all illegal drugs combined. Cigarette smoking is the largest preventable cause of illness and premature death in the United States. When considering all related deaths, smoking is responsible for more than 450,000 unnecessary deaths each year, enough deaths to wipe out the entire population of Miami and Miami Beach in a single year.

Death rates from heart disease, cancer, stroke, aortic aneurysm, chronic bronchitis, emphysema, and peptic ulcers have increased noticeably. Figure 12.1 illustrates normal air sacs in the lung (alveoli) and diseased alveoli seen with emphysema. Cigarette smoking by pregnant women has been linked to retarded fetal growth, higher risk for spontaneous abortion, and prenatal death. Smoking also is the most prevalent cause of injury and death from fire. The average life expectancy for a chronic smoker is as much as 18 years shorter than for a nonsmoker, and the death rate among chronic smokers during the most productive years of life, between ages 25 and 65, is twice that of the national average.

According to a 1993 report by U.S. government physicians, each cigarette shortens life by 7 minutes. This figure represents 5 million years of potential life that Americans lose to smoking each year.

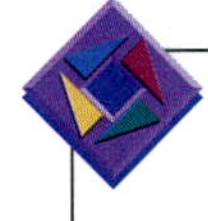

*Cigarette smoking is the largest preventable cause of illness and premature death in the United States.*

The American Heart Association estimates that more than 30% of fatal heart attacks, or 120,000 annually, results from smoking. The risk for heart attack is 50% to 100% higher for smokers than for nonsmokers. The mortality rate following heart attacks also is higher for smokers, as the attacks usually are more severe and the risk for deadly arrhythmias is much greater.

Cigarette smoking affects the cardiovascular system by increasing the heart rate, blood pressure, susceptibility to atherosclerosis, and potential for blood clots. Evidence also indicates that smoking

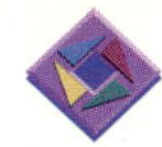

decreases high-density lipoprotein (HDL) cholesterol, the "good" cholesterol that lowers the risk for heart disease. Finally, the carbon monoxide in smoke hinders the capacity of the blood to carry oxygen to body tissues.

The American Cancer Society reports that 83% of lung cancer and 30% of all cancers are attributable to smoking. It kills about 142,000 people each year. Lung cancer is the leading cancer killer, responsible for 30% of all cancer deaths.

The largest carcinogenic exposure in the workplace is cigarette smoke. Based on a 1990 report by the Environmental Protection Agency (EPA), secondhand smoke also is a killer. Secondhand smoke is responsible for 3,000 or more lung cancer deaths each year.

Research presented at the 1990 World Conference on Lung Health also reveals that nonsmokers who live with smokers have a 20% to 30% greater risk of dying from heart disease than do other nonsmokers. Results of this research further suggest that the number of deaths from heart disease attributed to passive smoking is 10 times that of cancer.

Although half of all cancers are now curable, the 5-year survival rate for lung cancer is less than 13%. Tobacco use also increases the risk for cancer of the oral cavity, larynx, esophagus, bladder, pancreas, and kidneys.

Even though many tobacco users are aware of the health consequences of cigarette smoking, they may not realize the risk of pipe smoking, cigar smoking, and tobacco chewing. As a group in general, the risk for heart disease and lung cancer is lower than for cigarette smokers. Nevertheless, blood nicotine levels in pipe and cigar smokers have been shown to approach those of cigarette smokers, as nicotine still is absorbed through the membranes of the mouth. Therefore, these tobacco users still have a higher risk for heart disease than nonsmokers do.

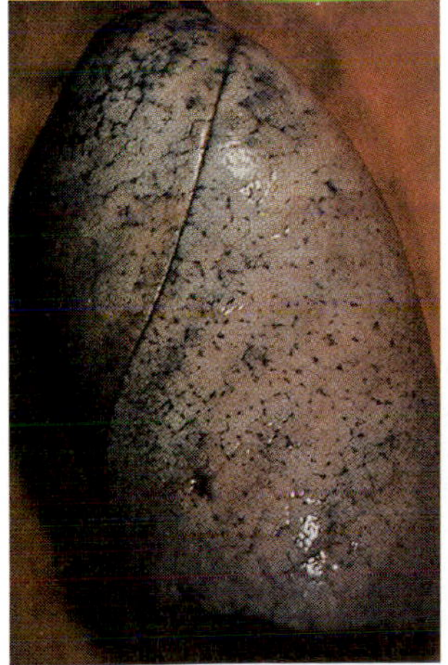

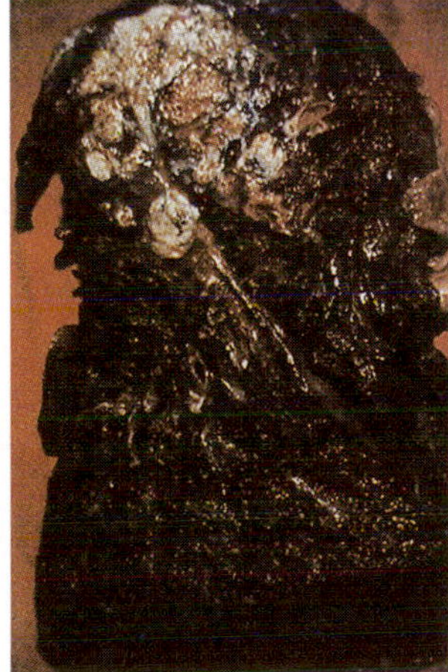

Reproduced by permission from "If You Smoke" slide show by Gordon Hewlett.

*Normal lung (left) contrasted with diseased lung (right). The white growth near the top of the diseased lung is cancer; the dark appearance on the bottom half is emphysema.*

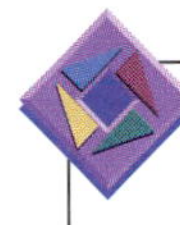

*Approximately 450,000 people die each year in the United States from smoking-related conditions.*

Cigarette smokers who substitute pipe or cigar smoking for cigarettes usually continue to inhale the smoke, which actually brings more nicotine and tar into the lungs. Consequently, the risk for disease is even higher if pipe or cigar smoke is inhaled. The risk and mortality rates for lip, mouth, and larynx cancer for pipe smoking, cigar smoking, and tobacco chewing are higher than for cigarette smoking.

The economic impact of cigarette smoking on American business and industry also is staggering. Companies pay more than $16 billion each year as a direct result of smoking in the workplace, and another $37 billion in lost productivity and earnings because of illness, disability, and death.

Heavy smokers use the health care system, especially hospitals, twice as much as nonsmokers do. The yearly cost to a given company has been estimated at between $624 and $4,611 per smoking employee. These costs include employee health care, absenteeism, additional health insurance, morbidity/disability and early mortality, on-the-job lost time, property damage/maintenance and depreciation, Workers Compensation, and the impact of secondhand smoke.

In the summer of 1985, more than 1,500 people worldwide died in major airplane accidents. These accidents generated a tremendous amount of media attention, and planes were grounded for safety reasons. Now imagine the coverage and concern if 450,000 people each year were to die in the United States alone because of airplane accidents. People would not even consider flying any more. Most would think of it as a form of suicide. Or think of the public outrage if close to 450,000 Americans were to die annually in a meaningless war, or if a single nonprescription drug would cause more than

138,000 cancer deaths and 120,000 fatal heart attacks. The American public never would tolerate these situations. We probably would mount an intense fight to prevent these deaths.

Yet, are we not committing a form of slow suicide by smoking cigarettes? Isn't tobacco, a nonprescription drug, available to almost anyone who wishes to smoke, killing some 450,000 people each year? If cigarettes were invented today, the tobacco industry would be put on trial for mass murder.

The fight against all forms of tobacco use has been gaining momentum in the last few years. This was not always the case. First, it is difficult to fight an industry that has as much financial and political influence as the tobacco industry has in the United States. Tobacco is the sixth largest cash crop in the United States, producing 2.5% of the gross national product. It has influenced elections cleverly by emphasizing the individual's right to smoke, avoiding the fact that so many people die because of its use.

In 1990 Philip Morris, one of the largest tobacco-producing companies in the world, ranked seventh among Fortune 500 companies. Nearly 70% of the profits came from cigarette sales. In 1992 Philip Morris donated about $17 million to "bribing" leading organizations, so they no longer question the detrimental effects of tobacco use. Among the organizations receiving donations from Philip Morris in 1992 were: United Way, YMCA, Salvation Army, Pediatric AIDS Foundation, Red Cross, Cystic Fibrosis Foundation, March of Dimes, Easter Seals, Muscular Dystrophy Association, Multiple Sclerosis Society, Hemophilia Foundation, United Cerebral Palsy, American Civil Liberties Union, American Bar Association, Task Force for Battered Women, Boy Scouts, Boys and Girls Club, and Big Brothers and Big Sisters. "We call Colombian drug runners uncivilized scums (for about 19,100 illegal drug-related deaths per year), but we welcome Philip Morris with glee and we call it civic pride."[1]

Second, tobacco had been socially accepted for so many years that many people simply have learned to live with it. In the 1980s, however, cigarette smoking no longer was acceptable in many social circles. Nonsmokers and ex-smokers alike are fighting for clean air and health. If every smoker were to give up cigarettes, in one year alone sick time would drop by approximately 90 million days, heart conditions would decrease by 280,000, chronic bronchitis and emphysema would number 1 million fewer cases, and total death rates from cardiovascular disease, cancer, and peptic ulcers would fall off drastically.

Many smokers are unaware of, or simply do not care to realize, how much cigarette smoke bothers nonsmokers. These smokers think it really is not that bad and if they themselves can put up with it, it should not bother nonsmokers that much. In many instances smokers think that blowing the smoke off to the side is enough to get it out of the way. As a matter of fact, it is not enough. Smokers do not comprehend this until they quit and later find themselves in that situation. At times, ex-smokers even are bothered by someone else smoking several yards away and all of a sudden come to recognize why cigarette smoke is so unpleasant and undesirable to most people.

## SMOKELESS TOBACCO

Smokeless tobacco often is promoted as a safe alternative to cigarette smoking. According to the Advisory Committee to the U. S. Surgeon General, smokeless tobacco represents a significant health risk and is just as addictive as cigarette smoking. Unlike smoking, the use of smokeless tobacco has increased during the last 15 years. Currently, some 15 million Americans use tobacco in this form. The greatest concern is the increase in use of "spit" tobacco, especially by young people.

More than 2 million people under age 25 use spit tobacco, including nearly 20% of all males in grades 9 through 12. One-third of those who use spit tobacco started at age 5, and the average starting age was 9. Spit tobacco contains 2.5 times as much nicotine as a similarly priced pack of cigarettes.

Using smokeless tobacco leads to gingivitis, periodontitis, a fourfold increase in oral cancer, and in some cases even premature death. People who chew or dip also have a higher rate of cavities, sore gums, bad breath, and stained teeth. They can't smell or taste as well. Consequently, they frequently add sugar and salt to food. These practices alone increase the risk for overweight and high blood pressure.

Nicotine addiction and its related health risks hold true for smokeless tobacco users. Nicotine blood levels approach those of cigarette smokers, increasing the risk for diseases of the cardiovascular system. Further, research has revealed changes in heart rate and blood pressure similar to those of cigarette smokers.

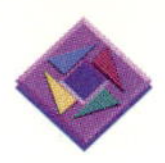

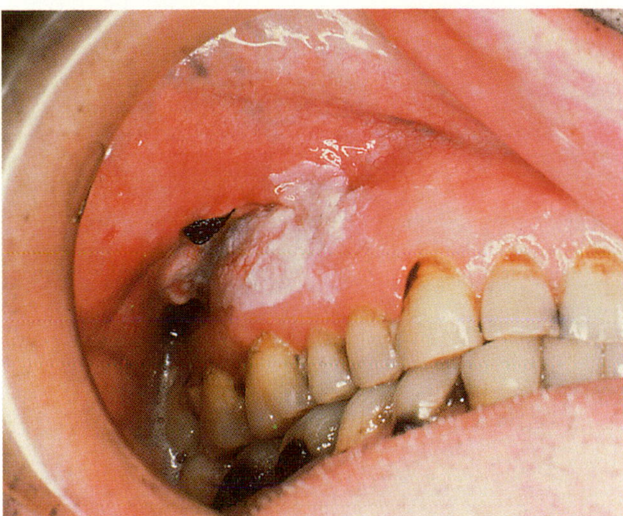

*Oral cancer (white growth) and gum and teeth damage caused by smokeless tobacco.*

Using tobacco in any form is addictive and poses a serious threat to health and well-being. Completely eliminating it in any form is the single most important lifestyle change a tobacco user can make to improve health, quality of life, and longevity.

## WHY DO PEOPLE SMOKE?

People typically begin to smoke without realizing its detrimental effects on their health and life in general. Although people start to smoke for many different reasons, the three most common instigators are peer pressure, the desire to appear "grown up," and rebellion against authority. Unfortunately, smoking only three packs of cigarettes is enough to cause physiological addiction, turning smoking into a nasty habit that has become the most widespread example of drug dependency in the country.

When tobacco leaves are burned, hot air and gases containing tar (chemical compounds) and nicotine are released in the smoke. More than 1,200 toxic chemicals have been found in tobacco smoke. Tar contains about 30 chemical compounds that are proven *carcinogens*, or cancer-producing agents.

The drug *nicotine* has strong addictive properties. Within seconds after inhalation, nicotine affects the central nervous system and can act simultaneously as a tranquilizer and a stimulant. The stimulating effect produces strong physiological and psychological dependency. The physical addiction to nicotine is six to eight times more powerful than the addiction to alcohol and most likely is greater than for some of the hard drugs currently used.

The psychological dependency develops over a longer time. People smoke to help themselves relax, and they also gain a certain amount of pleasure from the ritual of smoking. Smokers automatically associate many activities of daily life with cigarettes. Typical associated activities are: coffee drinking, alcohol drinking, social gatherings, after a meal, talking on the telephone, driving, reading, watching television. In many cases the social rituals of smoking are the most difficult to eliminate. This psychological dependency is so strong that even years after people have stopped smoking, they still may crave cigarettes when they engage in some of these activities.

Most people smoke for a variety of reasons. To find out why people smoke, the National Clearinghouse for Smoking and Health developed a simple "Why-Do-You-Smoke Test" (see Figure 12.2). The scores obtained on this test give an indication for each of six factors that describe people's feelings when they smoke. The first three factors point out the positive feelings people derive from smoking. The fourth factor relates to reducing tension and relaxing. The fifth reveals the extent of dependence on cigarettes. The last factor differentiates habit smoking and purely automatic smoking.

### Why-Do-You-Smoke Test

The "Why-Do-You-Smoke Test," contained in Figure 12.2, lists some statements by people describing what they get out of smoking cigarettes. Smokers are to indicate how often they have the feelings described in each statement when smoking. This test, as well as much of the remaining information in this chapter, is presented in the same format as it is given to smokers.

### Interpreting Results of "Why-Do-You-Smoke Test"

The "Why-Do-You-Smoke Test" elicits reasons you smoke. A score of 11 or above on any factor indicates that smoking is an important source of satisfaction for you. The higher you score (15 is the highest), the more important a given factor is in your smoking and the more useful the discussion of that factor can be in your attempt to quit.

## WHY-DO-YOU-SMOKE TEST

| | Always | Fre-quently | Occa-sionally | Seldom | Never |
|---|---|---|---|---|---|
| A. I smoke cigarettes to keep myself from slowing down. | 5 | 4 | 3 | 2 | 1 |
| B Handling a cigarette is part of the enjoyment of smoking it. | 5 | 4 | 3 | 2 | 1 |
| C. Smoking cigarettes is pleasant and relaxing. | 5 | 4 | 3 | 2 | 1 |
| D. I light up a cigarette when I feel angry about something. | 5 | 4 | 3 | 2 | 1 |
| E. When I have run out of cigarettes, I find it almost unbearable until I can get them. | 5 | 4 | 3 | 2 | 1 |
| F. I smoke cigarettes automatically without even being aware of it. | 5 | 4 | 3 | 2 | 1 |
| G. I smoke cigarettes to stimulate me, to perk myself up. | 5 | 4 | 3 | 2 | 1 |
| H. Part of the enjoyment of smoking a cigarette comes from the steps I take to light up. | 5 | 4 | 3 | 2 | 1 |
| I. I find cigarettes pleasurable. | 5 | 4 | 3 | 2 | 1 |
| J. When I feel uncomfortable or upset about something, I light up a cigarette. | 5 | 4 | 3 | 2 | 1 |
| K. I am very much aware of the fact when I am not smoking a cigarette. | 5 | 4 | 3 | 2 | 1 |
| L I light up a cigarette without realizing I still have one burning in the ashtray. | 5 | 4 | 3 | 2 | 1 |
| M. I smoke cigarettes to give me a "lift." | 5 | 4 | 3 | 2 | 1 |
| N. When I smoke a cigarette, part of the enjoyment is watching the smoke as I exhale it. | 5 | 4 | 3 | 2 | 1 |
| O. I want a cigarette most when I am comfortable and relaxed. | 5 | 4 | 3 | 2 | 1 |
| P. When I feel "blue" or want to take my mind off cares and worries, I smoke cigarettes. | 5 | 4 | 3 | 2 | 1 |
| Q. I get a real gnawing hunger for a cigarette when I I haven't smoked for a while. | 5 | 4 | 3 | 2 | 1 |
| R. I've found a cigarette in my mouth and didn't remember putting it there. | 5 | 4 | 3 | 2 | 1 |

**Scoring Your Test:**

Enter the numbers you have circled on the test questions in the spaces provided below, putting the number you circled for question A on line A, for question B on line B, etc. Add the three scores on each line to get a total for each factor. For example, the sum of your scores for lines A, G, and M gives you your score on "Stimulation," lines B, H, and N give the score on "Handling," etc. Scores can vary from 3 to 15. Any score 11 and above is high; any score 7 and below is low.

A ________ + G ________ + M ________ = ________ Stimulation
B ________ + H ________ + N ________ = ________ Handling
C ________ + I ________ + O ________ = ________ Pleasure/Relaxation
D ________ + J ________ + P ________ = ________ Crutch: Tension Reduction
E ________ + K ________ + Q ________ = ________ Craving: Psychological Addiction
F ________ + L ________ + R ________ = ________ Habit

From *A Self-Test for Smokers*. Washington, DC: (U.S. Department of Health and Human Services, 1983).

**FIGURE 12.2** ◆

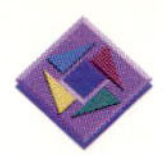

If you do not score high on any of the six factors, chances are that you do not smoke much or have not been smoking very many years. If so, giving up smoking, and staying off, should be fairly easy.

1. **Stimulation.** If you score high or fairly high on this factor, you are one of those smokers who is stimulated by a cigarette; you feel that it helps wake you up, organize your energies, and keep you going. If you try to give up smoking, you may want a safe substitute — a brisk walk or moderate exercise, for example — whenever you feel the urge to smoke.
2. **Handling.** Handling things can be satisfying, but you can keep your hands busy in many ways without lighting up or playing with a cigarette. Why not toy with a pen or pencil? Try doodling. Play with a coin, a piece of jewelry, or some other harmless object.
3. **Accentuation of pleasure/pleasurable relaxation.** Finding out whether you use the cigarette to feel good — get real, honest pleasure out of smoking (Factor 3) — or to keep from feeling bad (Factor 4) is not always easy. About two-thirds of smokers score high or fairly high on accentuation of pleasure, and about half of those also score as high or higher on reduction of negative feelings. Those who do get real pleasure from smoking often find that honest consideration of the harmful effects of their habit is enough to help them quit. They substitute social and physical activities and find they do not miss their cigarettes seriously.
4. **Reduction of negative feelings, or "crutch."** Many smokers use cigarettes as a kind of crutch in moments of stress or discomfort. Ironically, the heavy smoker — the person who tries to handle severe personal problems by smoking many times a day — is apt to discover that cigarettes do not help in dealing with problems effectively. This kind of smoker may stop smoking readily when everything is going well but may be tempted to start again in a time of crisis. Again, physical exertion or social activity may be useful substitutes for cigarettes, even in times of tension.
5. **Craving or dependence.** Quitting smoking is difficult for people who score high on this factor. The craving for a cigarette begins to build up the moment the cigarette is put out, so tapering off is not likely to work. This smoker must go "cold turkey." If you are dependent on cigarettes, you may try smoking more than usual for a day or two so the taste for cigarettes is spoiled, then isolating yourself completely from cigarettes until the craving is gone.
6. **Habit.** If you are smoking out of habit, you no longer get much satisfaction from the cigarettes. You just light them frequently without even realizing you are doing so. You may have an easy time quitting and staying off if you can break the habitual patterns you have built up. Cutting down gradually may be effective if you change the way you smoke cigarettes and the conditions under which you smoke them. The key to success is to become aware of each cigarette you smoke. You can do this by asking yourself, "Do I really want this cigarette?" You may be surprised at how many you do not want.

## SMOKING CESSATION

Quitting cigarette smoking is not easy. Only about 20% of smokers who try to quit the first time succeed each year. The addictive properties of nicotine and smoke make quitting difficult.

The American Psychiatric Association and the National Institute on Drug Abuse have indicated that nicotine is perhaps the most addictive drug known to humans. Smokers develop a tolerance to nicotine and smoke. They become dependent on both and get physical and psychological withdrawal symptoms when they stop smoking. Even though giving up smoking can be extremely difficult, it by no means is impossible.

During the last several years cigarette smoking in the United States has been declining gradually among smokers of all ages with the exception of young women. Surveys have shown that between 75% and 90% of all smokers would like to quit. Forty percent of the adult population — 53% of men and 32% of women — smoked in 1964 when the U. S. Surgeon General first reported the link between smoking and increased risk for disease and mortality. By 1991, only 25.7%, or 46.3 million adults, smoked. Among men, 24 million (28.1%) were smokers, and 22.2 million (23.5%) women smoked. Approximately 43.5 million Americans have given up cigarettes.

More than 95% of successful ex-smokers have been able to do it on their own, either by quitting cold turkey or by using self-help kits available from organizations such as the American Cancer Society, the American Heart Association, and the American Lung Association. Only 3% of ex-smokers have quit as a result of formal cessation programs. Smokers' information and treatment centers commonly are listed in the yellow pages of the telephone book.

## Do-You-Want-To-Quit Test

The most important factor in quitting cigarette smoking is the person's sincere desire to do so. Although some smokers can simply quit, this is not the case in most cases. Those who can quit easily tend to be light or casual smokers. They realize that the pleasure of an occasional cigarette is not worth the added risk for disease and premature death. For heavy smokers, quitting probably will be a difficult battle. Even though many do not succeed the first time around, the odds of quitting are much better for those who try to stop repeatedly.

To find out a smoker's preparedness to quit, the "Do-You-Want-To-Quit Test" contained in Figure 12.3, developed by the National Clearinghouse for Smoking and Health, will measure a person's attitude toward the four primary reasons people want to quit smoking. The results will give an indication of whether the person is really ready to start the program. On this test the higher you score in any category, say "Health," the more important that reason is to you. A score of 9 or above in one of these categories indicates that this is one of the most important reasons you may want to quit.

1. **Health.** Knowing the harmful consequences of cigarettes, many people have stopped smoking

### DO-YOU-WANT-TO-QUIT TEST

| | Strongly Agree | Mildly Agree | Mildly Disagree | Strongly Disagree |
|---|---|---|---|---|
| A. Cigarette smoking might give me a serious illness. | 4 | 3 | 2 | 1 |
| B. My cigarette smoking sets a bad example for others. | 4 | 3 | 2 | 1 |
| C. I find cigarette smoking to be a messy kind of habit. | 4 | 3 | 2 | 1 |
| D. Controlling my cigarette smoking is a challenge to me. | 4 | 3 | 2 | 1 |
| E. Smoking causes shortness of breath. | 4 | 3 | 2 | 1 |
| F If I quit smoking cigarettes, it might influence others to stop. | 4 | 3 | 2 | 1 |
| G. Cigarettes damage clothing and other personal property. | 4 | 3 | 2 | 1 |
| H. Quitting smoking would show that I have willpower. | 4 | 3 | 2 | 1 |
| I. My cigarette smoking will have a harmful effect on my health. | 4 | 3 | 2 | 1 |
| J. My cigarette smoking influences others close to me to take up or continue smoking. | 4 | 3 | 2 | 1 |
| K. If I quit smoking, my sense of taste or smell would improve. | 4 | 3 | 2 | 1 |
| L. I do not like the idea of feeling dependent on smoking. | 4 | 3 | 2 | 1 |

**Scoring Your Test:**

Write the number you have circled after each statement on the test in the corresponding space to the right. Add the scores on each line to get your totals. For example, the sum of your scores A, E, I gives you your score for the Health factor. Scores can vary from 3 to 12. Any score of 9 or over is high, and a score of 6 or under is low.

A ________ + G ________ + M ________ = ________ Health
B ________ + H ________ + N ________ = ________ Example
C ________ + I ________ + O ________ = ________ Aesthetics
D ________ + J ________ + P ________ = ________ Mastery

From *A Self-Test for Smokers* by National Clearinghouse for Smoking and Health, Washington, DC: (U.S. Department of Health and Human Services, 1983).

**FIGURE 12.3** ◆

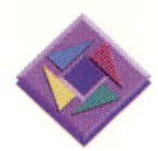

and many others are considering it. If your score on the health factor is 9 or above, the health hazards of smoking may be enough to make you want to quit now. If your score on this factor is low (6 or below), consider the hazards of smoking. You may be lacking important information or even may have incorrect information. If so, health considerations are not playing the role they should be in your decision to keep smoking or to quit.

2. **Example.** Some people stop smoking because they want to set a good example for others. Parents quit to make it easier for their children to resist starting to smoke. Doctors quit to be role models for their patients. Teachers quit to discourage their students from smoking. Sports stars want to set an example for their young fans. Husbands quit to influence their wives to quit, and vice versa. Examples have a significant influence on our behavior. Almost twice as many high school students smoke if both parents are smokers, compared to those whose parents are nonsmokers or former smokers.

   If your score is low (6 or lower), you might not be interested in giving up smoking to set an example for others. Perhaps you do not realize how important your example could be.

3. **Aesthetics.** People who score high (9 or above) in this category recognize and are disturbed by some of the unpleasant aspects of smoking. The smell of stale smoke on their clothing, bad breath, and stains on their fingers and teeth might be reason enough to consider quitting.

4. **Mastery.** If you score 9 or above on this factor, you are bothered by the knowledge that you cannot control your desire to smoke. You are not your own master. Awareness of this challenge to your self-control may make you want to quit.

## Breaking the Habit

The following seven-step plan has been developed as a guide to help you quit smoking. The total program should be completed in 4 weeks or less. Steps one through four should take no longer than 2 weeks. A maximum of 2 additional weeks is allowed for the rest of the program.

### Step One

Decide positively that you want to quit. Avoid negative thoughts of how difficult this can be. Think positive. You can do it. Prepare a list of the reasons you smoke and why you want to quit (see Figure 12.4). Make several copies of the list and keep them in places where you commonly smoke. Frequently review the reasons for quitting, as this will motivate and prepare you psychologically for cessation. When the reasons for quitting outweigh the reasons for smoking, you will have an easier time quitting. Try to read as much information as possible on the detrimental effects of tobacco and the benefits of quitting.

### Step Two

Begin a personal diet and exercise program. About one-third of the people who quit smoking gain weight. This could be caused by one or a combination of several reasons: (a) Food becomes a substitute for cigarettes; (b) appetite increases; (c) basal metabolism may slow down.

If you start an exercise and weight-control program prior to quitting smoking, weight gain should not be a problem. If anything, exercise and lower body weight create more awareness of healthy living and strengthen the motivation for giving up cigarettes. Further, a recent study conducted at the 6.2-mile Peachtree Road Race in Atlanta indicated that over 75% of those who smoked when they started running had quit before the race date.

Even if you do gain some weight, the harmful effects of cigarette smoking are much more detrimental to human health than a few extra pounds of body weight. Experts have indicated that, as far as the extra load on the heart is concerned, giving up

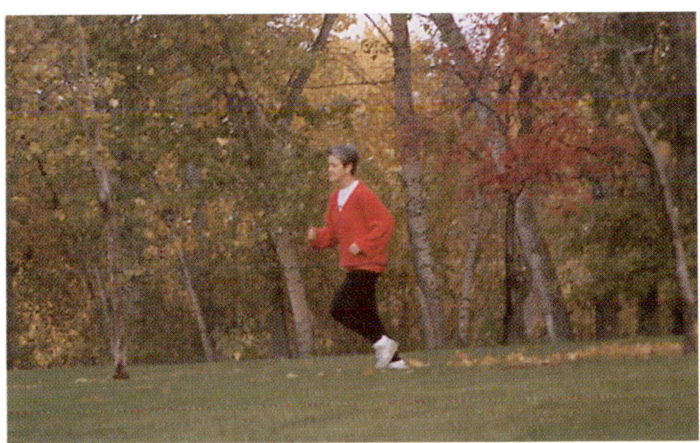

*Starting an exercise program prior to giving up cigarettes motivates toward cessation and helps with weight control during this process.*

## SMOKING VERSUS QUITTING REASONS

Name: ______________________ Date: ______________

Reasons for Smoking Cigarettes

1. ______________________
2. ______________________
3. ______________________
4. ______________________
5. ______________________
6. ______________________
7. ______________________
8. ______________________

Reasons for Quitting Cigarette Smoking

1. ______________________
2. ______________________
3. ______________________
4. ______________________
5. ______________________
6. ______________________
7. ______________________
8. ______________________

**FIGURE 12.4** ◆

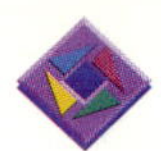

one pack of cigarettes a day is the equivalent of losing between 50 and 75 pounds of excess body fat!

### Step Three

Decide on the approach you will use to stop smoking. You may quit cold turkey or gradually cut down the number of cigarettes you smoke daily. Base your decision on your scores obtained on the "Why-Do-You-Smoke Test" (Figure 12.2). If you scored 11 points or higher in either the "Crutch: Tension Reduction" or the "Craving: Psychological Addiction" categories, your best chance for success is quitting cold turkey. For any of the other four categories, you may choose either approach.

People still argue about which approach is more effective. Quitting cold turkey may cause fewer withdrawal symptoms than gradually tapering off. When cutting down, the fewer the cigarettes you smoke, the more important each one becomes. Therefore, you have a greater chance for relapse and returning to the original number of cigarettes smoked. When the cutting-down approach is accompanied by a definite target date for quitting, the technique has been shown to be quite effective. Smokers who taper off without a target date for quitting are the most likely to relapse.

### Step Four

Keep a daily log of your smoking habit for a few days. This will help you understand the situations in which you smoke. To assist you in doing this, make copies of Figure 12.5 or develop your own form. Keep this form with you, and every time you smoke, record the required information. Keep track of the number of cigarettes you smoke, times of day you smoke them, events associated with smoking, amount of each cigarette smoked, and a rating of how badly you needed that cigarette. Rate each cigarette from 1 to 3. A 1 means "desperately needed," a 2 means "moderately needed," and a 3 means "no real need." This daily log will assist you in three ways: (a) You will get to know your habit; (b) it will help you eliminate cigarettes you really do not need; (c) it will aid you in finding positive substitutes for situations that trigger your desire to smoke.

### Step Five

Set the target date for quitting. If you are going to taper off gradually, read the instructions under the Cutting Down section of this chapter before you proceed to Step Six. In setting the target date, a special date may add a little extra incentive. An upcoming birthday, anniversary, vacation, graduation, family reunion — all are examples of good dates to free yourself from smoking. Dates when you are going to be away from events that trigger your desire to smoke may be especially helpful. Once you have set the date, do not change it. Do not let anyone or anything interfere with this date.

Let your friends and relatives know of your intentions, and ask for their support. Consider asking someone else to quit with you. This way, you can support each other in your efforts to stop. Avoid anyone who will not support you in your effort to quit. Unfortunately, other people can be a prime obstacle when you are attempting to quit. Many smokers can get quite intolerable when they first stop smoking, so some friends and relatives prefer that the person continue to smoke rather than make the extra effort and be more patient for a few days.

### Step Six

Stock up on low-calorie foods — carrots, broccoli, cauliflower, celery, popcorn (butter- and salt-free), fruits, sunflower seeds (in the shell), sugarless gum — and drink plenty of water. Keep the food handy on the day you stop and the first few days following cessation. Substitute this food for a cigarette when you want one.

### Step Seven

On your quit day and the first few days thereafter, do not keep cigarettes handy. Stay away from friends and events that trigger your desire to smoke, and drink large amounts of water and fruit juices. To replace the old behavior with new behavior, replace smoking time with new, positive substitutes that will make smoking difficult or impossible.

When you want a cigarette, take a few deep breaths and then occupy yourself by doing any of a number of things such as talking to someone else, washing your hands, brushing your teeth, eating a healthy snack, chewing on a straw, doing dishes, playing sports, going for a walk or bike ride, going swimming, and so on. Engage in activities that require the use of your hands. Try gardening, sewing, writing letters, drawing, doing household chores, or washing the car. Visit nonsmoking places

## DAILY CIGARETTE SMOKING LOG

Today's Date: ______________ Quit Date: ______________ Decision Date: ______________

Cigarettes to be Smoked Today: ______________ Brand: ______________

| No. | Time | Activity | Rating[a] | Amount Smoked[b] | Remarks/Substitutes |
|---|---|---|---|---|---|
| 1. | | | | | |
| 2. | | | | | |
| 3. | | | | | |
| 4. | | | | | |
| 5. | | | | | |
| 6. | | | | | |
| 7. | | | | | |
| 8. | | | | | |
| 9. | | | | | |
| 10. | | | | | |
| 11. | | | | | |
| 12. | | | | | |
| 13. | | | | | |
| 14. | | | | | |
| 15. | | | | | |
| 16. | | | | | |
| 17. | | | | | |
| 18. | | | | | |
| 19. | | | | | |
| 20. | | | | | |

Additional comments, list of friends and/or activities to avoid

. ______________

. ______________

. ______________

. ______________

. ______________

. ______________

[a] Rating: 1 = desperately needed, 2 = moderately needed, 3 - no real need

[b] Amount smoked: entire cigarette, two-thirds, half, etc.

**FIGURE 12.5** ◆

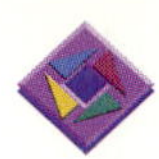

such as libraries, museums, stores, or theaters. Plan an outing or a trip away from home. All of these activities have been shown to keep your mind away from cigarettes. Record your choice of activity or substitute under the Remarks/Substitute column in Figure 12.5.

## Quitting Cold Turkey

Many people have found that quitting all at once is the easiest way to do it. Most smokers have tried this approach at least once. Even though it may not work the first time, they do not allow themselves to get discouraged, and they succeed eventually. After several attempts, all of a sudden they are able to overcome the habit without too much difficulty.

On the average, as few as three smokeless days are enough to break the physiological addiction to nicotine. The psychological addiction may linger for years but will get weaker as time goes by.

## Cutting Down Gradually

Tapering off cigarettes can be done in several ways. You might start by eliminating cigarettes you do not necessarily need (those ranked numbers 3 and 2 on your daily log). You may switch to a brand lower in nicotine/tar every couple of days. You can smoke less of each cigarette. Or you can simply smoke fewer cigarettes each day. Most people prefer a combination of these four suggestions.

When planning your strategy, set a target date for quitting before you start cutting down. Once the date is set, do not change it. The total time until your quit date should be no longer than 2 weeks. Reduce the total number of cigarettes smoked each day by 10% to 25%. As you smoke less, be careful not to take more puffs or inhale more deeply as you smoke, as this would offset the principle of cutting down.

As an aid in tapering off, make several copies of Figure 12.5. (By now you already should have completed the initial daily log of your smoking habit — see Step Four under Breaking the Habit.) Start a new daily log, and every night review your data and set goals for the following day.

Decide which cigarettes will be easiest to give up, what brand you will smoke, the total number of cigarettes to be smoked, and how much of each you will smoke. Write down any comments or situations you may want to avoid, as well as any substitutes you could use to help you in the program. For example, if you always smoke with coffee, substitute juice for coffee. If you smoke while driving, arrange for a ride or take a bus to work. If you smoke with a certain friend at lunch, avoid having lunch with that friend for a week or so. Continue using this log until you have stopped smoking completely.

# LIFE AFTER CIGARETTES

When you first quit smoking, you can expect a series of withdrawal symptoms. Among the typical physiological and psychological reactions during the first few days are lower heart rate and blood pressure, headaches, gastrointestinal discomfort, mood changes, irritability, aggressiveness, and difficulty sleeping.

The physiological addiction to nicotine is broken only 3 days following your last cigarette. Therefore, you should not crave cigarettes as much. For the habitual smoker, the psychological dependency could be the most difficult to break. The first few days may not be as difficult as the first few months. Any of the activities in daily life that have been associated with smoking — stress or relaxation, joy or unhappiness — may trigger a relapse even months, or at times years, after quitting.

Ex-smokers should realize that even though some harm may have been done already, it is never too late to quit. The greatest early benefit is a lower risk for sudden death. Furthermore, the risk for illness starts to decrease the moment you stop smoking. You will have fewer sore throats and sores in the mouth, less hoarseness, no more cigarette cough, and less risk for peptic ulcers.

Circulation to the hands and feet will improve, as will gastrointestinal and kidney and bladder functions. Everything will taste and smell better. You will have more energy, and you will gain a sense of freedom, pride, and well-being. You no longer will have to worry whether you have enough cigarettes to last you through a day, a party, a meeting, a weekend, a trip.

When you first quit and you think how tough it is and how miserable you feel because you cannot have a cigarette, try the opposite: Think of the benefits and how great it is not to smoke! The ex-smoker's risk for heart disease approaches that of a lifetime nonsmoker 10 years following cessation, and cancer 15 years after cessation.

If you have been successful in stopping smoking, a lot of events can trigger your urge to smoke. When confronted with these events, people rationalize and think, "One cigarette won't hurt. I've been off for months (years in some cases)" or, "I can handle it. I'll smoke just today." It won't work! Before you know it, you will be back to the regular nasty habit. Be prepared to take action in those situations. Find substitutes. In addition to the many things that have been discussed in this chapter, the tips given in Figure 12.6 should help you in retraining yourself to live without cigarettes.

Start thinking of yourself as a nonsmoker — no "buts" about it. Remind yourself of how difficult it has been and how long it has taken you to get to this point. If you have come this far, you certainly can resist "but" small moments of temptation. It will get easier rather than worse as time goes on.

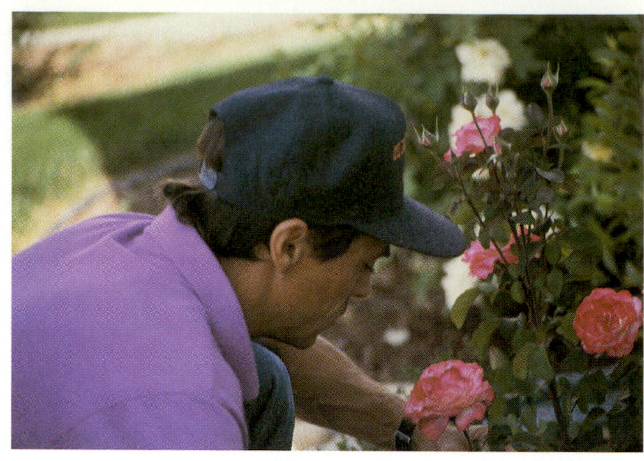

*Simple pleasures of life, such as smell and taste, improve with smoking cessation.*

## NOTES

1. American Cancer Society, *World Smoking & Health* (Atlanta: ACS, 1993).

## SELECT BIBLIOGRAPHY

American Cancer Society. *Cancer Facts & Figures – 1994*. New York: ACS, 1994.

American Cancer Society. *Fifty Most Often Asked Questions About Smoking and Health and the Answers*. New York: ACS, 1982.

American Cancer Society. *Quitter's Guide: Seven-Day Plan to Help You Stop Smoking Cigarettes*. New York: ACS, 1978.

American Heart Association. *Heart at Work: Smoking Reduction Program — Coordinator's Guide*. Dallas: AHA, 1984.

American Heart Association. *How to Quit*. Dallas: AHA, 1984.

American Heart Association. *Smoking and Heart Disease*. Dallas: AHA, 1981.

American Heart Association. *The Good Life: A Guide to Becoming a Nonsmoker*. Dallas: AHA, 1984.

Carroll, C. R. *Drugs in Modern Society*. Dubuque, IA: Wm. C. Brown, 1985.

Channing L. Bete Co. *Smoking and Your Heart*. South Deerfield, MA: Author, 1982.

Girdano, D. A., D. Dusek, and G. S. Everly. *Experiencing Health*. Englewood Cliffs, NJ: Prentice Hall, 1985.

Halper, M. S. *How to Stop Smoking: A Preventive Medicine Institute/Strang Clinic Health Action Plan*. New York: Holt Rinehart and Winston, 1980.

Hodgson, R. J., and P. Miller. *Self-Watching: Addictions, Habits, Compulsions, What to Do*. New York: Facts on File, 1982.

National Cancer Institute. *Clearing the Air: A Guide to Quitting Smoking*. Bethesda, MD: NCI, 1979.

Public Health Service. *A Self-Test for Smokers*. Rockville, MD: U.S. Department of Health and Human Services, 1983.

Public Health Service. *Chronic Obstructive Lung Disease: A Report of the Surgeon General*. Rockville, MD: U.S. Department of Health and Human Services, 1984.

Public Health Service. *Why People Smoke Cigarettes*. Rockville, MD: U.S. Department of Health and Human Services, 1982.

Public Health Service. *Smoking Tobacco and Health: A Fact Book*. Rockville, MD: U.S. Department of Health and Human Services, 1981.

U.S. Office on Smoking and Health. *Smoking and Health: A Report of the Surgeon General*. Washington, DC: U.S. Department of Health, Education and Welfare, 1979.

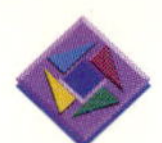

## TIPS TO HELP STOP SMOKING

The following are different ways smokers retrained themselves to live without cigarettes. Any one or several of these methods in combination might be helpful to you. Check the ones you like and from these develop your own retraining program.

- ☐ Before you quit smoking, try wrapping your cigarettes with a sheet of paper like a Christmas present. Every time you want a cigarette, unwrap the pack and write down what you are doing, how you feel, and how important this cigarette is to you. Do this for two weeks and you'll have cut down as well as developed new insights into your smoking.
- ☐ If cigarettes give you an energy boost, try gum, modest exercise, a brisk walk, or a new hobby. Avoid eating new foods that are high in calories.
- ☐ If cigarettes help you relax, try eating, drinking new beverages, or social activities within reasonable bounds.
- ☐ When you crave cigarettes, you must quit suddenly. Try smoking an excess of cigarettes for a day or two before you quit so the taste of cigarettes is spoiled. Or, an opportune time to quit is when you are ill with a cold or influenza and have lost your taste for cigarettes.
- ☐ On a 3" X 5" card, make a list of what you like and dislike about smoking. Add to it and read it daily.
- ☐ Make up a short list of luxuries you have wanted or items you would like to purchase for a loved one. Next to each item, write down the cost. Now convert the cost to "packs of cigarettes." If you save the money each day from packs of cigarettes, you will be able to purchase these items. Use a special "piggy" bank for saving your money or start a "Christmas Club" account at your bank.
- ☐ Never smoke after you get a craving for a cigarette until three minutes have passed since you got the urge. During those three minutes, change your thinking or activity. Telephone an ex-smoker or somebody you can talk to until the craving subsides.
- ☐ Plan a memorable day for stopping. You might choose your vacation, New Year's Day, your birthday, a holiday, the birthday of your child, your anniversary. But don't make the date so distant that you lose momentum.
- ☐ If you smoke under stress at work, pick a date for stopping when you will be away from your work.
- ☐ Decide whether you are going to stop suddenly or gradually. If it is to be gradual, work out a tapering system so that you have intermediate goals on your way to an "I.Q." day.
- ☐ Don't store up cigarettes. Never buy a carton. Wait until one pack is finished before you buy another.
- ☐ Never carry cigarettes about with you at home or at work. Keep your cigarettes as far from you as possible. Leave them with someone or lock them up.
- ☐ Until you quit, make yourself a "smoking corner" that is far from anything interesting. If you like to smoke with others, always smoke alone. If you like to smoke alone, always smoke with others, preferably if they are nonsmokers. Never smoke while watching television.
- ☐ Never carry matches or a lighter with you.
- ☐ Put away your ashtrays or fill them with objects so they cannot be used for ashes. Plant flowers in them or fill them with walnuts. The latter will give you something to do with your hands.
- ☐ Change your brand of cigarettes weekly so that you are always smoking a brand of lower tar and nicotine content than the week before.
- ☐ Never say, "I quit smoking," because your resolution is broken if you have a cigarette. Better to say, "I don't want to smoke." This way you maintain your resolution even if you accidentally have a cigarette.
- ☐ Try to help someone else quit smoking, particularly your spouse.
- ☐ Always ask yourself, "Do I need this cigarette or is this just a reflex?"
- ☐ Each day try to put off lighting your first cigarette.
- ☐ Decide arbitrarily that you will smoke only on even- or odd-numbered hours of the clock.
- ☐ Try going to bed early and rising a half hour earlier than usual to avoid hurrying through breakfast and rushing to work.
- ☐ Keep your hands occupied. Try playing a musical instrument, knitting, or fiddling with hand puzzles.

*(Continued)*

**FIGURE 12.6** ◆

## TIPS TO HELP STOP SMOKING

- ☐ Take a shower. You cannot smoke in the shower.
- ☐ Brush your teeth frequently to get rid of the tobacco taste and stains.
- ☐ If you have a sudden craving for a cigarette, take ten deep breaths, holding the last breath while you strike a match. Exhale slowly, blowing out the match. Pretend the match was a cigarette by crushing it out in an ashtray. Now immediately get busy on some work or activity.
- ☐ Smoke only half a cigarette.
- ☐ After you quit, start using your lungs. Increase your activities and indulge in moderate exercise, such as short walks before or after a meal.
- ☐ Bet with someone that you can quit. Put the cigarette money in a jar each morning and forfeit it if you smoke. Keep the money if you don't smoke by the end of the week. Try to extend this period for a month.
- ☐ If you gain weight because you are not smoking, wait until you get over the craving before you diet. Dieting is easier then.
- ☐ If you are depressed or have physical symptoms that might be related to your smoking, relieve your mind by discussing this with your physician. It is easier to quit when you know your health status.
- ☐ Visit your dentist after you quit and have your teeth cleaned to get rid of the tobacco stains.
- ☐ If the cost of cigarettes is your motivation for quitting, try purchasing a money order equivalent to a year's supply of cigarettes. Give it to a friend. If you smoke in the next year, he cashes the money order and keeps the money. If you don't smoke, he gives back the money order at the end of the year.
- ☐ After you quit, never face the confusion of "craving a cigarette" alone. Find someone you can call or visit at this critical time.
- ☐ When you feel irritable or tense, shut your eyes and count backward from ten to zero as you imagine yourself descending a flight of stairs, or imagine that you are looking at the horizon as the sun sets in the west.
- ☐ Get out of your old habits. Seek new activities or perform old activities in a new way. Don't rely on the old ways of solving problems. Do things differently.
- ☐ If you are a "kitchen smoker" in the morning, volunteer your services to schools or nonprofit organizations to get you out of the house.
- ☐ Stock up on light reading materials, crossword puzzles, and vacation brochures that you can read during your coffee breaks.
- ☐ Frequent places where you can't smoke, such as libraries, buses, theatres, swimming pools, department stores, or just going to bed during the first weeks you are off cigarettes.
- ☐ Give yourself time to think and get fit by walking one-half hour each day. If you have a dog, take it for a walk with you.

From *TIPS*. American Cancer Society, Texas Division, Inc., with permission.

**FIGURE 12.6** ◆ *(continued)*

# Addictive Behavior and Sexually Transmitted Diseases

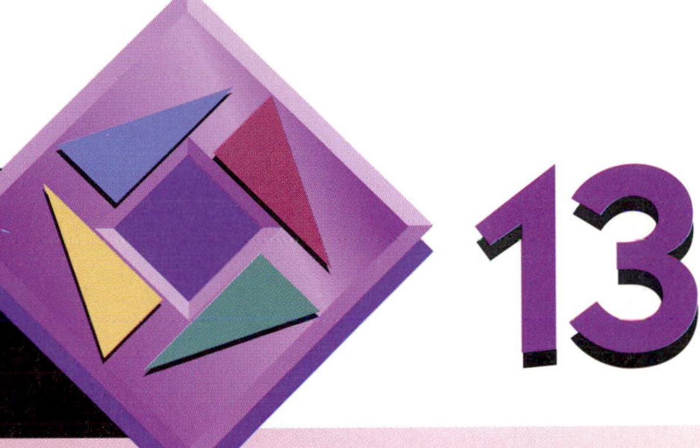


## Key Concepts

Addiction
Chemical dependency
Marijuana
Amotivational syndrome
Cocaine
Alcohol (ethyl alcohol)
Synergistic action
STDs
Chlamydia
Gonorrhea
Pelvic inflammatory disease (PID)
Genital warts
Herpes
Syphilis
AIDS
HIV
Opportunistic infections
HIV antibody test
Risky behaviors
AIDS clinical trials
Monogamous relationship
Nonoxynol-9

## Objectives

- Address the detrimental effects of addictive behavior, including marijuana, cocaine, and alcohol.
- Describe the most common sexually transmitted diseases.
- Outline the health consequences of sexually transmitted disease, including HIV infection (AIDS)
- Define the difference between HIV and AIDS.
- Introduce guidelines for the prevention of sexually transmitted diseases.

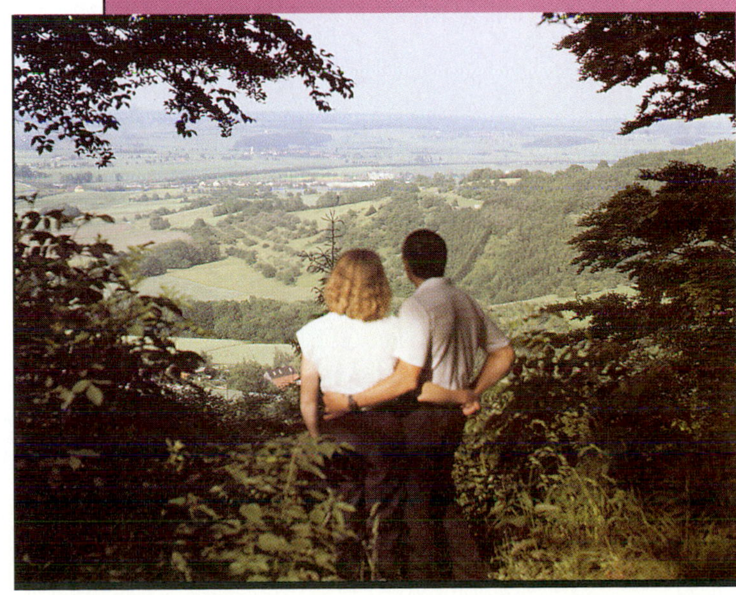

As we head into the 21st century, two of the most serious problems that afflict society are chemical dependency (addictive behavior) and the epidemic of sexually transmitted diseases. Addictive behavior and unprotected sex are extremely destructive behaviors that have ruined and ended millions of lives.

People need to understand that perhaps more so than with any other unhealthy behavior, when addiction and sexually transmitted diseases (especially HIV infection) are concerned, "An ounce of prevention is worth a pound of cure." The time to make healthy choices is now. The information in this chapter can help you make informed decisions before it is too late. Education on these subjects may help in the search for answers, treatment, and, hopefully, a more productive and happier life.

## ADDICTION

When most people think of addiction, they probably think of dark and dirty alleys, an addict shooting drugs into the veins, or the "junkie" passed out next to a garbage can after spending an evening with alcohol. Jacquelyn Small, psychotherapist and author, defines addiction as *a problem of imbalance or unease within the body and mind.*

Although some addictive behaviors are more detrimental than others, addiction has many forms including food, television, work, compulsive shopping, even exercise. The most serious type of addiction is *chemical dependency* to drugs such as tobacco, coffee, alcohol, cocaine, heroin, marijuana, and even prescription drugs.

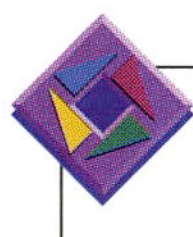

*Addictive behavior and unprotected sex are destructive behaviors that have ruined and ended millions of lives.*

Some people become addicted to *food*. They eat to release stress or boredom or to reward themselves for every small personal achievement. Great numbers of people are addicted to television. Estimates indicate that the average adult in the United States spends 7 hours a day watching television.

Other individuals become addicted to their *jobs* to the extent that all they think about is work. Although work starts out as an enjoyable leisure activity, it can become an unhealthy behavior when it totally consumes a person's life. If you find that you are irritated readily, moody, grouchy, constantly tired, not as alert as you used to be, or making more mistakes than usual, you probably are becoming a workaholic and need to slow down or take time off work.

Exercise has enhanced the health and quality of life of millions of people, but for a very small group of individuals, *exercise* can become an obsessive behavior with potential addictive and overuse properties. Compulsive exercisers often express feelings of guilt and discomfort when they miss a day's workout. Often these individuals continue to exercise even during periods of injury and sickness that require proper rest for adequate recovery. People who exceed the recommended guidelines for fitness development and maintenance (see Chapters 3, 4, and 5) are exercising for reasons other than health, including addictive behavior.

Addiction to *caffeine* can produce undesirable side effects. Caffeine doses in excess of 200 to 500 mg can produce an abnormally rapid heart rate, abnormal heart rhythms, higher blood pressure, birth defects, higher body temperature, and increased secretion of gastric acids leading to stomach problems. It also may induce symptoms of anxiety, depression, nervousness, and dizziness.

The caffeine content of different drinks varies with the product. The content of 6 ounces of coffee varies from 65 mg for instant coffee to as high as 180 mg for drip coffee. Soft drinks, mainly colas, range in caffeine content from 30 to 60 mg per 12-ounce can.

The previous examples, as well as more serious forms of chemical dependency, are by no means the only types of addiction but are used only to illustrate addictive behaviors. Other examples include gambling, pornography, sex, people, places, and on and on.

Recognizing that all forms of addiction are unhealthy, this chapter focuses on three of the most self-destructive forms of addiction in our society: marijuana, cocaine, and alcohol. The fourth one, addiction to cigarette smoking and tobacco, has been discussed in detail already in Chapter 12.

## DRUGS AND DEPENDENCE

Approximately 60% of the world's production of illegal drugs is consumed in the United States. Each year Americans spend more than $100 billion on

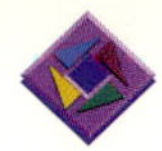

illegal drugs, an amount that surpasses the total amount taken in from all crops by U.S. farmers. According to the U.S. Department of Education, today's drugs are stronger, more addictive, and pose a greater risk than ever before.

Drugs lead to physical and psychological dependence. If they are used regularly, they integrate into the body's chemistry, increasing drug tolerance and forcing the user to increase the dosage constantly to obtain similar results. In addition to serious health problems, more than half of all adolescent suicides are drug-related.

## Marijuana

Marijuana (pot or grass) is the most widely used illegal drug in the United States. According to estimates, 64% of Americans between ages 18 and 25 and 23% of those 26 and older have smoked marijuana. Approximately 20 million people in the country use marijuana regularly.

This psychoactive drug is prepared from a mixture of crushed leaves, flowers, small branches, stems, and seeds from the hemp plant, *cannabis sativa*. In small doses marijuana has a sedative effect. Larger doses produce physical and psychic changes.

Earlier studies in the 1960s indicated that the potential effects of marijuana were exaggerated and that the drug was relatively harmless. The drug as it is used today, however, is as much as 10 times stronger than it was when the initial studies were conducted. Ninety percent of research today shows marijuana to be a dangerous and harmful drug.

The major and most active psychoactive and mind-altering ingredient of marijuana is thought to be delta-9-tetrahydrocannabinol (THC). In the 1960s THC content in marijuana ranged from .02% to 2%. Users called the latter "real good grass." Today's THC content averages 4% to 6%, although it has been reported as high as 20%. The THC content in *sinsemilla*, a seedless variety of high-potency marijuana grown from the seedless female cannabis plant, is approximately 8% THC.

THC reaches the brain within 30 seconds after inhalating marijuana smoke, and the psychic and physical changes reach their peak in about 2 or 3 minutes. THC then is metabolized in the liver to waste metabolites, but 30% of it remains in the body a week after marijuana was first smoked.

Studies indicate that 30 days or longer are required to eliminate THC completely following an initial dose of the drug. The drug always remains in the system of regular users.

Some of the short-term effects of marijuana include tachycardia (a fast heart rate, sometimes as rapid as 180 beats per minute), dryness of the mouth, reddening of the eyes, enhanced appetite, less coordination and tracking (following a moving stimulus), difficulty concentrating, intermittent confusion, impairment of short-term memory and continuity of speech, and interference with the physical and mental learning process during periods of intoxication. Another effect commonly seen with marijuana use is the *amotivational syndrome*, characterized by loss of motivation, dullness, apathy, and no interest in the future. This syndrome persists even after periods of intoxication but usually disappears a few weeks after the individual stops using the drug.

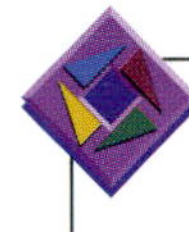

*Marijuana, the most widely used illegal drug in the United States, can cause irreversible brain damage.*

Long-term harmful effects include atrophy of the brain, leading to irreversible brain damage, decreased resistance to infectious diseases, chronic bronchitis, lung cancer (marijuana may contain as much as 50% more cancer-producing hydrocarbons than cigarette smoke), and possible sterility and impotence.

One of the most common myths about using marijuana is that it does not lead to addiction. To the contrary, ample scientific evidence shows clearly that regular marijuana users do develop physical and psychological dependence. Similar to cigarette smoking, when regular users do without the drug, they crave the substance, go through changes in mood, are irritable and nervous, and become obsessed with getting more "pot."

## Cocaine

Similar to marijuana, cocaine was thought for many years to be a relatively harmless drug. This misconception came to an abrupt halt in 1986 when two well-known athletes, Len Bias (basketball) and Don Rogers (football), died suddenly following a cocaine overdose. An estimated 4 to 8 million Americans use cocaine, 96% of whom had used marijuana previously.

Cocaine (2-beta-carbomethoxy-3-betabenozoxy-tropane) is the primary psychoactive ingredient derived from coca plant leaves. Over the years it has been given several different names, including coke, C, snow, blow, toot, flake, Peruvian lady, white girl, and happy dust. The drug is typically sniffed or snorted, but it can be smoked or injected.

An expensive drug, some users pay more than $2,000 per ounce for cocaine. Cocaine used in medical therapy sells for about $100 per ounce. Because of the high cost, cocaine is viewed as a luxury drug. Many users are well-educated, affluent, upwardly mobile professionals who otherwise are law-abiding citizens.

Cocaine has become the fastest growing drug problem in the United States. About 5,000 people try cocaine for the first time each day. The addiction begins with a desire to get high, often at social gatherings, with the assurance that occasional use is harmless. About one in five will continue to use the drug now and then, and for some it's the beginning of a lifetime nightmare.

The popularity of cocaine is based on the almost universal guarantee that the user will enter an immediate state of euphoria and well-being. When cocaine is snorted, it is absorbed quickly through the mucous membranes of the nose into the bloodstream. The drug usually is arranged in fine powder lines one to two inches long. Each line results in about 30 minutes of stimulation to the autonomic nervous system.

Cocaine seems to help relieve fatigue and increase energy levels, as well as decrease the need for appetite and sleep. Following this stimulation comes a "crash," a state of physiological and psychological depression, often leaving the user with the desire to get more. This can lead to a constant craving for the drug.

Addiction becomes a lifetime illness, and, similar to alcoholism, the individual recovers only by completely abstaining from the drug. A single pitfall often results in renewed addiction.

Light to moderate use of cocaine usually is associated with feelings of pleasure and well-being. Sustained cocaine snorting can lead to a constant runny nose, nasal congestion and inflammation, and perforation of the nasal septum. Long-term consequences of cocaine use in general include loss of appetite, digestive disorders, weight loss, malnutrition, insomnia, confusion, anxiety, and cocaine psychosis. *Cocaine psychosis* is characterized by paranoia and hallucinations. In a particular type of hallucination, referred to as formication or "coke bugs," the chronic user perceives imaginary insects or snakes crawling on or underneath the skin.

High doses of cocaine can cause nervousness, dizziness, blurred vision, vomiting, tremors, seizures, high blood pressure, strokes, angina, and cardiac arrhythmias. Freebase (a purer, more potent smokable form of cocaine) users have a higher risk for lung disease, and intravenous users are at risk for hepatitis, AIDS, and other infectious diseases.

Large overdoses of cocaine end in sudden death from respiratory paralysis, cardiac arrhythmias, and severe convulsions. Some individuals, however, may lack an enzyme used in metabolizing cocaine, and as few as two to three lines of cocaine may be fatal.

Chronic users who crave the drug constantly often turn to crime, including murder, to sustain their habit. Some users view suicide as the only solution to this sad syndrome.

## Alcohol

Drinking alcohol has been socially acceptable for centuries. Alcohol is an accepted accompaniment at parties, ceremonies, dinners, sport contests, the establishment of kingdoms or governments, and the signing of peace treaties. Alcohol also has been used for medical reasons as a mild sedative or as a pain killer accompanying surgery.

For a short period of 14 years, from 1920 to 1933, by constitutional amendment, the sale and use of alcohol were declared illegal in the United States. This amendment was repealed because drinkers and nondrinkers alike questioned the right of the government to pass judgment on individual moral

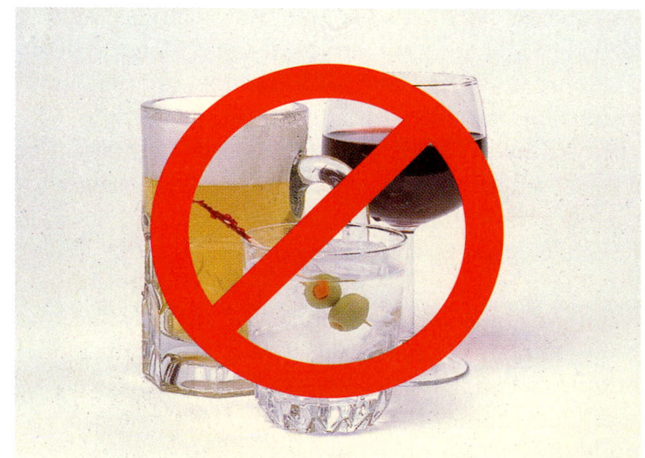

*Between 1920 and 1933 the sale of alcohol was illegal in the United States.*

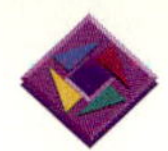

standards. In addition, organized crime to smuggle and sell alcohol illegally expanded enormously.

The alcohol contained in drinks is known as *ethyl alcohol*, a depressant drug that affects the brain and slows down central nervous system activity. As with most drugs that affect the brain, it has strong addictive properties and therefore can be abused easily.

Alcohol abuse is one of the most significant health-related drug problems in the United States today. Estimates indicate that six in 10 adults, or more than 100 million Americans 18 years and older, are drinkers. Approximately 10 million of them will have a drinking problem, including alcoholism, sometime during their life. Another 3 million teenagers are thought to have a drinking problem.

The addiction to alcohol develops slowly. Most people feel that they are in control of their drinking habits and do not realize they have a problem until they become alcoholics — when they develop a physical and emotional dependence on the drug, characterized by excessive use and constant preoccupation with drinking. Alcohol abuse in turn leads to mental, emotional, physical, and social problems.

Alcohol intake reduces peripheral vision, decreases visual and hearing acuity, slows reaction time, impairs concentration and motor performance (including more swaying and impaired judgment of distance and speed of moving objects). Further, it dissipates fear, increases risk-taking behaviors, stimulates urination, and induces sleep.

A single large dose of alcohol also may decrease sexual function. One of the most unpleasant, dangerous, and life-threatening effects of drinking is the *synergistic action* of alcohol when combined with other drugs, particularly central nervous system depressants. The effects of mixing alcohol with another drug can be much greater than the sum of two drug actions by themselves. Although people react differently to a combination of alcohol and other drugs, the effects range from loss of consciousness to death.

Long-term effects of alcohol abuse may be life-threatening. Some of these detrimental effects are cirrhosis of the liver (scarring of the liver, which is often fatal); higher risk for oral, esophageal, and liver cancer; cardiomyopathy (a disease that affects the heart muscle); higher blood pressure; greater risk for strokes; inflammation of the esophagus, stomach, small intestine, and pancreas; stomach ulcers; sexual impotence; malnutrition; brain cell damage inducing loss of memory; psychosis; depression; and hallucinations.

### Alcohol on Campuses

Alcohol is the number-one drug problem among college students. According to a 1992 national survey, 86.9% of college students reported using alcohol, and 41% of them had engaged in binge drinking (five or more drinks in a row) at least once in the 2 weeks preceding the survey. Alcohol is a factor in about 28% of all college dropouts, costing the federal government more than $3 billion in taxes. Today's student spends more on alcohol than on books.

A second 1992 survey, involving 56,000 college students, showed that grade-point average (GPA) is related to the average number of drinks per week (see Figure 13.1). Students with a "D" or "F" GPA reported a weekly consumption of 11 drinks. Students with "A" GPAs consumed only 3.5 drinks per week. Of greater concern is that 36% indicated driving while intoxicated. This figure translates to about 20,000 college student deaths related to automobile accidents each year. Of the current 12 million college students in the United States, between 2% and 3% will die from alcohol-related

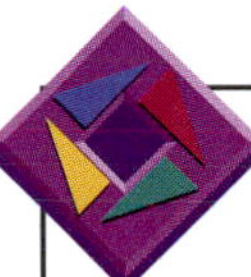

**DO'S AND DON'TS WHEN YOUR DATE DRINKS**

- **Don't** make excuses for his/her behavior, no matter how embarrassing.
- **Don't** allow embarrassment to put you in a situation with which you are uncomfortable.
- **Do** be sure that body language and tone of voice match verbal messages you send.
- **Do** make your position clear. "No!" is much more effective than "Please stop!" or "Don't!"
- **Do** make it clear that you will call the police if rape is attempted.
- **Do** leave as quickly as you can, without your date. **Don't** stop to argue. Intoxicated people can't listen to reason.
- **Do** call a cab, a friend, or your parents. **Don't** ride home with your date.

Source: "Sexuality Under the Influence of Alcohol." *Human Sexuality Supplement to Current Health*, 2 (October 1990), p. 3.

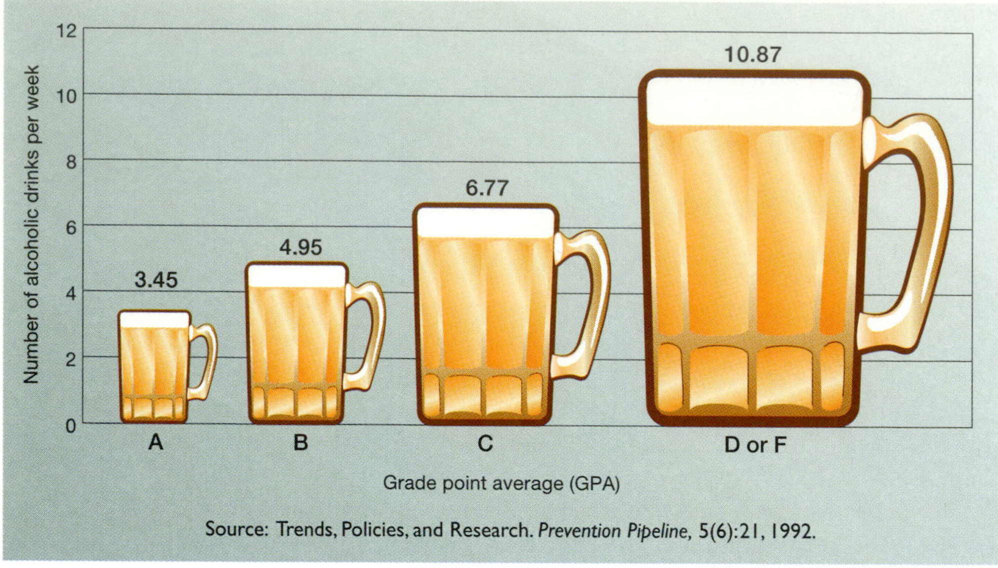


**FIGURE 13.1** ◆ Average number of drinks by college students per week by grade-point average.

causes. This represents approximately the same number as those who will receive advanced degrees (master's and doctorate degrees combined).

Another major concern is that over 50% of college students participate in games that involve heavy drinking (6 to 10 drinks) in a very short period of time. Often students participate because of fear of rejection and peer pressure. Further, up to 48% report getting drunk at least once a month. Excessive drinking can lead to unplanned and unprotected sex (risking HIV infection) or even date rape. Practice common sense when your date drinks.

## How to Cut Down Your Drinking*

To find out if drinking is a problem in your life, refer to the questionnaire "Alcohol Abuse: Are You Drinking Too Much," given in Figure 13.2. If you answer "yes" twice or more on this questionnaire, you may be jeopardizing your health through excessive consumption of alcohol.

Many people who are determined to control the problem find that it is not that hard to do. The first and most important step is to want to cut down. If you want to cut down but find you cannot, you had better accept the probability that alcohol is becoming a serious problem for you, and you should seek guidance from your physician or from an organization such as Alcoholics Anonymous. The next few suggestions also may help you cut down on alcohol intake.

1. **Set reasonable limits for yourself.** Decide not to exceed a certain number of drinks on a given occasion, and stick to your decision. No more than two beers or two cocktails a day is a reasonable limit. You have proven to yourself that you can control your drinking if you set such a target and regularly do not exceed it.
2. **Learn to say no.** Many people have "just one more" drink because others in the group are having one or because someone puts pressure on them, not because they really want a drink. When you reach the sensible limit you have set for yourself, politely but firmly refuse to exceed it. If you are being the generous host, pour yourself a glass of water or juice "on the rocks." Nobody will notice the difference.
3. **Drink slowly.** Never gulp down a drink. Choose your drinks for their flavor, not their "kick," and savor the taste of each sip.
4. **Dilute your drinks.** If you prefer cocktails to beer, try having long drinks. Instead of downing your gin or whiskey neat or nearly so, drink it diluted with a mixer such as tonic, water, or soda water, in a tall glass. That way, you can enjoy the flavor as well as the act of drinking, but it will take longer to finish each drink. Also, you can make your two-drink limit last all evening or switch to the mixer by itself.

* Reproduced by permission from *Family Medical Guide* by American Medical Association (New York: Random House, 1982).

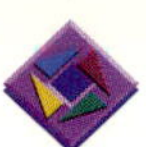

## ALCOHOL ABUSE: ARE YOU DRINKING TOO MUCH?

1. When you are holding an empty glass at a party, do you always actively look for a refill instead of waiting to be offered one?
2. If given the chance, do you frequently pour out a more generous drink for yourself than seems to be the "going" amount for others?
3. Do you often have a drink or two when you are alone, either at home or in a bar?
4. Is your drinking ever the direct cause of a family quarrel, or do quarrels often seem to occur, if only by coincidence, when you have had a drink or two?
5. Do you feel that you must have a drink at a specific time every day — right after work, for instance?
6. When worried or under unusual stress, do you almost automatically take a stiff drink to "settle your nerves?"
7. Are you untruthful about how much you have had to drink when questioned on the subject?
8. Does drinking ever cause you to take time off work, or to miss scheduled meetings or appointments?
9. Do you feel physically deprived if you cannot have at least one drink every day?
10. Do you sometimes crave a drink in the morning?
11. Do you sometimes have "mornings after" when you cannot remember what happened the night before?

**Evaluation**

You should regard a "yes" answer to any one of the above questions as a warning sign. Do not increase your consumption of alcohol. Two "yes" answers suggest that you already may be becoming dependent on alcohol. Three or more "yes" answers indicate that you may have a serious problem, and you should get professional help.

**FIGURE 13.2** ◆

5. **Do not drink on your own.** Confine your drinking to social gatherings. Sometimes resisting the urge to pour a relaxing drink at the end of a hard day is difficult but many formerly heavy drinkers have found that a cup of coffee or a soft drink satisfies the need as well as alcohol did and that it was just a habit. What may help you really to unwind, even with no drink at all, is a comfortable chair, loosened clothing, and perhaps soothing music, a television program, or a good book to read.

## Treatment of Addiction

Treatment of drug (including alcohol) addiction seldom is accomplished without professional guidance and support. Of course the first step is to recognize that a problem exists. The questionnaire given in Figure 13.3 can help you recognize possible addictive behavior either in yourself or in someone you know. If you answer "yes" to more than half of these questions, you may have a problem and should speak to your doctor or contact the local mental health clinic for a referral (see the Yellow Pages in your phone book).

## ADDICTIVE BEHAVIOR QUESTIONNAIRE: COULD YOU BE AN ADDICT?

**Directions**

The following test, designed by Dr. Lawrence J. Hatterer, is not a way to diagnose whether you are in the early, middle, or chronic stage of addictive disease. It is meant merely to help you understand addictive behavior better so you can recognize it in yourself or perhaps in people you know.

1. I am a person of excesses. I can't regulate what I do for pleasure and often use a substance or indulge in an activity heavily to get high.
2. I am an extremely self-involved person. People tell me I am into myself too much.
3. I am compulsive. I must have what I want when I want it, regardless of the consequences.
4. I am excessively dependent on or independent of others.
5. I am preoccupied. I spend a lot of time thinking or fantasizing about a particular activity or substance. Also, I will work my day around doing it or go to pains to make sure it's available.
6. I deny that I do this, and lie about it to others who ask me.
7. I have been involved in this behavior for at least a year.
8. I've told myself I could easily stop, even though I've shown no signs of slowing down.
9. Once I start indulging in this behavior or substance, I find I have trouble stopping.
10. One or more members of my family also are involved in some kind of excessive behavior or substance abuse.
11. I find I gravitate mostly toward people who have the same behavior or take the same substance as I do.
12. I seem to be developing a tolerance of the behavior or substance. I have had a need to steadily increase the amounts I take or the time I spend doing it.
13. I have found that my excessive use of highs has, in fact, only made my problems worse.
14. If someone tries to keep me from obtaining the substance or practicing the activity, I get angry and reject or abuse that person.
15. I experience withdrawal symptoms if I cannot indulge in the substance or activity.
16. This has gotten in the way of my functioning. I have missed something important — days at work, time with my friends, family, children — because of it.
17. The substance/activity is destroying my home life. I know I am hurting those closest to me.
18. I have failed in many goals in life, lost money, given up many social and occupational contacts, all because of my excessive behavior.
19. I have tried to stop or cut down on my excesses but have been unsuccessful.
20. I have physically endangered myself or others in accidents that were a direct result of my excessive behavior.

**Evaluation**

If you answer "yes" to half or more of the questions, you may have a problem with addictive disease and should seek immediate professional help. For a referral, contact your local mental health clinic (look in the Yellow Pages) or speak to your doctor.



**FIGURE 13.3** ◆

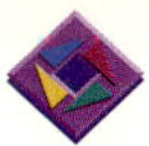

## SEXUALLY TRANSMITTED DISEASES

Sexually transmitted diseases (STDs) have reached epidemic proportions in the United States. Of the more than 25 known STDs, some are still incurable. The American Social Health Association stated that 25% of all Americans will acquire at least one STD in their lifetime. Each year more than 12 million people are newly infected with STDs, including 4.6 million cases of chlamydia, 1.8 million of gonorrhea, 1 million of genital warts, half a million of herpes, and nearly 100,000 cases of syphilis. Attracting most of the attention because of its life-threatening potential were more than 46,648 new cases of AIDS in 1992 alone.

### Chlamydia

Chlamydia is a bacterial infection that spreads during vaginal, anal, or oral sex, or from the vagina to a newborn baby during childbirth. Chlamydia can damage the reproductive system seriously.

This disease is considered to be a major factor in male and female infertility. Because it may have no symptoms, three of four people don't realize they have the disease until it is quite serious. According to the Centers for Disease Control, about 20% of all college students have chlamydia.

When symptoms are present, they tend to mimic other STDs, so the disease can be easily mistreated. Symptoms of serious infection include abdominal pain, fever, nausea, vaginal bleeding, and arthritis. It can be treated successfully with oral antibiotics but will not reverse any damage already done to the reproductive system.

### Gonorrhea

One of the oldest STDs, gonorrhea also is caused by a bacterial infection. Gonorrhea is transmitted through vaginal, anal, and oral sex. Typical symptoms in men include a puslike secretion from the penis and painful urination. Most infected women don't have any symptoms until the infection is fairly serious. At this stage, women develop fever, severe abdominal pain, and pelvic inflammatory disease (see below).

If untreated, gonorrhea can produce infertility, widespread bacterial infection, heart damage, arthritis, and also blindness in children born to infected women. Gonorrhea is treated successfully with penicillin and other antibiotics.

### Pelvic Inflammatory Disease

Each year approximately 750,000 women incur pelvic inflammatory disease (PID). This disease is caused most frequently by chlamydia and gonorrhea. Typical symptoms of PID include fever; nausea; vomiting; chills; spotting, heavy bleeding during menstrual periods; and pain in the lower abdomen during sexual intercourse, between menstrual periods, or urination. Many women do not know they have PID because they have no symptoms.

PID often develops when the STD spreads to the fallopian tubes, uterus, and ovaries. If the women becomes pregnant, it may result in an ectopic or tubal pregnancy. That pregnancy destroys the embryo and can kill the patient.

PID is treated with antibiotics, bed rest, and sexual abstinence. Surgery also may be required to remove infected or scarred tissue or to repair or remove the fallopian tubes or uterus.

### Genital Warts

Genital warts are caused by a viral infection and show up anywhere from 1½ months to 8 months after exposure. These warts may be flat or raised and usually are found on the penis or around the vulva and the vagina, but they also can appear in the mouth, throat, and rectum, on the cervix, or around the anus.

Of sexually active people in the United States 20% to 30% are infected with the virus that causes this STD. In some cities, almost half of all sexually active teenagers have genital warts. Similar to chlamydia, the virus is spread through vaginal, anal, and oral sex, or from the vagina to a newborn baby.

Health problems associated with genital warts include higher risk for cancers of the cervix, vulva, or penis and enlargement and spread of the warts leading to obstruction of the urethra, vagina, and anus. Babies born to infected mothers typically develop warts over their bodies; therefore, Cesarean sections are recommended.

Treatment requires completely removing all warts, which can be done by freezing them with liquid nitrogen, dissolving them with chemicals, or removing them through electrosurgery or laser surgery. Infected patients may have to be treated more than once because genital warts can recur.

## Herpes

Herpes, too, is caused by a viral infection (herpes simplex virus types I and II), and it still has no known cure. Sores appear on the mouth, genitals, rectum, or other parts of the body. The symptoms usually disappear within a few weeks, causing some people to believe they are cured. Herpes, however, is presently incurable, and its victims do remain infected. Repeated outbreaks are common.

Herpes is highly contagious and can be transmitted through simple finger contact from the mouth to the genitals. Victims are most contagious during an outbreak. In conjunction with the sores, victims usually have a mild fever, swollen glands, and headaches.

## Syphilis

Another common type of STD, also caused by bacterial infection, is syphilis. Approximately 3 weeks after infection, a painless sore appears where the bacteria entered the body. This sore disappears on its own in a few weeks. If untreated, more sores may appear within 6 months of the initial outbreak but will again disappear by themselves.

A latent stage, during which the victim is not contagious, may last up to 30 years, lulling victims into thinking they are healed. During the last stage of the disease, some people develop paralysis, crippling, blindness, heart disease, brain damage, insanity, and even may die. One of the oldest known STDs, syphilis used to end up killing its victims. Penicillin and other antibiotics now are used to treat it.

If you test positive for any type of STD, you need to tell anyone with whom you have had sex so he or she can be tested, and treated if necessary. Unless you do this, you run the risk of being infected again, permanently damaging your partner(s), and spreading the disease to others.

## HIV and AIDS

AIDS is the most frightening of all STDs because it has no known cure and none predicted for the near future. AIDS, which stands for *acquired immunodeficiency syndrome*, is the end stage of infection by the *human immunodeficiency virus* HIV.

HIV is a chronic infectious disease that spreads among individuals who choose to engage in risky behavior such as unprotected sex or the sharing of hypodermic needles. When a person becomes infected with HIV, the virus multiplies, and attacks and destroys white blood cells. These cells are part of the immune system, and their function is to fight off infections and diseases in the body.

As the number of white blood cells killed increases, the body's immune system gradually breaks down or may be totally destroyed. Without the immune system, a person becomes susceptible to *opportunistic infections* or cancers not ordinarily seen in healthy people.

HIV is a progressive disease. At first, people who become infected with HIV may not know they are infected. An incubation period of weeks, months, or years may go by during which time no symptoms appear. The virus may live in the body 10 years or longer before symptoms emerge.

As the infection progresses to the point at which certain diseases develop, the person is said to have AIDS. HIV itself doesn't kill. Nor do people die of AIDS. AIDS is the term used to define the final stage of HIV infection. Death is caused by a weakened immune system that is unable to fight off opportunistic diseases.

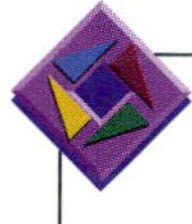

*One the average, 7 to 8 years elapse after infection before the individual develops the symptoms that fit the case definition of AIDS.*

Earliest symptoms of the disease include unexplained weight loss, constant fatigue, mild fever, swollen lymph glands, diarrhea, and sore throats. Advanced symptoms include loss of appetite, skin diseases, night sweats, and deterioration of the mucous membranes.

Most of the illnesses that AIDS patients develop are harmless and rare in the general population but are fatal to the AIDS victim. The two most common fatal conditions in AIDS patients are *pneumocystis carinii pneumonia* (a parasitic infection of the lungs) and *kaposis sarcoma* (a type of skin cancer). The AIDS virus also may attack the nervous system, causing brain and spinal cord damage.

On the average, 7 to 8 years elapse after infection before the individual develops the symptoms that fit the case definition of AIDS. From that point on, the person may live another 2 to 3 years. In essence, from the point of infection, the individual may endure a chronic disease for 8 to 10 years.

The only means to determine whether someone has HIV is through an HIV antibody test. Being

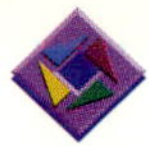

HIV-positive does not necessarily mean the person has AIDS. Again, several years may pass before the person actually develops the diseases that fit the case definition of AIDS.

Upon HIV infection the immune system's line of defense against the virus is the formation of antibodies that bind to the virus. On the average, the body requires 3 months to manufacture enough antibodies to show positive in an HIV antibody test. Sometimes this may take 6 months or longer.

If HIV infection is suspected, a prudent waiting period of 3 to 6 months should be observed before testing. During this waiting period, and from there on, these individuals should refrain from endangering themselves and others further through risky behaviors. Some people choose to be tested to be reassured that their risky behaviors are acceptable. Even if the test shows negative for HIV, however, this does not represent a "license" to continue risky behaviors.

No one has to become infected with HIV. Once infected with the virus, a person will never become uninfected. There is no second chance. Everyone must protect himself or herself against this chronic disease. No one should be so ignorant as to believe that it can never happen to him or her!

Although professionals disagree as to how many carriers actually will develop AIDS, sooner or later most HIV-infected persons will be diagnosed with AIDS. Even if a person has not developed AIDS, the virus still can be passed on to others who could easily develop AIDS.

### HIV Transmission

HIV is transmitted by the exchange of cellular body fluids — blood, semen, vaginal secretions, and maternal milk. These fluids may be exchanged during sexual intercourse, by using hypodermic needles used previously by infected individuals, between a pregnant woman and her developing fetus, babies from an infected mother during childbirth, less frequently during breast feeding, and rarely from a blood transfusion or organ transplant.

The risk of being infected with HIV from a blood transfusion today is slight. Prior to 1985 several cases of HIV were transmitted through blood transfusions because the blood was donated by HIV-infected persons. Today, all individuals who donate blood are tested for HIV.

A myth regarding HIV is that it can be transmitted by donating blood. People cannot get HIV from giving blood. Health professionals use a brand-new needle every time they withdraw blood. These needles are used only once and are destroyed and thrown away immediately after each individual has donated blood.

People do not get HIV because of who they are, but, rather, because of what they do. HIV and AIDS can threaten anyone, anywhere: men, women, children, teenagers, young people, older adults, Whites, Blacks, Hispanics, Orientals, homosexuals, heterosexuals, bisexuals, druggies, Americans, Africans, Europeans. Nobody is immune to HIV.

HIV can be transmitted between males, between females, from male to female, or from female to male. Although HIV infection is largely preventable, almost all of the people who get HIV do so because they choose to engage in risky behaviors.

### Risky Behaviors

You cannot tell if people are infected with HIV or have AIDS simply by looking at them or taking their word. Not you, not a nurse, not even a doctor can tell, unless an HIV antibody test is done. Therefore, every time you engage in risky behavior, you run the risk of contracting HIV. The two most basic risky behaviors are:

1. **Having unprotected vaginal, anal, or oral sex with an HIV-infected person.** Unprotected sex means having sex without using a condom properly. Only latex (rubber or prophylactic) condoms that state "disease prevention" on the package should be used. Although a person may have unprotected sex with an infected person and not get the virus, that person can also get it by having unprotected sex only once with an infected individual.

   Rubbing during sexual intercourse often damages mucous membranes and causes unseen bleeding (even in the mouth). During vaginal, anal, or oral sexual contact, infected blood, semen, or vaginal fluids can penetrate the mucous membranes that line the vagina, the penis, the rectum, the mouth, or the throat. From the membrane, HIV can travel into the previously uninfected person's blood.

   Health experts believe that unprotected anal sex is the riskiest type of sex. Although in most cases bleeding is not visible, anal sex almost always causes tiny tears and bleeding in the rectum. This happens because the rectum does not stretch easily, the mucous membrane is quite thin, and small blood vessels lie directly beneath the membrane. Condoms also are more likely to break during anal intercourse because of the greater friction produced in a smaller cavity. All of these factors magnify the risk of HIV transmission.

Although, if used correctly, a latex condom provides for "safer" sex, *it is not 100% fool-proof*. Abstaining from sex is the only 100% sure way to protect yourself from HIV infection and other STDs.

2. **Sharing hypodermic needles or other drug paraphernalia with someone who is infected.** Following an injection, a small amount of blood remains in the needle and sometimes in the syringe itself. If the person who used the syringe is infected with HIV and someone else uses that same syringe to shoot up, regardless of the drug used (legal or illegal), that small amount of blood is enough to spread the virus. All used syringes should be destroyed and disposed of immediately after their use.

   In addition, caution must be taken when getting acupuncture, a tattoo, or the ears pierced. If the needle used on you was previously used on someone who is HIV infected, and it was not properly disinfected, you risk getting HIV as well.

Infrequent drug (including alcohol) use also increases the risk of spreading HIV. Otherwise prudent people often act irrationally and engage in risky behaviors when they are under the influence of drugs. Getting high can make you willing to have sex when you really didn't plan to, and thereby run the risk of HIV infection.

**VANESSA WAS IN A FATAL CAR ACCIDENT LAST NIGHT. ONLY SHE DOESN'T KNOW IT YET.**

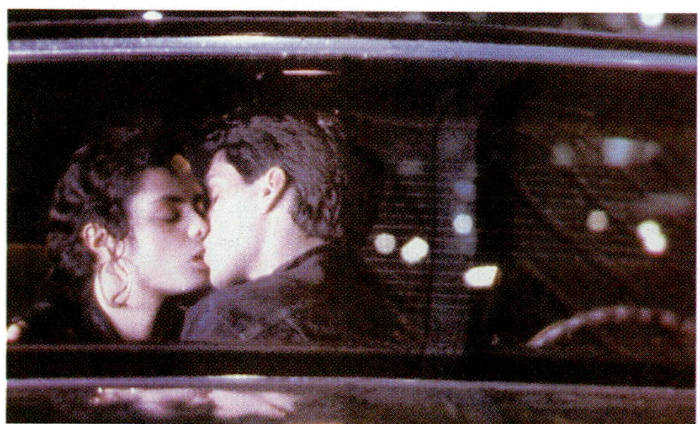

*Drug and alcohol use can make people more willing to have unplanned and unprotected sex, thereby risking HIV infection.*

Photo courtesy of the National Institute on Drug Abuse, U.S. Department of Health & Human Services.

As pointed out earlier, HIV can be transmitted through a blood transfusion, an organ transplant, pregnancy (mother to fetus), and maternal milk (usually mother to child). Even though the nation's blood supply is quite safe (because all donors are tested for HIV), a small risk exists for getting infected from previously tested blood. Because of the 3- to 6-month incubation period, a donor recently infected with HIV tested negative at the time of donating blood (or an organ). Anyone who is planning to have surgery should store his or her own blood in advance to make sure that safe blood is available if it becomes necessary.

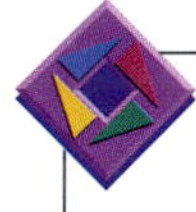

*No one should be so ignorant as to believe that HIV infection can never happen to him or her. Once infected, a person will never become uninfected.*

Small concentrations of the virus have been found in saliva and teardrops, but no record exists of anyone getting HIV through French-kissing or from someone else's tears, coughs, or sneezes. In principle, if both people have open cuts in the lips, mouth, or gums, HIV could be transmitted through open-mouthed kissing, but such a case never has been documented.

The virus cannot be transmitted through perspiration (sweat) either. Sporting activities involving physical contact pose no risk to uninfected individuals unless there are open wounds through which blood from an infected person can come in direct contact with the open wound of the uninfected person. The skin is an excellent line of defense against HIV. Blood from an infected person cannot penetrate the skin except through an opening in the skin. As an extra precaution, anyone who performs work that requires direct contact with someone else's blood or open wound should use vinyl or latex gloves.

Some people fear getting HIV from health-care professionals. The chances of getting infected during physical or medical procedures are practically nil. Health-care workers take extra care to protect themselves and their patients from HIV.

HIV is not transmitted through casual contact. HIV cannot be caught by spending time, shaking hands, or hugging an infected person; from a toilet seat, dishes, or silverware used by an HIV patient; or by sharing a drink, food, a towel or clothes with a person who has HIV.

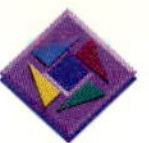

What about dating? Dating and getting to know other people is a normal part of life. Dating, however, does not mean the same thing as having sex. Sexual intercourse as a part of dating can be risky, and one of the risks is AIDS. You can't tell if someone you are dating or would like to date has been exposed to HIV. The good news, though, is that as long as you avoid sexual activity and don't share drug needles, it doesn't matter whom you date.

Another myth regarding HIV transmission is that you can get it from insects or animals. The H in HIV stands for *human* and you cannot catch HIV from insects or animals. Animals do not get infected with HIV.

### HIV and AIDS Statistics

The Centers for Disease Control estimate that 1 million Americans are infected with HIV. Around the world an estimated 12 million people are infected. Because of the lengthy incubation period (7 to 8 years to develop AIDS), about 20% of the AIDS patients today are believed to have been infected as teenagers.

By the end of 1993, a total of 357,916 AIDS cases had been diagnosed in the United States (see Figure 13.4) and 171,980 had died from the diseases caused by HIV. The number of deaths is expected to double in three years. Most of the people who die are in the 20- to 45-year-old age group. By the year 2000, deaths from HIV infection will become the third leading cause of death, behind cardiovascular disease and cancer.

Approximately 66% of all AIDS cases in the United States have occurred in gay or bisexual men. AIDS among heterosexuals, nonetheless, is on the rise. In fact, HIV is now spreading at a faster rate among heterosexuals. Many heterosexuals practice unprotected sex because they don't believe it can happen to their segment of the population. HIV is an epidemic that does not discriminate by sexual orientation. Worldwide, about 75% of the AIDS cases have been reported in heterosexuals.

As with any other serious illness, AIDS patients deserve respect, understanding, and support. Rejection and discrimination are traits of immature,

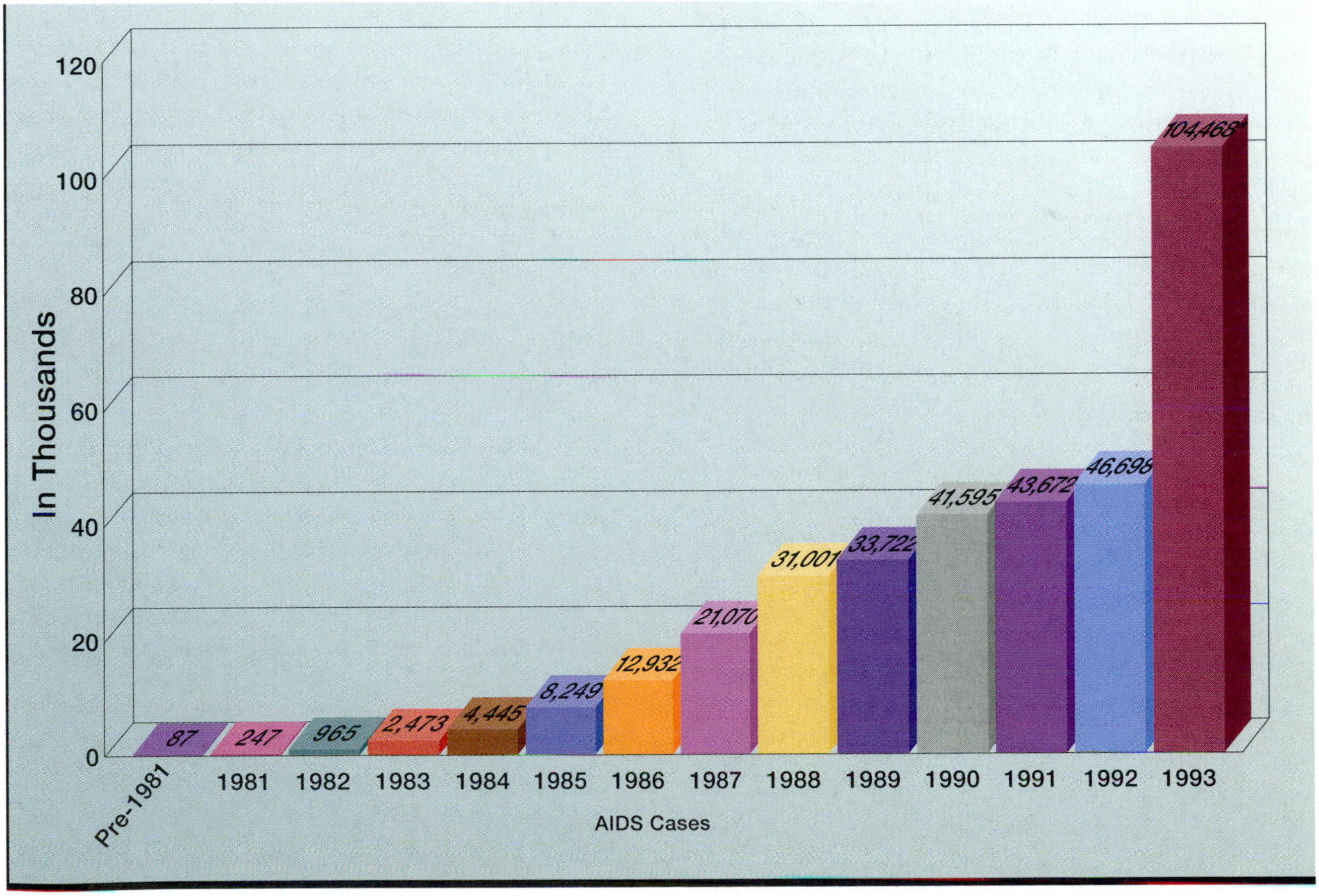

**FIGURE 13.4** ♦ Reported U.S. AIDS Cases Between 1981 and 1993 (the large increase between 1992 and 1993 was due to the implementation of the new case definition of AIDS in 1993).

hateful, and ignorant people. Education, knowledge, and responsible behaviors are the best ways to minimize fear and discrimination.

### HIV Testing

A person can be tested for HIV in several ways. The local Public Health Department or AIDS Information Service (or related names) are listed in the phone book. Testing usually is free of charge, and the results are kept confidential.

Many states also conduct anonymous testing. The person's name is never recorded. Several toll-free hotlines are available for more information on anonymous testing, treatment programs, support services, HIV and AIDS information, and STDs in general. All information discussed during a phone call to these hotlines is strictly confidential. The numbers to call are:

- The National AIDS Hotline: 1-800-342-AIDS or La Linea Nacional de SIDA: 1-800-344-SIDA for Spanish speaking persons.
- The STD Hotline: 1-800-227-8922.
- The National Institute on Drug Abuse (NIDA) Information and Treatment Referral: 1-800-662-HELP or 1-800-66-AYUDA for Spanish-speaking only. (NIDA also provides information on drug abuse and addictive behavior).

### HIV Treatment

Even though several drugs are being tested to treat and slow down the disease process, AIDS has no known cure. Approximately 30 different approaches to an AIDS vaccine are being explored, with two approved for testing in humans. The best advice at this point is to a preventive approach. In the absence of a cure, medications are available that allow HIV-infected patients to live longer. The sooner the treatment is begun following infection, the better are the chances of delaying the onset of AIDS.

Development of a vaccine to prevent HIV infection or AIDS seems highly unlikely in the next few years. People should not expect a medical breakthrough. Treatment modalities, however, should continue to improve and allow HIV-infected individuals and AIDS patients to live longer and lead more productive lives.

Presently several AIDS clinical trials are available in the United States. These projects are co-sponsored by the Centers for Disease Control, the Food and Drug Administration, the National Institute of Allergy and Infectious Diseases, and the National Library of Medicine. The purpose of AIDS clinical trials is to evaluate experimental drugs and various therapies for people at all stages of HIV infection. Interested individuals can call 1–800–TRIALS–A. As with all HIV testing, these calls are completely confidential. Eligibility to participate in an AIDS clinical trial varies, and all applicants are evaluated individually. Interested individuals receive information on the purpose and location of the trials that are open, eligibility requirements and exclusion criteria, and names and telephone numbers of contact persons.

### Economic Impact of HIV and AIDS

Federal government spending for AIDS-related projects gradually increased to more than $900 million between 1982 and 1988. Costs continued to escalate to $1.3 billion in 1989 and $4.3 billion in 1992, and were expected to be in excess of $10.4 billion in 1994.

As of 1993, the annual U. S. health-care cost to care for an HIV-positive individual who had not reached the AIDS stage was approximately $5,150. The yearly cost to treat an individual who had developed AIDS was about $32,000. The average cost from the onset of AIDS until death was $85,333. Assuming an incubation period of 7 years and an additional 3 years of AIDS, the direct treatment costs per person would average $121,383. This represents in excess of $43.4 billion dollars to treat the 357,916 AIDS cases reported as of December 1993.

If the estimated 1 million people infected with HIV in the United States develop AIDS, the direct health-care costs for the disease would equal $121.383 billion. To place this figure in perspective, a person would have to spend $1 million per day for the next 332.5 years to spend the $121.382 billion. Every American will help pay for these costs through taxes and a more expensive health care system. In the words of Dr. Russell Centanni, Professor of Biology at Boise State University, "rather sobering for a preventable disease."

## GUIDELINES FOR PREVENTING SEXUALLY TRANSMITTED DISEASES

With all the grim news about STDs, there is also some good news: You can do some things to

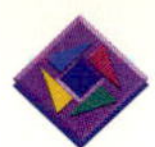

prevent their spread, and take some precautions to keep yourself from becoming a victim.

The facts are in: The best prevention technique is a mutually monogamous sexual relationship, one in which two people have sexual relationships only with each other. That one behavior, says Dr. James Mason, director of the Centers for Disease Control in Atlanta, will almost completely remove you from any risk of developing an STD.

Unfortunately, in today's society, to know at what point you can truly trust a person is increasingly difficult. You may be led to believe that you are in a monogamous relationship, when in reality your partner: (a) may be cheating on you and gets infected, (b) ends up having a one-night stand with someone who is infected, (c) got the virus several years ago, before the present relationship and still doesn't know of the infection, (d) may not be honest with you and chooses not to tell you about the infection, or (e) is shooting up drugs and becomes infected. In any of these cases, HIV can be passed on to you.

Because your future and your life are at stake, and because you never may know if your partner is infected, you should give serious and careful consideration to postponing sex until you believe you have found a lifetime monogamous relationship. In this way, you will not have to live with the fear of catching HIV or other STDs or deal with an unplanned pregnancy.

As strange as it may seem to some, many people still postpone sexual activity until they are married. This is the best guarantee against HIV. Young people have plenty of time for fulfilling and rewarding sex throughout married life.

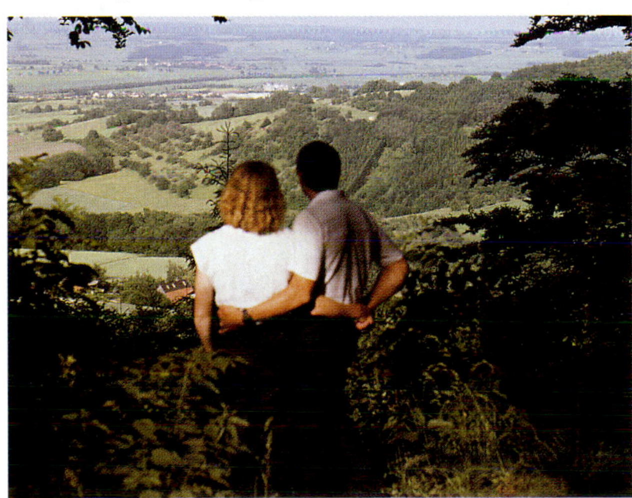

*A monogamous sexual relationship almost completely removes people from risking HIV infection and the danger of developing other sexually transmitted diseases.*

If you choose to delay sex, peers may try to pressure you into having sex. Some people would have you believe that you are not a real man or woman if you don't have sex. Manhood and womanhood are not proven during sexual intercourse but, instead, through mature, responsible, and healthy choices.

Other people lead you to believe that love can't exist apart from sex. In the early stages of a relationship, sex is not the product of love but is simply the fulfillment of a physical, and often selfish, drive. A loving relationship develops over a long time with mutual respect for each other.

Teenagers are especially susceptible to peer pressure leading to premature sexual intercourse. The result is more than a million teenage pregnancies per year and a 43% pregnancy rate for all girls at least once as a teenager. Too many young people wish they had postponed sex and silently admire those who do. Sex lasts only a few minutes. The consequences of irresponsible sex, however, may last a lifetime. And in some cases they are fatal!

Then there are those who enjoy bragging about their sexual "conquests" and attempt to mock people who choose to wait. In essence, many of these conquests are only fantasies to gain popularity with peers. Sexual promiscuity never leads to a trusting, loving, and lasting relationship. Mature people respect others' choices. If someone does not respect your choice to wait, he or she certainly does not deserve your friendship or, for that matter, anything else.

There is no greater sex than that between two loving and responsible individuals who have mutual trust and admiration for each other. Contrary to many beliefs, such relationships are possible. They are built upon unselfish attitudes and behaviors. As you look around, you will find that many believe the same way you do. Seek them out, and build your friendships and future around people who respect you for what you are and what you believe. You don't have to compromise your choices or values. In the end you will reap the greater rewards of a choice and lasting relationship, free of AIDS and other STDs.

What about those who do not have — or do not desire — a monogamous relationship? Some other things can be done to lower, but never completely eliminate, the risk of developing STDs in general:

1. Know your partner. The days are gone when anonymous bathhouse or singles-bars sex is

safe. Limit your sexual relationships, and always practice safer sex.

2. Limit the number of sexual partners you have. Having one partner lowers your chance of infection. The more partners you have, the greater is your chance of infection.

3. If you are sexually promiscuous, consider having periodic physical check-ups. You can get exposed to an STD easily by a person who does not have any symptoms and who is unaware of the infection. Sexually promiscuous men and women between the ages 15 and 35 are considered to be in a particularly high-risk group for developing STDs.

4. Use "barrier" methods of contraception to help prevent the disease from spreading. Condoms, diaphragms, the contraceptive sponge, and spermicidal suppositories, foams, and jellies can all deter the spread of certain STDs. Spermicidal agents may help act as a disinfectant as well.

   Many physicians are especially encouraging promiscuous teenagers to use condoms. Traditionally, teenagers do not use any birth-control methods at all and remain at high risk for STDs.

5. Be responsible enough to abstain from sexual activity if you know you have an infection. Go to a physician or a clinic for treatment, and ask your doctor when you can resume sexual activity safely. Abstain until then. Just as you want to be protected in a sexual relationship, you have to protect your partner as well.

6. Urinate immediately after sexual intercourse. This is not a very reliable method, but it may help (especially men) flush bacteria and viruses from the urinary tract.

7. Wash thoroughly immediately after sexual activity. Washing with hot, soapy water will not guarantee safety against STDs, but it can prevent you from spreading certain germs on your fingers and may wash away bacteria and viruses that have not yet entered the body.

8. If you suspect your partner is infected with a STD, ask. He or she may not even be aware of the infection, so look for signs of infection, such as sores, redness, inflammations, a rash, growths, warts, or discharge. If you are unsure, abstain.

9. Consider abstaining from sexual relations if you have any kind of an illness or disease, even a common cold. Any kind of illness makes you more susceptible to other illnesses, and lowered immunity can make you extra vulnerable to STDs. The same holds true for times when you are under extreme stress, when you are fatigued, and when you are overworked. Drugs and alcohol also can lower your resistance to disease.

10. Wear loose-fitting clothes made of natural fibers; tight-fitting clothing made of synthetic fibers (especially underwear and nylon pantyhose) can create conditions that encourage bacterial growth and actually can aggravate STDs.

### HIV Risk Reduction

Based upon recommendations from health experts, observing the following precautions can reduce your risk for getting HIV and subsequently AIDS:

1. Postpone sex until you and your uninfected partner are prepared to enter in a lifetime monogamous relationship. In his book, *What You Can Do to Avoid AIDS*, Magic Johnson stated:[1]

   > *But if I had known what I do now when I was younger, I would have postponed sex as long as I could, and I would have tried to have it the first time with somebody that I knew I wanted to spend the rest of my life with. I certainly want my children to postpone sex. Now, the rest of my life may be a lot shorter than I thought it was going to be, and I may not be around to see my son, Andre, grow up and to see what happens to the baby Cookie and I are having in the summer of '92, and of course I may not have the long life I want with Cookie.*[1]

2. Unless you are in a monogamous relationship and you know your partner is not infected (which you may never know for sure), practice safer sex every single time you have sex. This means: Use a latex condom from start to finish for each sexual act. If you think your partner should use a condom but refuses to do so, say NO to sex with that person.

   Many experts believe that greater protection can be obtained by placing a small amount of the spermicide *nonoxynol-9* inside the condom at its tip and then lubricating the

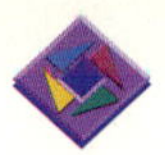

outside with additional spermicide. Nonoxynol-9 is used to kill the man's sperm for birth-control purposes. In test tubes it has been shown to kill STDs germs and HIV. This spermicide, however, should not be used in place of a condom because it will not offer the same protection as the condom does by itself.

3. Avoid having multiple partners and anonymous partners. Keep in mind that anyone you have sex with could be infected with HIV.
4. Don't have sexual contact with anyone who does not practice safer sex.
5. Avoid sexual contact with anyone who has had sex with people at risk for getting HIV, even if they now are practicing safer sex.
6. Don't have sex with prostitutes.
7. If you do have sex with someone who might be infected with HIV or whose history is unknown to you, avoid exchange of body fluids.
8. Don't share toothbrushes, razors, or other implements that could become contaminated with blood, with anyone who is, or who might be, infected with HIV.
9. Be cautious regarding procedures such as acupuncture, tattooing, and ear piercing, in which needles or other nonsterile instruments may be used again and again to pierce the skin or mucous membranes. These procedures are safe if proper sterilization methods or disposable needles are used. Before undergoing the procedure, ask what precautions are being taken.
10. If you are planning to undergo artificial insemination, insist on frozen sperm obtained from a laboratory that tests all donors for infection with HIV. Donors should be tested twice before the sperm is accepted, once at the time of donation and again a few months later.
11. If you know you will be having surgery in the near future, and if you are able, consider donating blood for your own use. This will eliminate completely the already small risk of contracting HIV through a blood transfusion. It also will eliminate the more substantial risk of contracting other blood-borne diseases, such as hepatitis, from a transfusion.

Avoidance of risky behaviors that destroy quality of life and life itself are critical components of a healthy lifestyle. Learning the facts so you can make responsible choices can protect you and those around you from startling and unexpected conditions. Moderately using alcohol (or not at all), refraining from substance abuse, and preventing sexually transmitted diseases are keys to averting both physical and psychological damage.

## NOTES

1. E. M. Johnson, *What You Can Do to Avoid AIDS*. New York: Random House, 1992.

## SELECT BIBLIOGRAPHY

"Addiction." *Aerobics News*. Dallas: Institute for Aerobics Research, July 1987.

American Medical Association. *Family Medical Guide*. New York: Random House, 1982.

Bennett, E. G., and D. Woolf (Editors). *Substance Abuse*. Albany, NY: Delmar Publishers, 1991.

Carroll, C. R. *Drugs in Modern Society*. Dubuque, IA: Wm. C. Brown Publishers, 1985.

Channing L. Bete Co. *About AIDS and Shooting Drugs*. South Deerfield, MA: Author, 1986.

Hafen, B. Q., A. L. Thygerson, and K. J. Frandsen. *Behavioral Guidelines for Health & Wellness*. Englewood, CO: Morton Publishing, 1988.

Schlaadt, R. G., and P. T. Shannon. *Drugs*. Englewood Cliffs, NJ: Prentice Hall, 1990.

# Healthy Lifestyle Issues and Wellness Guidelines for the Future

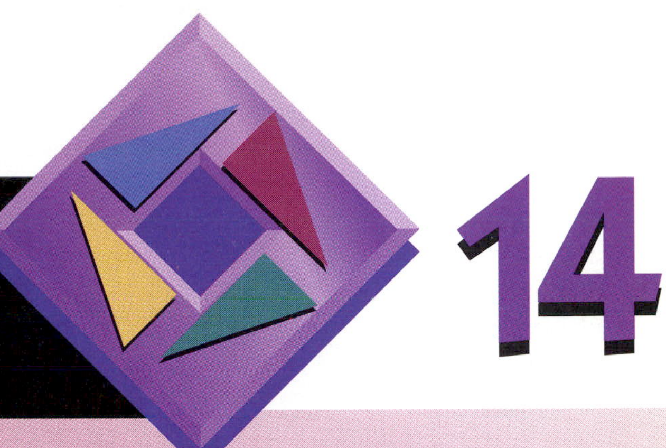


## Key Concepts

Spirituality
Altruism
Aging
Functional capacity
Prevention Index
Consumer fraud
Behavioral objectives
Quality of life

## Objectives

- Define spiritual well-being and its relationship to a healthy lifestyle.
- Describe the relationship between fitness and aging.
- Learn guidelines for preventing consumer fraud.
- Understand factors to consider when selecting a health/fitness club.
- Become acquainted with the Prevention Index, a measure of the effort the American people are making to prevent disease and improve total well-being.
- Review health/fitness accomplishments and chart a wellness program for the future.

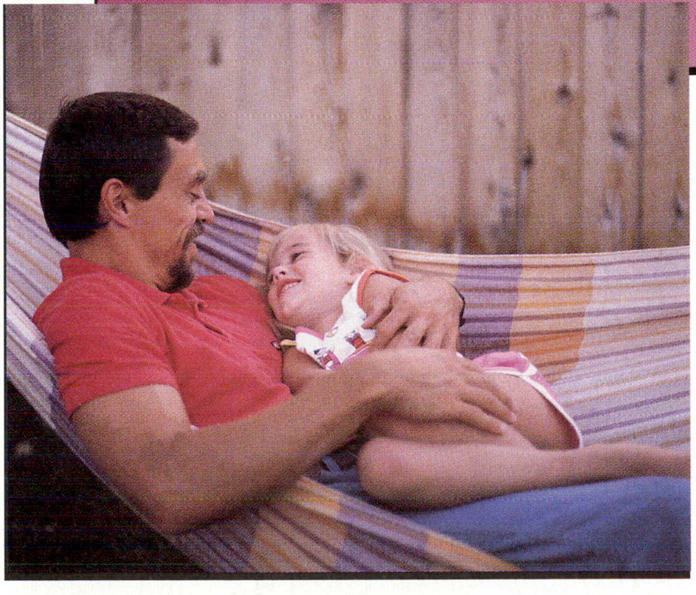

Throughout this book you have had an opportunity to assess various components of fitness and wellness. Better health, higher quality of life, and longevity are the three most vital benefits derived from a lifetime physical fitness program. Physical fitness in itself does not always lower the risk for chronic diseases and ensure better health, but the importance of a healthy lifestyle is one means to attain the highest potential for total well-being.

In addition to the wellness issues already discussed, three factors that are a part of daily living and may influence your well-being directly are: (a) spirituality, (b) exercise and aging, and (c) health-promoting behaviors. These components of wellness are the focus of this chapter.

Guidelines for preventing consumer fraud and selecting a health/fitness club also are presented in this last chapter. Further, you will have the opportunity to determine how well you are achieving your wellness objectives. Finally, you will receive instructions to help you chart a personal wellness program for the future.

## SPIRITUAL WELL-BEING

The National Interfaith Coalition on Aging defines spiritual well-being as *an affirmation of life in a relationship with God, self, community, and environment that nurtures and celebrates wholeness* (see Figure 14.1). Because this definition encompasses Christians and non-Christians alike, it assumes that all people are spiritual in nature. Spiritual health provides a unifying power that integrates the other dimensions of wellness. Basic characteristics of spiritual people include a sense of meaning and direction in life, a relationship to a higher being, freedom, prayer, faith, love, closeness to others, peace, joy, fulfillment, and altruism (service to others).

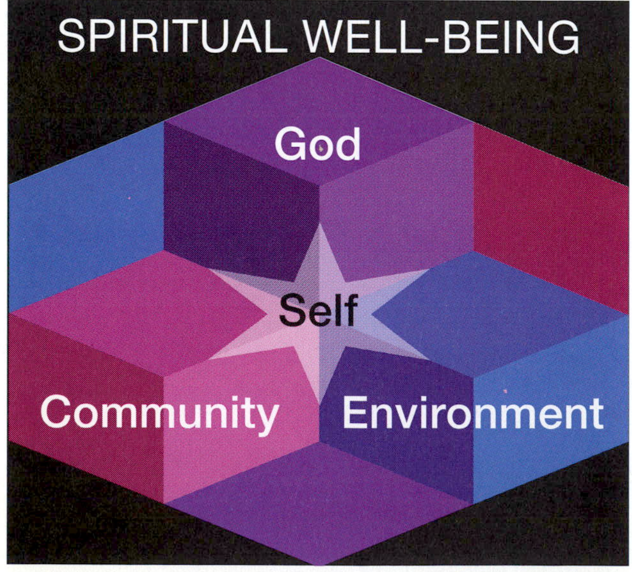


**FIGURE 14.1** ◆ Components of spiritual well-being.

Religion has been a major part of cultures since the beginning of time. Although not everyone in the United States claims affiliation with a certain religion or denomination, current surveys indicate that 94% of the U. S. population believes in God or a universal spirit functioning as God.

People, furthermore, believe to a varying extent that (a) a relationship with God is meaningful; (b) God can grant help, guidance, and assistance in daily living; and (c) mortal existence has a purpose. If we accept any or all of these statements, attaining spirituality will have a definite effect on our happiness and well-being.

### Spirituality and Health

The scientific association between spirituality and health is more difficult to establish than that of other lifestyle factors such as alcohol use, smoking, physical inactivity, seat belt use, and so on. Several research studies, nonetheless, have reported positive relationships among spiritual well-being, emotional well-being, and life's satisfaction. Further, people who attend church and participate in religious organizations regularly enjoy better health, have a lower incidence of chronic diseases, handle stress more effectively, and seem to live longer.

Although the reasons why religious affiliation enhances wellness are difficult to determine, possible reasons include the promotion of healthy lifestyle behaviors, social support, assistance in times of crisis and need, and counseling to overcome one's weaknesses.

Researchers have found that most successful men and women have strong spiritual values. Furthermore, almost all of these people experienced a crisis early in life. Spiritual beliefs seemed to help them overcome the crisis and aided in developing better coping techniques to deal with future trauma.

*Altruism*, a key attribute of spiritual people, seems to enhance health and longevity. Altruism is defined as *true concern for the welfare of others* (opposite of egoism) or a sincere desire to serve

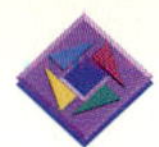

others above one's personal needs. Altruism has been the focus of several studies in recent years. Researchers believe that doing good for others is good for oneself, especially for the immune system. The health benefits of altruism could be so powerful, researchers at Harvard found, that even just watching films of altruistic endeavors enhances the formation of an immune system chemical that helps fight disease.[1]

In a study of more than 2,700 people in Michigan,[2] the investigators found that people who did regular volunteer work lived longer. People who did not perform regular volunteer work (at least once a week) had a 250% greater mortality risk during the course of the study.

Wellness requires a balance between physical, mental, spiritual, emotional, and social well-being. The relationship between spirituality and wellness, therefore, is meaningful in our quest for a better quality of life. As with other parameters of wellness, optimum spirituality requires development of the spiritual nature to its fullest potential.

## EXERCISE AND AGING

Unlike any prior time in American society, the elderly population constitutes the fastest growing segment. In 1880, less than 3% of the total population, or fewer than 2 million people, was older than 65. By 1980 the elderly population had reached approximately 25 million, more than 11.3% of the population. According to estimates, the elderly will make up more than 20% of the total population by the year 2035.

Historically, older adults have been neglected when developing fitness programs. Nevertheless, fitness is just as important for older people as it is for young people. Although much research remains to be done in this area, studies indicate that older individuals who are physically fit also enjoy better health and a higher quality of life.

The main objective of fitness programs for older adults should be to help them improve their functional health status. This implies the ability to maintain independent living status and avoiding disability. A committee of the American Alliance of Health, Physical Education, Recreation and Dance (AAHPERD) recently defined functional fitness for older adults as *the physical capacity of the individual to meet ordinary and unexpected demands of daily life safely and effectively*.[3] This definition clearly indicates the need for fitness programs that closely relate to activities this population normally encounters. The AAHPERD committee encourages participation in programs that will help develop cardiovascular endurance, localized muscular endurance, muscular flexibility, agility and balance, and motor coordination. A copy of the battery of fitness tests for older adults can be obtained from AAHPERD, Reston, Virginia.

### Relationship Between Fitness and Aging

Although previous research studies have documented declines in physiological functioning and motor capacity as a result of aging, no hard evidence at present proves that declines in physical work capacity are related primarily to the aging process. Lack of physical activity — a common phenomenon seen in our society as people age — may be accompanied by decreases in physical work capacity that are greater by far than the effects of aging itself.

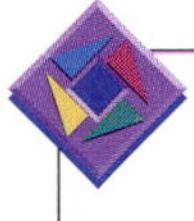

*Sedentary people often stop living at age 60 but choose to be buried at age 70!*

Data on individuals who have taken part in systematic physical activity throughout life indicate that these groups of people maintain a higher level of functional capacity and do not experience the typical declines in later years. From a functional point of view, the typical sedentary American is about 25 years older than his or her chronological age indicates. Thus, an active 60-year-old person can have a work capacity similar to that of a sedentary 35-year-old.

Unfortunately, unhealthy behaviors precipitate premature aging. For sedentary people, productive life ends at about age 60. Most of these people hope to live to be 65 or 70 and often must cope with serious physical ailments. These people stop living at age 60 but choose to be buried at age 70 (see Figure 14.2).

Scientists believe a healthy lifestyle allows people to live a vibrant life — a physically, intellectually, emotionally, socially active and functionally independent existence — to age 95. When death comes to active people, it usually is rather quick and not as a result of prolonged illness (see Figure

14.2). Such are the rewards of a wellness way of life.

## Physical Training in the Older Adult

The trainability of elderly men and women alike and the effectiveness of physical activity for health enhancement have been demonstrated in prior research. Older adults who increase their level of physical activity experience significant changes in cardiovascular endurance, strength, and flexibility. The extent of the changes depends on their initial fitness level and the types of activities selected for their training (walking, cycling, strength training, and so on).

Improvements in maximal oxygen uptake in older adults are similar to those of younger people, although older people seem to require a longer training period to achieve these changes. Declines in endurance (maximal oxygen uptake) per decade of life after age 25 seem to be about 9% for sedentary adults and 5% or less in active people.

Results of a recent study on the effects of aging on the cardiovascular system of male exercisers versus nonexercisers showed that the maximal oxygen uptake of regular exercisers was almost twice that of the nonexercisers (see Table 14.1).[4] Between ages 50 and 68 the study revealed a decline in maximal oxygen uptake of only 13% in the active group, compared to 41% in the inactive group. These changes indicate that about one-third of the loss in maximal oxygen uptake results from aging and two-thirds of the loss comes from inactivity. Blood pressure, heart rate, and body weight also were remarkably better in the exercising group.

**TABLE 14.1**
**Effects of Physical Activity and Inactivity on Older Men**

| | Exercisers | Non-exercisers |
|---|---|---|
| Age (yrs) | 68.0 | 69.8 |
| Weight (lbs) | 160.3 | 186.3 |
| Resting heart rate (bpm) | 55.8 | 66.0 |
| Maximal heart rate (bpm) | 157.0 | 146.0 |
| Heart rate reserve** (bpm) | 101.2 | 80.0 |
| Blood pressure (mmHg) | 120/78 | 150/90 |
| Maximal oxygen uptake (ml/kg/min) | 38.6 | 20.3 |

From "The Effect of Physical Activity on Aerobic Power in Older Men (A Longitudinal Study)," by F. W. Kash, J. L. Boyer, S. P. Van Camp, L. S. Verity, and J. P. Wallace, *Physician and Sports Medicine* 18:4 (1990), 73–83.

*Heart rate reserve = maximal heart rate − resting heart rate.

In strength development older adults can increase their strength levels, but the amount of muscle hypertrophy achieved decreases with age. Strength gains close to 200% have been found in previously inactive adults over age 90. In terms of body composition, inactive adults continue to gain body fat after age 60 despite the tendency toward lower body weight.

Older adults who wish to initiate or continue an exercise program are encouraged strongly to have a complete medical exam, including a stress electrocardiogram test (see Chapter 9). Recommended activities for older adults include calisthenics, walking, jogging, swimming, cycling, and water aerobics.

Isometric and other intense weight-training exercises should be avoided. Activities that require all-out effort or require participants to hold their breath (valsalva maneuver) tend to lessen blood flow to the heart and cause a significant increase in blood pressure and the load placed on the heart. Older adults should participate in activities that require continuous and rhythmic muscular activity (about 50% to 70% of functional capacity). These

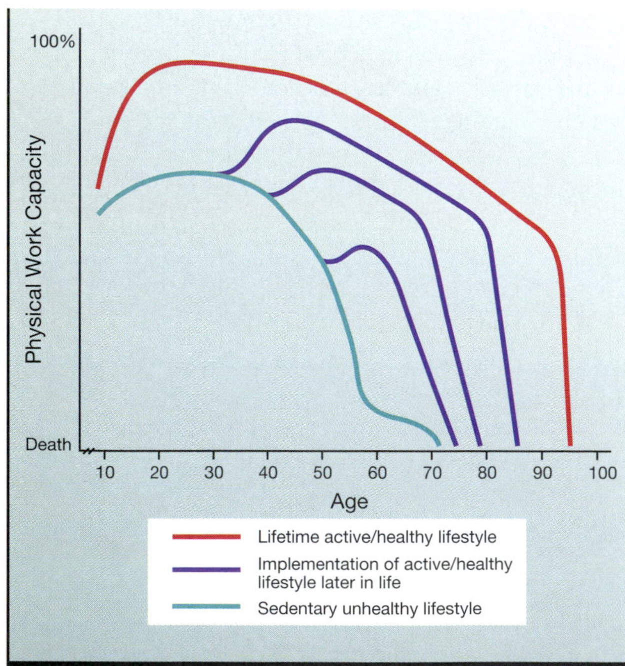


**FIGURE 14.2** ◆ Relationships between physical work capacity, aging, and lifestyle habits.

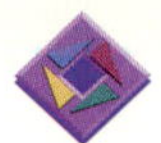

activities do not cause large increases in blood pressure or place an intense overload on the heart.

## THE PREVENTION INDEX

The Prevention Index is an annual measure of the effort adults in the U.S. are making to prevent disease and accidents and to promote good health and longevity. This nationwide index of the American public, commissioned by *Prevention Magazine*, has been developed from information collected by Louis Harris and Associates in two national surveys:

1. Self-reported practice of preventive health and safety behaviors based on a national probability sample of 1,250 adults in the continental United States 18 years of age and older.
2. Ratings on the relative importance of each of these behaviors for preventing disease and disability in the general population (on a scale of 1 to 10), as determined by a sample of 103 representative experts in disease prevention and health promotion.

In the Harris national probability survey of adults, 21 of the behaviors were selected for inclusion in the Prevention Index according to the following criteria:

1. A documented relationship between the health behavior and disease or disability, as published in the professional literature.
2. Behaviors that are relevant to the entire adult population.
3. Behaviors that individuals can control or affect (thus the exclusion of important environmental determinants of health such as exposure to air pollution or industrial toxins).

Currently accepted standards of practice for each behavior were determined by thorough review of the professional literature and consultation with experts. In the case of continuous variables (for example, moderate alcohol consumption, exercise, frequency of dental examination), practice was ascertained by the prevailing consensus in the relevant professional literature and from personal consultation with researchers and spokespersons of professional organizations. For behaviors with no clear consensus on a minimum compliance level (for example, taking steps to control stress or restricting cholesterol intake), practice was defined in terms of always engaging in the behavior (taking steps to control stress) or trying a lot (restricting cholesterol intake). The 1994 percentages of the adult population practicing these 21 major health-promoting behaviors are given in Table 14.2.[5]

A detailed description of the development and computation of the Prevention Index and related analyses is presented in the technical report, "The Prevention Index: A Report Card on the Nation's Health," available from *Prevention Magazine*.[5] You can score your own prevention profile by taking the test provided in Figure 14.3.

**TABLE 14.2**
**1994 Prevention Index Results**

| Health-Promoting Behavior | % of Adults Practicing |
|---|---|
| 1. Annual blood pressure test | 82 |
| 2. Annual dental exam | 73 |
| 3. Limit sodium in the diet | 50 |
| 4. Limit fat in the diet | 52 |
| 5. Consume adequate fiber | 61 |
| 6. Limit cholesterol in the diet | 47 |
| 7. Adequate vitamins/minerals | 61 |
| 8. Limit sugar in the diet | 42 |
| 9. Maintain proper weight | 19 |
| 10. Frequent strenuous exercise | 40 |
| 11. Do not smoke | 75 |
| 12. Control stress | 68 |
| 13. Sleep 7-8 hours per night | 65 |
| 14. Socialize regularly | 87 |
| 15. Drink alcohol moderately | 90 |
| 16. Wear seat belts | 73 |
| 17. Obey speed limit | 51 |
| 18. Avoid driving after drinking | 85 |
| 19. Smoke detector in home | 92 |
| 20. Avoid smoking in bed | 93 |
| 21. Avoid home accidents | 80 |
| Average | 66 |

Data from Consumers' Survey conducted for *Prevention Magazine* by Louis Harris & Associates. *Summary Report — The Prevention Index 1994: A Report Card on the Nation's Health* (Emmaus, PA: *Prevention Magazine*, 1994).

## THE PREVENTION INDEX

**Please carefully check "YES" or "NO" to each of the following questions.**

| Yes | No | | |
|---|---|---|---|
| ☐ | ☐ | 1 | Do you have a blood pressure reading at least once a year? |
| ☐ | ☐ | 2. | Do you go to the dentist at least once a year for treatment or a checkup? |
| ☐ | ☐ | 3. | Do you avoid eating too much salt or sodium? |
| ☐ | ☐ | 4. | Do you avoid eating too much fat? |
| ☐ | ☐ | 5. | Do you eat enough fiber from whole grains, cereals, fruits, and vegetables? |
| ☐ | ☐ | 6. | Do you avoid eating too many high cholesterol foods, such as eggs, dairy products, and fatty meats? |
| ☐ | ☐ | 7. | Do you get enough vitamins and minerals in your diet? |
| ☐ | ☐ | 8. | Do you avoid getting too much sugar and sweet food? |
| ☐ | ☐ | 9. | Is your body weight within the recommended range for your sex, height, and bone structure? |
| ☐ | ☐ | 10. | Do you exercise strenuously (that is, so you breathe heavily and your heart and pulse rate are accelerated for a period lasting at least 20 minutes) 3 days or more a week? |
| ☐ | ☐ | 11. | Do you smoke cigarettes now? |
| ☐ | ☐ | 12. | Do you consciously take steps to control or reduce stress in your life? |
| ☐ | ☐ | 13. | Do you usually sleep a total of 7 to 8 hours during each 24-hour day? (If you usually sleep either more or less than this, please mark "no.") |
| ☐ | ☐ | 14. | Do you socialize with close friends, relatives, or neighbors at least once a week? |
| ☐ | ☐ | 15. | In general, when you drink alcoholic beverages, do you consume fewer than 14 drinks per week and fewer than two on any single day? (Mark "yes" only if the answer to both parts of this question is "yes." If you never drink at all, also mark "yes." A "drink" means a drink with a shot of hard liquor, a can or bottle of beer, or a glass of wine.) |
| ☐ | ☐ | 16. | Do you wear a seat belt all the time when you are in the front seat of a car? |
| ☐ | ☐ | 17. | Do you drive at or below the speed limit all the time? (If you don't drive, please mark "yes.") |
| ☐ | ☐ | 18. | Do you ever drive after drinking? (If you don't drink, please mark "no.") |
| ☐ | ☐ | 19. | Do you have a smoke detector in your home? |
| ☐ | ☐ | 20. | Does anyone in your household smoke in bed? |
| ☐ | ☐ | 21. | Do you take any special steps or precautions to avoid accidents in and around your home? |

**Interpreting The Prevention Index (PI)**

The correct answer for questions 11, 18, and 20 is "no." The correct answer for all other questions is "yes." Add up your total number of correct responses. Then divide that number by 21 to obtain the percentage of the 21 Prevention Index behaviors that you practice.

$$PI = \frac{\text{Number of correct answers}}{21} = \frac{\_\_\_\_}{21} = \boxed{\quad}$$

**RATINGS**

| **Prevention Index** | **Category** |
|---|---|
| 90> | Excellent |
| 70-89 | Good |
| 60-69 | Average |
| <59 | Poor |

The Prevention Index: A Louis Harris & Associates, Inc. survey conducted for *Prevention Magazine*.

**FIGURE 14.3**

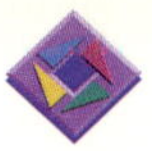

## AN EDUCATED WELLNESS CONSUMER

The rapid growth in fitness and wellness programs during the last two decades has spurred the promotion of fraudulent products that deceive consumers into "miraculous," quick, and easy ways toward total well-being. Quackery and fraud have been defined as the *conscious promotion of unproven claims for profit.*

Today's market is saturated with "special" foods, diets, supplements, pills, cures, equipment, books, and videos that promise quick, dramatic results. Advertisements for these products often are based on testimonials, unproven claims, secret research, half-truths, and quick-fix statements that the uneducated consumer wants to hear. In the meantime, the organization or enterprise making the claims stands to make a large profit from the consumers' willingness to pay for astonishing and spectacular solutions to problems related to their unhealthy lifestyle.

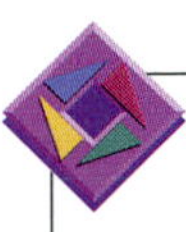

*Quick-fix, miraculous, special, secret, mail orders only, money-back guarantee, and testimonials often are used in advertisements of fraudulent promotions.*

Television, magazine, and newspaper advertisements are not necessarily reliable. For instance, one piece of equipment sold through television and newspaper advertisements promised to "bust the gut" through 5 minutes of daily exercise that appeared to target the abdominal muscle group. This piece of equipment consisted of a metal spring attached to the feet on one end and held in the hands on the other end. According to handling and shipping distributors, the equipment was "selling like hotcakes," and companies could barely keep up with the consumer's demands.

Three problems became apparent to the educated consumer. First, there is no such thing as spot-reducing; therefore, the claims could not be true. Second, 5 minutes of daily exercise burn hardly any calories and, therefore, have no effect on weight loss. Third, the intended abdominal (gut) muscles were not really involved during the exercise. The exercise engaged mostly the gluteal and lower back muscles. This piece of equipment now can be found at garage sales for about a tenth of its original cost!

Although people in the United States tend to be firm believers in the benefits of physical activity and positive lifestyle habits as a means to promote better health, most do not reap these benefits because they simply do not know how to put into practice a sound fitness and wellness program that will give them the results they want. Unfortunately, many uneducated wellness consumers are targets of deception by organizations making fraudulent claims for their products.

Even though deceit is all around us, we can protect ourselves from consumer fraud. The first step, of course, is education. You have to be an informed consumer of the product you intend to purchase. If you do not have or cannot find the answers, seek the advice of a reputable professional. Ask someone who understands the product but does not stand to profit from the transaction. As examples, a physical educator or an exercise physiologist can advise you regarding exercise equipment; a registered dietitian can provide information on nutrition and weight control programs; a physician can offer advice on nutritive supplements. Also, be alert to those who bill themselves as "experts." Look for qualifications degrees, professional experience, certifications, reputation.

Another clue to possible fraud is that if it sounds too good to be true, it probably is. Quick-fix, miraculous, special, secret, mail orders only, money-back guarantee, and testimonials often are heard in advertisements of fraudulent promotions. When claims are made, ask where the claims are published. Newspapers, magazines, and trade books are apt to be unreliable sources of information. Refereed scientific journals are the most reliable sources of information. When a researcher submits information for publication in a refereed journal, at least two qualified and reputable professionals in the field conduct blind reviews of the manuscript. A blind review means the author does not know who will review the manuscript and the reviewers do not know who submitted the manuscript. Acceptance for publication is based on this input and relevant changes.

If you have questions or concerns about a health product, you may write to the National Council Against Health Fraud (NCAHF), P. O. Box 1276, Loma Linda, CA 92354. The purpose of this organization is to monitor deceitful advertising, investigate complaints, and offer the public information regarding fraudulent health claims.

## HEALTH/FITNESS CLUB MEMBERSHIPS

As you follow a lifetime wellness program, you may want to consider joining a health/fitness facility. Or, if you have mastered the contents of this book and your choice of fitness activity is one you can pursue on your own (walking, jogging, cycling), you may not need to join a health club. Barring injuries, you may continue your exercise program outside the walls of a health club for the rest of your life. You also can conduct strength training and stretching programs within the walls of your own home (see Chapters 4 and 5).

To stay up to date on fitness and wellness developments, you probably should buy a reputable and updated fitness/wellness book every 4 to 5 years. You also might subscribe to a credible health, fitness, nutrition, or wellness newsletter (see Table 14.3) to stay current.

If you are contemplating membership in a fitness facility:

- Examine all exercise options in your community: health clubs/spas, YMCAs, gyms, colleges, schools, community centers, senior centers, and the like.
- Check to see if the facility's atmosphere is pleasurable and nonthreatening to you. Will you feel comfortable with the instructors and other people who go there? Is it clean and well kept up? If the answer is no, this may not be the right place for you.
- Analyze costs versus facilities, equipment, and programs. Take a look at your personal budget. Will you really use the facility? Will you exercise there regularly? Many people obtain memberships and permit dues to be withdrawn automatically from a local bank account, yet seldom attend the fitness center.
- Find out what types of facilities are available: running track, basketball/tennis/racquetball courts, aerobic exercise room, strength training room, pool, locker rooms, saunas, hot tubs, handicapped access, and so on.
- Check the aerobic and strength training equipment available. Does the facility have treadmills, bicycle ergometers, Stair Masters, cross-country skiing simulators, free weights, Universal Gym, Nautilus? Make sure the facilities and equipment meet your activity interests.
- Consider the location. Is the facility close, or do you have to travel several miles to get there? Distance often discourages participation.
- Check on times the facility is accessible. Is it open during your preferred exercise time (for example, early morning or late evening)?
- Work out at the facility several times before becoming a member. Are people standing in line to use the equipment, or is it readily available during your exercise time?
- Inquire about the instructors' qualifications. Do the fitness instructors have college degrees or professional certifications from organizations such as the American College of Sports Medicine (ACSM) or the International Dance Exercise Association (IDEA)? These organizations have rigorous standards to ensure professional preparation and quality of instruction.
- Consider the approach to fitness (including all health-related components of fitness). Is it well-rounded? Do the instructors spend time with members, or do members have to seek them out constantly for help and instruction?
- Ask about supplementary services. Does the facility provide or contract out for regular health and fitness assessments (cardiovascular

**TABLE 14.3**
**Reliable Sources of Health, Fitness, Wellness, and Nutrition Information**

| Newsletter | Yearly Issues | Approx. Annual Cost |
|---|---|---|
| *Consumer Reports Health Letter*<br>P.O. Box 56356<br>Boulder, CO 80323–2148 | 12 | $24 |
| *Executive Health's Good Health Report*<br>P.O. Box 8880<br>Chapel Hill, NC 27515 | 12 | $34 |
| *Tufts University Diet & Nutrition Letter*<br>P.O. Box 57857<br>Boulder, CO 80322–7857 | 12 | $20 |
| University of California<br>Berkeley *Wellness Letter*<br>P.O. Box 420148<br>Palm Coast, FL 32142 | 12 | $20 |

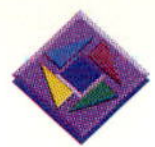

endurance, body composition, blood pressure, blood chemistry analysis)? Are wellness seminars (nutrition, weight control, stress management) offered? Do these have hidden costs?

A final consideration is that of purchasing your own exercise equipment. Many people buy expensive equipment only to find out they really do not enjoy that mode of activity. Stationary bicycles (lower body only) and rowing ergometers were among the most popular pieces of equipment sold in the 1980s. Many of them are seldom used and now are stored away in basements. Actually try out the piece of equipment several times before you buy it.

Quality also is important. Some cheaper brands of equipment may not be durable, so your investment would be wasted. Ask for references — people or clubs that have used the equipment extensively. Are they satisfied? Have they enjoyed the activity (the equipment)? You also may want to talk with professionals at colleges, sports medicine clinics, or health clubs.

## SELF-EVALUATION AND BEHAVIORAL OBJECTIVES FOR THE FUTURE

The main objective of this book is to provide the information and experiences necessary to implement your personal fitness and wellness program. If you have implemented the programs in this book, including exercise, you should be convinced that a wellness lifestyle is the only way to attain a higher quality of life.

Most people who engage in a personal fitness and wellness program experience this new quality of life after only a few weeks of training and practicing healthy lifestyle patterns. In some cases, however, especially individuals who have led a poor lifestyle for a long time, a few months may be required to establish positive habits and feelings of well-being. In the end, though, everyone who applies the principles of fitness and wellness will reap the desired benefits.

### Self-Evaluation

Throughout this course you may have had an opportunity to assess various fitness and wellness components and write behavioral objectives to improve your quality of life. You now should take the time to evaluate how well you have achieved your own objectives. Ideally, if time allows and facilities and technicians are available, you should reassess the health-related components of physical fitness. If you are unable to reassess these components, determine subjectively how well you accomplished your objectives. You will find a self-evaluation form in Figure A.1 of Appendix A.

### Behavioral Objectives for the Future

The real challenge will come now that you are about to finish this course: a lifetime commitment to fitness and wellness. Adhering to a program in a structured setting is a lot easier, but from now on you will be on your own. Realizing that you may not have achieved all of your objectives during this course, or perhaps you need to reach beyond your current achievements, a final assignment will help you chart the future. You can do this by referring to the Wellness Scale provided in Figure 14.4. This guide provides a list of various wellness components, each illustrating a scale from poor to excellent. Using the Wellness Scale, rate yourself for each component according to the following instructions:

1. Indicate with an "I" (I = Initial) the category from poor to excellent where you stood on each component at the beginning of the semester. For example, if at the start of this course, you rated poor in cardiovascular endurance, place an "I" under the poor column for this component.
2. Mark with a "C" (C = Current) a second column (between poor and excellent) to indicate where you stand on each component at the current time. If your level of cardiovascular endurance improved to average by the end of the semester, write a "C" under this column. If you were not able to work on a given component, simply make a "C" out of the "I."
3. Select one or two components you intend to work on in the next 2 months. Developing new behavioral patterns takes time, and trying to work on too many components at once most likely will lower your chances for success. Start with components in which you think you will have a high chance for success.

Name: ______________________ Course: __________ Section: __________ Date: __________

| Wellness Components | Wellness Rating | | | | |
|---|---|---|---|---|---|
| | Poor | Fair | Average | Good | Excellent |
| Cardiovascular Endurance | | | | | |
| Muscular Strength/Endurance | | | | | |
| Muscular Flexibility | | | | | |
| Body Composition | | | | | |
| Nutrition | | | | | |
| Cardiovascular Disease Prevention | | | | | |
| Cancer Prevention | | | | | |
| Stress Control | | | | | |
| Tobacco Use | | | | | |
| Substance Abuse Control* | | | | | |
| Sexuality* | | | | | |
| Accident Prevention and Personal Safety | | | | | |
| Spirituality* | | | | | |
| Health Education | | | | | |

*These components are personal, and you are not required to reveal this information. If you think that counseling is necessary, you are encouraged to seek professional help.

**FIGURE 14.4** ◆ The Wellness Scale.

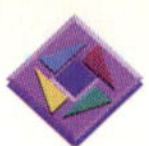

Next, place an "F" (F = Future) under the Intended Objectives column to accomplish by the end of this period. If your objective in the next 2 months is to achieve a "good" level of cardiovascular endurance, place an "F" under the good column for this objective in the Wellness Scale. When you achieve this level, make an "A" (A = Achieved) out of the "F" and mark your next objective (excellent column) with an "F."

After you have completed the previous exercise, use Figure 14.5 to write behavioral objectives for the two components you intend to work on during the next 2 months. As you write and work on these objectives, keep in mind the following guidelines:

1. **Set both general and specific objectives.** The general objective is the ultimate goal you intend to achieve. The specific objectives are the steps required to reach this general objective. For example, a general objective might be to achieve recommended body weight. Several specific objectives could be to: (a) lose an average of one pound (or one fat percentage point) per week, (b) monitor body weight before breakfast every morning, (c) assess body composition every two weeks, (d) limit fat intake to less than 30% of total calories, (e) eliminate all pastries from the diet during this time, and (f) exercise in the proper target zone for 40 minutes, five times per week.
2. **Whenever possible, set objectives (general and specific) that are measurable.** For example, "to lose weight" is not measurable. In the previous general objective, recommended body weight implies lowering your body weight (fat) to the recommended percent body fat standards

Select two components from the Wellness Scale and write general objectives to achieve in 2 months. Next, write the specific objectives that will lead to the accomplishment of the general objectives.

General Objective: ______________________

Specific Objectives: ______________________

1. ______________________
2. ______________________
3. ______________________
4. ______________________
5. ______________________
6. ______________________
7. ______________________
8. ______________________

General Objective: ______________________

Specific Objectives: ______________________

1. ______________________
2. ______________________
3. ______________________
4. ______________________
5. ______________________
6. ______________________
7. ______________________
8. ______________________

**FIGURE 14.5** ◆ Behavioral objectives for the future.

given in Chapter 6. If this person is a 19-year-old female, the high fitness recommended fat percent would be in the range of 17% to 27%.

To be more descriptive, the general objective could be reworded as: Reduce body weight to 22% body fat. The sample specific objectives given in Item 1 also are measurable. For instance, you can figure out easily whether you are losing a pound (a percentage point) per week. You could conduct a nutrient analysis to assess the average fat intake, or you can monitor your weekly exercise sessions to make sure you are meeting this specific objective.

3. **Make objectives realistic.** If you currently weigh 170 pounds and your target weight at 22% is 120 pounds, implementing a weight loss program to lose 50 pounds in 2 months would be unsound if not impossible. This program would not allow implementation of adequate behavior modification techniques and ensure weight maintenance at the target weight.

4. **Write either short-term or long-term objectives.** If the general objective is to attain recommended body weight and you are 50 pounds overweight, setting a general short-term objective of losing 10 pounds and writing specific objectives to accomplish this goal is best. Then the task will not seem as overwhelming and will be easier to do.

5. **Set a specific date to achieve your objective.** To simply state "I will lose weight" is not time-specific. It is much easier to work toward a deadline.

6. **Educate yourself about the objective you plan to work on.** You cannot lose weight if you do not know the principles governing weight loss and maintenance. This is the reason only three in 10 individuals achieve the target weight loss and only one in those three is able to keep it off thereafter.

7. **Think positive, and reward yourself for your accomplishments.** As difficult as some tasks may seem, where there's a will, there's a way. If you prepare a plan of action according to these guidelines, you should be able to achieve your objective. Reward yourself for your accomplishments. Buy yourself new clothing, exercise shoes, or something special you have wanted for some time.

8. **Seek support from those around you.** Losing weight is difficult if you share meal planning and cooking with a roommate who enjoys foods that are high in fat and sweets. It can be even worse if the roommate also has a weight problem and does not desire or have the willpower to lose weight. Surround yourself with people who will help and encourage you along the way. If necessary, plan and prepare your own meals.

9. **Recognize that you will face obstacles and make mistakes.** Making mistakes is human and does not mean failure. Failure comes only to those who give up. Use your mistakes and learn from them by creating a plan that will help you get around self-defeating behaviors in the future.

10. **Monitor your progress regularly.** You will not always be meeting the specific objectives. If you are not, you will need to evaluate your objectives and perhaps make changes in the general or the specific objectives, or both. People are different, and you may not be able to progress as fast as someone else. Be flexible with yourself, and reconsider your plan of action.

## THE FITNESS/WELLNESS EXPERIENCE AND A CHALLENGE FOR THE FUTURE

The process of change is never easy. Lifestyle behaviors are developed over many years. For most, to improve functional capacity and quality of life requires change in behaviors, which takes time and an ongoing, conscious effort to do so.

For instance, for someone who has not been on a regular aerobic program, the process of starting and adhering to exercise requires knowledge (exercise prescription guidelines), commitment, support, action, and perseverance. Although health and self-esteem benefits can be reaped immediately upon the start of exercise, considerable improvements in fitness may take months or longer.

Prior to her marriage a young lady who never had been on a jogging program became convinced that aerobic exercise would improve her fitness and help her maintain recommended body weight. Her fiancé believed in fitness and had been jogging

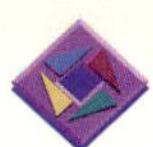

regularly for several years. An exercise prescription was written, and they started jogging together.

Exercise helped accomplish her goals through her first two pregnancies. The feeling of being physically fit was a reward in itself, but being able to jog 2 consecutive miles was seldom truly enjoyable. With young children at home, the couple was forced to take turns jogging so that one always could be home. Her jogging program consisted of a 20-minute jog: 1 mile out and 1 mile back.

One day 25 minutes went by and she had not returned home. At 30 minutes, there was a knock on the door: "Honey, I feel great, I'll be back in 10 minutes." This same event was repeated at 40 and 50 minutes. That young lady had jogged for a full 60 minutes for the first time in her life, and the experience was genuinely joyful. That day, this lady finally reached "the top of the mountain" and experienced the joy of being physically fit. She has not stopped jogging in more than 18 years! It wasn't easy at first, but knowledge, commitment, support, action, and perseverance paid off.

Fitness also was the factor that led to improvements in other wellness components in the lives of this couple (continuing health education, proper nutrition, stress reduction, and chronic disease prevention). Fitness is the daily "bread and butter" that enhances their quality of life. Their children now also follow the parents' active lifestyle. This has prompted the parents to say: "The family that exercises together stays together."

Perhaps the new quality of life that fitness provided was explained best by the late Dr. George Sheehan, cardiologist, avid runner, and health and fitness promoter, when he wrote:

> *For every runner who tours the world running marathons, there are thousands who run to hear the leaves and listen to the rain, and look to the day when it is all suddenly as easy as a bird in flight. For them, sport is not a test but a therapy, not a trial but a reward, not a question but an answer.*[6]

If you have read and successfully completed all of the assignments set out in this book, including a regular exercise program, you should be convinced of the value of exercise and healthy lifestyle habits in helping achieve a new quality of life.

The real challenge will come now: a lifetime commitment to fitness and wellness. To make the commitment easier, enjoy yourself and have fun along the way. Implement your program based on

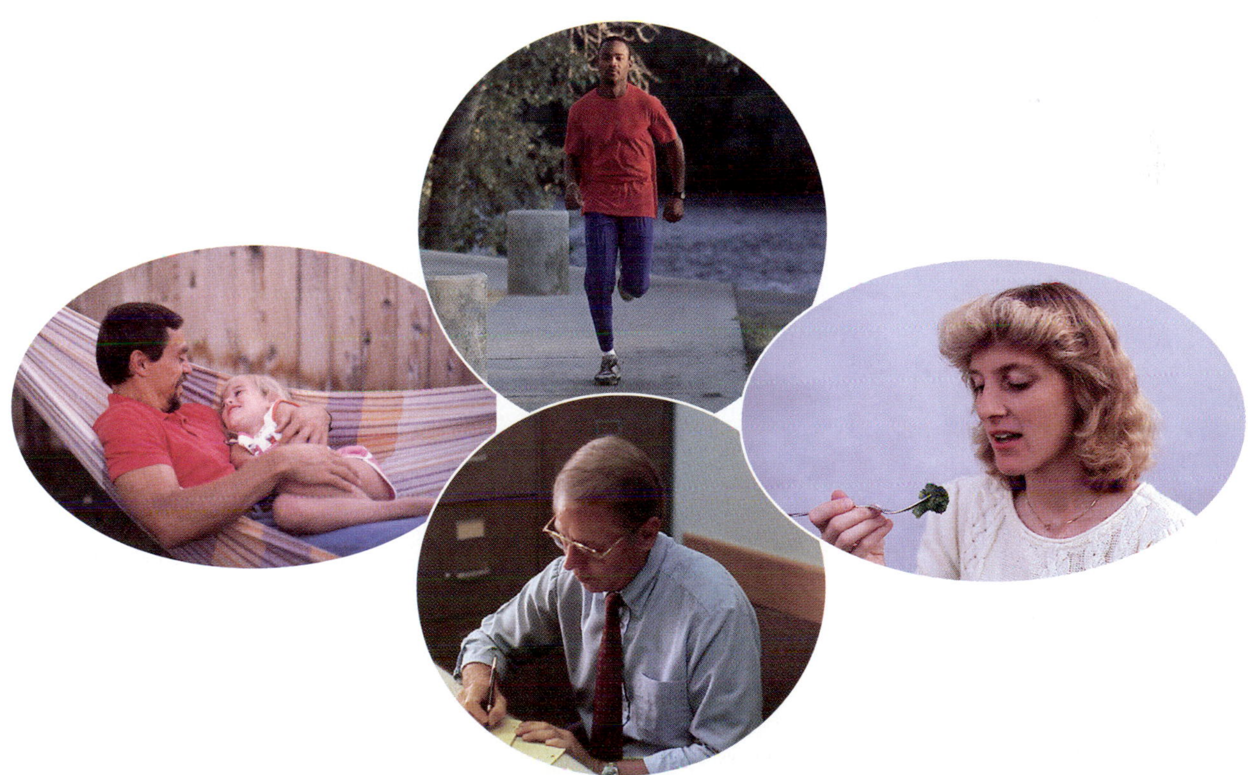

*Fitness and healthy lifestyle habits lead to improved health, quality of life, and wellness.*

your interests and what you enjoy doing most. Then, adhering to your new lifestyle will not be difficult.

Your activities over the last few weeks or months may have helped you develop positive "addictions" that will carry on throughout life. If you truly experience the feelings Dr. Sheehan expressed, there will be no looking back. If you don't get there, you won't know what it's like. Fitness and wellness is a process, and you need to put forth a constant and deliberate effort to achieve and maintain a higher quality of life. Improving the quality of your life, and most likely your longevity, is in your hands. Only you can take control of your lifestyle and thereby reap the benefits of wellness.

## NOTES

1. E. R. Growald and A. Lusks. "Beyond Self," *American Health*, March 1988, pp. 51-53.
2. Growald and Lusks.
3. W. Osness, M. Adrian, B. Clark, W. W. K. Hoeger, D. Raab, and R. Wiswell. "The AAHPERD Fitness Task Force, History and Philosophy," *Journal of Physical Education, Recreation and Dance* 60:3 (1989), 64-65.
4. F. W. Kash, J. L. Boyer, S. P. Van Camp, L. S. Verity, and J. P. Wallace. "The Effect of Physical Activity on Aerobic Power in Older Men (A Longitudinal Study)," *The Physician and Sports Medicine,* 18:4 (1990), 73–83.
5. Prevention Magazine. *The Prevention Index 1994: A Report Card on the Nation's Health* (Emmaus, PA: Prevention Magazine, 1994).
6. Human Relations Media, "What is Fitness?" *Dynamics of Fitness: The Body in Action* (Pleasantville, NY: Author, 1980).

## SELECT BIBLIOGRAPHY

Clark, B., W. Osness, W. W. K. Hoeger, M. Adrian, D. Raab, and R. Wiswell. "Tests for Fitness in Older Adults: AAHPERD Fitness Task Force." *Journal of Physical Education, Recreation, and Dance* 60:3 (1989), 66-71. A copy of the battery of tests can be obtained from AAHPERD.

Food and Drug Administration (FDA). "Foods, Drugs or Frauds." *FDA Consumer*, May 1985.

Hafen, B. Q., and W. W. K. Hoeger. *Wellness: Guidelines for a healthy Lifestyle*. Englewood, CO: Morton Publishing, 1994.

Hagberg, J. M., J. E. Graves, and M. Limacher et al. "Cardiovascular Responses of 70–79 Year Old Men and Women to Exercise Training." *Journal of Applied Physiology*, 66 (1989), 2589-2594.

Health Quackery. *Consumer Reports Books*. Mount Vernon, NY: Consumer's Union, 1980.

Hoeger, W. W. K., and S. A. Hoeger. *Principles and Labs for Physical Fitness and Wellness*. Englewood, CO: Morton Publishing, 1994.

Levy, M., and J. Shafran. *Gym Psych: The Insider's Guide to Health Clubs*. New York: Fawcett Columbine, 1986.

APPENDIX A

# Physical Fitness and Wellness Profile

Fill out the following profile as you obtain the results for each fitness and wellness component. Attempt to determine the fitness components (cardiovascular endurance, muscular strength/endurance, muscular flexibility, and body composition) during the first two or three weeks so you may proceed with your exercise program. After determining each component, discuss with your instructor the objectives to be accomplished and the date of completion.

**Name:** ______________________ **Course:** ____________ **Section:** ____________ **Date:** ____________

| **Item** | **Pre-Assessment** | | | **Objective** | **Post-Assessment** | | |
|---|---|---|---|---|---|---|---|
| | **Date** | **Test Results** | **Classification** | | **Date** | **Test Results** | **Classification** |
| Cardiovascular Endurance | | | | | | | |
| Muscular Strength | | | | | | | |
| Muscular Flexibility | | | | | | | |
| Body Composition | | | | | | | |
| Cardiovascular Risk | | | | | | | |
| Cancer Risk<br>Lung | | | | | | | |
| Colon-Rectum | | | | | | | |
| Skin | | | | | | | |
| Breast[b] | | | | | | | |
| Cervical[b] | | | | | | | |
| Endometrial[b] | | | | | | | |
| Prostate[c] | | | | | | | |
| Testicular[c] | | | | | | | |
| Pancreatic | | | | | | | |
| Kidney & Bladder | | | | | | | |
| Esophageal & Stomach | | | | | | | |
| Ovarian[b] | | | | | | | |
| Thyroid | | | | | | | |
| Leukemia | | | | | | | |
| Lymphomas | | | | | | | |
| Stress | | | | | | | |
| Life Exp. Survey | | | | | | | |
| Vulnerability Scale | | | | | | | |
| Tobacco Use[d] | | | | | | | |

Instructor's Signature: ______________________ Student's Signature: ______________________

[a] Indicate specific objective and date of completion.
[b] Women only
[c] Men only
[d] For test results indicate type and amount smoked; for classification indicate smoker, ex-smoker, nonsmoker.

**FIGURE A.1** ◆ Personal Fitness and Wellness Profile.

APPENDIX

# B

# Nutritive Value of Selected Foods

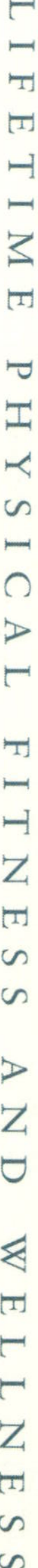

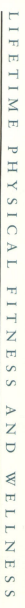

| Code | Food | Amount | Weight gm | Calo-ries | Pro-tein gm | Fat gm | Sat. Fat gm | Cho-les-terol mg | Car-bohy-drate gm | Cal-cium mg | Iron mg | Sodium mg | Vit A I.U. | Thia-min (Vit $B_1$) mg | Ribo-flavin (Vit $B_2$) mg | Niacin mg | Vit C mg |
|---|---|---|---|---|---|---|---|---|---|---|---|---|---|---|---|---|---|
| 1. | Almond Joy, candy bar | 1.5 oz. | 42 | 227 | 2.5 | 12 | 10.2 | 0 | 28 | 3 | 1.2 | 0 | 0 | 0.00 | 0.00 | 0.0 | 0 |
| 2. | Almonds, shelled | 1/4 c | 36 | 213 | 6.6 | 19 | 1.4 | 0 | 9 | 83 | 1.7 | 2 | 0 | 0.09 | 0.33 | 1.3 | 0 |
| 3. | Apple, raw, unpared | 1 med | 150 | 80 | 0.3 | 1 | 0.0 | 0 | 20 | 10 | 0.4 | 1 | 120 | 0.04 | 0.03 | 0.1 | 6 |
| 4. | Apple juice, canned or bottled | 1/2 c | 124 | 59 | 0.1 | 0 | 0.0 | 0 | 15 | 8 | 0.7 | 1 | 0 | 0.01 | 0.03 | 0.1 | 1 |
| 5. | Apple Pie, McDonald's | 1 | 307 | 260 | 2 | 15 | 10.0 | 6 | 30 | 0 | 0.48 | 240 | 0 | 0.06 | 0 | 0 | 12 |
| 6. | Applesauce, canned, sweetened | 1/2 c | 128 | 116 | 0.3 | 0 | 0.0 | 0 | 31 | 5 | 0.7 | 3 | 50 | 0.02 | 0.01 | 0.0 | 2 |
| 7. | Apricots, canned, heavy syrup | 3 halves; 1¾ tbsp liq. | 85 | 73 | 0.5 | 0 | 0.0 | 0 | 19 | 9 | 0.3 | 1 | 1,480 | 0.02 | 0.02 | 0.3 | 3 |
| 8. | Apricots, dried, sulfured, uncooked | 10 med halves | 35 | 91 | 1.8 | 0 | 0.0 | 0 | 23 | 23 | 1.9 | 9 | 3,820 | 0.00 | 0.06 | 1.2 | 4 |
| 9. | Apricots, raw | 3 (12 per lb) | 114 | 55 | 1.1 | 0 | 0.0 | 0 | 14 | 18 | 0.5 | 1 | 2,890 | 0.06 | 0.04 | 0.6 | 11 |
| 10. | Arby Q, Arby's | 1 | 190 | 389 | 18 | 15 | 5.5 | 29 | 48 | 84 | 6.1 | 1,268 | 0 | 0.27 | 0.41 | 9.2 | 0 |
| 11. | Arby Sauce, Arby's | .5 oz. | 14 | 15 | 0 | 0 | 0.0 | 0 | 3 | 0 | 0.2 | 113 | 0 | 0.00 | 0.00 | 0.0 | 0 |
| 12. | Asparagus, cooked green spears | 4 med | 60 | 12 | 1.3 | 0 | 0.0 | 0 | 2 | 13 | 0.4 | 1 | 540 | 0.10 | 0.11 | 0.8 | 16 |
| 13. | Avocado, raw | 1/2 med | 120 | 185 | 2.4 | 19 | 3.2 | 0 | 7 | 11 | 0.6 | 4 | 310 | 0.12 | 0.22 | 1.7 | 15 |
| 14. | Bacon, cooked, drained | 2 slices | 15 | 86 | 3.8 | 8 | 2.7 | 30 | 1 | 2 | 0.5 | 153 | 0 | 0.08 | 0.05 | 0.8 | 0 |
| 15. | Bacon, lettuce, tomato sandwich | 1 | 130 | 327 | 11.6 | 19 | 4.7 | 21 | 31 | 84 | 2.5 | 661 | 426 | 0.42 | 0.28 | 4.1 | 12 |
| 16. | Bagel | 1 3½ in. | 68 | 180 | 7.0 | 1 | 0.2 | 0 | 35 | 20 | 2.1 | 124 | 0 | 0.26 | 0.20 | 2.4 | 0 |
| 17. | Banana, raw | 1 sm (7¼") | 140 | 81 | 1.0 | 0 | 0.0 | 0 | 21 | 8 | 0.7 | 1 | 180 | 0.05 | 0.06 | 0.7 | 10 |
| 18. | Banana, nut bread | 1 slice | 50 | 169 | 3.0 | 8 | 1.5 | 33 | 22 | 18 | 0.9 | 172 | 49 | 0.09 | 0.09 | 0.8 | 1 |
| 19. | BBQ Sauce, McDonald's | 1.12 oz. | 32 | 50 | 0 | 0.6 | 0.2 | 0 | 12 | 0.0 | 0.0 | 350 | 200 | 0.00 | 0.00 | 0 | 2.4 |
| 20. | Beans, green snap, cooked | 1/2 c | 65 | 16 | 1.0 | 0 | 0.0 | 0 | 3 | 32 | 0.4 | 4 | 340 | 0.05 | 0.06 | 0.3 | 8 |
| 21. | Beans, lentils | 1/4 c | 50 | 53 | 3.9 | 0 | 0.0 | 0 | 10 | 12 | 1.0 | 0 | 10 | 0.03 | 0.04 | 0.4 | 0 |
| 22. | Beans, lima (Fordhook), froz., cooked | 1/2 c | 85 | 84 | 6.0 | 0 | 0.0 | 0 | 17 | 40 | 2.1 | 1 | 240 | 0.15 | 0.08 | 1.1 | 15 |
| 23. | Beans, red kidney, cooked | 1 c | 185 | 218 | 14.4 | 1 | 0.0 | 0 | 40 | 70 | 4.4 | 6 | 10 | 0.20 | 0.11 | 1.3 | 0 |
| 24. | Beans, refried | 1/2 c | 145 | 148 | 9.0 | 1 | 0.2 | 0 | 25 | 71 | 2.6 | 614 | 0 | 0.07 | 0.08 | 0.7 | 9 |
| 25. | Bean sprouts, mung, raw | 1/2 c | 52 | 18 | 2.0 | 0 | 0.0 | 0 | 4 | 10 | 0.7 | 3 | 10 | 0.07 | 0.07 | 0.4 | 10 |
| 26. | Beef, chuck, cooked, | 3 oz. | 85 | 212 | 25.0 | 12 | 7.8 | 80 | 0 | 11 | 3.1 | 43 | 20 | 0.05 | 0.19 | 3.8 | 0 |
| 27. | Beef, corned, canned | 3 oz. | 85 | 163 | 21.0 | 10 | 8.0 | 70 | 0 | 22 | 5.0 | 802 | 0 | 0.02 | 0.27 | 3.9 | 0 |
| 28. | Beef, ground, lean | 3 oz. | 85 | 186 | 23.3 | 10 | 5.0 | 81 | 0 | 10 | 3.0 | 57 | 20 | 0.08 | 0.20 | 5.1 | 0 |
| 29. | Beef, Lite Roast Deluxe, Arby's | 1 | 182 | 294 | 18 | 10 | 3.5 | 42 | 33 | 156 | 3.0 | 826 | 200 | 0.27 | 0.52 | 8.4 | 8 |
| 30. | Beef, meatloaf | 1 piece | 111 | 246 | 20.0 | 15 | 6.1 | 125 | 6 | 37 | 2.4 | 434 | 181 | 0.08 | 0.23 | 4.1 | 1 |
| 31. | Beef N' Cheddar, Arby's | 1 | 194 | 508 | 25 | 27 | 7.7 | 52 | 43 | 180 | 4.1 | 1,166 | 0 | 0.42 | 0.67 | 9.8 | 1 |
| 32. | Beef, round steak, cooked, trimmed | 3 oz. | 85 | 222 | 24.3 | 13 | 6.0 | 77 | 0 | 10 | 3.0 | 60 | 20 | 0.07 | 0.20 | 4.8 | 0 |
| 33. | Beef, rump roast | 3 oz. | 85 | 177 | 24.7 | 9 | 4.0 | 80 | 0 | 10 | 3.1 | 61 | 10 | 0.06 | 0.19 | 4.4 | 0 |
| 34. | Beef, sirloin, cooked | 3 oz. | 85 | 329 | 19.6 | 27 | 13.0 | 77 | 0 | 9 | 2.5 | 48 | 50 | 0.05 | 0.15 | 4.0 | 0 |
| 35. | Beef, T-bone steak | 3 oz. | 85 | 403 | 16.7 | 37 | 15.6 | 66 | 0 | 7 | 2.2 | 40 | 23 | 0.07 | 0.14 | 3.5 | 0 |
| 36. | Beef, thin, sliced | 3 oz. | 85 | 105 | 18.5 | 3 | 1.4 | 36 | 0 | 11 | 1.8 | 1,409 | 0 | 0.07 | 0.16 | 4.5 | 0 |
| 37. | Beer | 12 fl. oz. | 360 | 151 | 1.1 | 0 | 1.1 | 0 | 14 | 18 | 0.0 | 25 | 0 | 0.01 | 0.11 | 2.2 | 0 |
| 38. | Beer, light | 12 fl. oz. | 354 | 96 | 0.7 | 0 | 0.0 | 0 | 4 | 17 | 0.1 | 10 | 0 | 0.03 | 0.10 | 1.3 | 0 |
| 39. | Beets, red, canned, drained | 1/2 c | 80 | 32 | 0.8 | 0 | 0.0 | 0 | 8 | 15 | 0.6 | 164 | 15 | 0.01 | 0.02 | 0.1 | 2 |
| 40. | Beet greens, cooked | 1/2 c | 73 | 13 | 1.3 | 0 | 0.0 | 0 | 2 | 72 | 1.4 | 55 | 3,700 | 0.05 | 0.11 | 0.2 | 11 |
| 41. | Biscuits, baking powder | 1 med | 35 | 114 | 2.5 | 6 | 1.1 | 0 | 18 | 60 | 0.8 | 272 | 0 | 0.06 | 0.06 | 0.7 | 0 |
| 42. | Blueberries, fresh cultivated | 1/2 c | 73 | 45 | 0.5 | 0 | 0.0 | 0 | 11 | 10 | 0.8 | 1 | 75 | 0.02 | 0.05 | 0.4 | 10 |

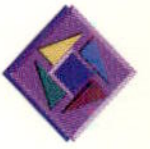

| | | | | | | | | | | | | | | | | | |
|---|---|---|---|---|---|---|---|---|---|---|---|---|---|---|---|---|---|
| 43. | Bologna | 1 slice (1 oz.) | 28 | 86 | 3.4 | 8 | 3.0 | 15 | 0 | 2 | 0.5 | 369 | 0 | 0.05 | 0.06 | 0.7 | 0 |
| 44. | Bologna, turkey | 2 slices | 57 | 113 | 7.8 | 9 | 3.0 | 56 | 1 | 47 | 0.9 | 498 | 0 | 0.03 | 0.09 | 2.1 | 0 |
| 45. | Bouillon, broth | 1 cube | 4 | 5 | 0.8 | 0 | 0.0 | 0 | 0 | 0 | 0.0 | 960 | 0 | 0.00 | 0.00 | 0.0 | 0 |
| 46. | Brandy | 1 oz. | 28 | 69 | 0.0 | 0 | 0.0 | 0 | 11 | 0 | 0.0 | 1 | 0 | 0.00 | 0.00 | 0.0 | 0 |
| 47. | Bread, Corn | 1 slice | 78 | 161 | 5.8 | 6 | 0.1 | 0 | 23 | 94 | 0.9 | 490 | 120 | 0.10 | 0.15 | 0.5 | 1 |
| 48. | Bread, Cracked wheat | 1 slice | 25 | 65 | 2.3 | 1 | 0.2 | 0 | 12 | 16 | 0.7 | 106 | 0 | 0.10 | 0.10 | 0.8 | 0 |
| 49. | Bread, French enriched | 1 slice | 35 | 102 | 3.2 | 1 | 0.2 | 0 | 19 | 15 | 0.8 | 203 | 0 | 0.10 | 0.08 | 0.9 | 0 |
| 50. | Bread, Oatmeal | 1 slice | 25 | 65 | 2.1 | 1 | 0.2 | 0 | 12 | 15 | 0.7 | 124 | 0 | 0.12 | 0.07 | 0.9 | 0 |
| 51. | Bread, Pita pocket | 1 piece | 60 | 165 | 6.2 | 1 | 0.1 | 0 | 33 | 49 | 1.5 | 339 | 0 | 0.27 | 0.13 | 2.3 | 0 |
| 52. | Bread, Pumpernickel | 1 slice | 32 | 80 | 2.9 | 1 | 0.2 | 0 | 15 | 23 | 0.9 | 277 | 0 | 0.11 | 0.17 | 1.1 | 0 |
| 53. | Bread, Rye (American) | 1 slice | 25 | 61 | 2.3 | 0 | 0.0 | 0 | 13 | 19 | 0.4 | 139 | 0 | 0.05 | 0.02 | 0.4 | 0 |
| 54. | Bread, white enriched | 1 slice | 25 | 68 | 2.2 | 1 | 0.2 | 0 | 13 | 21 | 0.6 | 127 | 0 | 0.06 | 0.05 | 0.6 | 0 |
| 55. | Bread, whole wheat | 1 slice | 25 | 61 | 2.6 | 1 | 0.6 | 0 | 12 | 25 | 0.8 | 132 | 0 | 0.06 | 0.03 | 0.7 | 0 |
| 56. | Broccoli, cooked drained | 1 sm stalk | 140 | 36 | 4.3 | 0 | 0.0 | 0 | 6 | 123 | 1.1 | 14 | 3,500 | 0.13 | 0.28 | 1.1 | 126 |
| 57. | Broccoli, raw | 1 sm stalk | 114 | 38 | 4.1 | 0 | 0.0 | 0 | 7 | 117 | 1.3 | 17 | 2,835 | 0.10 | 0.23 | 0.9 | 125 |
| 58. | Brownies, with nuts | 1 | 20 | 95 | 1.3 | 6 | 2.3 | 18 | 11 | 9 | 0.4 | 51 | 20 | 0.05 | 0.05 | 0.3 | 0 |
| 59. | Brussels sprouts, froz., cooked, drained | 1/2 c | 78 | 28 | 3.2 | 0 | 0.0 | 0 | 5 | 25 | 0.8 | 8 | 405 | 0.06 | 0.11 | 0.5 | 63 |
| 60. | Bulgur, wheat | 1 c | 135 | 227 | 8.4 | 1 | 0.0 | 0 | 47 | 27 | 1.8 | 809 | 0 | 0.07 | 0.04 | 3.2 | 0 |
| 61. | Burrito, bean | 1 | 166 | 307 | 12.5 | 9.5 | 3.6 | 14 | 45 | 173 | 2.4 | 983 | 283 | 0.15 | 0.22 | 2.3 | 5 |
| 62. | Burrito, combination, Taco Bell | 1 | 175 | 404 | 21.0 | 16 | 0.0 | 0 | 43 | 91 | 3.7 | 300 | 1,666 | 0.34 | 0.31 | 4.6 | 15 |
| 63. | Butter | 1 tsp | 5 | 36 | 0.0 | 4 | 0.4 | 12 | 0 | 1 | 0.0 | 46 | 160 | 0.00 | 0.00 | 0.0 | 0 |
| 64. | Buttermilk, cultured | 1 c | 245 | 88 | 8.8 | 0 | 1.3 | 5 | 12 | 296 | 0.1 | 319 | 10 | 0.10 | 0.44 | 0.2 | 2 |
| 65. | Cabbage, boiled, drained wedge | 1/2 c | 85 | 16 | 0.9 | 0 | 0.0 | 0 | 3 | 36 | 0.3 | 10 | 100 | 0.02 | 0.02 | 0.1 | 21 |
| 66. | Cabbage, raw chopped | 1/2 c | 45 | 11 | 0.6 | 0 | 0.0 | 0 | 3 | 22 | 0.2 | 9 | 60 | 0.03 | 0.03 | 0.2 | 21 |
| 67. | Cake, Angel food, plain | 1 piece | 60 | 161 | 4.3 | 0 | 0.0 | 0 | 36 | 5 | 0.1 | 170 | 0 | 0.01 | 0.08 | 0.1 | 0 |
| 68. | Cake, Carrot | 1 piece | 96 | 385 | 4.2 | 21 | 4.1 | 74 | 48 | 44 | 1.3 | 279 | 75 | 0.11 | 0.12 | 0.9 | 1 |
| 69. | Cake, Cheesecake | 1 piece (3½") | 85 | 257 | 4.6 | 16 | 9.0 | 150 | 24 | 48 | 0.4 | 189 | 216 | 0.03 | 0.11 | 0.4 | 4 |
| 70. | Cake, Chocolate, w/icing | 1 piece | 69 | 235 | 3.0 | 8 | 3.6 | 37 | 40 | 41 | 1.4 | 181 | 100 | 0.07 | 0.10 | 0.6 | 0 |
| 71. | Cake, Coffee | 1 piece | 72 | 230 | 4.5 | 7 | 2.5 | 47 | 38 | 44 | 1.2 | 310 | 120 | 0.14 | 0.15 | 1.3 | 0 |
| 72. | Cake, Devil's food, iced | 1 piece | 99 | 365 | 4.5 | 16 | 5.0 | 68 | 55 | 69 | 1.0 | 233 | 160 | 0.02 | 0.10 | 0.2 | 0 |
| 73. | Cake, Pound | 1 piece | 30 | 120 | 2.0 | 5 | 1.0 | 32 | 15 | 20 | 0.5 | 98 | 200 | 0.05 | 0.06 | 0.5 | 0 |
| 74. | Cake, White, choc. icing | 1 piece | 71 | 268 | 3.5 | 11 | 3.7 | 2 | 48 | 35 | 0.3 | 162 | 40 | 0.19 | 0.14 | 1.6 | 0 |
| 75. | Candy, hard | 1 oz. | 28 | 109 | 0.0 | 0 | 0.0 | 0 | 28 | 6 | 0.5 | 9 | 0 | 0.00 | 0.00 | 0.0 | 0 |
| 76. | Cantaloupe | 1/4 melon 5" diam. | 239 | 35 | 2.0 | 0 | 0.0 | 0 | 10 | 20 | 0.8 | 17 | 4,620 | 0.06 | 0.04 | 0.6 | 45 |
| 77. | Caramel (candy, plain or choc.) | 1 oz. | 28 | 113 | 1.1 | 3 | 1.6 | 0 | 22 | 42 | 0.4 | 64 | 0 | 0.01 | 0.05 | 0.1 | 0 |
| 78. | Carrots, cooked, drained | 1/2 c | 73 | 23 | 0.7 | 0 | 0.0 | 0 | 5 | 24 | 0.5 | 10 | 7,615 | 0.04 | 0.04 | 0.4 | 5 |
| 79. | Carrots, raw | 1 carrot 7½" long | 81 | 30 | 0.8 | 0 | 0.0 | 0 | 7 | 27 | 0.5 | 34 | 7,930 | 0.04 | 0.04 | 0.4 | 6 |
| 80. | Cashew, roasted, unsalted | 2 oz. | 57 | 326 | 9.2 | 27 | 5.4 | 0 | 16 | 23 | 2.3 | 10 | 0 | 0.24 | 0.10 | 1.0 | 0 |
| 81. | Cauliflower, cooked, drained | 1/2 c | 63 | 14 | 1.5 | 0 | 0.0 | 0 | 3 | 13 | 0.5 | 6 | 40 | 0.06 | 0.05 | 0.4 | 35 |
| 82. | Celery, green, raw, long | 1 outer stalk 8" | 40 | 7 | 0.4 | 0 | 0.0 | 0 | 2 | 16 | 0.1 | 50 | 110 | 0.01 | 0.01 | 0.1 | 4 |
| 83. | Cereal, All-Bran | 1/4 c | 21 | 53 | 3.0 | 0 | 0.1 | 0 | 16 | 17 | 3.4 | 242 | 947 | 0.28 | 0.33 | 3.8 | 11 |
| 84. | Cereal, Alpha Bits | 1 c | 28 | 111 | 2.2 | 1 | 0.0 | 0 | 25 | 8 | 1.8 | 219 | 1,875 | 0.40 | 0.40 | 5.0 | 0 |
| 85. | Cereal, Bran | 1/2 c | 30 | 72 | 3.8 | 1 | 0.0 | 0 | 22 | 25 | 3.0 | 247 | 2,000 | 1.00 | 0.80 | 3.0 | 20 |
| 86. | Cereal, Cheerios | 1 c | 23 | 89 | 3.4 | 1 | 1.2 | 0 | 16 | 38 | 3.6 | 246 | 949 | 0.32 | 0.32 | 4.0 | 12 |
| 87. | Cereal, Corn Chex | 1 c | 28 | 111 | 2.0 | 0 | 0.1 | 0 | 25 | 3 | 1.8 | 271 | 75 | 0.40 | 0.07 | 5.0 | 15 |
| 88. | Cereal, Corn Flakes | 1 c | 25 | 97 | 2.0 | 0 | 0.0 | 0 | 21 | 3 | 0.6 | 251 | 180 | 0.29 | 0.55 | 2.9 | 9 |
| 89. | Cereal, Cream of Wheat | 1 c | 244 | 140 | 3.6 | 1 | 0.1 | 0 | 29 | 54 | 10.9 | 5 | 0 | 0.24 | 0.07 | 1.5 | 0 |
| 90. | Cereal, Frosted Mini-Wheats | 4 biscuits | 31 | 111 | 3.2 | 0 | 0.0 | 0 | 26 | 10 | 2.0 | 9 | 2,050 | 0.40 | 0.50 | 5.5 | 16 |

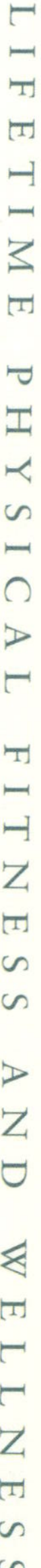

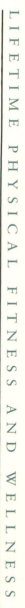

| Code | Food | Amount | Weight gm | Calories | Protein gm | Fat gm | Sat. Fat gm | Cholesterol mg | Carbohydrate gm | Calcium mg | Iron mg | Sodium mg | Vit A I.U. | Thiamin (Vit $B_1$) mg | Riboflavin (Vit $B_2$) mg | Niacin mg | Vit C mg |
|---|---|---|---|---|---|---|---|---|---|---|---|---|---|---|---|---|---|
| 91. | Cereal, Fruit & Fibre w/dates | 1 c | 56 | 180 | 6.0 | 2 | 0.3 | 0 | 42 | 20 | 9.0 | 340 | 3,780 | 0.75 | 0.85 | 10.0 | 0 |
| 92. | Cereal, Granola, Nature Valley | 1/2 c | 57 | 252 | 5.8 | 10 | 7.0 | 0 | 38 | 36 | 1.9 | 116 | 41 | 0.20 | 0.10 | 0.4 | 0 |
| 93. | Cereal, Grape Nuts | 1/2 c | 57 | 202 | 6.6 | 0 | 0.0 | 0 | 47 | 22 | 2.5 | 394 | 3,815 | 0.80 | 0.80 | 10.0 | 0 |
| 94. | Cereal, Life | 1 c | 44 | 162 | 8.1 | 1 | 0.1 | 0 | 32 | 154 | 11.6 | 229 | 0 | 0.95 | 1.00 | 11.6 | 0 |
| 95. | Cereal, Nutri-Grain Wheat | 1 c | 44 | 158 | 3.8 | 1 | 0.1 | 0 | 37 | 12 | 1.2 | 299 | 2,915 | 0.60 | 0.70 | 7.7 | 23 |
| 96. | Cereal, Oatmeal, quick, cooked | 1/2 c | 120 | 66 | 2.4 | 1 | 0.2 | 0 | 12 | 11 | 0.7 | 262 | 0 | 0.10 | 0.03 | 0.1 | 0 |
| 97. | Cereal, Raisin Bran | 1 c | 49 | 160 | 4.0 | 1 | 0.2 | 0 | 40 | 25 | 24.0 | 293 | 2,500 | 0.51 | 0.57 | 6.7 | 0 |
| 98. | Cereal, Rice Krispies | 3/4 c | 22 | 85 | 1.4 | 0 | 0.0 | 0 | 19 | 3 | 1.4 | 255 | 971 | 0.30 | 0.30 | 3.8 | 11 |
| 99. | Cereal, Shredded Wheat | 1 c | 19 | 65 | 2.1 | 0 | 0.0 | 0 | 11 | 8 | 0.6 | 1 | 0 | 0.06 | 0.05 | 0.9 | 0 |
| 100. | Cereal, Special K | 1 c | 21 | 83 | 4.2 | 0 | 0.0 | 0 | 16 | 6 | 3.4 | 199 | 1,430 | 0.30 | 0.30 | 3.8 | 11 |
| 101. | Cereal, Sugar Corn Pops | 1 c | 28 | 108 | 1.4 | 0 | 0.0 | 0 | 26 | 1 | 1.8 | 103 | 1,875 | 0.40 | 0.40 | 5.0 | 15 |
| 102. | Cereal, Sugar Frosted Flakes | 1 c | 35 | 133 | 1.8 | 0 | 0.0 | 0 | 32 | 1 | 2.2 | 284 | 2,315 | 0.50 | 0.50 | 6.2 | 19 |
| 103. | Cereal, Sugar Smacks | 1 c | 37 | 141 | 2.7 | 1 | 0.1 | 0 | 32 | 4 | 2.4 | 100 | 2,500 | 0.49 | 0.57 | 6.7 | 20 |
| 104. | Cereal, Total | 1 c | 33 | 116 | 3.3 | 1 | 0.1 | 0 | 26 | 56 | 21.0 | 409 | 8,845 | 1.70 | 2.00 | 23.3 | 70 |
| 105. | Cereal, Wheat Chex | 1 c | 46 | 169 | 4.5 | 1 | 0.2 | 0 | 38 | 18 | 7.3 | 308 | 0 | 0.60 | 0.17 | 8.1 | 24 |
| 106. | Cereal, whole wheat, cooked | 1/2 c | 123 | 55 | 2.2 | 0 | 0.0 | 0 | 12 | 9 | 0.06 | 260 | 0 | 0.08 | 0.03 | 0.8 | 0 |
| 107. | Cereal, whole wheat flakes, ready-to-eat | 1 c | 30 | 106 | 3.1 | 1 | 0.0 | 0 | 24 | 12 | 2.0 | 310 | 1,410 | 0.35 | 0.42 | 3.5 | 11 |
| 108. | Cereal, 40% Bran Flakes | 1 c | 39 | 125 | 4.9 | 1 | 0.1 | 0 | 31 | 19 | 11.2 | 363 | 2,610 | 0.51 | 0.59 | 6.9 | 0 |
| 109. | Cereal, 100% Bran | 1/2 c | 33 | 89 | 4.2 | 2 | 0.3 | 0 | 24 | 23 | 4.1 | 229 | 0 | 0.80 | 0.90 | 10.4 | 31 |
| 110. | Champagne | 4 oz. | 113 | 87 | 0.2 | 0 | 0.1 | 0 | 2 | 6 | 0.4 | 7 | 0 | 0.00 | 0.01 | 0.1 | 0 |
| 111. | Cheese, American | 1 oz. slice | 28 | 100 | 6.0 | 8 | 5.6 | 27 | 0 | 188 | 0.1 | 307 | 343 | 0.01 | 0.10 | 0.0 | 0 |
| 112. | Cheese, Bleu | 1 oz. | 28 | 100 | 6.0 | 8 | 5.3 | 25 | 1 | 89 | 0.1 | 510 | 204 | 0.01 | 0.11 | 0.3 | 0 |
| 113. | Cheese, Cheddar | 1 oz. | 28 | 114 | 7.0 | 9 | 6.0 | 30 | 0 | 204 | 0.2 | 171 | 300 | 0.01 | 0.11 | 0.0 | 0 |
| 114. | Cheese, Cottage, 2% | 1/2 c | 113 | 103 | 15.5 | 2 | 1.4 | 10 | 4 | 78 | 0.2 | 459 | 79 | 0.03 | 0.21 | 0.2 | 0 |
| 115. | Cheese, Cottage, creamed | 1/2 c | 105 | 112 | 14.0 | 5 | 6.4 | 15 | 3 | 99 | 0.3 | 241 | 180 | 0.03 | 0.26 | 0.1 | 0 |
| 116. | Cheese, Creamed | 1 oz. | 28 | 99 | 6.0 | 8 | 3.0 | 31 | 1 | 167 | 0.3 | 71 | 320 | 0.02 | 0.14 | 0.0 | 0 |
| 117. | Cheese, Feta | 1 oz. | 28 | 75 | 4.5 | 6 | 4.2 | 25 | 1 | 140 | 0.2 | 316 | 180 | 0.04 | 0.23 | 0.3 | 0 |
| 118. | Cheese, Monterey jack | 1 oz. | 28 | 106 | 6.9 | 9 | 5.4 | 26 | 0 | 212 | 0.2 | 152 | 405 | 0.00 | 0.11 | 0.0 | 0 |
| 119. | Cheese, Mozzarella, skim | 1 oz. | 28 | 80 | 7.6 | 5 | 3.1 | 15 | 1 | 207 | 0.1 | 150 | 216 | 0.01 | 0.10 | 0.0 | 0 |
| 120. | Cheese, Parmesan | 1 tbsp | 5 | 23 | 2.1 | 2 | 1.0 | 4 | 0 | 69 | 0.1 | 93 | 45 | 0.00 | 0.02 | 0.0 | 0 |
| 121. | Cheese, Ricotta, part skim | 1 oz. | 28 | 39 | 3.2 | 2 | 1.4 | 9 | 1 | 77 | 0.1 | 35 | 160 | 0.01 | 0.05 | 0.0 | 0 |
| 122. | Cheese, Souffle | 1 portion | 110 | 240 | 10.9 | 19 | 9.5 | 189 | 7 | 221 | 1.1 | 400 | 880 | 0.06 | 0.26 | 0.2 | 0 |
| 123. | Cheese, Swiss | 1 oz. | 28 | 107 | 8.0 | 8 | 5.0 | 26 | 1 | 272 | 0.1 | 74 | 360 | 0.01 | 0.10 | 0.0 | 0 |
| 124. | Cheese puffs, Cheetos | 1 oz. | 28 | 158 | 2.2 | 10 | 4.8 | 5 | 14 | 17 | 0.4 | 344 | 130 | 0.01 | 0.03 | 0.2 | 0 |
| 125. | Cheeseburger, McDonald's | 1 | 115 | 321 | 15.2 | 16 | 6.7 | 40 | 29 | 170 | 2.9 | 736 | 353 | 0.30 | 0.24 | 4.4 | 2 |
| 126. | Cherries | 10 | 75 | 47 | 0.9 | 0 | 0.0 | 0 | 12 | 15 | 0.3 | 8 | 450 | 0.20 | 0.24 | 1.6 | 41 |
| 127. | Chicken, BK Broiler sandwich, Burger King | 1 sandwich | 168 | 379 | 24.0 | 18 | 3.0 | 53 | 31 | 48 | 2.3 | 764 | 350 | 0.42 | 0.22 | 9.2 | 5 |
| 128. | Chicken Breast Filet, Arby's | 1 | 204 | 445 | 22 | 23.0 | 3.0 | 45 | 52 | 72 | 1.9 | 958 | 0 | 0.23 | 0.58 | 9.0 | 5 |
| 129. | Chicken breast, roast w/skin | 1 | 98 | 193 | 29.2 | 8 | 2.1 | 83 | 0 | 14 | 1.0 | 69 | 91 | 0.07 | 0.12 | 12.5 | 0 |
| 130. | Chicken chow mein | 1 c | 250 | 255 | 31.0 | 11 | 3.6 | 75 | 10 | 58 | 2.5 | 718 | 250 | 0.08 | 0.23 | 4.3 | 10 |
| 131. | Chicken club sandwich, Wendy's | 1 | 220 | 520 | 30 | 25 | 6.0 | 75 | 44 | 120 | 9.6 | 980 | 100 | 0.60 | 0.45 | 16.0 | 9 |
| 132. | Chicken Cordon Bleu, Arby's | 1 | 225 | 518 | 30 | 27 | 5.3 | 92 | 52 | 204 | 2.1 | 1,463 | 0 | 0.42 | 0.68 | 10.2 | 5 |
| 133. | Chicken, drumstick Kentucky Fried | 1 | 54 | 136 | 14.0 | 8 | 2.2 | 73 | 2 | 20 | 0.9 | 320 | 30 | 0.04 | 0.12 | 2.7 | 0 |
| 134. | Chicken, drumstick, roasted | 1 | 52 | 112 | 14.1 | 6 | 1.6 | 48 | 0 | 6 | 0.7 | 47 | 52 | 0.04 | 0.11 | 3.1 | 0 |

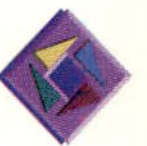

| | | | | | | | | | | | | | | | | |
|---|---|---|---|---|---|---|---|---|---|---|---|---|---|---|---|---|
| 135. Chicken McNuggets | 6 | 111 | 329 | 19.5 | 21 | 5.2 | 64 | 15 | 11 | 1.3 | 521 | 92 | 0.16 | 0.14 | 7.7 | 2 |
| 136. Chicken Nuggets, Wendy's | 6 pc. | 94 | 280 | 14 | 20 | 5.0 | 50 | 12 | 48 | 0.48 | 600 | 0 | 0.09 | 0.11 | 6.0 | 0 |
| 137. Chicken, patty sandwich | 1 | 157 | 436 | 24.8 | 23 | 6.1 | 68 | 34 | 44 | 1.9 | 2,732 | 47 | 0.13 | 0.26 | 9.2 | 4 |
| 138. Chicken, wing, Kentucky Fried | 1 | 45 | 151 | 11.0 | 10 | 2.9 | 70 | 4 | 0 | 0.6 | 300 | 0 | 0.03 | 0.07 | 0.0 | 0 |
| 139. Chicken, roast, light meat without skin | 3 oz. | 85 | 141 | 27.0 | 3 | 0.4 | 45 | 0 | 10 | 1.2 | 54 | 51 | 0.03 | 0.09 | 9.9 | 0 |
| 140. Chicken, roast, dark meat without skin | 3 oz. | 85 | 149 | 24.0 | 5 | 0.8 | 50 | 0 | 11 | 1.5 | 54 | 127 | 0.06 | 0.19 | 4.7 | 0 |
| 141. Chicken, Roast Deluxe, Arby's | 1 | 195 | 276 | 24 | 7 | 1.7 | 33 | 33 | 156 | 1.9 | 777 | 200 | 0.44 | 0.80 | 9.4 | 7 |
| 142. Chicken Sandwich, breaded Wendy's | 1 | 208 | 450 | 26 | 20 | 4.0 | 60 | 44 | 120 | 9.6 | 740 | 100 | 0.45 | 0.36 | 14.0 | 6 |
| 143. Chicken Sandwich, Grilled, Wendy's | 1 | 177 | 290 | 24 | 7 | 1.0 | 60 | 35 | 120 | 2.4 | 670 | 100 | 0.38 | 0.27 | 10.0 | 6 |
| 144. Chicken Sandwich, McChicken | 1 | 187 | 415 | 19 | 19 | 9.0 | 50 | 39 | 180 | 1.8 | 830 | 100 | 0.90 | 0.18 | 9.0 | 2.4 |
| 145. Chili con carne | 1 c | 255 | 339 | 19.1 | 16 | 5.8 | 28 | 31 | 82 | 4.3 | 1,354 | 150 | 0.08 | 0.18 | 3.3 | 8 |
| 146. Chocolate fudge | 1 oz. | 28 | 115 | 0.6 | 3 | 2.1 | 1 | 21 | 22 | 0.3 | 54 | 0 | 0.01 | 0.03 | 0.1 | 0 |
| 147. Chocolate, milk | 1 oz. | 28 | 147 | 2.0 | 9 | 3.6 | 5 | 16 | 65 | 0.3 | 27 | 80 | 0.02 | 0.10 | 0.1 | 0 |
| 148. Chocolate, milk w/almonds | 1 oz. | 28 | 150 | 2.9 | 10 | 4.4 | 5 | 15 | 61 | 0.6 | 23 | 30 | 0.03 | 0.13 | 0.3 | 0 |
| 149. Clam, canned, drained | 3 oz. | 85 | 83 | 13.0 | 2 | 0.2 | 50 | 2 | 46 | 3.5 | 750 | 93 | 0.01 | 0.09 | 0.9 | 9 |
| 150. Cocoa, hot, with whole milk | 1 c | 250 | 218 | 9.1 | 9 | 6.1 | 33 | 26 | 298 | 0.8 | 123 | 318 | 0.10 | 0.44 | 0.4 | 2 |
| 151. Cocoa, plain, dry | 1 tbsp | 5 | 14 | 0.9 | 1 | 0.0 | 0 | 3 | 7 | 0.6 | 0 | 0 | 0.01 | 0.02 | 0.1 | 0 |
| 152. Coconut, shredded, packed | 1/2 c | 65 | 225 | 2.3 | 23 | 20.0 | 0 | 6 | 8 | 1.1 | 165 | 0 | 0.03 | 0.01 | 0.3 | 2 |
| 153. Cod, batter fried | 3.5 oz. | 100 | 199 | 19.6 | 10 | 3.9 | 55 | 8 | 80 | 0.5 | 100 | 2 | 0.02 | 0.02 | 1.8 | 0 |
| 154. Cod, cooked | 3 oz. | 85 | 144 | 24.3 | 4 | 1.5 | 60 | 0 | 27 | 0.9 | 63 | 150 | 0.06 | 0.09 | 2.7 | 0 |
| 155. Cod, poached | 3.5 oz. | 100 | 94 | 20.9 | 1 | 0.3 | 60 | 0 | 29 | 0.5 | 110 | 2 | 0.08 | 0.08 | 3.0 | 0 |
| 156. Coffee | 3/4 cup | 180 | 1 | 0.0 | 0 | 0.0 | 0 | 0 | 1 | 0.2 | 2 | 0 | 0.00 | 0.00 | 0.1 | 0 |
| 157. Coleslaw | 1 c | 120 | 173 | 1.6 | 17 | 1.0 | 5 | 6 | 53 | 0.5 | 144 | 190 | 0.06 | 0.06 | 0.4 | 35 |
| 158. Collards, leaves without stems, cooked, drained | 1/2 c | 95 | 32 | 3.4 | 1 | 2.0 | 0 | 5 | 178 | 0.8 | 28 | 7,410 | 0.01 | 0.19 | 1.2 | 72 |
| 159. Cookies, Chocolate chip homemade | 2 2¼" diam. | 20 | 103 | 1.0 | 6 | 1.7 | 14 | 12 | 7 | 0.4 | 70 | 20 | 0.02 | 0.02 | 0.2 | 0 |
| 160. Cookies, Fig bars | 4 bars | 56 | 210 | 2.0 | 4 | 1.0 | 27 | 42 | 40 | 1.4 | 180 | 31 | 0.08 | 0.07 | 0.7 | 0 |
| 161. Cookies, Oatmeal raisin | 2 2" diam. | 26 | 122 | 1.5 | 5 | 1.3 | 1 | 18 | 9 | 0.6 | 74 | 20 | 0.04 | 0.04 | 0.5 | 0 |
| 162. Cookies, Peanut butter, homemade | 2 cookies | 24 | 123 | 2.0 | 7 | 2.0 | 11 | 14 | 10 | 0.5 | 71 | 12 | 0.03 | 0.03 | 0.9 | 0 |
| 163. Cookies, sandwich, all | 4 cookies | 40 | 195 | 2.0 | 8 | 2.0 | 0 | 29 | 12 | 1.4 | 189 | 0 | 0.90 | 0.07 | 0.8 | 0 |
| 164. Cookies, Shortbread | 4 cookies | 32 | 155 | 2.0 | 8 | 2.9 | 27 | 20 | 13 | 0.8 | 123 | 40 | 0.10 | 0.09 | 0.9 | 0 |
| 165. Cookies, Vanilla | 5 1¾" diam. | 20 | 93 | 1.0 | 3 | 0.8 | 10 | 15 | 8 | 0.1 | 50 | 25 | 0.00 | 0.01 | 0.0 | 0 |
| 166 Cookies, Vanilla wafers | 10 wafers | 40 | 185 | 2.0 | 7 | 1.8 | 25 | 29 | 16 | 0.8 | 150 | 70 | 0.07 | 0.10 | 1.0 | 0 |
| 167. Corn, boiled on cob | 1 ear 5" long | 140 | 70 | 2.5 | 1 | 0.0 | 0 | 16 | 2 | 0.5 | 1 | 310 | 0.09 | 0.08 | 1.1 | 7 |
| 168. Corn, canned, drained | 1/2 c | 83 | 70 | 2.2 | 1 | 0.0 | 0 | 16 | 4 | 0.4 | 195 | 290 | 0.03 | 0.04 | 0.8 | 4 |
| 169. Corn chips | 1 oz. | 28 | 155 | 2.0 | 9 | 1.8 | 0 | 16 | 35 | 0.5 | 233 | 110 | 0.04 | 0.05 | 0.4 | 1 |
| 170. Cornmeal, degermed, yellow, enriched, cooked | 1/2 c | 120 | 60 | 1.3 | 0 | 0.0 | 0 | 13 | 1 | 0.5 | 264 | 70 | 0.07 | 0.05 | 0.6 | 0 |
| 171. Crab, canned | 1 c | 135 | 135 | 23.0 | 3 | 0.5 | 135 | 1 | 61 | 1.1 | 1,350 | 70 | 0.11 | 0.11 | 2.6 | 0 |
| 172. Crackers, Cheese | 10 crackers | 10 | 50 | 1.0 | 3 | 0.9 | 6 | 5 | 11 | 0.4 | 112 | 25 | 0.05 | 0.04 | 0.4 | 0 |
| 173. Crackers, Graham | 2 squares | 14 | 55 | 1.1 | 1 | 0.3 | 0 | 10 | 6 | 0.2 | 95 | 0 | 0.01 | 0.03 | 0.2 | 0 |
| 174. Crackers, Ritz | 1 cracker | 3 | 15 | 0.2 | 1 | 0.2 | 0 | 2 | 3 | 0.1 | 30 | 0 | 0.01 | 0.01 | 0.1 | 0 |
| 175. Crackers, Ryewafers, whole grain | 2 crackers | 14 | 55 | 1.0 | 1 | 0.3 | 0 | 10 | 7 | 0.5 | 115 | 0 | 0.06 | 0.03 | 0.5 | 0 |
| 176. Crackers, Saltines | 4 squares | 11 | 48 | 1.0 | 1 | 0.3 | 0 | 8 | 2 | 0.1 | 123 | 0 | 0.00 | 0.00 | 0.1 | 0 |
| 177. Crackers, Soda | 1 | 3 | 13 | 0.3 | 0 | 0.1 | 0 | 2 | 1 | 0.1 | 39 | 0 | 0.02 | 0.01 | 0.1 | 0 |

| Code | Food | Amount | Weight gm | Calories | Protein gm | Fat gm | Sat. Fat gm | Cholesterol mg | Carbohydrate gm | Calcium mg | Iron mg | Sodium mg | Vit A I.U. | Thiamin (Vit $B_1$) mg | Riboflavin (Vit $B_2$) mg | Niacin mg | Vit C mg |
|---|---|---|---|---|---|---|---|---|---|---|---|---|---|---|---|---|---|
| 178. | Crackers, Triscuits | 1 | 5 | 23 | 0.4 | 1 | 0.3 | 0 | 3 | 0 | 0.0 | 0 | 0 | 0.00 | 0.00 | 0.0 | 0 |
| 179. | Crackers, Wheat Thins | 1 | 2 | 9 | 0.2 | 0 | 0.1 | 0 | 1 | 1 | 0.1 | 17 | 0 | 0.01 | 0.01 | 0.1 | 0 |
| 180. | Cranberry juice | 1 c | 253 | 145 | 0.1 | 0 | 0.0 | 0 | 36 | 8 | 0.4 | 5 | 5 | 0.02 | 0.02 | 0.1 | 90 |
| 181. | Cream, light coffee or table | 1 tbsp | 15 | 20 | 0.5 | 2 | 0.5 | 5 | 1 | 16 | 0.0 | 7 | 70 | 0.00 | 0.02 | 0.0 | 0 |
| 182. | Cream, heavy whipping | 1 tbsp | 15 | 53 | 0.3 | 6 | 1.3 | 12 | 1 | 11 | 0.0 | 5 | 230 | 0.00 | 0.02 | 0.0 | 0 |
| 183. | Croissant | 1 | 57 | 235 | 4.7 | 12 | 4.0 | 13 | 27 | 20 | 2.1 | 452 | 50 | 0.17 | 0.13 | 1.3 | 0 |
| 184. | Croissants (Sara Lee) | 1 roll | 18 | 59 | 1.6 | 2 | 0.3 | 0 | 8 | 22 | 0.6 | 105 | 0 | 0.14 | 0.09 | 0.8 | 0 |
| 185. | Croissan'wich, egg, cheese Burger King | 1 sandwich | 110 | 315 | 13.0 | 20 | 7.0 | 222 | 19 | 112 | 1.8 | 607 | 500 | 0.22 | 0.37 | 1.4 | 0 |
| 186. | Cucumbers, raw pared | 9 sm slices | 28 | 4 | 0.3 | 0 | 0.0 | 0 | 1 | 7 | 0.3 | 2 | 70 | 0.01 | 0.01 | 0.1 | 3 |
| 187. | Danish, Apple, McDonald's | 1 | 115 | 390 | 6 | 17 | 11.0 | 25 | 51 | 0 | 1.0 | 370 | 0 | 0.30 | 0.18 | 2.0 | 15 |
| 188. | Danish, Cinnamon Raisin | 1 | 110 | 440 | 6 | 21 | 13.0 | 34 | 58 | 48 | 0.12 | 430 | 0 | 0.30 | 0.27 | 3.0 | 4 |
| 189. | Dates hydrated | 5 | 46 | 110 | 0.9 | 0 | 0.0 | 0 | 29 | 24 | 1.2 | 1 | 20 | 0.04 | 0.04 | 0.9 | 0 |
| 190. | Doughnut, plain | 1 | 42 | 164 | 1.9 | 8 | 2.0 | 19 | 22 | 17 | 0.6 | 210 | 30 | 0.07 | 0.07 | 0.5 | 0 |
| 191. | Doughnut, yeast raised | 1 | 27 | 235 | 4.0 | 13 | 5.2 | 21 | 26 | 17 | 1.4 | 222 | 2 | 0.28 | 0.12 | 1.8 | 0 |
| 192. | Dressing, Bleu cheese | 1 tbsp | 15 | 77 | 0.7 | 8 | 1.9 | 4 | 1 | 12 | 0.0 | 8 | 32 | 0.00 | 0.02 | 0.0 | 0 |
| 193. | Dressing, French | 1 tbsp | 16 | 83 | 0.1 | 9 | 1.4 | 0 | 1 | 2 | 0.1 | 184 | 0 | 0.00 | 0.00 | 0.0 | 0 |
| 194. | Dressing, French, low cal | 1 tbsp. | 15 | 24 | 0.0 | 2 | 0.2 | 0 | 2 | 6 | 0.1 | 306 | 0 | 0.00 | 0.00 | 0.0 | 0 |
| 195. | Dressing, Italian | 1 tbsp. | 15 | 69 | 0.1 | 9 | 1.3 | 0 | 2 | 1 | 0.0 | 73 | 29 | 0.00 | 0.00 | 0.0 | 0 |
| 196. | Dressing, Italian, low cal | 1 tbsp. | 15 | 10 | 0.0 | 1 | 0.0 | 0 | 1 | 1 | 0.0 | 136 | 1 | 0.00 | 0.00 | 0.0 | 0 |
| 197. | Dressing, Ranch style | 1 tbsp. | 15 | 54 | 0.4 | 6 | 0.9 | 6 | 1 | 15 | 0.0 | 65 | 36 | 0.01 | 0.02 | 0.0 | 0 |
| 198. | Dressing, Thousand island | 1 tbsp. | 15 | 60 | 0.2 | 6 | 1.0 | 4 | 2 | 2 | 0.1 | 110 | 75 | 0.00 | 0.01 | 0.0 | 1 |
| 199. | Dressing, Thousand island, low cal | 1 tbsp. | 15 | 25 | 0.1 | 2 | 0.2 | 2 | 3 | 2 | 0.1 | 153 | 70 | 0.00 | 0.00 | 0.0 | 0 |
| 200. | Egg, hard cooked | 1 large | 50 | 72 | 6.0 | 5 | 1.6 | 212 | 1 | 24 | 1.0 | 113 | 520 | 0.05 | 0.13 | 0.0 | 0 |
| 201. | Egg, fried with butter | 1 | 46 | 95 | 5.4 | 7 | 2.4 | 240 | 1 | 28 | 0.9 | 162 | 320 | 0.04 | 0.13 | 0.0 | 0 |
| 202. | Egg McMuffin | 1 | 138 | 327 | 18.5 | 15 | 5.9 | 259 | 31 | 226 | 2.9 | 885 | 591 | 0.47 | 0.44 | 3.8 | 1 |
| 203. | Egg salad sandwich | 1 | 111 | 325 | 10.0 | 19 | 3.9 | 215 | 28 | 95 | 2.5 | 461 | 242 | 0.29 | 0.29 | 2.1 | 0 |
| 204. | Egg, scrambled, with milk, butter | 1 egg | 64 | 95 | 6.0 | 7 | 3.0 | 244 | 1 | 54 | 0.9 | 176 | 510 | 0.04 | 0.18 | 0.0 | 0 |
| 205. | Egg, white | 1 large | 33 | 17 | 3.6 | 0 | 0.0 | 0 | 0 | 3 | 0.0 | 48 | 0 | 0.00 | 0.09 | 0.0 | 0 |
| 206. | Egg, yolk, raw | 1 yolk | 17 | 63 | 2.8 | 5 | 1.6 | 212 | 0 | 26 | 1.0 | 8 | 390 | 0.04 | 0.07 | 0.0 | 0 |
| 207. | Enchilada, beef | 1 | 200 | 487 | 21.8 | 23 | 8.8 | 63 | 26 | 425 | 2.9 | 262 | 595 | 0.02 | 0.27 | 3.5 | 5 |
| 208. | Enchilada, cheese | 1 | 230 | 632 | 25.3 | 34 | 17.6 | 82 | 31 | 876 | 2.6 | 596 | 1,672 | 0.13 | 0.40 | 1.2 | 15 |
| 209. | Figs, dried | 1 large | 21 | 60 | 1.0 | 0 | 0.0 | 0 | 15 | 26 | 0.6 | 1 | 20 | 0.16 | 0.17 | 3.9 | 0 |
| 210. | Filet of Fish, McDonald's | 1 | 131 | 402 | 15.0 | 23 | 7.9 | 43 | 34 | 105 | 1.8 | 709 | 152 | 0.28 | 0.28 | 3.9 | 4 |
| 211. | Fish sandwich, Wendy's | 1 | 182 | 460 | 16 | 25 | 5.0 | 55 | 42 | 120 | 1.8 | 780 | 0 | 0.60 | 0.45 | 4.0 | 1 |
| 212. | Fish, sticks | 2 | 56 | 140 | 12.0 | 6 | 1.6 | 52 | 8 | 22 | 0.6 | 106 | 40 | 0.06 | 0.10 | 1.2 | 0 |
| 213. | Flounder | 3 oz. | 85 | 171 | 25.5 | 7 | 1.0 | 60 | 0 | 21 | 1.2 | 201 | 0 | 0.06 | 0.06 | 2.1 | 3 |
| 214. | Flour, all purpose enriched | 1 c | 125 | 455 | 13.0 | 1 | 0.0 | 0 | 95 | 20 | 3.6 | 3 | 0 | 0.55 | 0.33 | 4.4 | 0 |
| 215. | Flour, whole wheat | 1 c | 120 | 400 | 16.0 | 2 | 0.0 | 0 | 85 | 49 | 4.0 | 4 | 0 | 0.66 | 0.14 | 5.2 | 0 |
| 216. | Frankfurter, cooked | 1 | 57 | 176 | 7.0 | 16 | 5.6 | 45 | 1 | 4 | 1.1 | 627 | 0 | 0.09 | 0.11 | 1.5 | 0 |
| 217. | Frankfurter, turkey, cooked | 1 | 45 | 102 | 6.4 | 8 | 2.7 | 39 | 1 | 58 | 0.8 | 454 | 60 | 0.04 | 0.08 | 1.7 | 0 |
| 218. | French Dip, Arby's | 1 | 154 | 368 | 22 | 15 | 5.6 | 43 | 35 | 60 | 2.8 | 1,018 | 0 | 0.20 | 0.50 | 8.4 | 0 |
| 219. | French toast | 1 piece | 65 | 123 | 4.9 | 4 | 1.1 | 73 | 15 | 79 | 1.1 | 189 | 285 | 0.15 | 0.17 | 1.1 | 0 |
| 220. | Fries, Curly, Arby's | 1 small | 99 | 337 | 4 | 18 | 7.4 | 0 | 43 | 24 | 1.0 | 167 | 0 | 0.06 | 0.07 | 2.0 | 0 |
| 221. | Fruit cocktail | 1 c | 245 | 91 | 1.0 | 0 | 0.0 | 0 | 24 | 22 | 1.0 | 12 | 370 | 0.05 | 0.02 | 1.2 | 5 |
| 222. | Fruit cocktail, juice pack | 1 c | 248 | 115 | 1.1 | 0 | 0.0 | 0 | 29 | 20 | 0.5 | 10 | 380 | 0.03 | 0.04 | 1.0 | 7 |
| 223. | Grapefruit, raw white | 1/2 med | 301 | 56 | 1.0 | 0 | 0.0 | 0 | 15 | 22 | 0.5 | 1 | 10 | 0.05 | 0.03 | 0.3 | 52 |
| 224. | Grapefruit juice, unsweet. canned | 1/2 c | 124 | 50 | 0.6 | 0 | 0.0 | 0 | 12 | 11 | 0.2 | 2 | 10 | 0.05 | 0.03 | 0.3 | 46 |

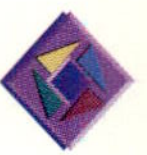

| Food | Amount | | | | | | | | | | | | | | | |
|---|---|---|---|---|---|---|---|---|---|---|---|---|---|---|---|---|
| 225. Grapes, seedless, European | 10 grapes | 50 | 34 | 0.3 | 0 | 0.0 | 0 | 9 | 6 | 0.2 | 2 | 50 | 0.03 | 0.03 | 0.2 | 2 |
| 226. Grape juice, unsweetened bottled | 1/2 c | 127 | 84 | 0.3 | 0 | 0.0 | 0 | 21 | 14 | 0.4 | 3 | 0 | 0.05 | 0.03 | 0.3 | 0 |
| 227. Gravy, beef, homemade | 1 tbsp | 17 | 19 | 0.3 | 2 | 1.0 | 1 | 1 | 1 | 0.1 | 49 | 0 | 0.01 | 0.01 | 0.2 | 0 |
| 228. Haddock, fried (dipped in egg, milk, bread crumbs) | 3 oz. | 85 | 141 | 17.0 | 5 | 1.0 | 54 | 5 | 33 | 0.9 | 150 | 0 | 0.03 | 0.06 | 2.7 | 3 |
| 229. Halibut, broiled with butter or margarine | 3 oz. | 85 | 144 | 21.0 | 6 | 2.1 | 55 | 0 | 15 | 0.6 | 114 | 570 | 0.03 | 0.06 | 7.2 | 1 |
| 230. Ham (cured pork) | 3 oz. | 85 | 318 | 20.0 | 26 | 9.4 | 77 | 0 | 9 | 2.6 | 48 | 0 | 0.43 | 0.20 | 3.8 | 0 |
| 231. Ham, lunch meat | 1 slice | 28 | 37 | 5.5 | 1 | 0.5 | 13 | .3 | 2 | 0.2 | 405 | 0 | 0.26 | 0.06 | 1.4 | 7 |
| 232. Hamburger, Big Classic, Wendy's | 1 | 251 | 480 | 27 | 23 | 7.0 | 75 | 44 | 180 | 4.2 | 850 | 300 | 0.45 | 0.27 | 7.0 | 12 |
| 233. Hamburger, Big Mac | 1 | 204 | 581 | 25.1 | 36 | 12.0 | 85 | 40 | 207 | 5.0 | 999 | 388 | 0.49 | 0.39 | 7.3 | 3 |
| 234. Hamburger bun | 1 bun | 40 | 129 | 3.7 | 2 | 1.0 | 0 | 23 | 61 | 1.3 | 271 | 2 | 0.22 | 0.15 | 1.8 | 0 |
| 235. Hamburger, Jr. Bacon Cheeseburger, Wendy's | 1 | 170 | 440 | 22 | 25 | 8.0 | 65 | 33 | 240 | 3.0 | 870 | 300 | 0.45 | 0.27 | 6.0 | 9 |
| 236. Hamburger, McDonald's | 1 | 99 | 257 | 13.0 | 9 | 3.7 | 26 | 30 | 63 | 3.0 | 526 | 231 | 0.23 | 0.23 | 5.1 | 2 |
| 237. Hamburger, McLean Deluxe | 1 | 206 | 320 | 22 | 10 | 5.0 | 60 | 35 | 180 | 2.4 | 670 | 500 | 0.38 | 0.36 | 7.0 | 6 |
| 238. Hamburger, McLean Deluxe, w/cheese | 1 | 219 | 370 | 24 | 14 | 8.0 | 75 | 35 | 240 | 2.4 | 890 | 750 | 0.38 | 0.36 | 7.0 | 6 |
| 239. Hamburger, Quarter pounder | 1 burger | 160 | 427 | 24.6 | 24 | 9.1 | 80 | 29 | 98 | 4.3 | 718 | 115 | 0.35 | 0.32 | 7.2 | 3 |
| 240. Hamburger, Quarter pounder, with cheese | 1 burger | 186 | 525 | 29.6 | 32 | 12.8 | 107 | 31 | 255 | 4.8 | 1,195 | 640 | 0.37 | 0.41 | 7.1 | 3 |
| 241. Hamburger, Wendy's | 1 | 219 | 440 | 26 | 23 | 7.0 | 75 | 36 | 120 | 3.6 | 850 | 300 | 0.38 | 0.18 | 7.0 | 9 |
| 242. Ham N' Cheese, Arby's | 1 | 169 | 355 | 25 | 14 | 5.1 | 55 | 35 | 204 | 1.8 | 1400 | 0 | 0.83 | 0.40 | 7.8 | 0 |
| 243. Honey | 1 tbsp | 21 | 64 | 0.0 | 0 | 0.0 | 0 | 17 | 1 | 0.1 | 1 | 0 | 0.00 | 0.01 | 0.1 | 0 |
| 244. Honeydew melon | 1 slice (1/10 melon) | 129 | 45 | 0.6 | 0 | 0.0 | 0 | 12 | 8 | 0.1 | 13 | 25 | 0.10 | 0.02 | 0.8 | 32 |
| 245. Horsey Sauce, Arby's | .5 oz. | 14 | 55 | 0 | 5 | 2.0 | 0 | 3 | 24 | 0.0 | 105 | 0 | 0.00 | 0.00 | 0.0 | 0 |
| 246. Hotcakes w/Margarine & Syrup, McDonald's | 1 serving | 174 | 440 | 8 | 12 | 5.0 | 8 | 74 | 120 | 1.2 | 685 | 200 | 0.30 | 0.36 | 3.0 | 0 |
| 247. Hotdog bun | 1 bun | 40 | 115 | 3.3 | 2 | 1.0 | 0 | 20 | 54 | 1.2 | 241 | 2 | 0.20 | 0.13 | 1.6 | 0 |
| 248. Ice cream, vanilla | 1/2 c | 67 | 135 | 3.0 | 7 | 4.4 | 27 | 14 | 97 | 0.1 | 42 | 295 | 0.03 | 0.14 | 0.1 | 1 |
| 249. Ice cream cone | 1 small | 115 | 185 | 4.3 | 5 | 2.2 | 24 | 30 | 183 | 0.1 | 109 | 218 | 0.06 | 0.36 | 0.4 | 1 |
| 250. Ice cream cone, Dairy Queen | medium | 142 | 230 | 6.0 | 7 | 4.6 | 15 | 35 | 200 | 0.0 | 150 | 300 | 0.09 | 0.26 | 0.0 | 0 |
| 251. Ice cream, hot fudge sundae | 1 | 164 | 357 | 7.0 | 11 | 5.4 | 27 | 58 | 215 | 0.6 | 170 | 233 | 0.07 | 0.31 | 1.1 | 2 |
| 252. Ice milk, vanilla | 1/2 c | 61 | 100 | 3.0 | 3 | 1.8 | 13 | 15 | 102 | 0.1 | 45 | 140 | 0.04 | 0.15 | 0.1 | 1 |
| 253. Instant breakfast, whole milk | 1 c | 281 | 280 | 15.0 | 8 | 5.1 | 33 | 34 | 301 | 8.0 | 286 | 2,057 | 0.39 | 0.46 | 5.2 | 29 |
| 254. Instant breakfast, skim milk | 1 c | 282 | 216 | 15.4 | 0 | 0.0 | 4 | 35 | 312 | 8.0 | 292 | 1,635 | 0.39 | 0.41 | 5.2 | 29 |
| 255. Jams or preserves | 1 tbsp | 7 | 18 | 0.0 | 0 | 0.0 | 0 | 5 | 1 | 0.1 | 1 | 1 | 0.00 | 0.00 | 0.0 | 0 |
| 256. Jelly | 1 tbsp | 18 | 49 | 0.0 | 0 | 0.0 | 0 | 13 | 4 | 0.3 | 3 | 0 | 0.00 | 0.01 | 0.0 | 1 |
| 257. Kale, fresh cooked, drained | 1/2 c | 55 | 22 | 2.5 | 0 | 0.0 | 0 | 3 | 103 | 0.9 | 24 | 4,565 | 0.06 | 0.10 | 0.9 | 51 |
| 258. Kiwi fruit, raw | 1 med | 76 | 46 | 1.0 | 0 | 0.0 | 0 | 11 | 20 | 0.3 | 4 | 65 | 0.02 | 0.04 | 0.4 | 75 |
| 259. Kool Aid, with sugar | 1 c | 240 | 100 | 0.0 | 0 | 0.0 | 0 | 25 | 0 | 0.0 | 0 | 0 | 0.00 | 0.00 | 0.0 | 6 |
| 260. Lamb leg, roast, trimmed | 3 oz. | 85 | 237 | 22.0 | 16 | 7.3 | 60 | 0 | 9 | 1.4 | 53 | 0 | 0.13 | 0.23 | 4.7 | 0 |
| 261. Lamb loin chop, broiled, lean | 3 oz. | 84 | 183 | 25.0 | 8 | 3.4 | 78 | 0 | 16 | 1.7 | 70 | 7 | 0.10 | 0.23 | 5.7 | 0 |
| 262. Lasagna, homemade | 1 piece | 220 | 357 | 23.6 | 18 | 8.3 | 50 | 27 | 413 | 2.8 | 703 | 1,008 | 0.19 | 0.30 | 3.3 | 6 |
| 263. Lemon juice, fresh | 1 tbsp | 15 | 4 | 0.1 | 0 | 0.0 | 0 | 1 | 1 | 0.0 | 0 | 0 | 0.00 | 0.00 | 0.0 | 7 |
| 264. Lemonade (concentrate) | 12 oz. | 340 | 137 | 0.2 | 0 | 0.1 | 0 | 36 | 11 | 0.6 | 11 | 73 | 0.02 | 0.07 | 0.1 | 13 |
| 265. Lentils, cooked | 1/2 c | 100 | 106 | 8.0 | 0 | 0.0 | 0 | 19 | 25 | 2.1 | 0 | 20 | 0.07 | 0.06 | 0.6 | 0 |
| 266. Lettuce, crisp head | 1 c sm chunks | 75 | 10 | 0.7 | 0 | 0.0 | 0 | 2 | 15 | 0.4 | 7 | 250 | 0.05 | 0.05 | 0.2 | 5 |
| 267. Lettuce, cos or romaine | 1 c chopped | 55 | 10 | 0.7 | 0 | 0.0 | 0 | 2 | 37 | 0.8 | 5 | 1,050 | 0.08 | 0.04 | 0.2 | 10 |
| 268. Liver, beef, fried | 1 slice 3 oz. | 85 | 195 | 22.0 | 9 | 2.5 | 345 | 5 | 9 | 7.5 | 156 | 45,390 | 0.22 | 3.56 | 14.0 | 23 |
| 269. Liverwurst, fresh | 1 slice 1 oz. | 28 | 87 | 5.0 | 7 | 3.5 | 50 | 1 | 3 | 1.5 | 0 | 1,800 | 0.06 | 0.37 | 1.6 | 0 |
| 270. Lobster | 1 c | 145 | 138 | 27.0 | 2 | 1.0 | 293 | 0 | 94 | 1.2 | 305 | 0 | 0.15 | 0.10 | 0.0 | 0 |
| 271. M&M's, Chocolate, plain | 1 oz. | 28 | 140 | 1.9 | 6 | 3.3 | 0 | 19 | 47 | 0.5 | 24 | 30 | 0.01 | 0.07 | 0.2 | 0 |

| Code | Food | Amount | Weight gm | Calo-ries | Pro-tein gm | Fat gm | Sat. Fat gm | Cho-les-terol mg | Car-bohy-drate gm | Cal-cium mg | Iron mg | Sodium mg | Vit A I.U. | Thia-min (Vit $B_1$) mg | Ribo-flavin (Vit $B_2$) mg | Niacin mg | Vit C mg |
|---|---|---|---|---|---|---|---|---|---|---|---|---|---|---|---|---|---|
| 272. | M&M's, Chocolate, w/peanuts | 1 oz. | 28 | 145 | 3.2 | 7 | 3.2 | 0 | 17 | 36 | 0.4 | 17 | 15 | 0.02 | 0.05 | 0.9 | 0 |
| 273. | Macaroni, enriched, cooked | 1/2 c | 70 | 78 | 2.4 | 0 | 0.0 | 0 | 16 | 6 | 0.7 | 1 | 0 | 0.10 | 0.06 | 0.8 | 0 |
| 274. | Macaroni and cheese | 1/2 c | 100 | 215 | 8.2 | 11 | 4.0 | 21 | 20 | 181 | 0.9 | 543 | 430 | 0.10 | 0.20 | 0.9 | 0 |
| 275. | Margarine | 1 tsp | 5 | 34 | 0.0 | 4 | 0.7 | 2 | 0 | 1 | 0.0 | 46 | 160 | 0.00 | 0.00 | 0.0 | 0 |
| 276. | Mars bar | 1 bar | 50 | 240 | 4.0 | 11 | 4.8 | 0 | 30 | 85 | 0.6 | 85 | 1 | 0.02 | 0.16 | 0.5 | 0 |
| 277. | Matzo | 1 piece | 30 | 117 | 3.0 | 0 | 0.0 | 0 | 25 | * | * | 0 | * | * | * | * | * |
| 278. | Mayonnaise | 1 tsp | 5 | 36 | 0.0 | 4 | 0.7 | 3 | 0 | 1 | 0.0 | 28 | 13 | 0.00 | 0.00 | 0.0 | 0 |
| 279. | Milk, chocolate, 2% | 1 c | 250 | 180 | 8.0 | 5 | 3.1 | 17 | 26 | 284 | 0.6 | 151 | 143 | 0.09 | 0.41 | 0.3 | 2 |
| 280. | Milk, evaporated whole | 1/2 c | 126 | 172 | 9.0 | 10 | 5.8 | 40 | 13 | 329 | 0.2 | 149 | 405 | 0.05 | 0.43 | 0.2 | 2 |
| 281. | Milk, lowfat 2% fat | 1 c | 246 | 145 | 10 | 5 | 3.1 | 5 | 15 | 352 | 0.1 | 150 | 200 | 0.10 | 0.52 | 0.2 | 2 |
| 282. | Milk shake, chocolate | 1 (10 fluid oz.) | 340 | 433 | 11.5 | 13 | 7.8 | 45 | 70 | 383 | 1.1 | 328 | 312 | 0.20 | 0.83 | 0.5 | 0 |
| 283. | Milk shake, Frosty, Wendy's | 16 oz. | 324 | 460 | 13 | 13 | 7.0 | 55 | 76 | 480 | 1.0 | 260 | 500 | 0.15 | 1.08 | 0.8 | 0 |
| 284. | Milk shake, strawberry | 1 (10 fluid oz.) | 340 | 383 | 11.4 | 10 | 6.0 | 37 | 64 | 384 | 0.4 | 281 | 418 | 0.14 | 0.61 | 0.5 | 4 |
| 285. | Milk shake, vanilla, McDonald's | 1 | 289 | 323 | 10 | 8 | 5.1 | 29 | 52 | 346 | 0.2 | 250 | 346 | 0.12 | 0.66 | 0.6 | 3 |
| 286. | Milk, skim | 1 c | 245 | 88 | 9.0 | 0 | 0.3 | 5 | 12 | 296 | 0.1 | 126 | 10 | 0.09 | 0.44 | 0.2 | 2 |
| 287. | Milk, whole 3.5% fat | 1 c | 244 | 159 | 9.0 | 9 | 5.1 | 34 | 12 | 288 | 0.1 | 120 | 350 | 0.07 | 0.40 | 0.2 | 2 |
| 288. | Milky Way bar | 1 bar | 60 | 260 | 3.2 | 9 | 5.4 | 14 | 43 | 86 | 0.5 | 140 | 125 | 0.03 | 0.15 | 0.2 | 1 |
| 289. | Molasses, medium | 1 tbsp | 20 | 50 | 0.0 | 0 | 0.0 | 0 | 13 | 33 | 0.9 | 3 | 0 | 0.01 | 0.01 | 0.0 | 0 |
| 290. | Muffin, apple bran, fat free, McDonald's | 1 | 75 | 180 | 5 | 0 | 0.0 | 0 | 40 | 48 | 0.7 | 200 | 0 | 0.15 | 0.18 | 2.0 | 0 |
| 291. | Muffin, blueberry | 1 | 45 | 135 | 3.0 | 5 | 1.5 | 19 | 20 | 54 | 0.9 | 198 | 40 | 0.10 | 0.11 | 0.9 | 1 |
| 292. | Muffin, bran | 1 | 45 | 125 | 3.0 | 6 | 1.4 | 24 | 19 | 60 | 1.4 | 189 | 230 | 0.11 | 0.13 | 1.3 | 3 |
| 293. | Muffin, cornmeal | 1 | 45 | 145 | 3.0 | 5 | 1.5 | 23 | 21 | 66 | 0.9 | 169 | 80 | 0.11 | 0.11 | 0.9 | 0 |
| 294. | Muffin, English, plain | 1 | 57 | 140 | 4.5 | 1 | 0.3 | 0 | 26 | 96 | 1.7 | 378 | 0 | 0.26 | 0.18 | 2.1 | 0 |
| 295. | Muffin, English w/butter | 1 | 63 | 186 | 5.0 | 5 | 2.3 | 15 | 30 | 117 | 1.5 | 310 | 164 | 0.28 | 0.49 | 2.6 | 1 |
| 296. | Mushrooms, fresh cultivated | 1/2 c sliced | 35 | 12 | 1.0 | 0 | 0.0 | 0 | 2 | 4 | 0.5 | 4 | 0 | 0.04 | 0.12 | 2.4 | 1 |
| 297. | Mustard greens, cooked drained | 1/2 c | 70 | 16 | 1.7 | 0 | 0.0 | 0 | 3 | 96 | 1.2 | 13 | 4,060 | 0.05 | 0.10 | 0.4 | 33 |
| 298. | Noodles, egg, enriched cooked | 1/2 c | 80 | 100 | 3.3 | 1 | 0.0 | 0 | 19 | 8 | 0.7 | 2 | 55 | 0.11 | 0.07 | 1.0 | 0 |
| 299. | Nuts, Brazil | 1 oz. (6-8 nuts) | 28 | 185 | 4.1 | 19 | 4.8 | 0 | 3 | 53 | 1.0 | 0 | 0 | 0.27 | 0.03 | 0.5 | 0 |
| 300. | Nuts, Pecans | 1 oz. | 28 | 195 | 2.6 | 20 | 1.4 | 0 | 4 | 21 | 0.7 | 0 | 40 | 0.24 | 0.04 | 0.3 | 1 |
| 301. | Nuts, Walnuts | 1 oz. (14 halves) | 28 | 185 | 4.2 | 18 | 1.0 | 0 | 5 | 28 | 0.9 | 1 | 10 | 0.09 | 0.04 | 0.3 | 1 |
| 302. | Oil, Corn | 1 tbsp. | 15 | 125 | 0.0 | 14 | 1.8 | 0 | 0 | 0 | 0.0 | 0 | 0 | 0.00 | 0.00 | 0.0 | 0 |
| 303. | Oil, Olive | 1 tbsp. | 15 | 125 | 0.0 | 14 | 1.9 | 0 | 0 | 0 | 0.0 | 0 | 0 | 0.00 | 0.00 | 0.0 | 0 |
| 304. | Oil, Safflower | 1 tbsp. | 15 | 125 | 0.0 | 14 | 1.3 | 0 | 0 | 0 | 0.0 | 0 | 0 | 0.00 | 0.00 | 0.0 | 0 |
| 305. | Oil, Soybean | 1 tsp. | 5 | 44 | 0.0 | 5 | 2.0 | 0 | 0 | 0 | 0.0 | 0 | 0 | 0.00 | 0.00 | 0.0 | 0 |
| 306. | Okra, cooked, drained | 1/2 c | 80 | 23 | 1.6 | 0 | 0.0 | 0 | 5 | 74 | 0.4 | 2 | 390 | 0.11 | 0.15 | 0.7 | 16 |
| 307. | Olives, black, ripe | 10 extra large | 55 | 61 | 0.5 | 7 | 1.0 | 0 | 1 | 40 | 0.8 | 385 | 30 | 0.00 | 0.00 | 0.0 | 0 |
| 308. | Onions, mature, | 1/2 c sliced | 105 | 31 | 1.3 | 0 | 0.0 | 0 | 7 | 25 | 0.4 | 8 | 40 | 0.03 | 0.03 | 0.2 | 8 |
| 309. | cooked, drained | | | | | | | | | | | | | | | | |
| 310. | Onion rings, fried | 3 | 30 | 122 | 1.6 | 8 | 2.3 | 0 | 11 | 9 | 0.5 | 113 | 68 | 0.08 | 0.04 | 1.1 | 0 |
| 311. | Onion rings (Brazier) Dairy Queen | 1 serving | 85 | 360 | 6.0 | 17 | 6.0 | 15 | 33 | 20 | 0.4 | 125 | 0 | 0.09 | 0.00 | 0.4 | 2 |
| 312. | Orange juice, froz. reconstituted | 1/2 c | 125 | 61 | 0.9 | 0 | 0.0 | 0 | 15 | 13 | 0.1 | 1 | 270 | 0.12 | 0.02 | 0.5 | 60 |
| 313. | Orange, raw (medium skin) | 1 med | 180 | 64 | 1.3 | 0 | 0.0 | 0 | 16 | 54 | 0.5 | 1 | 260 | 0.13 | 0.05 | 0.5 | 66 |

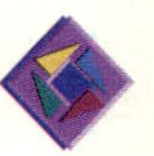

| | | | | | | | | | | | | | | | | |
|---|---|---|---|---|---|---|---|---|---|---|---|---|---|---|---|---|
| 314. Oysters, Eastern, breaded, fried | 1 oyster | 45 | 90 | 5.0 | 5 | 1.4 | 35 | 5 | 49 | 3.0 | 70 | 220 | 0.07 | 0.10 | 1.3 | 4 |
| 315. Oysters, raw, Eastern | 1/2 c (6-9 med) | 120 | 79 | 10.0 | 2 | 1.3 | 60 | 4 | 113 | 6.6 | 145 | 370 | 0.17 | 0.22 | 3.0 | 0 |
| 316. Pancakes | 1 6" diam x 1/2" thick | 73 | 169 | 5.2 | 5 | 1.0 | 36 | 25 | 74 | 0.9 | 310 | 90 | 0.12 | 0.16 | 0.9 | 0 |
| 317. Pancakes, buckwheat | 1 4 in. diam. | 27 | 55 | 2.0 | 2 | 0.9 | 20 | 6 | 59 | 0.4 | 125 | 17 | 0.04 | 0.05 | 0.2 | 0 |
| 318. Pancakes w/butter, syrup | 1 large | 100 | 250 | 4.0 | 5 | 1.9 | 24 | 47 | 1 | 1.1 | 535 | 160 | 0.13 | 0.18 | 1.1 | 2 |
| 319. Papaya, raw | 1/2 med | 227 | 60 | 0.9 | 0 | 0.0 | 0 | 15 | 31 | 0.5 | 5 | 2,660 | 0.06 | 0.06 | 0.5 | 85 |
| 320. Parsnips, cooked | 1 large 9" long | 160 | 106 | 2.4 | 1 | 0.0 | 0 | 24 | 72 | 1.0 | 13 | 50 | 0.11 | 0.13 | 0.2 | 16 |
| 321. Peaches, canned, heavy syrup | 1 half 2⅛ tbsp liq. | 96 | 75 | 0.4 | 0 | 0.0 | 0 | 19 | 4 | 0.3 | 2 | 410 | 0.01 | 0.02 | 0.6 | 3 |
| 322. Peaches, canned, juice pack | 1 half | 77 | 34 | 0.5 | 0 | 0.0 | 0 | 9 | 5 | 0.2 | 3 | 147 | 0.01 | 0.01 | 0.5 | 3 |
| 323. Peaches, raw, peeled | 1 2¾" diam. | 175 | 58 | 0.9 | 0 | 0.0 | 0 | 15 | 14 | 0.8 | 2 | 2,030 | 0.03 | 0.08 | 1.5 | 11 |
| 324. Peanut butter | 2 tbsp | 32 | 188 | 8.0 | 16 | 1.0 | 0 | 6 | 18 | 0.6 | 194 | 0 | 0.04 | 0.04 | 4.8 | 0 |
| 325. Peanut butter, jam sandwich | 1 | 100 | 340 | 11.4 | 14 | 2.6 | 0 | 45 | 87 | 2.3 | 414 | 1 | 0.32 | 0.22 | 5.3 | 0 |
| 326. Peanuts, roasted | 1 oz. | 28 | 166 | 7.0 | 14 | 1.0 | 0 | 5 | 21 | 0.6 | 119 | 0 | 0.09 | 0.04 | 4.9 | 0 |
| 327. Pears, canned, heavy syrup | 1 half 2¼ tbsp liq. | 103 | 78 | 0.2 | 0 | 0.0 | 0 | 20 | 5 | 0.2 | 1 | 0 | 0.01 | 0.02 | 0.1 | 1 |
| 328. Pears, canned, juice pack | 1 half | 77 | 38 | 0.3 | 0 | 0.0 | 0 | 10 | 7 | 0.2 | 3 | 3 | 0.01 | 0.01 | 0.2 | 1 |
| 329. Pears, raw | 1 pear | 180 | 100 | 1.1 | 1 | 0.0 | 0 | 25 | 13 | 0.5 | 2 | 30 | 0.03 | 0.07 | 0.2 | 7 |
| 330. Peas, canned, drained | 1/2 c | 85 | 75 | 4.0 | 0 | 0.0 | 0 | 14 | 22 | 1.6 | 200 | 585 | 0.08 | 0.05 | 0.7 | 7 |
| 331. Peas, frozen, cooked drained | 1/2 c | 80 | 55 | 4.1 | 0 | 0.0 | 0 | 10 | 15 | 1.5 | 92 | 480 | 0.22 | 0.07 | 1.4 | 11 |
| 332. Peppers, sweet, raw | 1 pepper 3¼" x 3" diam. | 200 | 36 | 2.0 | 0 | 0.0 | 0 | 8 | 15 | 1.1 | 21 | 690 | 0.13 | 0.13 | 0.8 | 210 |
| 333. Pickles, dill | 1 large 4" long | 135 | 15 | 0.9 | 0 | 0.0 | 0 | 3 | 35 | 1.4 | 1,928 | 140 | 0.00 | 0.03 | 0.0 | 8 |
| 334. Pickles, sweet | 1 large 3" long | 35 | 51 | 0.2 | 0 | 0.0 | 0 | 13 | 4 | 0.4 | 0 | 30 | 0.00 | 0.01 | 0.0 | 2 |
| 335. Pie, Apple | 1 piece (3½") | 118 | 302 | 2.6 | 13 | 3.5 | 120 | 45 | 9 | 0.4 | 355 | 40 | 0.02 | 0.02 | 0.5 | 1 |
| 336. Pie, Apple, fried | 1 pie | 85 | 255 | 2.2 | 14 | 5.8 | 14 | 32 | 12 | 0.9 | 326 | 15 | 0.09 | 0.06 | 1.0 | 1 |
| 337. Pie, Blueberry | 1 piece (3½") | 158 | 380 | 4.0 | 17 | 4.0 | 0 | 55 | 26 | 2.1 | 423 | 140 | 0.17 | 0.14 | 1.7 | 6 |
| 338. Pie, Cherry | 1 piece (3½") | 118 | 308 | 3.1 | 13 | 5.0 | 137 | 45 | 17 | 0.4 | 355 | 40 | 0.02 | 0.02 | 0.5 | 1 |
| 339 Pie, Cherry, fried | 1 pie | 85 | 250 | 2.0 | 14 | 5.8 | 13 | 32 | 11 | 0.7 | 371 | 95 | 0.06 | 0.06 | 0.6 | 1 |
| 340. Pie, Chocolate cream | 1 piece (1/6 pie) | 175 | 311 | 7.4 | 13 | 4.5 | 15 | 42 | 160 | 1.1 | 427 | 170 | 0.15 | 0.30 | 1.1 | 1 |
| 341. Pie, Lemon meringue | 1 piece (1/6 pie) | 140 | 355 | 4.7 | 14 | 3.5 | 137 | 53 | 25 | 1.4 | 395 | 330 | 0.10 | 0.14 | 0.8 | 4 |
| 342. Pie, Pecan | 1 piece (1/6 pie) | 138 | 583 | 6.3 | 24 | 3.9 | 13 | 92 | 35 | 1.9 | 304 | 206 | 0.22 | 0.17 | 1.1 | 0 |
| 343. Pie, Pumpkin | 1 (3½") | 114 | 241 | 4.6 | 13 | 3.0 | 70 | 28 | 58 | 0.6 | 244 | 2,810 | 0.03 | 0.11 | 0.6 | 0 |
| 344. Pineapple, canned, heavy syrup | 1/2 c | 128 | 95 | 0.4 | 0 | 0.0 | 0 | 25 | 14 | 0.4 | 2 | 65 | 0.10 | 0.03 | 0.3 | 9 |
| 345. Pineapple, canned, juice pack | 1/2 c | 125 | 75 | 0.5 | 0 | 0.0 | 0 | 20 | 17 | 0.3 | 1 | 24 | 0.12 | 0.24 | 0.3 | 12 |
| 346. Pineapple, raw | 1/2 c diced | 78 | 41 | 0.3 | 0 | 0.0 | 0 | 11 | 13 | 0.4 | 1 | 55 | 0.07 | 0.03 | 0.2 | 13 |
| 347. Pizza, Cheese, Thin 'n Crispy, Pizza Hut | 1/2 10" pie | * | 450 | 25.0 | 15 | 7.0 | 125 | 54 | 450 | 4.5 | 1,200 | 750 | 0.30 | 0.51 | 5.0 | 1 |
| 348. Pizza, Cheese, Thick 'n Chewy, Pizza Hut | 1/2 10" pie | * | 560 | 34.0 | 14 | 6.0 | 110 | 71 | 500 | 5.4 | 1,100 | 1,000 | 0.68 | 0.68 | 7.0 | 1 |
| 349. Plums, Japanese and hybrid, raw | 1 plum 2⅛" diam. | 70 | 32 | 0.3 | 0 | 0.0 | 0 | 8 | 8 | 0.3 | 1 | 160 | 0.02 | 0.02 | 0.3 | 4 |
| 350. Popcorn, cooked, oil | 1 c | 11 | 55 | 0.9 | 3 | 0.5 | 0 | 6 | 3 | 0.3 | 86 | 20 | 0.01 | 0.02 | 0.1 | 0 |
| 351. Popcorn, popped, plain, large kernel | 1 c | 6 | 12 | 0.8 | 0 | 0.0 | 0 | 5 | 1 | 0.2 | 0 | 0 | 0.00 | 0.01 | 0.1 | 0 |
| 352. Pork, roast, trimmed | 2 slices 3 oz. | 85 | 179 | 24.0 | 8 | 2.2 | 65 | 0 | 11 | 3.1 | 863 | 0 | 0.55 | 0.22 | 4.3 | 0 |
| 353. Pork, sausage, cooked | 1 sm link | 17 | 72 | 2.8 | 6 | 2.1 | 13 | 1 | 0 | 0.3 | 221 | 0 | 0.00 | 0.00 | 0.0 | 0 |
| 354. Potato, au gratin | 1 c | 245 | 228 | 5.6 | 10 | 6.3 | 12 | 32 | 203 | 0.8 | 1,076 | 380 | 0.05 | 0.20 | 2.3 | 8 |
| 355. Potato, baked in skin | 1 potato 2⅓ x 4¼" | 202 | 145 | 4.0 | 0 | 0.0 | 0 | 33 | 14 | 1.1 | 6 | 0 | 0.15 | 0.07 | 2.7 | 31 |
| 356. Potato chips | 10 chips | 20 | 114 | 1.1 | 8 | 2.1 | 0 | 10 | 8 | 0.4 | 150 | 0 | 0.04 | 0.01 | 1.0 | 3 |
| 357. Potato, French fried long | 10 strips 3½-4" | 78 | 214 | 3.4 | 10 | 1.7 | 0 | 28 | 12 | 1.0 | 5 | 0 | 0.10 | 0.06 | 2.4 | 16 |
| 358. Potato, Hashbrowns, McDonald's | 1 patty | 55 | 144 | 1.4 | 9 | 3.0 | 4 | 15 | 5 | 0.4 | 325 | 6 | 0.06 | 0.01 | 0.8 | 4 |

| Code | Food | Amount | Weight gm | Calo-ries | Pro-tein gm | Fat gm | Sat. Fat gm | Cho-les-terol mg | Car-bohy-drate gm | Cal-cium mg | Iron mg | Sodium mg | Vit A I.U. | Thia-min (Vit $B_1$) mg | Ribo-flavin (Vit $B_2$) mg | Niacin mg | Vit C mg |
|---|---|---|---|---|---|---|---|---|---|---|---|---|---|---|---|---|---|
| 359. | Potato, mashed, milk added | 1/2 c | 105 | 69 | 2.2 | 1 | 0.4 | 8 | 14 | 25 | 0.4 | 316 | 20 | 0.09 | 0.06 | 1.1 | 11 |
| 360. | Potato salad w/eggs, mayo | 1/2 c | 125 | 179 | 3.4 | 10 | 7.8 | 85 | 14 | 24 | 0.8 | 662 | 262 | 0.10 | 0.08 | 1.1 | 12 |
| 361. | Potato, hash brown | 1/2 c | 78 | 170 | 2.5 | 9 | 3.5 | 0 | 22 | 12 | 1.2 | 27 | 0 | 0.09 | 0.02 | 1.9 | 5 |
| 362. | Pretzel, thin, twists | 1 oz. | 28 | 113 | 2.8 | 1 | 0.3 | 0 | 23 | 8 | 0.6 | 456 | 0 | 0.09 | 0.07 | 1.2 | 0 |
| 363. | Prunes, dried “softenized” without pits | 5 prunes | 61 | 137 | 1.1 | 0 | 0.0 | 0 | 36 | 26 | 0.1 | 4 | 860 | 0.05 | 0.09 | 0.9 | 2 |
| 364. | Prune juice, canned or bottled | 1/2 c | 128 | 99 | 0.5 | 0 | 0.0 | 0 | 24 | 18 | 5.3 | 3 | 0 | 0.02 | 0.02 | 0.5 | 3 |
| 365. | Pudding, Chocolate, canned | 5 oz. | 142 | 205 | 3 | 11 | 9.5 | 1 | 30 | 74 | 1.2 | 285 | 155 | 0.04 | 0.17 | 0.6 | 0 |
| 366. | Pudding, Tapioca, canned | 5 oz. | 142 | 160 | 3 | 5 | 4.8 | 1 | 28 | 119 | 0.3 | 252 | 5 | 0.03 | 0.14 | 0.4 | 0 |
| 367. | Pudding, Vanilla, canned | 5 oz. | 142 | 220 | 2 | 10 | 9.5 | 1 | 33 | 79 | 0.2 | 305 | 1 | 0.03 | 0.12 | 0.6 | 0 |
| 368. | Quiche, Lorraine | 1 piece | 242 | 825 | 18 | 66 | 31.9 | 392 | 40 | 290 | 1.9 | 898 | 2,250 | 0.15 | 0.44 | 1.7 | 1 |
| 369. | Raisins, unbleached, seedless | 1 oz. | 28 | 82 | 0.7 | 0 | 0.0 | 0 | 22 | 18 | 1.0 | 8 | 10 | 0.03 | 0.02 | 0.1 | 0 |
| 370. | Raspberries, fresh | 1 c | 123 | 60 | 1.1 | 1 | 0.0 | 0 | 14 | 27 | 0.7 | 0 | 80 | 0.04 | 0.11 | 1.1 | 31 |
| 371. | Raspberries, frozen | 1 c | 250 | 255 | 1.7 | 1 | 0.0 | 0 | 62 | 38 | 1.6 | 3 | 75 | 0.05 | 0.11 | 1.5 | 41 |
| 372. | Rice, brown, cooked | 1/2 c | 96 | 116 | 2.5 | 1 | 0.0 | 0 | 25 | 12 | 0.5 | 275 | 0 | 0.09 | 0.02 | 1.3 | 0 |
| 373. | Rice, white enriched, cooked | 1/2 c | 103 | 113 | 2.1 | 0 | 0.0 | 0 | 25 | 11 | 0.9 | 384 | 0 | 0.12 | 0.01 | 1.1 | 0 |
| 374. | Rice, wild, cooked | 1/2 c | 100 | 92 | 3.6 | 0 | 0.0 | 0 | 19 | 5 | 1.1 | 2 | 0 | 0.11 | 0.16 | 1.6 | 0 |
| 375. | Roast Beef sand., Regular, Arby's | 1 | 155 | 383 | 22 | 18 | 7.0 | 43 | 35 | 72 | 3.2 | 936 | 0 | 0.28 | 0.50 | 11.0 | 0 |
| 376. | Roast Beef Sub, Arby's | 1 | 305 | 623 | 38 | 32 | 11.5 | 73 | 47 | 492 | 5.2 | 1,847 | 500 | 0.56 | 0.76 | 14.2 | 9 |
| 377. | Roll, hard, white | 1 roll | 50 | 155 | 5 | 2 | 0.0 | 0 | 30 | 24 | 1.4 | 313 | 0 | 0.20 | 0.12 | 1.7 | 0 |
| 378. | Reuben sandwich | 1 | 237 | 488 | 28.7 | 28 | 10.4 | 85 | 30 | 364 | 5.3 | 1,685 | 461 | 0.25 | 0.44 | 3.9 | 12 |
| 379. | Salad, Caesar side, Wendy's | 1 | 130 | 160 | 10 | 6 | 1.0 | 10 | 18 | 96 | 1.2 | 700 | 1,250 | 0.23 | 0.27 | 2.0 | 24 |
| 380. | Salad, Chef, Burger King | 1 serving | 273 | 178 | 17 | 9 | 4.0 | 103 | 7 | 128 | 1.6 | 568 | 4,750 | 0.35 | 0.26 | 3.6 | 15 |
| 381. | Salad, Chef, McDonald's | 1 | 265 | 170 | 17 | 9 | 4.0 | 111 | 8 | 180 | 1.0 | 400 | 5,000 | 0.30 | 0.27 | 4.0 | 21 |
| 382. | Salad, Chicken, Burger King | 1 serving | 258 | 142 | 20 | 4 | 1.0 | 49 | 8 | 32 | 1.3 | 443 | 4,600 | 0.14 | 0.17 | 8.5 | 20 |
| 383. | Salad, Chicken w/celery | 1/2 c | 78 | 266 | 10.5 | 25 | 4.1 | 48 | 1 | 16 | 0.7 | 199 | 153 | 0.03 | 0.08 | 3.3 | 1 |
| 384. | Salad, Deluxe Garden, Wendy's | 1 | 271 | 110 | 7 | 5 | 1.0 | 0 | 9 | 240 | 1.0 | 380 | 3,000 | 0.15 | 0.36 | 1.2 | 36 |
| 385. | Salad, Garden, Arby's | 1 | 330 | 117 | 7 | 5 | 2.7 | 12 | 11 | 192 | 1.1 | 134 | 4,900 | 0.17 | 0.20 | 1.2 | 52 |
| 386. | Salad, Grilled Chicken, Wendy's | 1 | 338 | 200 | 25 | 8 | 1.0 | 55 | 9 | 240 | 1.8 | 690 | 3,000 | 0.23 | 0.36 | 8.0 | 36 |
| 387. | Salad, Tuna | 1 c | 205 | 375 | 33 | 19 | 3.3 | 80 | 19 | 31 | 2.5 | 877 | 53 | 0.06 | 0.14 | 13.3 | 6 |
| 388. | Salami, dry | 1 oz. | 28 | 128 | 7.0 | 11 | 1.6 | 24 | 0 | 4 | 1.0 | 349 | 0 | 0.10 | 0.07 | 1.5 | 0 |
| 389. | Salmon, broiled with butter or margarine | 3 oz. | 85 | 156 | 23.0 | 6 | 2.2 | 53 | 0 | 0 | 0.9 | 99 | 150 | 0.15 | 0.06 | 8.4 | 0 |
| 390. | Salmon, canned Chinook | 3 oz. | 85 | 179 | 16.6 | 12 | 0.8 | 30 | 0 | 131 | 0.7 | 105 | 197 | 0.03 | 0.01 | 6.2 | 0 |
| 391. | Sardines, canned drained | 1 oz. | 28 | 58 | 7.0 | 3 | 1.0 | 20 | 0 | 124 | 0.8 | 233 | 60 | 0.01 | 0.06 | 1.5 | 0 |
| 392. | Sauerkraut, canned | 1/2 c | 118 | 21 | 1.2 | 0 | 0.0 | 0 | 5 | 43 | 0.6 | 878 | 60 | 0.04 | 0.05 | 0.3 | 17 |
| 393. | Sausage Biscuit w/Egg, McDonald's | 1 | 175 | 505 | 19 | 33 | 20.0 | 260 | 33 | 120 | 2.4 | 1,210 | 300 | 0.45 | 0.36 | 4.0 | 0 |
| 394. | Sausage McMuffin, McDonald's | 1 | 135 | 345 | 15 | 20 | 11.0 | 57 | 27 | 240 | 1.8 | 770 | 200 | 0.53 | 0.27 | 5.0 | 0 |
| 395. | Sausage McMuffin, w/Egg | 1 | 159 | 430 | 21 | 25 | 14.0 | 270 | 27 | 300 | 2.4 | 920 | 500 | 0.53 | 0.45 | 5.0 | 0 |
| 396. | Sausage, smoked link, pork | 1 | 68 | 265 | 15 | 22 | 7.7 | 46 | 1 | 20 | 0.8 | 1,020 | 0 | 1.04 | 0.29 | 5.0 | 14 |
| 397. | Scallops, breaded, cooked | 6 pieces | 90 | 195 | 15 | 10 | 2.5 | 70 | 10 | 39 | 2.0 | 298 | 105 | 0.11 | 0.11 | 1.6 | 0 |
| 398. | Sherbet | 1/2 c | 97 | 135 | 1.1 | 2 | 1.3 | 7 | 29 | 52 | 0.2 | 44 | 92 | 0.02 | 0.04 | 0.1 | 2 |
| 399. | Shrimp, boiled | 3 oz. | 85 | 99 | 18.0 | 1 | 0.1 | 128 | 1 | 99 | 2.7 | 0 | 60 | 0.00 | 0.03 | 1.5 | 0 |
| 400. | Shrimp, fried | 7 medium | 85 | 200 | 16.0 | 10 | 2.5 | 168 | 11 | 61 | 2.0 | 384 | 130 | 0.06 | 0.09 | 2.8 | 0 |
| 401. | Snickers bar | 1 bar | 61 | 290 | 6.6 | 4 | 5.4 | 0 | 37 | 70 | 0.5 | 170 | 25 | 0.03 | 0.11 | 1.8 | 0 |
| 402. | Soda pop, cola | 12 oz. | 369 | 144 | 0.0 | 0 | 0.0 | 0 | 37 | 27 | 0.0 | 30 | 0 | 0.00 | 0.00 | 0.0 | 0 |
| 403. | Soda pop, diet | 12 oz. | 340 | 2 | 0.1 | 0 | 0.0 | 0 | 0 | 13 | 0.1 | 31 | 0 | 0.00 | 0.00 | 0.0 | 0 |
| 404. | Soda pop, Ginger ale | 12 oz. | 366 | 113 | 0.0 | 0 | 0.0 | 0 | 29 | 0 | 0.0 | 45 | 0 | 0.00 | 0.00 | 0.0 | 0 |

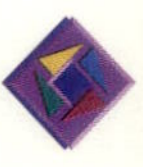

| Food | Measure | | | | | | | | | | | | | | | |
|---|---|---|---|---|---|---|---|---|---|---|---|---|---|---|---|---|
| 405. Soda pop, Lemon-lime | 12 oz. | 340 | 138 | 0.0 | 0 | 0.0 | 0 | 35 | 8 | 0.2 | 38 | 0 | 0.00 | 0.00 | 0.0 | 0 |
| 406. Soda pop, Root beer | 12 oz. | 340 | 140 | 0.0 | 0 | 0.0 | 0 | 36 | 17 | 0.2 | 45 | 0 | 0.00 | 0.00 | 0.0 | 0 |
| 407. Soup, Chicken, cream | 1 c | 248 | 191 | 7.5 | 12 | 4.6 | 27 | 15 | 180 | 0.7 | 1,046 | 710 | 0.07 | 0.26 | 0.9 | 1 |
| 408. Soup, Chicken noodle | 1 c | 241 | 75 | 4.0 | 2 | 0.7 | 7 | 9 | 17 | 0.8 | 900 | 711 | 0.05 | 0.06 | 1.4 | 0 |
| 409. Soup, Clam chowder, Manhattan | 1 c | 244 | 78 | 4.2 | 2 | 0.4 | 2 | 12 | 34 | 1.9 | 1,808 | 460 | 0.06 | 0.05 | 1.3 | 3 |
| 410. Soup, Clam chowder, north east | 1 c | 248 | 163 | 9.5 | 7 | 3.0 | 22 | 16 | 187 | 1.5 | 992 | 160 | 0.07 | 0.24 | 1.0 | 4 |
| 411. Soup, Cream of mushroom condensed, prepared with equal volume of milk | 1 c | 245 | 216 | 7.0 | 14 | 5.4 | 15 | 16 | 191 | 0.5 | 955 | 250 | 0.05 | 0.34 | 0.7 | 1 |
| 412. Soup, Minestrone | 1 c | 241 | 80 | 4.3 | 3 | 0.5 | 2 | 11 | 34 | 0.9 | 911 | 1,170 | 0.05 | 0.04 | 0.9 | 1 |
| 413. Soup, Split pea, condensed, prepared with equal volume of water | 1 c | 245 | 145 | 9.0 | 3 | 1.1 | 0 | 21 | 29 | 1.5 | 941 | 440 | 0.25 | 0.15 | 1.5 | 1 |
| 414. Soup, Tomato, condensed, prepared with equal volume of water | 1 c | 245 | 88 | 2.0 | 3 | 0.5 | 0 | 16 | 15 | 0.7 | 970 | 1,000 | 0.05 | 0.05 | 1.2 | 12 |
| 415. Soup, Tomato with milk | 1 c | 248 | 160 | 6.0 | 6 | 2.9 | 17 | 22 | 159 | 1.8 | 932 | 850 | 0.13 | 0.25 | 1.5 | 68 |
| 416. Soup, vegetable beef, condensed, prepared with equal volume of water | 1 c | 245 | 78 | 5.0 | 2 | 0.0 | 0 | 10 | 12 | 0.7 | 1,046 | 2,700 | 0.05 | 0.05 | 1.0 | 0 |
| 417. Soup, Vegetarian vegetable | 1 c | 250 | 70 | 2.1 | 2 | 0.3 | 0 | 12 | 21 | 1.1 | 823 | 1,505 | 0.05 | 0.05 | 0.9 | 1 |
| 418. Sour cream | 1 tbsp | 14 | 30 | 0.4 | 3 | 1.8 | 6 | 1 | 16 | 0.0 | 8 | 135 | 0.01 | 0.02 | 0.0 | 0 |
| 419. Soup cream, imitation | 1 tbsp. | 14 | 29 | 0.3 | 3 | 2.5 | 0 | 1 | 0 | 0.0 | 14 | 0 | 0.00 | 0.00 | 0.0 | 0 |
| 420. Spaghetti, in tomato sauce with cheese | 1 c | 250 | 260 | 8.8 | 9 | 2.0 | 10 | 37 | 80 | 2.3 | 955 | 1,080 | 0.25 | 0.18 | 2.3 | 13 |
| 421. Spaghetti, plain, cooked | 1 c | 140 | 155 | 5.0 | 1 | 0.1 | 0 | 32 | 11 | 1.7 | 1 | 0 | 0.20 | 0.11 | 1.5 | 0 |
| 422. Spaghetti, whole wheat, cooked | 1 c | 125 | 151 | 6.6 | 1 | 0.1 | 0 | 32 | 19 | 1.1 | 16 | 0 | 0.21 | 0.09 | 1.5 | 0 |
| 423. Spaghetti, with meatballs and tomato sauce | 1 c | 248 | 332 | 18.6 | 11.7 | 3.0 | 75 | 39 | 124 | 3.7 | 1,009 | 1,590 | 0.25 | 0.30 | 4.0 | 22 |
| 424. Spareribs, cooked | 3 oz. | 85 | 377 | 17.8 | 33 | 12.0 | 73 | 0 | 8 | 2.2 | 31 | 0 | 0.37 | 0.18 | 2.9 | 0 |
| 425. Spinach, canned, drained | 1/2 c | 103 | 25 | 2.3 | 1 | 0.0 | 0 | 4 | 121 | 2.6 | 242 | 8,200 | 0.02 | 0.12 | 0.3 | 15 |
| 426. Spinach, frozen, cooked, drained | 1/2 c | 103 | 24 | 3.1 | 0 | 0.0 | 0 | 4 | 116 | 2.2 | 54 | 8,100 | 0.07 | 0.16 | 0.4 | 20 |
| 427. Spinach, raw, chopped | 1 c | 55 | 14 | 1.8 | 0 | 0.0 | 0 | 2 | 51 | 1.7 | 39 | 4,460 | 0.06 | 0.11 | 0.3 | 28 |
| 428. Squash, summer, cooked | 1/2 c | 90 | 13 | 0.8 | 0 | 0.0 | 0 | 3 | 23 | 0.4 | 1 | 350 | 0.05 | 0.07 | 0.7 | 9 |
| 429. Squash, winter, baked mashed | 1/2 c | 103 | 70 | 1.9 | 0 | 0.0 | 0 | 18 | 41 | 1.0 | 1 | 6,560 | 0.05 | 0.14 | 0.7 | 8 |
| 430. Strawberries, frozen, sweetened | 1 c | 250 | 245 | 1.4 | 0 | 0.0 | 0 | 66 | 28 | 1.5 | 8 | 31 | 0.04 | 0.13 | 1.0 | 106 |
| 431. Strawberries, raw | 1 c | 149 | 55 | 1.0 | 1 | 0.0 | 0 | 13 | 31 | 1.5 | 1 | 90 | 0.04 | 0.10 | 0.9 | 88 |
| 432. Stuffing, bread, prepared | 1/2 c | 70 | 250 | 4.6 | 15 | 3.1 | 0 | 25 | 46 | 1.1 | 627 | 455 | 0.09 | 0.10 | 1.3 | 0 |
| 433. Sundae, choc. Dairy Queen | medium | 184 | 300 | 6.0 | 7 | 4.9 | 79 | 53 | 200 | 1.1 | 175 | 300 | 0.06 | 0.26 | 0.0 | 0 |
| 434. Sugar, brown granulated | 1 tsp | 5 | 17 | 0.0 | 0 | 0.0 | 0 | 5 | 4 | 0.1 | 0 | 0 | 0.00 | 0.00 | 0.1 | 0 |
| 435. Sugar, white granulated | 1 tsp | 4 | 15 | 0.0 | 0 | 0.0 | 0 | 4 | 0 | 0.0 | 0 | 0 | 0.00 | 0.00 | 0.0 | 0 |
| 436. Super Roast Beef, Arby's | 1 | 254 | 552 | 24 | 28 | 7.6 | 43 | 54 | 108 | 4.3 | 1,174 | 150 | 0.39 | 0.61 | 12.4 | 9 |
| 437. Sweet N' Sour Sauce, McDonald's | 1.12 oz. | 32 | 60 | 0 | 0.2 | 0.1 | 0 | 14 | 0 | 0 | 190 | 300 | 0.00 | 0.00 | 0.0 | 0 |
| 438. Sweet potato, baked | 1 potato 5" long | 146 | 161 | 2.4 | 1 | 0.0 | 0 | 37 | 46 | 1.0 | 14 | 9,230 | 0.10 | 0.08 | 0.8 | 25 |
| 439. Syrup (maple) | 1 tbsp | 20 | 50 | 0.0 | 0 | 0.0 | 0 | 13 | 33 | 0.2 | 3 | 0 | 0.00 | 0.00 | 0.0 | 0 |
| 440. Taco Salad, Wendy's | 1 | 510 | 640 | 34 | 30 | 12.0 | 80 | 70 | 540 | 5.4 | 960 | 1,750 | 0.23 | 0.45 | 3.0 | 27 |
| 441. Taco shell | 1 shell | 10 | 60 | 1.1 | 3 | 0.3 | 0 | 9 | 26 | 0.3 | 62 | 36 | 0.00 | 0.01 | 0.3 | 0 |
| 442. Taco, Taco Bell | 1 | 83 | 186 | 15.0 | 8 | 0.0 | 0 | 14 | 120 | 2.4 | 79 | 120 | 0.09 | 0.16 | 2.9 | 0 |
| 443. Tangerine | 1 med 2⅛" diam. | 116 | 39 | 0.7 | 0 | 0.0 | 0 | 10 | 34 | 0.3 | 2 | 360 | 0.05 | 0.02 | 0.1 | 27 |
| 444. Tartar sauce | 1 tbsp. | 14 | 74 | 0.2 | 8 | 1.2 | 4 | 1 | 3 | 0.1 | 182 | 54 | 0.00 | 0.00 | 0.0 | 0 |
| 445. Tea, brewed | 1/4 c | 180 | 0 | 0.0 | 0 | 0.0 | 0 | 0 | 0 | 0.0 | 0 | 0 | 0.00 | 0.00 | 0.0 | 0 |

| Code | Food | Amount | Weight gm | Calo-ries | Pro-tein gm | Fat gm | Sat. Fat gm | Cho-les-terol mg | Car-bohy-drate gm | Cal-cium mg | Iron mg | Sodium mg | Vit A I.U. | Thia-min (Vit $B_1$) mg | Ribo-flavin (Vit $B_2$) mg | Niacin mg | Vit C mg |
|---|---|---|---|---|---|---|---|---|---|---|---|---|---|---|---|---|---|
| 446. | Tomato juice, canned | 1 c | 244 | 42 | 1.9 | 0 | 0.1 | 0 | 10 | 22 | 1.4 | 881 | 1,357 | 0.12 | 0.08 | 1.6 | 45 |
| 447. | Tomato sauce (catsup) | 1 tbsp | 15 | 16 | 0.3 | 0 | 0.0 | 0 | 4 | 3 | 0.1 | 156 | 105 | 0.01 | 0.01 | 0.2 | 2 |
| 448. | Tomato, canned | 1/2 c | 121 | 26 | 1.2 | 0 | 0.0 | 0 | 5 | 7 | 0.6 | 157 | 1,085 | 0.06 | 0.04 | 0.9 | 21 |
| 449. | Tomato, raw | 1 tomato 3½ oz. | 100 | 20 | 1.0 | 0 | 0.0 | 0 | 4 | 12 | 0.5 | 3 | 820 | 0.05 | 0.04 | 0.6 | 21 |
| 450. | Tortilla chips | 1 oz. | 28 | 139 | 2.2 | 8 | 1.1 | 0 | 17 | 82 | 1.0 | 140 | 7 | 0.01 | 0.02 | 0.2 | 0 |
| 451. | Tortilla, corn, lime | 1 6" diam. | 30 | 63 | 1.5 | 1 | 0.0 | 0 | 14 | 60 | 0.9 | 0 | 6 | 0.04 | 0.02 | 0.3 | 0 |
| 452. | Tortilla, flour | 1 | 35 | 105 | 2.6 | 3 | 0.4 | 0 | 19 | 21 | 0.5 | 134 | 0 | 0.13 | 0.08 | 1.2 | 0 |
| 453. | Tostada | 1 | 148 | 206 | 9.2 | 18 | 3.0 | 14 | 25 | 167 | 1.8 | 200 | 445 | 0.06 | 0.13 | 0.8 | 6 |
| 454. | Trout, broiled w/butter, lemon | 3 oz. | 85 | 175 | 21.0 | 9 | 4.1 | 71 | 0 | 26 | 1.0 | 122 | 300 | 0.07 | 0.07 | 2.3 | 1 |
| 455. | Tuna, canned, oil pack, drained | 3 oz. | 85 | 167 | 25.0 | 7 | 1.7 | 60 | 0 | 7 | 1.6 | 0 | 70 | 0.04 | 0.10 | 10.1 | 0 |
| 456. | Tuna, canned, water pack, solids and liquid | 3½ oz. | 99 | 126 | 27.7 | 1 | 0.0 | 55 | 0 | 16 | 1.6 | 161 | 0 | 0.00 | 0.10 | 13.2 | 0 |
| 457. | Turkey, Lite Roast Deluxe, Arby' | 1 | 195 | 260 | 20 | 6 | 1.6 | 33 | 33 | 156 | 2.3 | 1,262 | 200 | 0.29 | 0.43 | 15.4 | 12 |
| 458. | Turkey, roast (light and dark mixed) | 3 oz. | 85 | 162 | 27.0 | 5 | 1.5 | 73 | 0 | 7 | 1.5 | 111 | 0 | 0.04 | 0.15 | 6.5 | 0 |
| 459. | Turnip, cooked, drained | 1/2 c cubed | 78 | 18 | 0.6 | 0 | 0.0 | 0 | 4 | 27 | 0.3 | 27 | 0 | 0.03 | 0.04 | 0.3 | 17 |
| 460. | Turnip greens, cooked drained | 1/2 c | 73 | 19 | 2.1 | 0 | 0.0 | 0 | 3 | 98 | 1.3 | 14 | 5,695 | 0.04 | 0.08 | 0.4 | 16 |
| 461. | Veal, cooked loin | 3 oz. | 85 | 199 | 22.0 | 11 | 4.0 | 90 | 0 | 9 | 2.7 | 55 | 0 | 0.06 | 0.21 | 4.6 | 0 |
| 462. | Veal cutlet, braised, broiled | 3 oz. | 85 | 185 | 23.0 | 9 | 4.0 | 109 | 0 | 9 | 0.8 | 56 | 5 | 0.06 | 0.21 | 4.6 | 0 |
| 463. | Vegetables, mixed, cooked | 1 c | 182 | 116 | 5.8 | 0 | 0.0 | 0 | 24 | 46 | 2.4 | 348 | 4,505 | 0.02 | 0.13 | 2.0 | 15 |
| 464. | Waffles | 1 waffle | 75 | 205 | 6.9 | 8 | 2.7 | 59 | 27 | 179 | 1.2 | 515 | 49 | 0.14 | 0.23 | 0.9 | 0 |
| 465. | Watermelon | 1 c diced | 160 | 42 | 0.8 | 0 | 0.0 | 0 | 10 | 11 | 0.8 | 2 | 940 | 0.05 | 0.05 | 0.3 | 11 |
| 466. | Wheat germ, plain toasted | 1 tbsp | 6 | 23 | 1.8 | 1 | 0.0 | 0 | 3 | 3 | 0.5 | 0 | 10 | 0.11 | 0.05 | 0.3 | 1 |
| 467. | Whiskey, gin, rum, vodka 90 proof | 1/2 11 oz (jigger) | 42 | 110 | 0 | 0 | 0.0 | 0 | 0 | 0 | 0.0 | 0 | 0 | 0.00 | 0.00 | 0.0 | 0 |
| 468. | Whopper, Burger King | 1 sandwich | 270 | 614 | 27.0 | 36 | 12.0 | 90 | 45 | 64 | 4.9 | 865 | 550 | 0.34 | 0.41 | 6.1 | 12 |
| 469. | Whopper with cheese, Burger King | 1 sandwich | 294 | 706 | 32.0 | 44 | 16.0 | 115 | 47 | 176 | 4.9 | 1,177 | 950 | 0.34 | 0.48 | 6.1 | 12 |
| 470. | Whopper, double, Burger King | 1 sandwich | 351 | 844 | 46.0 | 53 | 19.0 | 169 | 45 | 72 | 7.2 | 933 | 550 | 0.35 | 0.56 | 9.4 | 12 |
| 471. | Wine, dry table 12% alc. | 3½ fl. oz. | 102 | 87 | 0.1 | 0 | 0.0 | 0 | 4 | 9 | 0.4 | 5 | 0 | 0.00 | 0.01 | 0.1 | 0 |
| 472. | Wine, red dry 18.8% alc. | 2 oz. | 59 | 81 | 0.1 | 0 | 0.0 | 0 | 5 | 5 | 0.0 | 4 | 0 | 0.01 | 0.02 | 0.2 | 0 |
| 473. | Yeast, brewers | 1 tbsp | 8 | 23 | 3.1 | 0 | 0.0 | 0 | 3 | 17 | 1.4 | 10 | 0 | 1.25 | 0.34 | 3.0 | 0 |
| 474. | Yogurt, fruit | 1 c | 227 | 231 | 9.9 | 2 | 1.6 | 10 | 43 | 345 | 0.2 | 125 | 104 | 0.08 | 0.40 | 0.2 | 2 |
| 475. | Yogurt, nonfat, TCBY | 4 oz. | 113 | 110 | 4 | 0 | 0 | 0 | 23 | 96 | 0 | 45 | 0 | 0.03 | 0.14 | 0 | 0 |
| 476. | Yogurt, plain low fat | 1 8-oz. container | 226 | 113 | 7.7 | 4 | 2.3 | 15 | 12 | 271 | 0.1 | 115 | 150 | 0.09 | 0.41 | 0.2 | 2 |
| 477. | Yogurt, regular, TCBY | 4 oz. | 113 | 120 | 4 | 3 | 2.0 | 13 | 23 | 180 | 0.5 | 60 | 0 | 0.06 | 0.18 | 0 | 0 |
| 478. | Yogurt, sugar free, TCBY | 4 oz. | 113 | 80 | 4 | 0 | 0 | 0 | 18 | 96 | 0 | 40 | 200 | 0.06 | 0.18 | 0 | 0 |
| 479. | Yogurt, vanilla lowfat, McDonald's | 3 oz. | 85 | 105 | 4 | 1 | 0.3 | 3 | 22 | 120 | 0 | 80 | 100 | 0.03 | 0.18 | 0.4 | 0 |

"0" represents both less than 1 and 0

Sources:

Nutritive Value of American Foods in Common Units. *Agriculture Handbook No. 456*. U.S. Dept. of Agriculture. Washington, D.C. 1988.

Young, E. A., E. H. Brennan, and C. L. Irving, Guest Eds. Perspectives on Fast Foods. *Public Health Currents*, 19(1), 1979, Published by Ross Laboratories, Columbus, OH.

Dennison, D. *The Dine System: the Nutrition Plan For Better Health*. C. V. Mosby Company St. Louis, Missouri, 1982.

Pennington, S. A. T. and H. N. Church. *Food Values of Portions Commonly Used*. Harper and Row Publishers, New York, 1985.

Kullman, D. A. *ABC Milligram Cholesterol Diet Guide*. Merit Publications, Inc. North Miami Beach, Florida 1978.

Food Processor nutrient analysis software by Esha Corporation, P.O. Box 13028, Salem, Oregon, 97309. With permission.

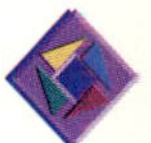

Date: ____________________

| Foods | Amount | Calories | Protein (gm) | Fat (total) (gm) | Sat. Fat (gm) | Cho-lesterol (mg | Carbo-hydrates (gm) | Cal-cium (mg) | Iron (mg) | Sodium (mg) | Vit. A (I.U.) | Vit. $B_1$ (I.U.) | Vit. $B_2$ (mg) | Niacin (mg) | Vit. C (mg) |
|---|---|---|---|---|---|---|---|---|---|---|---|---|---|---|---|
| | | | | | | | | | | | | | | | |
| | | | | | | | | | | | | | | | |
| | | | | | | | | | | | | | | | |
| | | | | | | | | | | | | | | | |
| | | | | | | | | | | | | | | | |
| | | | | | | | | | | | | | | | |
| | | | | | | | | | | | | | | | |
| | | | | | | | | | | | | | | | |
| | | | | | | | | | | | | | | | |
| | | | | | | | | | | | | | | | |
| | | | | | | | | | | | | | | | |
| | | | | | | | | | | | | | | | |
| | | | | | | | | | | | | | | | |
| | | | | | | | | | | | | | | | |
| | | | | | | | | | | | | | | | |
| | | | | | | | | | | | | | | | |
| | | | | | | | | | | | | | | | |
| | | | | | | | | | | | | | | | |
| | | | | | | | | | | | | | | | |
| | | | | | | | | | | | | | | | |
| | | | | | | | | | | | | | | | |
| | | | | | | | | | | | | | | | |
| Totals | | | | | | | | | | | | | | | |

(Make additional copies of this form for three-day analysis.)

**FIGURE B.1** ◆ Daily nutrient intake.

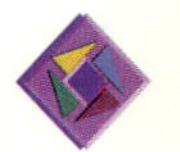

Name: ____________________

| Day | Calories | Protein (gm) | Fat (gm) | Sat. Fat (gm) | Chol-esterol (mg) | Carbo-hydrates (gm) | Calcium (mg) | Iron (mg) | Sodium (mg) | Vit. A (I.U.) | Thiamin Vit. $B_1$ (mg) | Riboflavin Vit. $B_2$ (mg) | Niacin (mg) | Vit. C (mg) |
|---|---|---|---|---|---|---|---|---|---|---|---|---|---|---|
| One | | | | | | | | | | | | | | |
| Two | | | | | | | | | | | | | | |
| Three | | | | | | | | | | | | | | |
| Totals | | | | | | | | | | | | | | |
| Average[a] | | | | | | | | | | | | | | |
| Percentages[b] | | | | | | | | | | | | | | |
| Recommended Dietary Allowances* | | | | | | | | | | | | | | |
| Men 15–18 yrs.below[c] | See below[d] | See | <30%[e] | <10%[e] | <300[e] | 58%>[e] | 1,200 | 12 | 2,400[e] | 5,000 | 1.5 | 1.8 | 20 | 60 |
| Men 19–24 yrs. | ↓ | ↓ | <30%[e] | <10%[e] | <300[e] | 58%>[e] | 1,200 | 10 | 2,400[e] | 5,000 | 1.5 | 1.7 | 19 | 60 |
| Men 25–50 yrs. | ↓ | ↓ | <30%[e] | <10%[e] | <300[e] | 58%>[e] | 800 | 10 | 2,400[e] | 5,000 | 1.5 | 1.7 | 19 | 60 |
| Men 51+ yrs. | ↓ | ↓ | <30%[e] | <10%[e] | <300[e] | 58%>[e] | 800 | 10 | 2,400[e] | 5,000 | 1.2 | 1.4 | 15 | 60 |
| Women 15–18 yrs. | ↓ | ↓ | <30%[e] | <10%[e] | <300[e] | 58%>[e] | 1,200 | 15 | 2,400[e] | 4,000 | 1.1 | 1.3 | 15 | 60 |
| Women 19–24 yrs. | ↓ | ↓ | <30%[e] | <10%[e] | <300[e] | 58%>[e] | 1,200 | 15 | 2,400[e] | 4,000 | 1.1 | 1.3 | 15 | 60 |
| Women 25–50 yrs. | ↓ | ↓ | <30%[e] | <10%[e] | <300[e] | 58%>[e] | 800 | 15 | 2,400[e] | 4,000 | 1.1 | 1.3 | 15 | 60 |
| Women 51+ yrs. | ↓ | ↓ | <30%[e] | <10%[e] | <300[e] | 58%>[e] | 800 | 10 | 2,400[e] | 4,000 | 1.0 | 1.2 | 13 | 60 |
| Pregnant | ↓ | ↓ | <30%[e] | <10%[e] | <300[e] | 58%>[e] | 1,200 | 30 | 2,400[e] | 4,000 | 1.5 | 1.6 | 17 | 70 |
| Lactating | ↓ | ↓ | <30%[e] | <10%[e] | <300[e] | 58%>[e] | 1,200 | 15 | 2,400[e] | 6,000 | 1.6 | 1.8 | 20 | 95 |

[a]Divide totals by 3 or number of days assessed.

[b]Percentages: Protein and Carbohydrates = multiply average by 4, divide by average calories, and multiply by 100,
Fat and Saturated Fat = multiply average by 9, divide by average calories, and multiply by 100.

[c]Use Table 8.1 (Chapter 8) for all categories.

[d]Protein intake should be .8 grams per kilogram of body weight. Pregnant women should consume an additional 15 grams of daily protein, while lactating women should have an extra 20 grams.

[e]Based on recommendations by nutrition experts.

*Adapted from *Recommended Dietary Allowances*, © 1989, by the National Academy of Sciences, National Academy Press, Washington, D.C.

**FIGURE B.2** ◆ Three-day nutritional analysis.

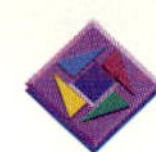

Date: ______________________

Name: ______________________ Age: __________ Weight: __________

Sex: Male–M, Female–F (Pregnant–P, Lactating–L, Neither–N)

Activity Rating: Sedentary (limited physical activity) = 1
Moderate physical activity = 2
Hard labor (strenuous physical activity = 3

Number of days to be analyzed: __________ Day: __________

| No. | Code* | Food | Amount |
|---|---|---|---|
| 1 | | | |
| 2 | | | |
| 3 | | | |
| 4 | | | |
| 5 | | | |
| 6 | | | |
| 7 | | | |
| 8 | | | |
| 9 | | | |
| 10 | | | |
| 11 | | | |
| 12 | | | |
| 13 | | | |
| 14 | | | |
| 15 | | | |
| 16 | | | |
| 17 | | | |
| 18 | | | |
| 19 | | | |
| 20 | | | |
| 21 | | | |
| 22 | | | |
| 23 | | | |
| 24 | | | |
| 25 | | | |
| 26 | | | |
| 27 | | | |
| 28 | | | |
| 29 | | | |
| 30 | | | |
| 31 | | | |

*When done, to advance to the next day or end, type 0 (zero).

**FIGURE B.3** ◆ Daily nutrient intake form for computer software use (make additional copies as necessary).

# Health Protection Plan for Environmental Hazards, Crime Prevention, and Personal Safety*

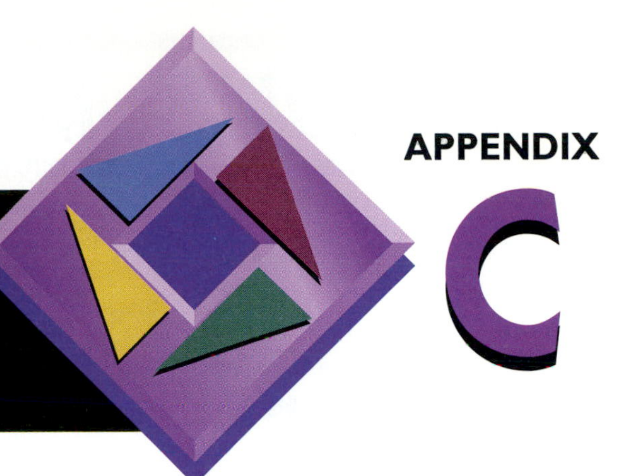


* Questionnaire published by the Preventive Medicine Institute/Strang Clinic. New York, 1982. Reproduced with permission.

# Personal Environment

*In addition to environmental problems in the community at large there are also important problems in our own immediate environment that affect our health, well-being, and comfort. These are problems we can control and improve ourselves.*

*The following self-assessment relates to environmental hazards dealing with water, wastes, noise and air pollution in our everyday lives.*

*All "no" answers are a cue to ACTION.*

| Concerning AIR POLLUTION, do you...? | YES | NO |
|---|---|---|
| ...Know the optimal conditions for temperature, humidity and air movement in your home? | ○ | ○ |
| ...Change the air filters once a year in your air conditioners or forced air heating systems? | ○ | ○ |
| ...Are your work areas ventilated so that fumes and dusts do not accumulate? | ○ | ○ |
| ...Do your throat or nasal passages feel moist and clear in the morning (not dry or stuffy)? | ○ | ○ |
| ...Know what to do when the weather report says the quality of the air is unsatisfactory? | ○ | ○ |
| ...Know what a "killer smog" is? | ○ | ○ |
| ...If you smoke, do you avoid smoking in a bedroom or areas where children play? | ○ | ○ |

## *RISK FACTORS:*

- *Bronchitis, asthma, emphysema, and heart disease are all aggravated by air pollution.*
- *Chronic exposure to dusts of metal or wood are risk factors for cancer of the respiratory passages.*
- *Children of cigarette smokers have a higher than usual incidence of respiratory infections.*
- *Many so-called allergies of the sinuses and upper respiratory tract are really due to air pollution.*

## *AWARENESS COUNTS:*

- **The optimal air comfort levels are 66-68°F temperature, 30-40% humidity, and air movement at 20-50 feet per minute. Lower humidity will lead to dryness of the respiratory passages, increase skin evaporation and make your home feel colder than it is.**
- **When the air quality is reported as "unsatisfactory" people with heart and lung disease should stay indoors.**
- **"Killer smog" refers to trapped air which cannot rise, with no available dispersing breeze, which accumulates industrial, auto and heating combustion products into a suffocating density. This may be fatal to those with cardiopulmonary disease, and uncomfortable for everyone.**

| Concerning WATER...? | YES | NO |
|---|---|---|
| ...Have you checked your home drinking water in the last year for clarity, color and taste? | ○ | ○ |
| ...If you shake up a glass of tap water does it remain clear (not foamy or frothy)? | ○ | ○ |
| ...Do you have a screen filter on your water tap? | ○ | ○ |
| ...Do you check restaurant water and ice for clarity and cleanliness? | ○ | ○ |
| ...Do you know the common water-borne diseases? | ○ | ○ |
| ...Do you know what kind of water purification tablets are best for traveling? | ○ | ○ |
| ...Do you take care when traveling in developing countries or in unsettled areas to drink bottled water, or coffee, tea, or soup made with boiling water, and to avoid ice cubes? | ○ | ○ |
| ...Do you think all wilderness water is safe? | ○ | ○ |
| ...Do you know what source of water is almost always safe to drink? | ○ | ○ |

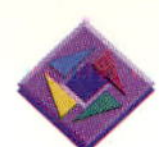

| Concerning WASTE...? | YES | NO |
|---|---|---|
| ...Do you place ordinary kitchen waste in plastic bags for disposal? | ○ | ○ |
| ...Do you know what kinds of wastes require special handling? | ○ | ○ |
| ...Are your garbage cans free from bad odors? | ○ | ○ |
| ...Is your sink or toilet bowl free from bad odors or back up of waste water in your drain? | ○ | ○ |
| ...If you live in a home with a septic tank do you know its location? | ○ | ○ |
| ...Do you know the last time the septic tank was cleaned? | ○ | ○ |

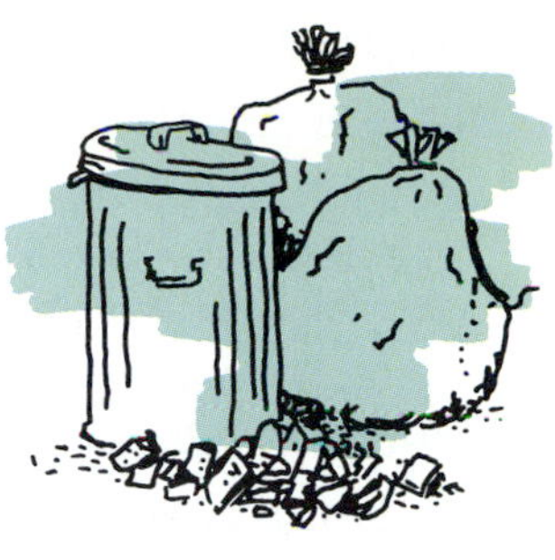

## *RISK FACTORS:* WATER AND WASTE

- *Diseases associated with water and waste include: typhoid fever, cholera, hepatitis, poliomyelitis, E. coli dysentery and amoebic dysentery.*
- *Very hard water containing large amounts of magnesium can cause diarrhea in children. It is difficult to wash with, and will cause deposits in water pipes.*
- *Chlorine is commonly used for water purification. An excess is harmful since it may be converted into chloroform, a toxic chemical.*
- *The presence of water supplies in proximity to industrial plants is a cause for concern since there are many instances of toxic chemicals leaking into local water supplies in this country.*

## *AWARENESS COUNTS:* WATER

- **All water taps should have screen filters to trap particulate material which may accidentally enter the water supply. These should be removed and cleaned regularly.**
- **Frothy water is due to detergents leaking into the water supply and this can cause intestinal upsets.**
- **Cloudy water may be due only to rusty pipes and while it may stain kitchen utensils it is not harmful; but turbid water with an odor may be due to seepage of sewage or industrial wastes into the water supply and this can be dangerous to health. Every state has a water supply agency that can give you information on the condition of your local water supply. However, if your water comes from a well, no one is checking it for purity. You must take the initiative and find out from the state agency how this can be done.**
- **The best type of water purification tablets is the iodine-releasing variety rather than the chlorine type. These are obtainable from your local pharmacy. Use these only if traveling in an area where bottled water is not available.**
- **Not all wilderness water is pure. It may come from springs which have toxic chemicals, or be contaminated by animal use upstream. If purified water is not available, the safest water to drink is rain water. (Make sure it is stored in a clean container.)**

## *AWARENESS COUNTS:* WASTE

- **Plastic bags for disposal of ordinary wastes have the advantage of keeping your garbage containers, indoor and outdoor, clean and free of odors. This helps prevent fly, roach, and rodent infestation, and the accidental contamination of food.**
- **Aerosol cans, solvents, and fuels should not be placed in plastic bags, and should not be disposed of with household wastes because of the hazards of fire and explosion; your local waste disposal service should be contacted regarding special handling.**
- **Bad odors or backup of waste water into your sink, tub, or toilet is a serious matter since this is untreated sewage and poses a health hazard. There may be an obstruction in the sewage system; check with your plumber first. If you have a septic tank, it may have to be cleaned. The frequency of cleaning of septic tanks depends on size and use. Three to four years of regular use is an average duration of time before cleaning is necessary.**
- **It's important to know the location of your septic tank and also those of your neighbors in relationship to your well water supply. There should be a distance of 100 feet between the septic tank and well. Your board of health can give you additional information about specific conditions in your area.**

| Concerning NOISE...? | YES | NO |
|---|---|---|
| ...Do you know how to tell if you are in an environment which could damage your hearing? | ○ | ○ |
| ...Do you know that permanent hearing loss can occur with a single exposure to a painfully loud noise? | ○ | ○ |
| ...Are you aware of the other effects on your health that noise can have other than hearing loss? | ○ | ○ |
| ...Do you know the accidents that can occur due to noise causing "warning concealment"? | ○ | ○ |
| ...Are you aware of "slow reaction time" as a noise associated danger? | ○ | ○ |
| ... Do you know what age group is especially susceptible to noise induced hearing loss? | ○ | ○ |

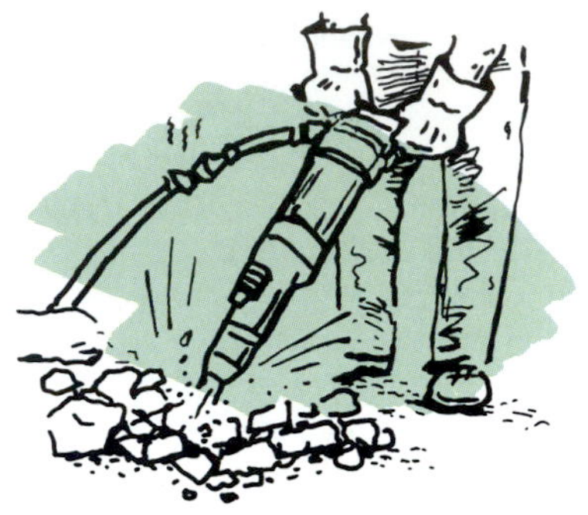

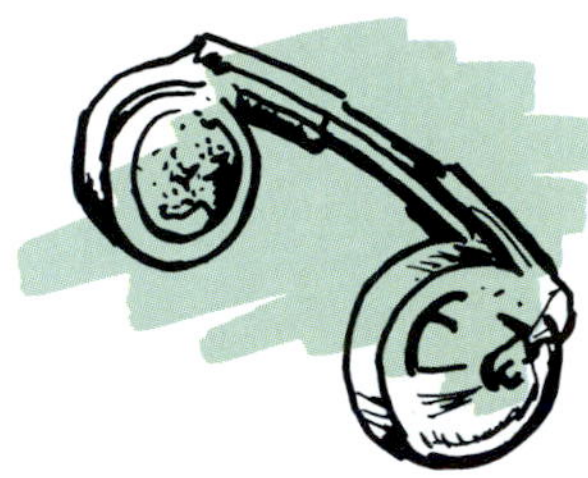

## RISK FACTORS:

NOISE

- *Noise hazards can lead not only to permanent hearing damage, but it has been established that noise can cause personality disorders, increase aggressive behavior and have an aggravating effect on headaches, hypertension, and peptic ulcers. It also lowers work efficiency and interferes with sleep patterns.*

## AWARENESS COUNTS:

- ***If you are in a noisy environment several hours a day where you have to raise your voice to be heard, you are in an area of potential danger for hearing loss. Noise that is painfully loud, such as pneumatic hammers or amplified rock music, has the greatest potential to damage hearing.***
- ***The age group in which there is particular susceptibility to hearing loss is adolescence.***
- ***It is particularly important to sleep in a quiet environment; use rugs, drapes, double windows, and finally ear plugs if necessary, to obliterate disturbing sound. (Cotton makes a poor plug unless saturated with wax or vaseline. Sponge plastic ear plugs are better.)***
- ***Pleasant background music can sometimes be used to mask disturbing sounds. However, background noise can conceal safety warnings, or lead to slow reaction time and thus contribute to accidents.***

## FOLLOW-THROUGH

*For information on all environmental hazards, write to:*

**The U.S. Environmental Protection Agency**
**Office of Public Affairs (A-107) Washington, D.C. 20460**

*For information about noise hazards, write to:*

**The National Information Center for Quiet**
**P.O. Box 57171 Washington, D.C. 20037**

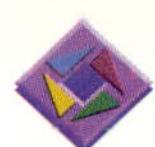

# Crime Prevention

*Through your own efforts, you can learn to reduce the opportunity and temptation for the criminal by accepting the responsibility to do everything possible for the protection of your personal well being and property.*
*All "no" answers are a cue to ACTION.*

| To protect yourself, do you...? | YES | NO |
|---|---|---|
| ...Always us a peephole or chain lock to identify your visitor? | ○ | ○ |
| ...Watch out for suspicious people or cars in your neighborhood? | ○ | ○ |
| ...Make an effort to get better acquainted with your neighbors, especially if you live in a large apartment building? | ○ | ○ |
| ...Avoid resisting the orders of a robber or purse snatcher? | ○ | ○ |
| ...List only your last name and initials in the phone directory and on the mailbox? | ○ | ○ |
| ...Always lock your doors during the day, even if you are at home? | ○ | ○ |
| ...Leave lights on doors you will be using when you return after dark? | ○ | ○ |
| ...Always have your key in your hand when you return home so you can open the door immediately? | ○ | ○ |

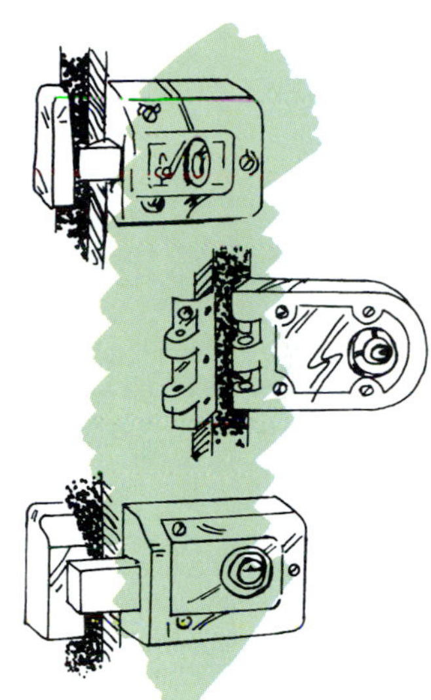

## RISK FACTORS:

PROTECTING YOURSELF

- *Women alone and the elderly are at highest risk at being victims of crime.*
- *People who are disabled are more vulnerable to crime.*
- *Certain areas of every large city are high crime areas and should be avoided if possible.*

## AWARENESS COUNTS:

- **List only your last name and initial in the phone directory and on the mailbox, particularly if you are a woman living alone.**
- **Always have your key ready when you return home.**
- **Always ask a visitor to identify himself before you let him in.**
- **Use automatic timers to turn on lights, radio, etc.**
- **If a window or lock has been forced or broken while you were out, use a neighbor's phone to call the police and wait outside until they arrive.**
- **Be cautious of unidentified phone callers. Hang up immediately if the caller will not identify himself.**
- **When traveling about at night, try to have a companion with you.**
- **Remember to ask for identification *before* you let repairmen, meter readers, or any other stranger into your home.**

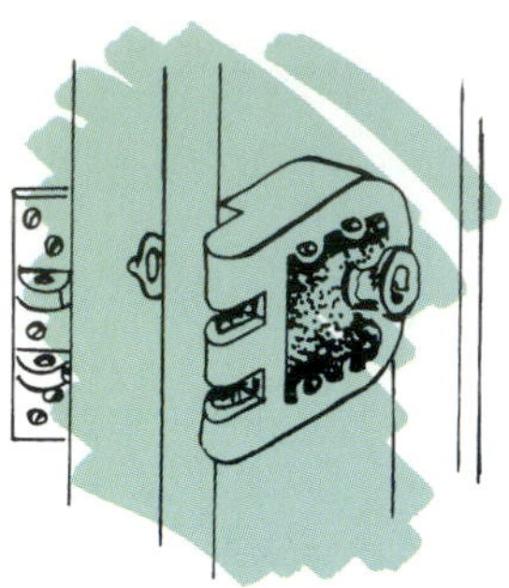

| To protect yourself, do you...? | YES | NO |
|---|---|---|
| ...Make specal plans for your home when you are away on vacation? | ○ | ○ |
| ...Avoid leaving a key under the doormat or in any accessible area? | ○ | ○ |
| ...Have you made sure that your door (s) have sturdy locks? | ○ | ○ |
| ...Check all windows and doors regularly for security? | ○ | ○ |
| ...Stop newspaper and milk deliveries when you go on vacation? | ○ | ○ |
| ...Keep especially valuable items in a safety deposit box away from home? | ○ | ○ |

## *RISK FACTORS:*

PROTECTING YOUR HOME

- Those at higher risk of home crime are people who leave their homes unattended for long periods of time and those who are nighttime travellers.
- Most crime takes place under cover of darkness.
- Letting mail and newspapers accumulate at your door announces the vulnerability of your home.

## *AWARENESS COUNTS:*

- **Keep your doors locked at all times.**
- **Have lights on an automatic timer while you are away.**
- **An alarm system is a useful crime deterrent.**
- **Make sure windows are secured.**
- **Make sure doorways and hallways are well lighted.**
- **Leave a radio on (a radio uses little electricity and gives the impression that your home is occupied).**

About Locks: Doors should be equipped with either a drop-bolt or dead-bolt lock. Do not use spring locks on any outside door. Spring locks work simply by closing the door and can be easily opened with a plastic card. Drop-bolt or dead-bolt locks can only be unlocked with a key.

## *FOLLOW-THROUGH*

Check with your local police department about joining the Operation Identification Program. You are provided with a sticker to display on your home and your valuable property is engraved with a non-removable code number. The police have a registered list of this property and statistics show that burglars avoid such homes because marked items are difficult to dispose of. Many police departments have crime prevention units and will give you personal advice.

Many states make available the Federal Crime Insurance Program – it provides federal crime insurance against burglary and robbery losses – rates depend upon the crime rate in the area where your home is located. For more information write to:

**Federal Crime Insurance, P.O. Box 11033**
**Washington, D.C. 20014 Toll Free (800) 638-8780**

*Review your homeowner's insurance coverage to make sure you have adequate coverage.*

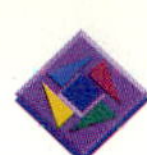

# Personal Safety

*While not all accidents are preventable, many are. Failure to take simple precautionary measures increases the risk of an avoidable accident. See if you can identify safety problem areas. All "yes" answers are a cue to Action.*

| Concerning PERSONAL SAFETY, | YES | NO |
|---|---|---|
| ...Have you had any accidents in the past years which could have been prevented? | ○ | ○ |
| ...If yes, where did this occur? at home? | ○ | ○ |
| in your automobile? | ○ | ○ |
| at work? | ○ | ○ |

| To ensure your SAFETY AT HOME, | YES | NO |
|---|---|---|
| ...Do you fail to go through your dwelling, room by room, deliberately looking for safety hazards once a year? | ○ | ○ |
| ...Does your dwelling have fewer than two means of escape in the event of an emergency? | ○ | ○ |
| ...If you smoke, do you ever smoke in bed? | ○ | ○ |
| ...Do you fail to keep a first aid kit, smoke alarm and fire extinguisher at home? | ○ | ○ |
| ...Are there loose electrical wiring or fixtures around your home? | ○ | ○ |
| ...Are carpets put down without non-skid backings? | ○ | ○ |
| ...Are poisons and pills in areas within reach of pre-school children? | ○ | ○ |

| In the BATHROOM, do you fail to... | YES | NO |
|---|---|---|
| ...Check the temperature of bath or shower water with your hand first? | ○ | ○ |
| ...Make sure electrical appliances are never used near water? | ○ | ○ |
| ...Use non-skid paste-ons or rubber mats for bathtub and shower surfaces? | ○ | ○ |

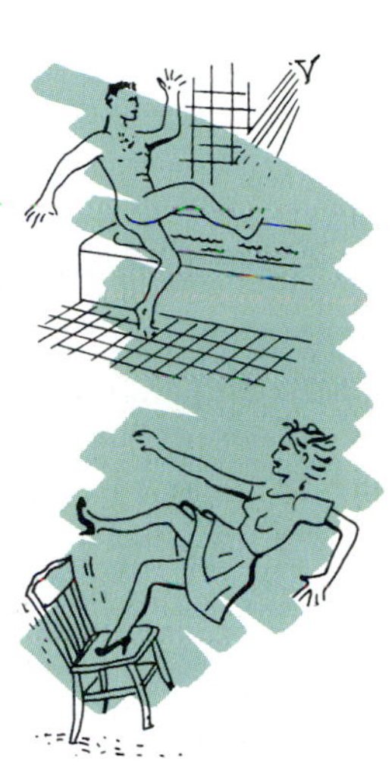

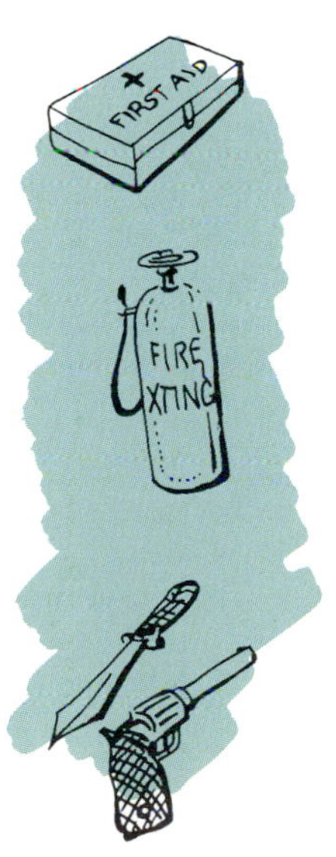


| In the KITCHEN, do you fail to... | YES | NO |
|---|---|---|
| ...Store knives with points away from the hand, or in special holders? | ○ | ○ |
| ...Keep curtains away from the cooking range? | ○ | ○ |
| ...Keep electrical appliances away from water? | ○ | ○ |
| ...Keep floors clean of grease and dirt? | ○ | ○ |
| ...Are you currently exposed to any of the material listed below? | ○ | ○ |
| dust (such as wood, leather, heavy metals, dyestuff)? | ○ | ○ |
| petroleum products? | ○ | ○ |
| radiation? | ○ | ○ |
| solvents? | ○ | ○ |
| ...If yes to any of the above...was your exposure usually indoors? | ○ | ○ |
| ...Did your exposure occur for an equivalent of at least one eight hour day per week for a period of five years? | ○ | ○ |
| ...If yes to dust, chemicals or petroleum products, was your skin or clothing regularly contacted by these materials? | ○ | ○ |

| To ensure your SAFETY IN YOUR AUTOMOBILE, do you...? | YES | NO |
|---|---|---|
| ...Neglect to <u>always</u> fasten your seat belts? | ○ | ○ |
| ...Ever drink alcoholic beverages before driving? | ○ | ○ |
| ...Drive even when you are sleepy? | ○ | ○ |
| ...Drive more than <u>40%</u> of the time in the dark? | ○ | ○ |
| ...Have you received more than <u>one</u> moving traffic violation this past year? | ○ | ○ |
| ...Have you had more than <u>one</u> accident this past year? | ○ | ○ |

## RISK FACTORS: PERSONAL SAFETY

- *Accidents are the leading cause of death among those under 44 years old.*
- *Accidents are the fourth most common cause of death in this country ranking behind heart disease, cancer and stroke.*

## AWARENESS COUNTS:

- **It is especially important that potential problem areas at home, on the road, and at work be identified so that you can create a relatively accident free environment. Improving your accident-prone behavior is the only way to decrease your risk of accidents.**
- **Your home or apartment should be regularly checked for safety hazards: ■ Slippery stairways ■ Unfastened carpets ■ Faulty fixtures or outlets ■ Store poisons, firearms in safe place ■ Have safety guard rails on upper level windows ■ Place smoke detectors in strategic areas ■ Have emergency numbers posted by the phone ■ Fire strikes more than 1,500 homes every day.**
- **Automobile accidents take more lives each year than any other type of accident or illness. Many of these can be prevented: ■ Make sure your car is in safe running condition, especially brakes and tires ■ Wear seat belts at all times. ■ Never drive while drinking. ■ Never drive while sleepy. ■ Always lock your car.**

| To ensure your SAFETY AT WORK, | YES | NO |
|---|---|---|
| ...Does your place of work fail to have regular safety checks? | ○ | ○ |
| ...Does your place of work fail to have regular emergency drills such as fire drills? | ○ | ○ |
| ...Does your place of work fail to have a current fire emergency plan? | ○ | ○ |
| ...Does your place of work fail to have rules governing the use of machinery and protective equipment? | ○ | ○ |

| ...Have you ever worked at a job where you were exposed to: asbestos? | ○○ | chemicals? | ○○ | coal dust? | ○○ |
|---|---|---|---|---|---|

## RISK FACTORS:
SAFETY AT WORK

- *13,000 accidental deaths per year occur on the job and over 2 million people are disabled or injured.*
- *Almost 30 billion dollars per year and about 25 million work days are lost due to accidents at work.*

## AWARENESS COUNTS:

- **Know where fire extinguishers are located.**
- **Is there a fire emergency plan in your office?**
- **Know the mandatory safety standards which apply to your business or industry.**
- **Use all protective clothing required.**
- **Know the names and hazards of all materials you are exposed to.**

## FOLLOW-THROUGH

*For information regarding safety procedures and requirements on the job write to:*
**The U.S. Department of Labor, Washington, D.C. 20212**
*Or get in touch with the Department of Labor office in your region. Or write to:*
**The National Institute for Occupational Safety and Health, Post Office Building, Cincinnati, Ohio 45202**
*For information regarding the safety of consumer products, write to:*
**U.S. Consumer Product Safety Commission Office of Washington, D.C. 20207**
*For information regarding all kinds of accidents, write to:*
**The National Safety Council, 444 N. Michigan Avenue, Chicago, Illinois 60611**

**Preventive Medicine Institute /Strang Clinic** 55 East 34 Street • New York, N.Y. 10016 • (212) 683-1000

APPENDIX

# D

# Blood Pressure Assessment

## BLOOD PRESSURE ASSESSMENT*

Blood pressure is assessed with a sphygmomanometer and a stethoscope. The sphygmomanometer consists of an inflatable bladder contained within a cuff and a mercury gravity manometer or an aneroid manometer from which the pressure is read (see Figure 8.12 and 8.13 in Chapter 8). The appropriate size cuff must be selected to get accurate readings. The size is determined by the width of the inflatable bladder, which should be about 40 percent of the circumference of the midpoint of the arm.

Measurement of blood pressure is usually done in the sitting position, with the forearm and the manometer at the same level as the heart. Initially, record the pressure from each arm, and subsequent pressures from the arm with the highest reading. Apply the cuff approximately one inch above the antecubital space (natural crease of the elbow), with the center of the bladder applied directly over the medial (inner) surface of the arm. Apply the stethoscope head firmly, but with little pressure, over the brachial artery in the antecubital space. The arm should be slightly flexed and placed on a flat surface. Inflate the bladder, while feeling the radial pulse, to about 30 to 40 mmHg above the disappearance of the pulse.

Do not overinflate the cuff, as it may cause blood vessel spasm, resulting in higher blood pressure readings. Release the pressure at a rate of 2 mmHg per second. As the pressure is released, determine the systolic blood pressure at the point where the initial pulse sound is heard. Determine the diastolic pressure at the point where the sound disappears. Make the recordings to the nearest 2 mmHg (even numbers), expressed as systolic over diastolic pressure (for example, 124/80).

**TABLE D.1**
**Blood Pressure Ratings in mmHg**

| Systolic | Diastolic | Rating* |
|---|---|---|
| ≤120 | ≤80 | Very Low Risk |
| 121–130 | 81–89 | Low Risk |
| 131–140 | 90–99 | Moderate Risk |
| 141–150 | 100–105 | High Risk |
| ≥151 | ≥106 | Very high Risk |

*Ratings expressed in terms of cardiovascular disease risk.

When taking more than one reading, completely deflate the bladder and allow at least one minute before making the next recording. Note whether the pressure was recorded from the left or the right arm. Resting blood pressure ratings are given in Table D.1.

In some cases, the loudness of the pulse sounds decreases in intensity (point of muffled sounds) and can still be heard at a lower pressure (50 or 40 mmHg) or even all the way down to zero. In this situation, record the diastolic pressure at the point where there is a clear/definite change in the loudness of the sound (also referred to as fourth phase), and at complete disappearance of the sound (fifth phase) (for example, 120/78/60 or 120/82/0).

Several readings by different people or at different times of the day should be taken to establish the real values. A single reading may not be an accurate value because of the various factors that can affect blood pressure.

*Recommendations for Human Blood Pressure Determination by Sphygmomanometers. American Heart Association, 1980.

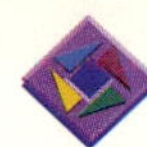

Name: ______________________ Course: __________ Section: __________ Date: __________

| Date | Arm | Blood Pressure | Recorder's Name |
|---|---|---|---|
| | | | |
| | | | |
| | | | |
| | | | |
| | | | |
| | | | |

**FIGURE D.1** ◆ Blood pressure recording form.

# Glossary of Terms

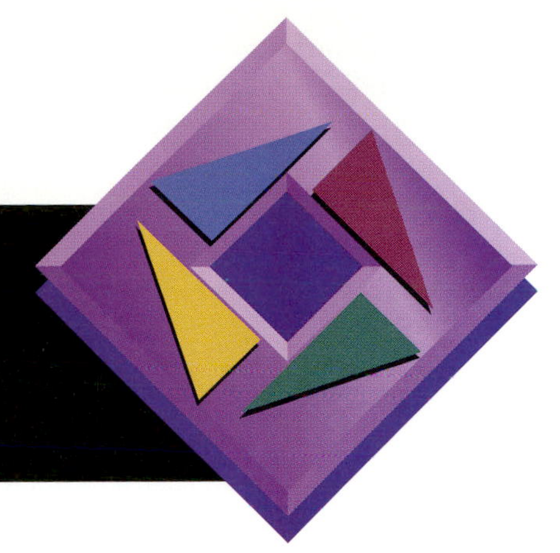

## A

**Accommodating resistance** Strength-training program that requires special equipment with mechanical devices that provide variable resistance, with the intent of overloading the muscle group maximally through the entire range of motion.

**Acquired immunodeficiency syndrome (AIDS)** Virus (HIV) that destroys the immune system.

**Addiction** Compulsive and uncontrollable behavior(s) or use of substance(s), most frequently drugs.

**Adenosine triphosphate (ATP)** A high-energy chemical compound used for immediate energy by the body.

**Adipose tissue** Fat cells.

**Aerobic exercise** Exercise that requires oxygen to produce the necessary energy (ATP) to carry out the activity.

**AIDS** *See* Acquired immunodeficiency syndrome.

**Alcohol (drinking alcohol)** Known as ethyl alcohol, a depressant drug that affects the brain and slows down central nervous system activity.

**Alcoholism** Disease in which an individual loses control over drinking alcoholic-containing beverages.

**Altruism** The act of providing service to others.

**Alveoli** Air sacs in the lungs where gas exchange (oxygen and carbon dioxide) takes place.

**Amenorrhea** Cessation of regular menstrual flow.

**Amino acids** Chemical compounds that contain nitrogen, carbon, hydrogen, and oxygen. Amino acids are the basic building blocks the body uses to build different types of protein.

**Anabolic steroids** Synthetic versions of the male sex hormone testosterone which promotes muscle development and hypertrophy.

**Anabolism** Process whereby simple substances are formed into more complex substances.

**Anaerobic exercise** Exercise that does not require oxygen to produce the necessary energy (ATP) to carry out the activity.

**Aneurysm** Weakness in the arterial wall allowing the formation of a balloon-like pouch.

**Angina pectoris** Chest pain.

**Angiogenesis** Capillary (blood vessel) formation into cancerous tumors.

**Anorexia nervosa** An eating disorder characterized by self-imposed starvation to lose and maintain very low body weight.

**Antioxidants** Compounds such as the vitamins C, E, beta-carotene (a precursor to vitamin A), and the mineral selenium, which prevent oxygen from combining with other substances to which it may cause damage. Antioxidants are thought to play a key role in the prevention of heart disease and cancer.

**Arteries** Major vessels that carry blood away from the heart to bodily tissues.

**Arteriosclerosis** Hardening of the arteries.

**Atherosclerosis** Type of arteriosclerosis characterized by plaque formation or the buildup of fatty tissue in the inner layers of the wall of the arteries.

**ATP** *See* Adenosine triphosphate.

**Atrophy** Decrease in size of a cell.

**Autogenic training** Stress management technique; a form of self-suggestion wherein an individual is able to place him/herself in an autohypnotic state by repeating and concentrating on feelings of heaviness and warmth in the extremities.

## B

**Ballistic or dynamic stretching (flexibility)** Exercises performed using jerky, rapid, and bouncy movements.

**Basal cell carcinoma** Type of skin cancer that occurs primarily on the face. It grows slowly and rarely spreads to other parts of the body.

**Basal metabolic rate** Lowest level of oxygen consumption (uptake) necessary to sustain life.

**Behavior modification** A process to permanently change destructive or negative behaviors and replace them with positive behaviors that will lead to better health and well-being.

**Benign** Noncancerous.

**Beta-carotene** Precursor to vitamin A.

**Bioelectrical impedance** Technique to assess body composition, including percent body fat, by running a weak electrical current (totally painless) through the body.

**Biofeedback** Stress management technique; a process in which a person learns to reliably influence physiological responses of two kinds: (a) responses that are not ordinarily under voluntary control or (b) responses that ordinarily are easily regulated but for which regulation has broken down because of trauma or disease.

**Blood pressure** Pressure of the blood exerted against the walls of the arteries.

**BMI** *See* Body Mass Index.

**Body composition** Term used in reference to the fat and nonfat components of the human body. Body composition is important in the assessment of recommended or "ideal" body weight.

**Body density** Weight of the body per unit volume.

**Body Mass Index (BMI)** Anthropometric technique used to determine potential risk for disease based on excessive thinness or fatness.

**Breathing techniques for relaxation** Stress management technique wherein the individual concentrates on "breathing away" the tension and inhaling fresh air to the entire body.

**Brown fat cells** Cells that produce body heat by burning fat.

**Bulimia** Eating disorder characterized by a pattern of binge eating and purging to attempt to lose and maintain low body weight.

## C

**CAD** (Coronary artery disease) *See* Coronary heart disease.

**Caffeine** A central nervous system stimulating drug most frequently found in coffee, tea, and colas.

**Calorie** (also referred to as "small calorie") The amount of heat necessary to raise the temperature of 1 gram of water 1° C. Short term for *kilocalorie*. Used to measure the energy value of food and cost of physical activity.

**Calorimeter** Equipment used to measure the caloric value of food or heat production of animals and humans.

**Cancer** Group of diseases characterized by uncontrolled growth and spread of abnormal cells into malignant tumors.

**Capillary** Smallest blood vessels carrying oxygenated blood in the body.

**Carbohydrates** Compounds containing carbon, hydrogen, and oxygen; the major source of energy for the human body.

**Carcinogens** Substances that contribute to the formation of cancers.

**Carcinoma in situ** Encapsulated malignant tumor (cancer) that is found at an early stage and has not spread.

**Cardiac output** Amount of blood ejected by the heart in 1 minute.

**Cardiovascular diseases** Conditions that affect the heart and the circulatory system (blood vessels). Examples of cardiovascular diseases are coronary heart disease, peripheral vascular disease, congenital heart disease, rheumatic heart disease, atherosclerosis, strokes, high blood pressure, and congestive heart failure.

**Cardiovascular endurance** Ability of the lungs, heart, and blood vessels to deliver adequate amounts of oxygen to the cells to meet the demands of prolonged (aerobic) physical activity.

**Catabolism** Process whereby complex substances are broken down into simpler substances.

**Catecholamines** Hormones; include epinephrine and norepinephrine.

**Cellulite** Term frequently used in reference to fat deposits that "bulge out." These deposits are nothing but enlarged fat cells from excessive accumulation of body fat.

**CHD** *See* Coronary heart disease.

**Chlamydia** Sexually transmitted disease caused by a bacterial infection that can cause significant damage to the reproductive system and may occur without symptoms.

**Cholesterol** A waxy substance that is technically a steroid alcohol found only in animal fats and oil.

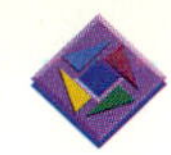

**Chronic diseases** Conditions that develop over a prolonged time, usually associated with unhealthy lifestyle factors (hypertension, atherosclerosis, coronary disease, strokes, diabetes, cancer).

**Chronic obstructive pulmonary disease (COPD)** An air flow-limiting condition that includes chronic bronchitis and emphysema, among others.

**Chronological age** Actual age of the individual (*See also* Functional age).

**Cocaine** 2-beta-carbomethoxy-3-betabenozoxytropane, the primary psychoactive ingredient derived from coca plant leaves. Also referred to as coke, C, snow, blow, toot, flake, Peruvian lady, white girl, and happy dust.

**Coenzyme** Nonprotein molecule required in enzyme reactions.

**Complex carbohydrates** Carbohydrates formed by three or more simple sugar molecules linked together; also referred to as polysaccharides. Commonly used to designate foods high in starch.

**Compound fats** A combination of simple fats with other chemicals. Examples are phospholipids, glucolipids, and lipoproteins.

**Concentric muscle contraction** Shortening of fibers during muscle contraction.

**Congenital heart disease** Heart defects present at birth.

**Coronary arteries** Arteries that supply the myocardium or heart muscle with oxygen and nutrients.

**Coronary heart disease** Condition caused by obstruction of coronary arteries by plaque formation (*See also* Atherosclerosis).

**Cruciferous vegetables** Plants that produce cross-shaped leaves (cauliflower, broccoli, cabbage, Brussels sprouts, kohlrabi), which seem to have a protective effect against cancer.

## D

**Dehydration** Loss of body water below normal volume.

**Deoxyribonucleic acid (DNA)** Genetic material, substance of which genes are made.

**Derived fats** A combination of simple and compound fats.

**Diabetes mellitus** Condition in which blood glucose is unable to enter cells because the pancreas either totally stops producing insulin or produces an insufficient amount for the body's needs.

**Diastolic blood pressure** Pressure exerted by the blood against the walls of the arteries during the relaxation phase (diastole) of the heart.

**Dietary fiber** Fiber in plant foods that cannot be digested by the human body.

**Dietary-induced thermogenesis (DIT)** Extra amount of heat production caused by metabolism of food.

**Disaccharides** Simple carbohydrates formed by two monosaccharide units linked together, one of which is glucose. Major disaccharides are sucrose, lactose, and maltose.

**Distress** Negative stress; unpleasant or harmful stress under which health and performance begin to deteriorate.

**DIT** *See* Dietary-induced thermogenesis.

**DNA** *See* Deoxyribonucleic acid.

**Dysmenorrhea** Painful menstruation.

## E

**Eccentric muscle contraction** Lengthening of fibers during muscle contraction.

**ECG** *See* Electrocardiogram.

**EKG** *See* Electrocardiogram.

**Elastic elongation (flexibility)** Temporary lengthening of soft tissue (muscles, tendons, and ligaments).

**Electrocardiogram (ECG or EKG)** Recording of electrical activity of the heart.

**Emphysema** Pulmonary disease caused by distention (overinflation) of the alveoli.

**Endorphines** Morphine-like substances released from pituitary gland in the brain during prolonged aerobic exercise. They are thought to induce feelings of euphoria and natural well-being.

**Endurance** *See* Cardiovascular endurance and muscular endurance.

**Energy** The ability to do work.

**Enzyme** Catalyst that facilitates chemical reactions.

**Epidemiology** Science that studies the relationship between diverse factors (lifestyle and environmental) and occurrence of disease.

**Essential amino acids** Amino acids that must be obtained in the diet because they cannot be produced in the body.

**Essential fat** Minimal amount of body fat needed for normal physiological functions; constitutes about 3% of total fat in men and 12% in women.

**Estrogen** Female sex hormone; essential for bone formation and bone density conservation.

**Eumenorrhea** Normal menstrual cycle.

**Eustress** Positive stress; health and performance continue to improve, even as stress increases.

**Exercise adherence** Initiating and participating in an exercise program for life.

**Exercise electrocardiogram** An exercise test during which workload is increased gradually (until the subject reaches maximal fatigue) with blood pressure and twelve-lead electrocardiographic monitoring throughout the test.

**Exercise intolerance** Inability to function during exercise, leading to symptoms such as very rapid or irregular heart rate, labored breathing, nausea, vomiting, lightheadedness, headaches, dizziness, pale skin, flushness, excessive weakness, lack of energy, shakiness, sore muscles, cramps, and tightness in the chest.

**Exercise tolerance test** *See* Exercise electrocardiogram.

## F

**Fatigue** Inability to maintain a given workload.

**Fats** Compounds made by a combination of triglycerides.

**Fiber** A form of complex carbohydrate made up of plant material that cannot be digested by the human body.

**Fight or flight mechanism** Physiological response of the body to stress, which prepares the individual to take action by stimulating the vital defense systems.

**Flexibility** Ability of a joint to move freely through its full range of motion.

**Fraud** *See* Quackery.

**Free fatty acids (FFA)** Fatty acids released by the breakdown of triglycerides.

**Free radicals** *See* Oxygen free radicals.

**Functional age** Physiological age; usually lower than chronological (actual) age in fit people and vice versa in unfit people.

## G

**Genetics** Science that studies genetic or hereditary conditions.

**Genital warts** Sexually transmitted disease caused by a viral infection. Genital warts increase the risk of cervical cancer. Enlargement and spread of the warts leads to obstruction of the urethra, vagina, and anus.

**Girth measurements technique** Method of assessing body composition, including percent body fat, by measuring circumferences at various body sites.

**Glucose** Blood sugar, type of carbohydrate (monosaccharide), a primary source of energy for the human body.

**Glucose intolerance** Inability to metabolize glucose properly.

**Glycogen** Form of carbohydrate (polysaccharide) storage in muscle.

**Glycolysis** Breakdown of glucose to pyruvic or lactic acid.

**Gonorrhea** Sexually transmitted disease caused by a bacterial infection that can lead to pelvic inflammation in women, infertility, widespread bacterial infection, heart damage, arthritis in men and women, and blindness in children born to infected women.

## H

**HDL** *See* High density lipoprotein.

**Health promotion** Programs aimed at helping people develop healthy lifestyle behaviors that will lead to a higher state of wellness.

**Health-related fitness** Refers to fitness components that, when enhanced, lead to better health (cardiovascular endurance, body composition, muscular strength and endurance, and muscular flexibility).

**Heart attack** *See* Myocardial infarct.

**Heart rate reserve** The difference between the maximal heart rate and the resting heart rate.

**Heat cramps** Muscle cramps caused by heat-induced changes in electrolyte balance in muscle cells.

**Heat exhaustion** Heat-related condition; symptoms include fainting, dizziness, profuse sweating, cold clammy skin, headaches, and a rapid, weak pulse.

**Heat stroke** Heat-related emergency; symptoms include serious disorientation, warm dry skin, no sweating, rapid full pulse, vomiting, diarrhea, unconsciousness, and high body temperature.

**Hemoglobin** Protein-iron compound in red blood cells that transports oxygen in the blood.

**Herpes** Sexually transmitted disease caused by viral infection (herpes simplex virus types I and II). Characterized by appearance of sores on mouth, genitals, rectum, or other parts of the body. Has no known cure.

**Hidden fat** Fat in food that can not be observed readily (lean meats contain about 30% to 40% fat calories).

**High density lipoprotein (HDL)** Cholesterol-transporting molecules in the blood. High HDL-cholesterol (good cholesterol) seems to offer protection against some forms of cardiovascular disease.

**HIV** *See* Human immunodeficiency virus.

**Human immunodeficiency virus (HIV)** Virus that causes acquired immunodeficiency syndrome (AIDS).

**Hydrostatic weighing** Underwater weighing technique to assess body composition, including percent body fat.

**Hyperglycemia** Elevated blood sugar (glucose).

**Hyperlipidemia** Elevated blood fats or lipids.

**Hyperplasia** An increase in the number of cells.

**Hypertension** Chronically elevated blood pressure.

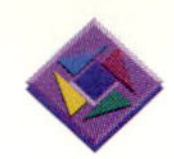

**Hypertrophy** An increase in the size of the cell (for example, muscle hypertrophy).

**Hypoglycemia** Low blood sugar (glucose).

**Hypokinetic disease** Condition associated with a lack of physical activity (for example, hypertension, coronary heart disease, obesity, and diabetes).

## I

**Insulin** Hormone secreted by the pancreas that increases the absorption and utilization of glucose by the body.

**Interval training** Method consisting of repeated bouts of exercise with rest intervals between each exercise bout.

**Ischemia** Lack of blood flow.

**Isokinetic contraction** Muscular contraction at a constant velocity.

**Isokinetic training** Strength-training method in which the speed of the muscle contraction is kept constant because the equipment (machine) provides an accommodating resistance to match the user's force (maximal) through the range of motion.

**Isometric training** Strength-training method that refers to a muscle contraction producing little or no movement, such as pushing or pulling against immovable objects.

**Isotonic training** Strength-training method that refers to a muscle contraction with movement, such as lifting an object over the head.

## K

**Kilocalorie** A unit to measure heat energy. A kilocalorie (kcal) or large calorie is the amount of heat necessary to raise the temperature of one kilogram of water one degree Centigrade. One kcal equals 1,000 calories.

## L

**Lactic acid** Strong acid, end product of anaerobic glycolysis (metabolism).

**Lactovegetarians** Vegetarians who also eat foods from the milk group.

**LDL** *See* Low density lipoprotein.

**Lean body mass** Body weight without body fat.

**Life Experiences Survey** Questionnaire used to assess sources of stress in life.

**Lipoprotein** A simple protein combined with a lipid group.

**Low density lipoprotein (LDL)** Bad cholesterol-transporting molecules in the blood (the "good" cholesterol). It increases the risk for some forms of cardiovascular disease.

## M

**Malignant melanoma** Deadliest of all types of skin cancer. Tumors grow rapidly and spread readily to other parts of the body if not treated at an early stage.

**Marijuana** A psychoactive drug prepared from a mixture of crushed leaves, flowers, small branches, stems, and seeds from the hemp plant cannabis sativa. Also referred to as pot and grass.

**Maximal oxygen uptake (Max $VO_2$)** The maximal amount of oxygen that the body is able to utilize per minute of physical activity, commonly expressed in ml/kg/min; the best indicator of cardiovascular or aerobic fitness.

**Meditation** Stress management technique used to gain control over one's attention, clearing the mind and blocking out the stressor(s) responsible for the increased tension.

**Megadose (of vitamins)** Large amount of vitamin(s) intake. For most vitamins, a megadose is ten times the RDA or more.

**Metabolism** All energy and material transformations that occur within living cells necessary to sustain life.

**Metastasis** Movement of bacteria or body cells from one part of the body to another. Often associated with cancer.

**METS (metabolic equivalents)** A measurement unit of resting energy expenditure. One MET is the equivalent of 3.5 ml/kg/min.

**Minerals** Inorganic elements found in the body and in food; essential for normal body functions.

**Mitochondria** Structures within the cells where energy transformations take place.

**Monosaccharides** The simplest carbohydrates (sugars) formed by five- or six-carbon skeletons. The three most common monosaccharides are glucose, fructose, and galactose.

**Monounsaturated fat** Fatty acids with only one double bond found along the carbon atom chain.

**Motor skill-related fitness** Fitness components that, when improved, lead to enhanced athletic performance (agility, balance, coordination, power, reaction time, and speed).

**Motor unit** The combination of a motor neuron and the muscle fibers that it innervates.

**Muscle fiber** A muscle cell.

**Muscular endurance (localized muscular endurance)** The ability of a muscle to exert submaximal force repeatedly over a period of time (for example, 30 repetitions on a bench press exercise). It usually implies a specific muscle group (chest, thighs, abdominals).

**Muscular strength** The ability of a muscle to exert maximum force against resistance (for example, 1 repetition maximum or 1 RM on the bench press exercise).

**Myocardial infarct** Death of part of the myocardium.

**Myocardium** Heart muscle.

**Myoglobin** Iron-containing compound that holds oxygen in muscle tissue.

## N

**Neuron** Nerve cell.

**Nicotine** Poisonous compound found in tobacco leaves.

**Nonmelanoma** Skin cancer that spreads or grows directly from the original site but does not metastasize to other regions of the body.

**Nonessential amino acids** Amino acids that can be manufactured in the body, and therefore, do not have to be obtained in the diet.

**Nulliparity** Never having had a child.

**Nutrient density** Ratio of nutrients to calories in food.

**Nutrient** Substance found in food that provides energy, regulates metabolism, and helps with growth and repair of body tissues.

**Nutrition** Science that studies the relationship of foods to optimal health and performance.

## O

**Obesity** An excessive accumulation of body fat, usually at least 30% above recommended body weight.

**Oligomenorrhea** Irregular menstrual cycles.

**Omega-3 fatty acids** Polyunsaturated fatty acids found primarily in cold water seafood and thought to be effective in lowering blood cholesterol and triglycerides.

**One repetition maximum (1 RM)** The maximal amount of resistance (weight) that an individual is able to lift in a single effort.

**Osteoporosis** Softening, deterioration, or loss of total body bone.

**Overload principle** Key training concept stating that the demands placed on a system (cardiovascular, muscular) must be increased systematically and progressively over time to cause physiologic adaptation (development or improvement).

**Ovolactovegetarians** Vegetarians who include egg and milk products in their diet.

**Ovovegetarians** Vegetarians who allow eggs in their diet.

**Oxygen free radicals** Substances formed during metabolism, which attack and damage proteins and lipids, in particular the cell membrane and DNA, leading to the development of diseases such as heart disease, cancer, and emphysema. Antioxidants are believed to exert a protective effect by absorbing free radicals before they can cause damage and also by interrupting the sequence of reactions once damage has begun.

## P

**Percent body fat** Ratio of fat in the body to total weight; includes both essential and storage fat. Used in body composition assessment.

**Peripheral vascular disease** Narrowing of the peripheral blood vessels (excluding cerebral and coronary arteries).

**Physical fitness** General capacity to adapt and respond favorably to physical effort, implying that individuals are physically fit when they can meet the ordinary as well as the unusual demands of daily life safely and effectively without being overly fatigued, and still have energy left for leisure and recreational activities.

**Phytochemicals** Chemical compounds thought to prevent and fight cancer; found in large quantities in fruits and vegetables.

**Plastic elongation (flexibility)** Permanent lengthening of soft tissue (capsules, tendons, and ligaments).

**Plyometrics** Strength training program designed to help increase speed and explosiveness.

**PNF** *See* Proprioceptive neuromuscular facilitation.

**Polyunsaturated fat** Fatty acids with two or more double bonds along the carbon atom chain.

**Prevention index** Annual measure of the effort Americans are making to prevent disease and accidents and to promote good health and longevity. The index is based on the 21 most significant health-promoting behaviors in the United States.

**Progressive muscle relaxation** Stress management technique involving progressive contraction and relaxation of muscle groups throughout the body.

**Progressive resistance training** *See* Strength training.

**Proprioceptive neuromuscular facilitation (PNF)** Stretching technique in which muscles are stretched out progressively with intermittent isometric contractions.

**Protein** Complex organic compounds containing nitrogen and formed by combinations of amino acids. The main substances used in the body to build and repair tissues such as muscles, blood, internal organs, skin, hair, nails, and bones; also part of hormones, antibodies, and enzymes.

## Q

**Quackery (fraud)** Conscious promotion of unproven claims for profit.

## R

**Rate of perceived exertion (RPE)** A perception scale to monitor or interpret the intensity of aerobic exercise.

**Recommended dietary allowances (RDA)** Daily recommended intakes of nutrients for normal, healthy people in the United States.

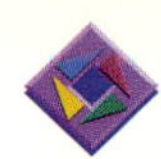

**Red muscle fibers (slow-twitch or type I)** Muscle fibers with greater aerobic potential and slow speed of contraction.

**Repetition (in strength training)** The number of times a given resistance is performed (for example, 12 repetitions on the bench press exercise).

**Repetition maximum (RM)** The most repetitions that can be performed with a specific resistance or weight (for example, 10 RM with 150 pounds) in strength training.

**Residual volume** Air left in the lungs following complete exhalation.

**Resistance** Amount of weight lifted in strength training.

**Ribonucleic acid (RNA)** Genetic material involved in formation of cell proteins.

**Risk factors** Lifestyle and genetic factors that may lead to disease.

**RNA** *See* Ribonucleic acid.

**RPE** *See* Rate of perceived exertion.

## S

**Saturated fat** Fatty acids with carbon atoms fully saturated with hydrogens; therefore, only single bonds link the carbon atoms on the chain. High intake of saturated fats increases the risk for coronary heart disease.

**Serum cholesterol** Blood cholesterol level.

**Set** Number of repetitions in strength training (e.g., 1 set of 12 repetitions).

**Setpoint theory** Weight control theory indicating that the body has an established weight and strongly attempts to maintain that weight.

**Sexually transmitted diseases (STDs)** Conditions spread through sexual contact.

**Shin Splints** Injury to the lower leg characterized by pain and irritation in the shin region or front of the leg.

**Simple carbohydrates** Carbohydrates formed by simple or double sugar units with little nutritive value (for example, candy, cakes). Divided into monosaccharides and disaccharides.

**Simple fats** A glyceride molecule linked to one, two, or three units of fatty acids (monoglycerides, diglycerides, and triglycerides).

**Skinfold thickness** Technique to assess body composition, including percent body fat, by measuring the thickness of a double fold of skin at different body sites.

**Slow-sustained or static stretching** Technique whereby the muscles are lengthened gradually through a joint's complete range of motion and the final position is held a few seconds.

**Specificity of training** Targeting the specific area the person is attempting to improve (aerobic, anaerobic, strength, flexibility).

**Sphygmomanometer** Equipment used to measure blood pressure; consists of an inflatable bladder contained within a cuff and a mercury gravity manometer or an aneroid manometer from which the pressure is read.

**Spiritual well-being** An affirmation of life in a relationship with God, self, community, and environment that nurtures and celebrates wholeness.

**Spot reducing** Theory that wrongly claims that exercising a specific body part (for example, abdominal or midsection of the body) will result in significant fat reduction in that area.

**Squamous cell carcinoma** Type of skin cancer that grows at a faster rate that basal cell carcinomas and seems to grow on sun-damaged areas. Squamous cell tumors spread to other parts of the body if not treated at an early stage.

**STDs** *See* Sexually transmitted diseases

**Storage fat** Body fat in excess of essential fat; stored in adipose tissue.

**Strength** *See* Muscular strength.

**Strength training** Conditioning program that requires weights to help increase muscular strength, endurance, power, or body size.

**Stress test** *See* Exercise electrocardiogram.

**Stress** The nonspecific response of the human organism to any demand placed upon it.

**Stress Vulnerability Scale** Questionnaire used to identify a number of factors that can help people decrease their vulnerability to stress.

**Stressor** Reaction of the organism to a stress-causing event.

**Stroke volume** Amount of blood ejected by the heart in one beat.

**Structured Interview** Assessment tool used in determining behavioral patterns (Type A and B personality).

**Syphilis** Sexually transmitted disease caused by bacterial infection. During the last stage of the disease, some people incur paralysis, crippling, blindness, heart disease, brain damage, insanity, and even death.

**Systolic blood pressure** Pressure exerted by the blood against walls of the arteries during forceful contraction (systole) of the heart.

## T

**Tar** Chemical compound that forms during the burning of tobacco leaves.

**Telomerase** Enzyme found in cancer cells that allows them to reproduce indefinitely.

**Telomeres** Strand of molecules found at both ends of chromosome. After many cell divisions, chromosomes eventually run out of telomeres and the cell dies.

Testosterone Male sex hormone.

Triglycerides Fats formed by glycerol and three fatty acids.

Type A personality Behavior pattern characteristic of a hard-driving, overambitious, aggressive, at times hostile, and overly competitive person.

Type B personality Behavior pattern characteristic of a calm, casual, relaxed, easy-going individual.

Type C personality Behavior pattern of individuals who are just as highly stressed as the Type A but do not seem to be at higher risk for disease than the Type B.

## U

U.S. RDA The United States recommended daily allowances. Derived from the RDA and developed as a standard for nutrition labeling.

## V

Vasoconstriction Narrowing or clamping down of blood vessels.

Vasodilation Widening or opening up of blood vessels.

Vegans Vegetarians who eat no animal products at all.

Vegetarians Individuals whose diet is of vegetable or plant origin.

Veins Major vessels that carry blood back to the heart.

Very low density lipoprotein (VLDL) Triglyceride, cholesterol and phospholipid-transporting molecules in the blood. Only a small amount of cholesterol is carried by the VLDL molecules.

Vitamins Organic substances essential for normal metabolism, growth, and development of the body.

VLDL *See* Very low density lipoprotein.

## W

Waist-to-Hip Ratio Test designed by a panel of scientists appointed by National Academy of Sciences and Dietary Guidelines Advisory Council for U.S. Departments of Agriculture and Health and Human Services to assess potential risk for diseases associated with obesity.

Weight training A conditioning program that requires weights to help increase muscular strength, endurance, power, and body size.

Weight-regulating mechanism Mechanism located in the hypothalamus of the brain that regulates how much the body should weigh (*See also* Setpoint theory).

Wellness The constant and deliberate effort to stay healthy and achieve the highest potential for well-being. Implies the adoption of healthy lifestyle factors that will decrease the risk for disease and enhance well-being.

White muscle fibers (fast-twitch or type II) Muscle fibers with greater anaerobic potential and fast speed of contraction.

Work Ability to utilize energy.

Workload Given level of exercise intensity or physical performance.

## Y

Yellow fat cells Cells used for fat storage (stores of energy in the form of fat).

# Index

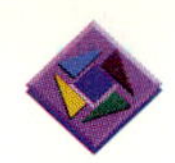

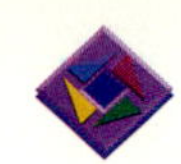